616.70754 MAN

 KU-160-882

**This book is to be returned on or before
the last date stamped below.**

8/2/17

WRIGHTINGTON
HOSPITAL LIBRARY

Wrightington Wigan &
Leigh NHS Trust Library

W00784

Musculoskeletal Imaging   THE REQUISITES

SERIES EDITOR **James H. Thrall,** M.D.
Radiologist-in-Chief
Department of Radiology
Massachusetts General Hospital
Boston, Massachusetts

OTHER VOLUMES IN THE REQUISITES SERIES

Gastrointestinal Radiology

Pediatric Radiology

Neuroradiology

Nuclear Medicine

Cardiac Radiology

Genitourinary Radiology

Ultrasound

Thoracic Radiology

Mammography

Musculoskeletal Imaging

THE REQUISITES

B. J. MANASTER, M.D., Ph.D.
Professor and Vice Chairman
Department of Radiology
University of Colorado Health Sciences Center
Denver, Colorado

DAVID G. DISLER, M.D.
Commonwealth Radiology
Richmond, Virginia
Associate Clinical Professor
Department of Radiology
Virginia Commonwealth University
Medical College of Virginia
Richmond, Virginia

DAVID A. MAY, M.D.
Radiology Associates
Richmond, Virginia
Associate Clinical Professor
Department of Radiology
Virginia Commonwealth University
Medical College of Virginia
Richmond, Virginia

Second Edition

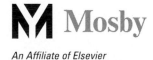

An Affiliate of Elsevier

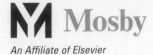

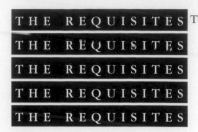

THE REQUISITES is a proprietary trademark of Mosby, Inc.

Library of Congress Cataloging-in-Publication Data

Manaster, B. J.
    Musculoskeletal imaging : the requisites / B.J. Manaster, David G. Disler, David A. May.—2nd ed.
        p. ; cm.—(Requisites series)
    Rev. ed. of: Musculoskeletal imaging / David J. Sartoris, C. 1996
    Includes bibliographical references and index.
    ISBN 0-323-01189-6
    1. Musculoskeletal system—Imaging. I. Disler, David G. II. May, David A. III. Sartoris, David J. Musculoskeletal imaging. IV. Title. V. Series.
    [DNLM: 1. Musculoskeletal System—radiography. 2. Musculoskeletal Diseases—physiopathology. WE 141 M267m 2002]
    RC925.7 M35 2002
    616.7′0754—dc21   2001037073

SECOND EDITION

Copyright © 2002, 1996 by Mosby, Inc.

All rights reserved. No part of this publication may be reproduced or transmitted in any form or by any means, electronic or mechanical, including photocopy, recording, or any information storage and retrieval system, without permission in writing from the publisher.

Permissions may be sought directly from Elsevier's Health Sciences Rights Department in Philadelphia, USA: phone: (+1)215-238-7869, fax: (+1)215-238-2239, email: healthpermissions@elsevier.com. You may also complete your request on-line via the Elsevier Science homepage (http://www.elsevier.com), by selecting 'Customer Support' and then 'Obtaining Permissions'.

Mosby, Inc.
11830 Westline Industrial Drive
St. Louis, Missouri 63146

Printed in the United States of America

Last digit is the print number   9 8 7 6 5 4 3 2

With love to
Steve, Tracy Joy, and Katy Rose
Robin, Mathew Joseph, and Emily Rose
Julie, Daniel Alden, and Kathryn Whitney
With deep gratitude to our many teachers and mentors

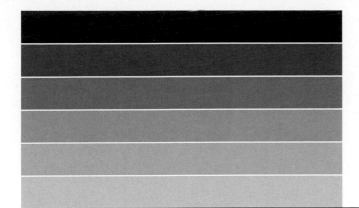

Preface

The Requisites series has almost become an institution in the field of radiology, and these authors are honored to offer the second edition of Musculoskeletal Imaging. This book is entirely new, with completely new and original text and figures. Musculoskeletal radiology is such an extensive field that it is difficult to narrow it down to "the requisites." Our book, in fact, covers two overlapping but different sets of requisites: those for the American Board of Radiology examinations and those for a radiology practitioner. Thus, we have eliminated many interesting but esoteric entities. We have endeavored to illustrate the book with examples of the "expected" appearance of the more common disease processes rather than spectacular but less informative or infrequently seen examples from our files.

"Key concepts" boxes are used liberally to remind readers of the key elements of the most common entities, but expanded discussion is readily accessible in the text. The book is designed for everyday use by diagnostic radiology residents and radiologists in a general practice. It is a complete source for musculoskeletal board review. Orthopaedic residents, as well as clinicians in rheumatology and rehabilitative medicine, will find pertinent information relating to their interests.

We hope that this is a welcome addition to The Requisites.

B.J. Manaster, M.D., Ph.D.

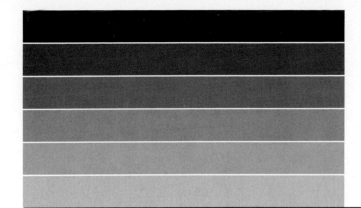

Acknowledgments

We greatly appreciate the professional help of Laurie Persson, artist, Julian Maack, artist, Sonia Crimaldi, M.D., MSK fellow and proofreader, the staff at Richmond Children's hospital, our many colleagues who contributed cases, and the technologists who skillfully obtained the studies. Most importantly, we thank Tina Kutsuma, COTA, administrative assistant, for her cheerful dedication and organization required in assembling this book.

NOTICE

Pharmacology is an ever-changing field. Standard safety precautions must be followed, but as new research and clinical experience broaden our knowledge, changes in treatment and drug therapy may become necessary or appropriate. Readers are advised to check the most current product information provided by the manufacturer of each drug to be administered to verify the recommended dose, the method and duration of administration, and contraindications. It is the responsibility of the treating physician, relying on experience and knowledge of the patient, to determine dosages and the best treatment for each individual patient. Neither the Publisher nor the editor assume any liability for any injury and/or damage to persons or property arising from this publication.

Contents

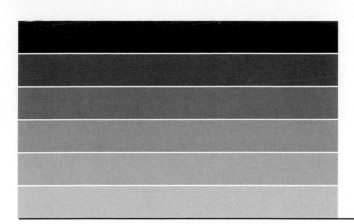

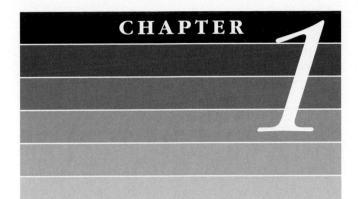

CHAPTER 1

Tumors

B.J. MANASTER M.D., Ph.D.

1

ANEURYSMAL BONE CYST
LANGERHANS' CELL HISTIOCYTOSIS
FIBROUS DYSPLASIA
BROWN TUMOR OF HYPERPARATHYROIDISM
MYOSITIS OSSIFICANS
METASTATIC DISEASE OF BONE

INTRODUCTION

Although musculoskeletal tumors are quite rare, these tumors can be problematic for the radiologist because they can be difficult to correctly characterize, which in turn can lead to devastating results. Radiologists should have three major goals for understanding musculoskeletal tumors. First, the radiologist should have sufficient knowledge to work up a newly discovered lesion. The lesion should be identified or provided a reasonable differential diagnosis, and it should be determined whether work-up beyond radiography is necessary. If so, the radiologist should assist in providing a cost-effective work-up that leads neither to overtreatment of a benign lesion or under treatment of an aggressive lesion. Second, the radiologist should play an active role in either providing the biopsy or guiding the open biopsy and/or surgical resection. The radiologist must understand the natural history of the lesion and must be knowledgeable of the surgeon's treatment options to give a complete assessment of tumor involvement. The radiologist, of course, must be aware of which diagnostic modality is most suitable for each tumor work-up. Third, the radiologist needs to provide knowledgeable posttreatment follow-up by knowing which diagnostic modality can most effectively monitor for recurrence and complications of tumor treatment. This chapter will acquaint the reader with the staging system used for musculoskeletal tumors, the surgical treatment options, and the philosophy of diagnostic management for both soft tissue and osseous lesions, including a discussion of the most commonly used modalities. It will conclude with a discussion of strategies for follow-up of these lesions.

SURGICAL STAGING OF SOLITARY BONE TUMORS AND SOFT TISSUE SARCOMAS

The Musculoskeletal Tumor Society has developed a staging system based on a combination of radiologic and histologic criteria in an attempt to reach an accurate prognosis and appropriate treatment for each individual lesion. This system, or a close variant, is universally used and relies on histology (grade), presence or absence of metastases, and evaluation of local site of involvement. Imaging is the crucial common denominator required for adequate staging, as it is used to evaluate site, detect metastases, and determine best location for obtaining

representative tissue in the biopsy. The staging is commonly referred to as the Enneking methodology.[1] Note that this staging does not apply to metastatic lesions or round cell lesions, although it does include Ewing's sarcoma. It is outlined in Table 1-1.

SURGICAL TREATMENT OPTIONS

There are four surgical treatment options. The first is intralesional excision (curettage). With this treatment, tumor is incompletely (partially) resected and tumor cells are found at the margin at histologic evaluation. This may be adequate for many benign tumors and, due to functional consideration, may even be considered in more aggressive lesions. The second surgical treatment option is marginal excision (excisional biopsy). With a marginal excision, the plane of dissection passes through the reactive tissue or pseudocapsule of the lesion. Satellites of residual tumor may be left behind. This is an inadequate treatment for malignant tumors or lesions with a high recurrence rate, but may occasionally be chosen for reasons of functionality if combined with other therapy. The third treatment option is wide excision. With wide excision, the entire lesion is removed, surrounded by an intact cuff of normal tissue. The plane of dissection is well beyond the reactive tissue surrounding the lesion, but the entire muscle or bone is not removed. This treatment is considered adequate for recurrent, aggressive benign tumors as well as most sarcomas. The fourth treatment option is radical resection, in which the lesion is removed along with the entire muscle, bone, or other involved tissues in the compartment. Radical resection is not commonly required for treatment of musculoskeletal tumors.

It is clear that a wide excision is required for optimal treatment of aggressive lesions. However, it should be noted that at times compromises may be made to retain limb functionality, achieving only a marginal excision but supplementing it with other therapy. Please note that the term "limb salvage" is not a specific treatment option. Rather, limb salvage procedures are simply those that offer tumor control without sacrifice of the limb. Most fall into the category of wide excisions. Consideration of limb salvage is based on the staging of the lesion, anatomic location, age and expected growth of the patient, extent of local disease, and expected function after the procedure.

MODALITIES USED FOR THE WORK-UP OF MUSCULOSKELETAL TUMORS

Radiography

The radiograph is the essential first step in evaluation of any musculoskeletal tumor. Although radiographs frequently appear normal in patients with soft tissue masses,

Table 1-1   Surgical staging of solitary bone tumors and soft tissue sarcomas

G: grade (histologic). Appropriate grading requires representative tissue sampling at biopsy, often guided by imaging.
(1) G_0–benign
(2) G_1–low-grade, malignant
(3) G_2–high-grade, malignant

S: site (radiographic and clinical features). This is determined by cross-sectional imaging (usually magnetic resonance [MR]).
(1) T_0–true capsule surrounds lesion (reactive rim of tissue).
(2) T_1–extracapsular, intracompartmental; compartments are defined as follows:
  a Skin–subcutaneous.
  b Parosseous–a potential compartment is seen when a lesion pushes muscle away from bone without invading either muscle or cortex.
  c Bone–intracortical; also a lesion in ray of the hand or foot is considered intracompartmental.
  d Muscle compartments–may contain more than one muscle if the muscle group is limited by a fascial plane:
    i Posterior compartment calf.
    ii Anterior compartment calf.
    iii Anterolateral compartment calf.
    iv Anterior thigh.
    v Medial thigh.
    vi Posterior thigh.
    vii Buttocks.
    viii Volar forearm.
    ix Dorsal forearm.
    x Anterior arm.
    xi Posterior arm.
    xii Deltoid.
    xiii Periscapula.

(3) T_2–extracapsular, extracompartmental extension from any of the above-named compartments or abutment of major neurovascular structures; in addition, some sites are extracompartmental by origin:
  a Midhand, dorsal or palmar.
  b Mid- or hindfoot.
  c Popliteal fossa.
  d Femoral triangle.
  e Obturator foramen.
  f Sciatic notch.
  g Antecubital fossa.
  h Axilla.
  i Periclavicular.
  j Paraspinal.
  k Periarticular, elbow or knee.

M: metastases, usually bone or lung.
(1) M_0–no metastases.
(2) M_1–metastases present.

Staging. Uses grade, site, and metastases as follows:
(1) *Benign*:

1 (Inactive)	2 (Active)	3 (Aggressive)
G_0	G_0	G_0
T_0	T_0	T_{1-2}
M_0	M_0	M_{0-1}

(2) *Malignant*:
Ia: Low-grade without metastases, intracompartmental.
Ib: Low-grade without metastases, extracompartmental.
IIa: High-grade without metastases, intracompartmental.
IIb: High-grade without metastases, extracompartmental.
III: Low- or high-grade with metastases.

Ia	Ib	IIa	IIb	III
G_1	G_1	G_2	G_2	G_2
T_1	T_2	T_1	T_2	T_2
M_0	M_0	M_0	M_0	M_1

they can be invaluable and must be included in the workup of any soft tissue mass. Although the mass itself may not be well characterized on radiographs, evaluation of the soft tissue planes can be helpful. Tumors usually displace soft tissue planes but their demarcation persists. On the other hand, infection (which can be mistaken for tumor) usually obliterates soft tissue planes. Radiographs also allow for the evaluation of the integrity of the adjacent bone. Finally, some soft tissue calcification patterns may be characteristic in diagnosing soft tissue tumors (for example, phleboliths in hemangiomas or the zonal calcification seen in myositis ossificans). Although soft tissue calcification is more characteristically seen in some lesions than in others, dystrophic calcification can in fact be seen in any soft tissue tumor. Noting its presence on the radiograph may help in interpretation of unusual signal characteristics seen on magnetic resonance imaging (MRI). Thus, the simple step of taking a radiograph should never be skipped in evaluating a soft tissue mass.

The radiograph is even more essential in the work-up of an osseous lesion. This is the most important imaging tool in determining biologic activity and, very often, histology. Although we occasionally can make a specific diagnosis based on the radiograph, more frequently we use it to place an osseous lesion in a category based on the degree of aggressiveness (Table 1-2). The first diagnostic category is that of a nonagressive "leave me alone lesion." These represent lesions of diagnostic certainty that should be ignored in terms of further work-up or even follow-up. The

Table 1-2   Diagnostic categories of osseous lesions

1. Benign "leave me alone" lesion
2. Benign lesion which can be safely watched
3. Benign symptomatic lesion which needs no further diagnostic workup
4. Lesion of uncertain diagnosis regarding benignancy or malignancy
5. Malignant lesion

Table 1-3   Ten criteria for categorizing of an osseous lesion on plain radiograph

Age of patient
Soft tissue involvement
Pattern of bone destruction
Size of lesion
Location of lesion
    Particular bone involved
    Location along the length of a long bone
    Location along the transverse axis of a long bone
Zone of transition
Margin of lesion
Visible tumor matrix
Host response
Polyostotic or monostotic

most notable example of a "leave me alone" lesion is a benign fibrous cortical defect. The second category of lesion is one that is felt, based on the radiograph, to be almost certainly benign, which can be followed with serial radiographs for confirmation of the diagnosis. Examples of this type of lesion include nonossifying fibroma, fibrous dysplasia, or myositis ossificans. The third category is that of a nonaggressive symptomatic lesion that needs no further diagnostic work-up before surgery. In some cases, a solitary bone cyst, chondroblastoma, or giant cell tumor might fit this category. The fourth category of lesions is one that has both aggressive and nonaggressive features. These lesions clearly require further work-up and biopsy. The fifth and final category is that of the aggressive lesions that require preoperative work-up and biopsy. In general, further work-up using other imaging modalities is required for staging purposes only if the lesion falls into category 4 or 5.

To correctly categorize an osseous tumor, radiologists have developed ten criteria (Table 1-3) that must be as-

Table 1-4   Age as a criterion for osseous tumor

Age (yr)	Lesion
1	Metastatic neuroblastoma
1-10	Ewing's sarcoma (tubular bones)
10-30	Aneurysmal bone cyst
10-30	Osteosarcoma, Ewing's sarcoma (flat bones)
Skeletally immature	Chondroblastoma
Skeletally mature-50	Giant cell tumor (GCT)
30-60	Chondrosarcoma, primary lymphoma, malignant fibrous histiocytoma, fibrosarcoma
50-80	Metastasis, multiple myeloma

sessed in each case. If these criteria are carefully and accurately assessed, the diagnosis, or at least a reasonable differential diagnosis, usually becomes apparent.

1. Age of patient. This parameter is essential for diagnosis, as some lesions are very typically found among certain age groups (Table 1-4). For example, a patient over the age of 50 with a solitary lesion should be considered most likely to have a metastasis or plasmacytoma rather than primary bone tumor. Similarly, between 30-60 years of age, the trio of chondrosarcoma, primary lymphoma, and malignant fibrous histiocytoma should be strongly considered. An aggressive lesion in a tubular bone in a child under the age of 10 is more likely Ewing sarcoma than osteosarcoma, but between the age of 10-20 years osteosarcoma is much more likely.

2. Soft tissue involvement. Not surprisingly, cortical breakthrough of a bone lesion to create a soft tissue mass generally suggests an aggressive lesion. There are, however, some benign lesions that can appear very aggressive and even show cortical breakthrough with soft tissue mass. It is interesting that infection can frequently mimic an aggressive osseous tumor in its destructive pattern of the bone and extend into the soft tissue as well. The appearance of the soft tissue fascial planes may help to distinguish infection from tumor, as tumor tends to displace fascial planes whereas infection tends to obliterate them.

3. Pattern of bone destruction. A geographic pattern is the least aggressive, with the lesion having a well-defined margin which is "maplike" (Fig. 1-1A).

Fig. 1-1   Patterns of bone destruction. **A,** Geographic destruction, where the mass is easily outlined in this giant cell tumor of the distal radius. **B,** An example of permeative bone destruction, with the tumor infiltrating among trabeculae, destroying some but leaving others. This metadiaphyseal lesion is an osteosarcoma arising in an 8-year-old male. **C,** A more subtle permeative lesion, with faintly seen destruction of trabeculae in the distal femoral metaphysis (*arrows*) on this lateral radiograph. Although the permeative pattern of bone destruction is much less obvious in Figure 1-1C than it was in Figure 1-1B, the aggressive nature of the lesion is still apparent. There is a very large soft tissue mass (*arrowheads*) and this is an osteosarcoma arising in a 16-year-old female. Figure **1-1D** demonstrates a lesion which is in large part geographic, with a sclerotic margin. However, the margin on the medial side of the tibial metaphysis shows cortical breakthrough (*arrow*). Despite the nonaggressive appearance of most of this lesion, the cortical destruction must be considered a "red-flag" and this lesion must be worked up as an aggressive lesion. At biopsy, this was an osteosarcoma in this 17-year-old male. (Figure 1-1C and 1-1D reprinted with permission from the ACR learning file.)

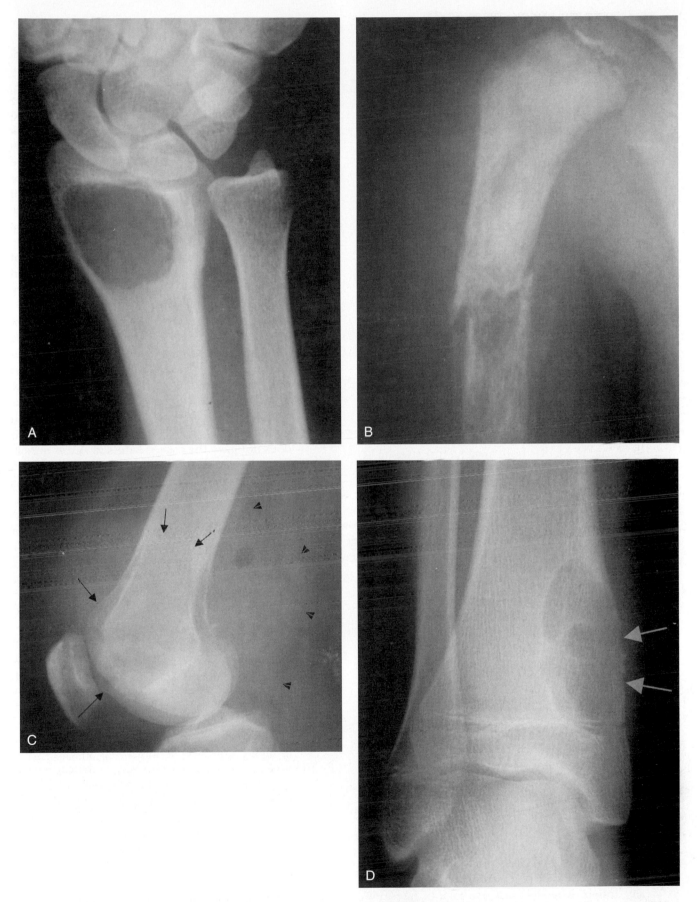

Fig. 1-1 For legend see opposite page

The opposite pattern of bone destruction, the permeative, is highly aggressive. A permeative pattern is poorly demarcated and often difficult to visualize (Fig. 1-1B and 1-1C). A subcategory of the permeative pattern is the moth-eaten pattern, which is also aggressive but with larger "holes," though still poorly marginated. The pattern of bone destruction is an extremely important parameter in determining aggressiveness of lesions. Although it would seem that this is a relatively easy pattern to distinguish, there are lesions that appear to be largely geographic in one part, but which appear more aggressive in another. This should be considered a red flag and these lesions should be worked up as if they fall into the more aggressive category (Fig. 1-1D).

4. Size of lesion. Generally, a large lesion is more likely to behave aggressively than a smaller lesion. This generalization, however, is of lesser importance than the pattern of bone destruction and other parameters relating to aggressiveness of lesions.

5. Location of lesion. There are three aspects of lesion location, any of which may be important in determining the probable histology of the lesion. First, the particular bone in which the lesion is found may be important. Although most lesions are found most frequently around the knee, certain tumors occur much more commonly in specific bones. Localization may refer to a specific bone such as the tibia (a favorite location of adamantinoma, ossifying fibroma, and chondromyxoid fibroma—all rare lesions), or a category of bones such as flat versus tubular, or appendicular versus axial. The second aspect of lesion location is location along the length of a tubular bone. Although most lesions are metaphyseal, some lesions are characteristically found in the region of the epiphysis (chondroblastoma) and others are more frequently found in a diaphyseal location (Ewing sarcoma). The third aspect related to location of lesion is location in the transverse plane of a long bone. Many lesions are centrally located, whereas others are usually eccentrically located or even cortically based or surface lesions (Fig. 1-2). Table 1-5 outlines examples of lesions that have characteristic transverse locations in long bones.

6. Zone of transition. This determinant refers to whether there is a wide or narrow zone of transition from abnormal to normal bone in an osseous tumor. A wide zone of transition implies an aggressive lesion, whereas a narrow zone of transition implies a nonaggressive lesion.

7. Margin sclerosis. A sclerotic margin generally suggests a nonaggressive lesion, whereas a lack of sclerotic margin suggests a more aggressive lesion. Please note that "margin" is a different entity than "zone of transition." Most nonaggressive lesions have a sclerotic margin as well as a narrow zone of transition, whereas most aggressive lesions do not have the sclerotic margin and have a wide zone of transition. There are, however, some lesions that typically have a narrow zone of transition but no sclerotic margin. This pattern can suggest the diagnosis of giant cell tumor, plasmacytoma, or enchondroma.

8. Presence of visible tumor matrix. One should not only identify the presence of tumor matrix, but try to categorize it (Fig. 1-3). Cartilage forming tumors produce a stippled matrix with C and J shapes (rings and arcs). The matrix of cartilage tends to be denser than normal bone. On the other hand, bone matrix demonstrates different characteristics depending on the aggressiveness of the lesion. Highly aggressive bone forming tumors such as osteosarcoma produce amorphous osteoid, which may be less dense than normal bone, or occasionally as dense as normal bone. It does not have the trabecular character of normal bone. Less aggressive bone-forming tumors such as parosteal osteosarcoma tend to produce better organized and denser appearing bone.

9. Host response. The character of transcortical and periosteal involvement should be noted, whether penetrated, expanded and thinned, or thickened. None of these characteristics specifically relate to aggressiveness or nonaggressiveness. For example, cortical thickening can be seen as a reaction to nonmalignant lesions such as infection or osteoid osteoma, but cortical thickening can also be seen in highly aggressive lesions such as Ewing sarcoma and primary lymphoma. Host response is also seen in the form of periosteal reaction. There are highly aggressive forms of periosteal reaction, that can have a sunburst character or be partially interrupted (Codman's triangle). However, a thin linear periosteal line also can be seen in highly aggressive lesions.

10. Polyostotic vs. monostotic lesion. This is a criterion that can be quite helpful. Although most primary bone tumors are monostotic, if one knows that the lesion is polyostotic one can assume that the disease process will fall into either the benign polyostotic category (fibrous dysplasia, Paget's disease, histiocytosis, multiple exostosis, multiple enchondromatosis) or the malignant category (metastases, multiple myeloma, or primary bone tumors with bony metastases such as Ewing sar-

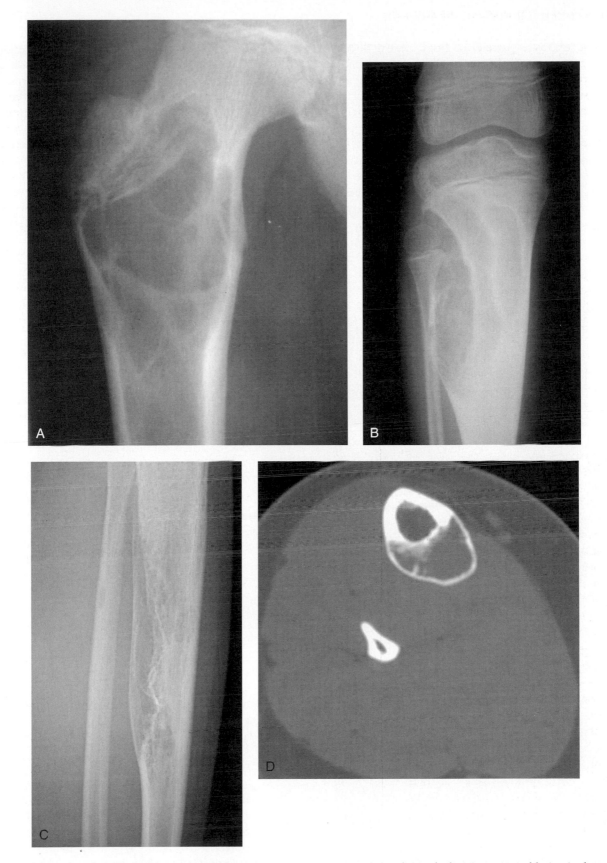

Fig. 1-2 Transverse locations of tumors in long bones. **A,** An AP (antero-posterior) radiograph showing a central lesion in the proximal femur, a solitary bone cyst in an 11-year-old male. **B,** An AP radiograph demonstrating an eccentric location of a metaphyseal lesion, in this case a chondromyxoid fibroma in an 18-year-old female. **C,** A cortically based lesion in the mid shaft of the tibia in a 14-year-old female. Although from the radiograph alone one may not be able to determine that the lesion is completely cortically based, CT **D,** confirms this. In this case, the lesion is an unusual manifestation of fibrous dysplasia, which can occasionally be cortically based.

Continued

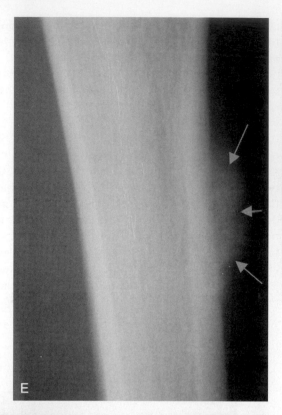

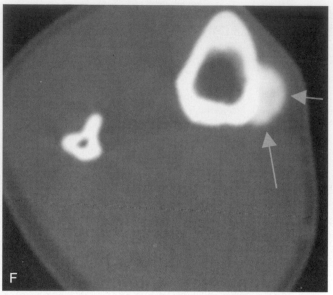

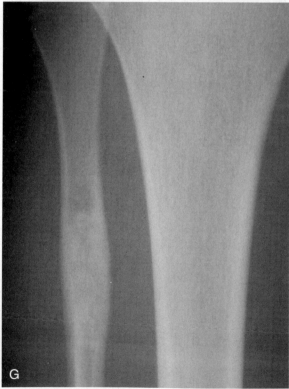

Fig. 1-2, cont'd   **E,** An AP radiograph of a surface lesion in the tibia of an 18-year-old male. The lesion arises from the surface of bone, forming tumor osteoid in the adjacent soft tissues (*arrows*). **F,** The surface location is confirmed on CT (*arrow*). **G,** An AP radiograph demonstrating a nonossifying fibroma that is sclerosing in. Although nonossifying fibroma is usually a cortically based lesion, when it occurs in very small bones such as the fibula, it fills the entire space and gives the appearance of being a central lesion.

Table 1-5	Transverse location in long bones
Central	Enchondroma
	Central chondrosarcoma
	Ewing sarcoma
	Primary lymphoma
	Malignant fibrous histiocytoma
	Solitary bone cyst
	Eosinophilic granuloma
	Fibrous dysplasia
Eccentric	Osteosarcoma
	Chondromyxoid fibroma
	Aneurysmal bone cyst
	Giant cell tumor
Cortical	Osteoid osteoma
	Ossifying fibroma
	Osteochondroma
	Adamantinoma
	Nonossifying fibroma
	Benign fibrous cortical defect
	Fibrous dysplasia (occasionally)
Surface	Parosteal osteosarcoma
	Periosteal osteosarcoma
	Juxtacortical chondroma
	Giant cell tumor of the tendon sheath

Please note that some lesions which are typically eccentrically or even cortically based can appear centrally located in bones of small diameter such as the fibula or ulna. Examples of these include: Nonossifying Fibroma and Aneurysmal Bone Cyst.

coma, osteosarcoma, and malignant fibrous histiocytoma).

After the 10 determinants are well described, a conclusion should be drawn that states whether the lesion is aggressive or nonaggressive. Please note that the conclusion specifically should not state whether the lesion is malignant or benign. There are several highly aggressive lesions that might be mistaken as malignant based on the ten criteria but are in fact benign. These radiographically aggressive lesions include histiocytosis, infection, and the occasional aneurysmal bone cyst or giant cell tumor.

Radionuclide Studies

Radionuclide studies are not generally used in the work-up of soft tissue tumors of the musculoskeletal system. However, bone scans (Technetium[99m]Tc MDP) are used if it is desirable to determine whether an osseous lesion is monostotic or polyostotic. In addition, bone scans are used to search for skip lesions in patients with osteosarcoma. Thus, they are helpful in staging a bone tumor. Although the degree of abnormal uptake sometimes is correlated to the aggressiveness of the lesion, it does not correlate with histologic grade. Some benign lesions show very significant uptake due to their hypervascularity and host bone reaction. Additionally, bone scan may not accurately demonstrate the extent of a lesion. Some lesions show "extended uptake," with the abnormal pattern extending beyond the margin of the tumor. Therefore, bone scans are used primarily to evaluate whether more than one lesion is present. This is helpful both in determining whether the lesion is polyostotic, which can lead one to a diagnosis, or whether there are metastatic bone lesions, an essential fact in staging a lesion.

Positron emitting tomography (PET) using 18F fluorodeoxyglucose (FDG) may be used to evaluate tumor metabolic activity, based on glucose uptake and retention. This is a promising method for tumor characterization and possibly even grading, but there is, at present, overlap between benign and malignant lesions and the technique's value has not been proven conclusively at this time.[2,3] There is also promising work suggesting that FDG imaging with PET may show better accuracy than MRI in differentiating recurrent or residual tumor from posttherapy changes.[4]

Computed Tomograpy (CT)

Generally, MRI is preferred for local staging both in osseous and soft tissue tumors. However, there may be a few circumstances in which CT is chosen. CT may clarify diagnostic features of the lesion. Matrix calcification is better seen and characterized by CT compared with MRI. In addition, a thin rim of calcification or cortical detail is seen better with CT than MRI. Extraosseous involvement, however, is difficult to evaluate with CT except in the pelvic or chest wall region.

Magnetic Resonance Imaging (MRI)

MRI is currently unequaled in soft-tissue contrast and therefore is considered the state-of-the-art requirement for local staging for both soft tissue and osseous tumors. Specific requirements for complete and cost effective MRI of musculoskeletal tumors are listed in Table 1-6. As can be seen from Table 1-6, axial imaging of the entire lesion, plus reactive tissue, using T1 and spin echo T2 sequences is an absolute requirement for true site evaluation. Coronal and/or sagittal sequences may be included, but are generally not necessary for complete site evaluation. These planes can be particularly helpful, however, if the tumor is adjacent to and involving a joint. Chemical fat suppression techniques are often favored as many feel they improve conspicuity of the lesion and can further characterize neoplasms of lipomatous origin. Similarly, the use of intravenous (IV) gadolinium contrast improves lesion conspicuity relative to T1 imaging and may subjectively (but not objectively) improve conspicuity relative to T2 imaging. If contrast is used, fat suppression should be used as well with the imaging sequence as tumor to fat contrast decreases markedly after contrast injection. Gadolinium is most useful in showing areas of tumor

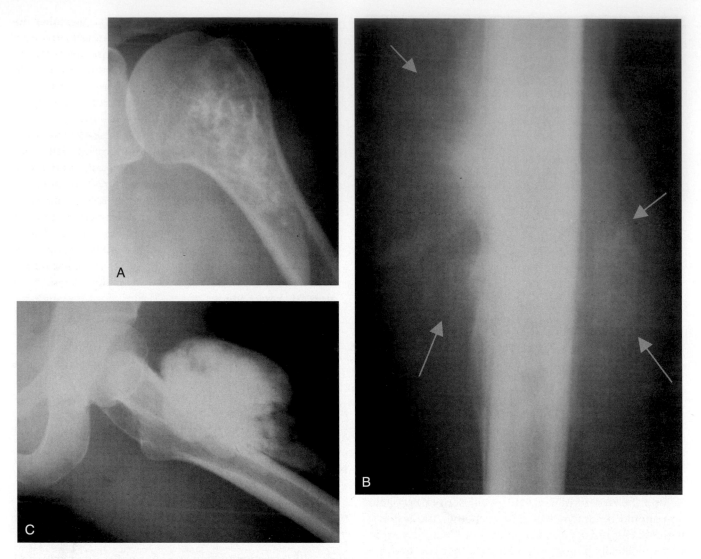

Fig. 1-3   Types of tumor matrix. **A,** An AP radiograph of the proximal humerus in a 42-year-old female that demonstrates the most typical appearance of cartilaginous matrix. Cartilaginous matrix is usually more dense than the underlying bone and has been described as being "spiculated," or having the shape of "rings and arcs" or "Cs and Js." The lesion in this case is an enchondroma. **B,** Amorphous osteoid matrix in the soft tissues of an osteosarcoma. The matrix is less dense than bone and shows no evidence of organized bone formation (*arrows*). **C,** A much more organized osteoid matrix, with denser bone formation that has a trabecular pattern in places. This is a parosteal osteosarcoma in a 22-year-old female.

necrosis, which in turn is useful in helping to guide biopsy.

Although we rely on MRI for site evaluation, it should be noted that many sequences exaggerate tumor size, as peritumoral edema signal cannot reliably be differentiated from adjacent tumor. This is the case with T2 spin echo sequences as well as inversion recovery imaging, and even postgadolinium imaging. It should also be remembered that hemorrhage, hematoma, and inflammatory change may produce abnormal signal intensity patterns that can be confused with tumor. Infection (Fig. 1-4) can involve several compartments, appear highly invasive, and incite prominent tissue reaction. Infections

may have nonspecific signal intensity on MRI unless there is an encapsulated abscess (which can be demonstrated with contrast injection). Similarly, hematoma, especially in a chronic stage, may be misdiagnosed as a malignant lesion by MRI. Chronic hematomas often incite tremendous adjacent tissue reaction and appear to involve many compartments with a highly inhomogeneous mass (see Fig. 1-4). Hematoma can mask an underlying tumor. If there is a question of whether a lesion thought to be hematoma is truly that lesion, biopsy is recommended.

As described above, MRI is used in musculoskeletal tumor evaluation primarily as a tool for tumor site evaluation. Thus, a complete report includes proximal and distal

Table 1-6   Requirements for musculoskeletal tumor MR imaging

1. Surface coils must be used if possible.
2. Axial images are required for evaluation of compartments as well as neurovascular bundles.
3. The entire extent of the lesion must be imaged with axial sequences. One longitudinal scan is also included for evaluation of skip metastases.
4. Inclusion of an externally palpable landmark is highly desirable, allowing measurement of distance to the lesion to be accurately translated from the MR scan to the surgical site.
5. T1 imaging must be included, as it shows high tumor to fat contrast.
6. T2 spin echo sequences are generally included, showing high tumor to muscle contrast.
7. Evaluation of joint involvement often requires coronal or sagittal imaging.
8. Inversion recovery or gadolinium enhanced imaging may subjectively enhance lesion conspicuity.
9. Gadolinum enhanced imaging may assist in guiding biopsy of necrotic lesions.

extent of soft tissue as well as osseous abnormality, located relative to an external landmark. Transverse extent of the lesion and specific compartmental involvement, as well as evaluation of neurovascular bundles and joint involvement is specified as well, including whether the lesion involves more than one compartment and whether it appears to be locally invasive or encapsulated. However, we also describe the different signal intensities and enhancement characteristics in an MRI report. The question then becomes how reliable these parameters are in predicting either the histology of the lesion, or whether the lesion is benign or malignant.[5,6] Parameters that have been considered useful by several investigators include signal intensity, tissue homogeneity, lesion size, lesion margins, peritumoral edema, involvement of adjacent tissues, and pattern of enhancement. None of these parameters alone is a reliable indicator of grade of lesion. In general, larger lesions are more likely to be malignant, but there is significant overlap between benign and malignant lesions using this parameter. Although one would teleologically expect that an appearance of encapsulation would indicate a benign lesion, malignant lesions can

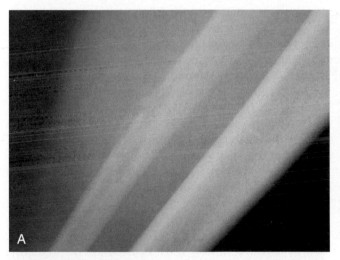

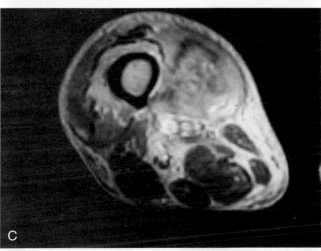

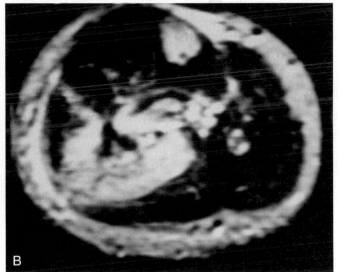

Fig. 1-4   Mimickers of aggressive tumors. **A,** A lateral radiograph of the fibula in a 48-year-old male that shows a highly aggressive lesion with permeative change and extensive periosteal reaction. **B,** The MR is an axial T2-weighted image of the leg (2000/80) showing an aggressive high signal lesion surrounding the fibula but extending into anterior, lateral, and posterior compartments and surrounding the neurovascular bundle. This gives the appearance of a highly aggressive lesion. At biopsy, this proved to be staphylococcal osteomyelitis. **C,** An axial T1-weighted (1000/30) gadolinium enhanced MR of a biopsy-proven hematoma in a 71-year-old male. Note the inhomogeneous enchancement and involvement of multiple muscle groups as well as neurovascular bundle. In this case, hematoma was not distinguishable by MRI from an aggressive tumor. (Reprinted with permission from the ACR learning file.)

acquire "pseudocapsules" that have well-defined margins. Additionally, several benign soft tissue tumors can be locally invasive with very ill-defined margins. This parameter of lesion margin is therefore of little reasonable predictive value. Peritumoral edema can be present in both benign and malignant lesions. Although increased vascularity tends to be present in malignant rather than benign tumors, the degree and pattern of enhancement does not relate reliably to tumor grade or malignancy, again because of significant overlap between these types of lesions. In addition, studies have attempted to classify soft tissue lesions using various combinations of the above parameters and multivariate analysis. One study of 225 soft tissue lesions (179 benign, 46 malignant) showed that no single feature or combination of features could reliably distinguish benign from malignant lesions.[7] For the entire cohort in this study, sensitivity of diagnosis of malignancy was 78% and specificity 89%. When benign tumors were excluded, sensitivity remained the same but specificity decreased to 76%. One concludes then that the accuracy of MRI parameters in determining whether a lesion is benign or malignant decreases to unacceptable levels when the typically benign tumors, such as lipomas, are excluded from the analysis.

If the accuracy of MRI in differentiating between benign and malignant tumors is disappointing, the accuracy of MRI in predicting histology is even more so. Most tumors have low T1 osseous signal, a T1 soft tissue signal that is isointense with muscle, and a high T2 signal. There are a few exceptions to the "isointense with muscle on T1" and "high signal intensity on T2" nonspecificity of tumors, where MRI does indeed aid in histologic diagnosis. These are outlined in Tables 1-7 and 1-8. One of the larger studies devoted to predicting histology of lesions was able to make an accurate histologic diagnosis using MRI alone in only 44% of 225 cases.[7] This discouragingly low accuracy decreases even further when the typically benign soft tissue lesions such as lipoma and hemangioma as well as pigmented villonodular synovitis and abscesses are excluded (as they do have fairly typical MRI appearances). It seems then that large studies confirm that, aside from a very few lesions, the histologic predictive value of MRI is poor. The reason for this is suggested by DeSchepper.[5] DeSchepper notes that soft

---

Table 1-7 Differential diagnosis for mass with short T1 (high signal intensity)

A. Lipoma
B. Hematoma (subacute): methemoglobin
C. Intralesional hemorrhage
D. Gadolinium enhancement
E. Dystrophic fat within another lesion
F. Fatty stroma of hemangioma
G. Proteinaceous material

Table 1-8 Differential diagnosis for mass with predominantly low signal intensity on T2

A. Hypocellular fibrous tumor
B. Scar tissue
C. Dense mineralization
D. Melanin
E. Acute hematoma
F. Vascular flow void
G. Gas
H. Foreign body
I. Hemosiderin or iron containing tissue
J. Pigmented villonodular synovitis
K. Giant cell tumor of the tendon sheath
L. Synovial pannus tissue
M. Gouty tophus
N. Amyloid

---

tissue tumors belonging to the same histologic group may have different proportions of tumor components, with high grade lesions being extremely cellular and showing virtually no hint by MRI of the cell of origin. An example here would be the spectrum ranging from lipoma through well differentiated liposarcoma to the polymorphic, poorly differentiated liposarcomas. DeSchepper also notes that some tumors have time-dependant changes in their cellular content. An example of differing MRI appearance over time of a single lesion would be of early desmoid tumors, which are highly cellular, with a high water content, but older desmoid tumors, which are more collagenous and less cellular, are classically described with low signal intensity in both T1 and T2 imaging. These observations also help to explain Kransdorf's statement that up to 20% of the "classic" appearances are absent in those lesions that have a typical specific appearance described.[8,9]

Kransdorf, using large volumes of material collected at the Armed Forces Institute of Pathology (AFIP), demonstrated the usefulness of tumor prevalence, patient age and gender, and lesion zonal distribution in predicting soft tissue tumor histology. Just as with skeletal lesions, these parameters give extremely useful information even without the addition of imaging.[8,9] This information is highly valuable. It is recommended that the tabular form be kept readily available for reference.[10] A brief summary of this information is as follows. Kransdorf's benign series showed that 70% of benign soft tissue tumors can be categorized into eight categories[8]: Lipomatous variants (16%), fibrous histiocytomas (13%), nodular fasciitis (11%), hemangioma (8%), fibromatosis (7%), neurofibroma (5%), schwannoma (5%), and giant cell tumor of the tendon sheath (4%). The other tables then group 80% of all benign tumors in the seven most common diagnoses for each age and location. Kransdorf's malignant series show that 80% of malignant soft tissue lesions can be classified into eight categories[9]: malignant fibrous histiocytoma (24%), liposarcoma (14%), leiomyosarcoma (8%), malignant schwannoma (6%), dermatofibrosarcoma protruberans (6%), synovial sarcoma (5%), fibrosarcoma (5%), and sarcoma not otherwise classified (12%). Kransdorf then uses tables to group 79% of all malignant tumors in the five most common diagnoses for each age and location.

The above information, particularly in the more detailed tabular form given by Kransdorf, can be used in combination with some other parameters to help suggest histologic diagnosis. Thus, although MRI alone has a poor record of histologic specificity for soft tissue tumors, when used in combination with statistical likelihood based on age, location, and prevalence, its histologic specficity improves.

SUGGESTED ALGORITHMS FOR MUSCULOSKELETAL TUMOR WORK-UP

Based upon the information that the treating clinician needs, algorithms can be suggested for the work-up of osseous as well as soft-tissue lesions. These algorithms

produce the information required of the work-up, and help make the package as cost efficient as possible. The osseous lesion work-up is pictured in Figure 1-5. Note that it always starts with a radiograph and with the evaluation of whether the lesion features are aggressive or nonaggressive. If the lesion is not aggressive, it is both logical and cost efficient to stop the work-up before obtaining an MRI or any other imaging. If the lesion is aggressive by plain film parameters, the algorithms work through the question of whether or not a bone scan is necessary, the timing of acquisition of the chest film and CT to evaluate for metastatic disease, and of MRI for local staging. The algorithm for soft tissue musculoskeletal lesion work-up is shown in Figure 1-6. This is a much simpler algorithm. It also starts with plain film, with the recognition that plain film will usually not add a significant amount of information. It proceeds directly to MRI, followed by biopsy. The reason for delaying the work-up for metastatic disease (chest film and CT) until after the biopsy relates to the fact that MRI parameters rarely are specific in predicting whether the primary tumor is benign or malignant.

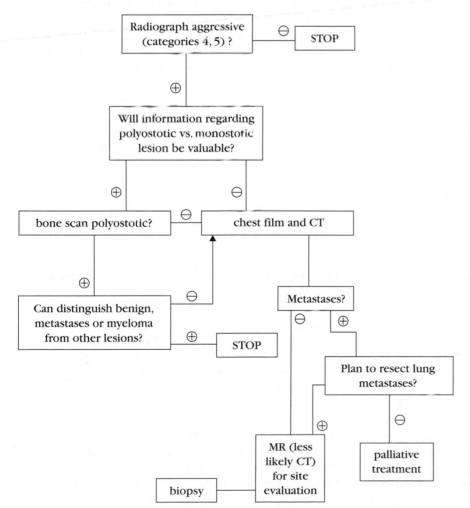

Fig. 1-5 Suggested algorithm for osseous lesion work-up. (Adapted from Manaster, B, Handbook of Skeletal Radiology, Second Edition, Mosby 1997, p 12.)

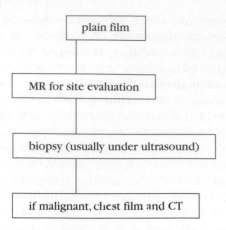

Fig. 1-6   Suggested algorithm for soft tissue musculoskeletal lesion work-up. (Adapted from Manaster, B, Handbook of Skeletal Radiology, Second Edition, Mosby 1997, p 13.)

BIOPSY OF THE TUMOR

Both tumor staging and treatment decisions require confidence that representative tissue is obtained in the biopsy. Whether the biopsy is obtained percutaneously by the radiologist or by surgical incision, imaging contributes significantly to the biopsy planning process. Imaging should help to direct sampling away from necrotic or less aggressive areas of tumor to obtain optimal tissue sampling. In addition, consideration of needle approach is crucial. One must work with the surgeon to determine the needle approach that will avoid contaminating more than one compartment or any of the soft tissues that the surgeon may require for reconstruction. There are two regions in the body that are frequently biopsied in a careless manner, compromising optimal treatment. The first is the region around the knee, where those obtaining a percutaneous biopsy may not recognize that the suprapatellar bursa extent is quite large, often resulting in contamination of the knee joint during placement of the needle for a biopsy nearby. The second site, which is occasionally biopsied in a suboptimal manner, is the region of the pelvis. It is important to avoid biopsying through the gluteal musculature if this soft tissue will be needed for coverage following resection of a pelvic lesion. Therefore, consultation with the surgical oncologist, combined with careful and thoughtful MRI, is a prerequisite to biopsy and eventual treatment of these musculoskeletal lesions.

TUMOR FOLLOW-UP

Follow-up examinations in patients with a musculoskeletal neoplasm are critical and must be planned ac-cording to a logical protocol. Timing and type of imaging used for follow-up examination is a crucial issue and ideally should be individualized for each tumor type and indeed each patient. It should relate to the hazard rate of the tumor in that individual (likelihood of timing of recurrence); the individual hazard rate is related to tumor type, grade, size, location, patient age, gender, stage, type of treatment, and surgical margins. The goal of a follow-up imaging protocol is to concentrate testing when the relapse is most likely to occur. However, models relating to the hazard rate and utility/risk analysis do not exist for most individual extremity tumor types, and the best the literature offers is to consider the sarcomas as a group. Most agree that approximately 80% of patients who recur locally or systemically will do so within 2 years of primary treatment. This suggests that the most frequent follow-up should occur in the first 2 years, with tapering of imaging frequency after that time. After an extensive review of the literature and development of a consensus, The American College of Radiology Appropriateness of Care committee came to the conclusion that local recurrence imaging should, for routine malignant musculoskeletal tumors, start with a baseline MRI evaluation 3 months postoperatively, followed by 6 month follow-up evaluation for the first 2 years. After the first 2 years of follow-up, it is recommended that imaging surveillance for local recurrence may decrease in frequency to yearly examinations and that follow-up examination beyond 5 years might occur only if the patient becomes symptomatic.[11] Note that follow-up examination for systemic disease includes chest CT, whereas follow-up for local recurrence uses MRI if possible. However, the presence of orthopedic hardware may preclude the use of MRI, in which case combinations of radiographs, CT, and ultrasound may be necessary.

When MRI is used to follow treated tumors, it is important to recognize that high signal intensity on T2-weighted MRI can be seen for a number of nonneoplastic lesions. These include the presence of postoperative seroma, hematoma, changes related to radiation therapy, fat necrosis, the presence of packing material, scar tissue, or even herniation of other tissue into the tumor bed. Although the timing of the study relative to the therapy and knowledge of details of the surgical treatment in individual cases can be highly valuable in trying to determine whether high signal on T2-weighted MRI is due to tumor recurrence, in many cases, biopsy will be necessary to rule out tumor recurrence. Very few specific protocols for follow-up examination of tumors have been advocated. However, in DeSchepper's book,[5] Vanel suggests an algorithm that begins with T2 imaging. If this demonstrates a mass with high signal, it is followed by T1 imaging, with and without contrast. This generally distinguishes hematoma and hygroma from tumors or inflammation. If necessary, this can by followed by dynamic subtraction contrast scanning that may help distinguish tumors from inflammation. In this algorithm, if a region of high signal intensity was seen on T2 imaging but there was no mass present, further imaging with contrast was not recommended. Although this sequence of imaging is logical, it is also recommended that biopsy should be considered with a finding of mass with high signal intensity on T2.

In addition to recurrence, there are other complications of tumor therapy (Table 1-9). Radiation therapy in a skeletally immature patient can result in growth cessation and/or deformities if the epiphyses or apophyses are included in the field of radiation (Fig. 1-7A). Before the early physeal fusion, epiphysial plate widening and metaphysial fraying may be seen, resembling rickets. In addition, skeletally immature patients undergoing radiation can develop radiation-induced osteochondromas (Fig. 1-7A). A patient of any age can develop radiation osteonecrosis, with the appearance of a permeative change, often with some sclerosis, in the bones, which is restricted to the radiation port (Fig. 1-7B). Radiation osteonecrosis often appears aggressive and may result in pathologic fracture. This necrotic bone is also more susceptible to infection. Therefore it may be quite difficult to differentiate radiation necrosis from infection or tumor recurrence. Finally, radiation induced sarcomas can occur (Fig. 1-7B). These most commonly result in development of osteosarcoma, malignant fibrous histiocytoma, fibrosarcoma, or chrondrosarcoma, which arises in a previously radiated field, usually 4–20 years after therapy. These sarcomas may be difficult to differentiate initially from radiation osteonecrosis, but a soft tissue mass and other aggressive features are soon demonstrated. The prognosis is very poor for radiation induced sarcomas.

Following tumors treated with chemotherapy to determine their response is difficult. The most important indicator determining response is a high percentage of tumor necrosis by pathologic evaluation. Clearly, histologic evaluation for necrosis is best, but imaging predictors are used as well. Size may be the best imaging predictor, with a 50% decrease in the product of the two largest diameters suggesting a good response. However, a patho-

logic fracture may falsely suggest increased size because of surrounding hemorrhage. In addition, osteosarcoma often shows little change in size despite good response as the soft tissue mass may evolve into a more mature, denser osteoid matrix, which itself does not decrease in size. If dynamic contrast enhanced MRI is available, then blood flow may differentiate between hypervascular viable tumor and inflammatory necrotic tissue response to therapy. However, this is subject to sampling error. Matrix does not represent a reliable parameter, as increasing reactive calcification only weakly correlates with tumor response. Similarly, the appearance of margins has a poor correlation with response, as a tumor-containing "pseudocapsule" may form. It is believed by many that P31 MR spectroscopy and PET imaging may show changes in metabolic rates indicating response, but these are neither proven nor in general use at this time.

During chemotherapy, reconversion to hematopoietic marrow in nonirradiated bones is often seen, especially if granulocyte/monocyte colony stimulating factor is given concurrently. This may be potentially confusing, as regions of previously normal appearing fatty marrow develop low signal intensity on T1 sequences.

Follow-up examination of a limb salvage with allograft is an art form as well. Because hardware is present, effective MR imaging may not be possible. If that is the case, tumor recurrence must be watched for on radiograph as a soft tissue mass, or subtle matrix formation, CT with contrast, or ultrasound may be useful in individual cases. Allografts are prone to an increased incidence of infection because of the presence of a large nonvascular piece of bone, in combination with hardware and an immunocompromised patient. Infection must be differentiated from tumor recurrence and certainly retards postoperative healing. Complications of limb salvage also include hardware failure. Graft resorption often occurs. Large osteoarticular allografts may show a pattern of early cortical graft resorption, followed by slow thickening over several months. Resorptive "cysts" may be prominent for the first 2 years. Late remodeling is manifest as a subcortical sclerotic rim. Late articular collapse also may occur. The allografts themselves may show a late fracture in 15%–20% of cases. These insufficiency fractures can be difficult to detect. Even with the presence of hardware, CT with reconstruction can be helpful. It may take up to 2 years for union with the graft to be demonstrated. Such "delay" should be expected, although vascularized fibular grafts may progress to union considerably faster.

CONCLUSION

Careful thought and planning is required in the workup and follow-up examination of musculoskeletal lesions. Consultation with the oncologist and surgeon is neces-

---

Table 1-9 Complications of radiation therapy for musculoskeletal tumors

A. Tumor recurrence
B. Early growth cessation
C. Growth deformities
D. Radiation induced osteochondroma
E. Infection
F. Radiation osteonecrosis
G. Radiation induced sarcoma

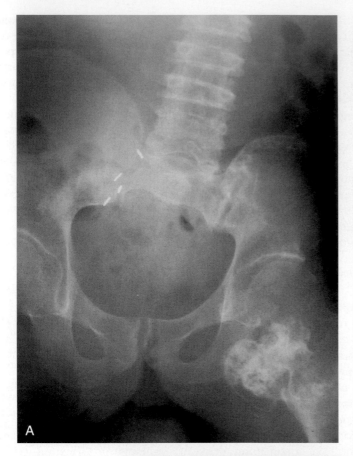

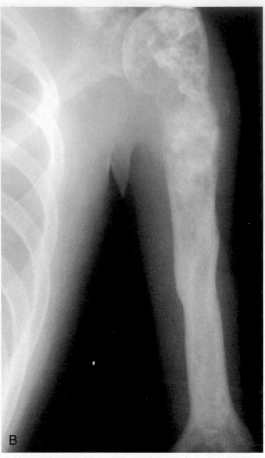

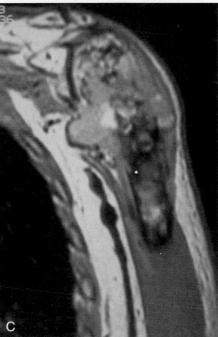

Fig. 1-7   Complications of radiation. **A,** An AP radiograph of the pelvis in a 20-year-old male. It demonstrates hypoplasia of the lower lumbar spine and left hemipelvis in a portlike distribution related to radiation for a Wilms tumor several years earlier. There is an additional finding of a large exostosis arising from the metaphyseal region of the proximal left femur. Exostoses can also be seen as a complication of radiation. (Fig. 1-7A is reprinted with permission from the ACR learning file.) **B,** An AP radiograph of the humerus in a 25-year-old male who had whole bone radiation for Ewing's sarcoma 12 years earlier. The proximal half of the humerus demonstrates mixed lytic and sclerotic bone, which is typical of radiation osteonecrosis. The bone is short relative to the patient's thorax, indicating arrested growth in this patient who was radiated before skeletal maturity. In addition, there is frank destruction of the bone at the proximal metaphysis, with a soft-tissue mass. **C,** This mass is confirmed on the coronal MRI (2200/20), indicating radiation sarcoma superimposed on the radiation necrosis.

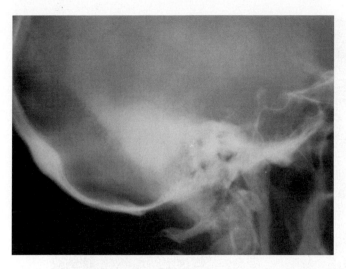

Fig. 1-8 Osteoma. This lateral radiograph of the skull demonstrates a calverial osteoma, with dense homogenous bone formation.

sary to provide optimal imaging and assist in optimal planning for these patients.

BONE-FORMING TUMORS: BENIGN

Osteoma

An osteoma is actually a hamartoma, an abnormal proliferation of compact bone without stromal cellular proliferation. Osteomas usually are found in membranous bones, either in the calvarium (usually arising from the external table), or in the paranasal sinuses (Fig. 1-8).

The entire lesion is sclerotic, with dense homogenous compact bone formation. The lesion is not aggressive, being geographic in nature and eliciting no host response except occasional expansion of adjacent bony margins. Osteomas may be multifocal, especially as part of Gardner syndrome, a disease of autosomal dominant inheritance that is associated with multiple colonic adenomatous polyps. Diagnosis is made by radiographic characteristics, and no treatment is necessary. If an osteoma is incidentally noted on MRI examination, it will appear with low signal on all sequences because of its dense bone formation. Differential diagnosis of an osteoma includes blastic metastasis, as well as calvarial hyperostosis adjacent to meningioma.

Enostosis (Bone Island)

Like the osteoma, a bone island is a hamartomatous proliferation of bone, with cortical bone density found in the medullary canal of any bone. At first glance, this dense bone appears geographic and generally rounded, but closer inspection demonstrates spicules at the margin of the lesion (Fig. 1-9) that blend into the normal surrounding trabeculae. Therefore they may not have a truly narrow zone of transition, but they also do not have an aggressive appearance. There is no host response to a bone island. The lesion is very common, usually noted incidentally. It can be highly variable in size, and if large enough will demonstrate increased uptake on bone scan due simply to the additional bone presence rather than implying any additional vascularity or activity. If a bone island is noted on MRI examination, it will appear with low signal intensity on all sequences, similar to cortical bone.

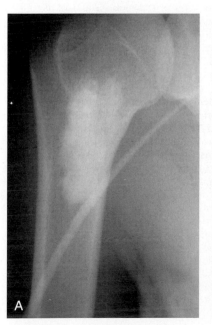
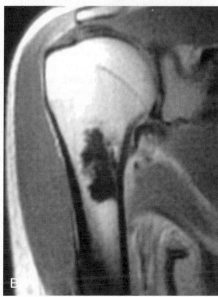

Fig. 1-9 Bone island. **A,** An AP radiograph of the humerus in a 23-year-old female, demonstrating a typical bone island in which dense bone formation is seen to be homogenous except at its peripheral edges where it blends into the underlying normal bone. A catheter is crossing the field. **B,** A coronal proton density MRI (2000/31) that shows the bone island to be low signal. It would have this appearance on any sequence.

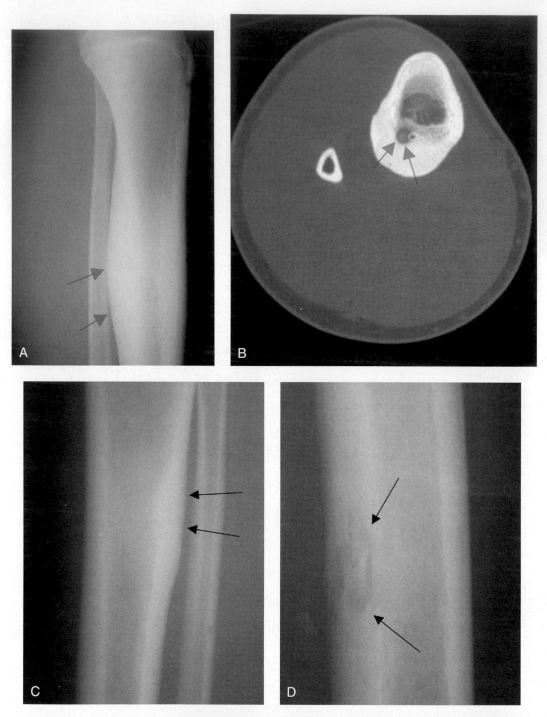

Fig. 1-10   Cortically based osteoid osteoma. **A,** A lateral radiograph demonstrating focal cortical thickening of the posterior diaphysis of the tibia in this 14-year-old male (*arrow*). The cortical reaction is so dense that the nidus of the osteoid osteoma is not seen. **B,** It is, however, easily seen on the CT (*arrows*). Note again the dense cortical thickening adjacent to the osteoid osteoma nidus. **C,** A lateral radiograph of the leg in a 16-year-old female, which demonstrates thickening of the cortex of the tibia in the posterior medial position in its proximal third (*arrows*). This is a typical position for a stress fracture, which it proved to be. However, the radiographic appearance is not always distinguishable from an osteoid osteoma with the nidus obscured. **D,** A lateral radiograph of the mid-diaphysis of the femur in a 15-year-old male. It also demonstrates thickening of the cortex, this time with a lytic lesion and central density (*arrows*). Although this could possibly represent an osteoid osteoma with central calcified nidus, the T1-weighted MRI **E,** (450/14) demonstrates that in fact the central density is a sequestrum within a focus of osteomyelitis in the femur (*arrows*).

Continued

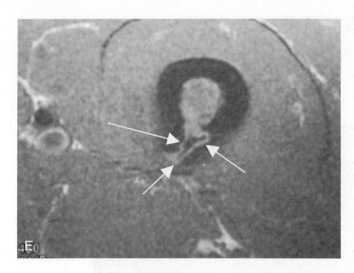

Fig. 1-10, cont'd   For legend see opposite page

Key Concepts   Osteoid Osteoma

- The lesion is lytic with or without a sclerotic nidus.
- Sclerotic host reaction may obscure the nidus on radiographs in a cortically based lesion of a tubular bone.
- Sclerotic host reaction may be located at some distance from the nidus if the lesion is intracapsular.
- Most common locations: Femoral diaphysis, tibial diaphysis, femoral neck, posterior elements of the spine.
- CT localization is most helpful in treatment.

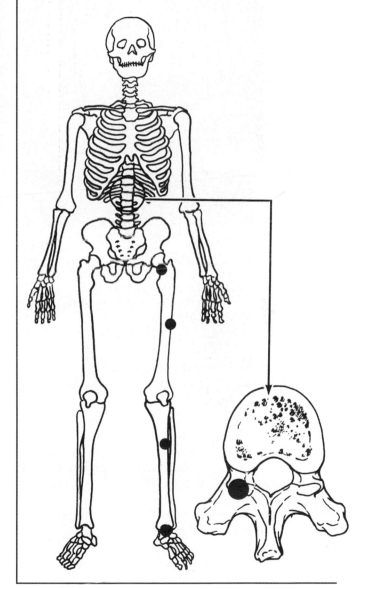

Bone islands may be polyostotic and in fact may be considered at one end of the spectrum of sclerosing dysplasias, which include the entity osteopoikilosis (multiple epiphysial bone islands). There is no treatment or further work-up examination required for bone island. Rarely, a bone island could be confused with other entities considered in a differential diagnosis, including blastic metastasis, a dense osteoid osteoma that obscures its nidus, osteoblastoma, or a sclerosing intramedullary osteosarcoma. Bone islands occasionally increase in size, further confusing the diagnosis.

Osteoid Osteoma

Osteoid osteoma is a small lytic lesion with a circumscribed nidus that may or may not contain a central site of mineralized osteoid. The nidus is, by definition, less than 2 cm in size, but elicits very prominent surrounding reactive bone formation. Osteoid osteoma may not be truly neoplastic as it has limited growth potential, unlike osteoblastoma, which is identical histologically, but has unlimited growth potential and may undergo malignant transformation.

The appearance of an osteoid osteoma may vary according to its location. Cortically based osteoid osteomas (the most common variety) are found in the tubular bones. These may elicit a densely sclerotic reaction so dense that the nidus may be masked on plain film (Figs. 1-10 and 1-11). If the nidus is not seen, these lesions could be confused with prominent healing bone formation about a stress fracture or possibly reactive bone formation about a small chronic cortically based abscess (see Fig. 1-10).

Another variety of osteoid osteoma is found in intracapsular locations, especially along the femoral neck. Unlike the cortical osteoid osteomas, these intracapsular lesions elicit little marginal sclerosis or periosteal bone formation. However, host reaction is often found at a considerable distance from the nidus, more distally along the cortex (Fig. 1-12). In addition, host reaction

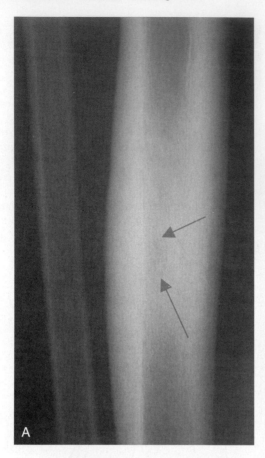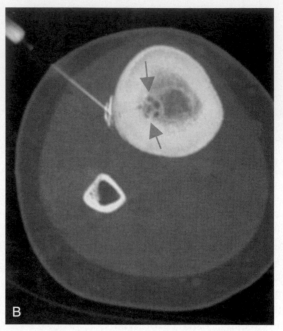

Fig. 1-11   Cortically based osteoid osteoma. **A,** Prominent circumferential cortical reactive bone formation with a faint suggestion of a nidus (*arrow*) in the mid diaphysis of the tibia of this 14-year-old male. **B,** The CT confirms the cicumferential nature of the cortical reaction and the cortically based nidus (*arrows*), with a pathologic fracture faintly seen. The best surgical access to the nidus has been localized with a needle and a drop of methyline blue mixed with radiographic contrast has been placed to guide the surgeon.

in the form of chronic synovitis can be intense and, over a long period of time, can result in lateral subluxation of the femoral head. In an adult, degenerative changes can ensue in the form of osteophytes or calcar buttressing (Fig. 1-12). If chronic synovitis and lateral subluxation of the femoral head occurs in a child with an intracapsular osteoid osteoma, irreversible limb length discrepancy and a valgus configuration of the femoral neck can result (see Fig. 1-12). Because the sclerotic bone reaction is found at some distance from the nidus and the articular reaction can be extreme, the actual culprit in this variety of osteoid osteoma, the nidus, can be easily missed.

The least common variety of osteoid osteoma is found in a subperiosteal location. These are manifest as a round, soft-tissue mass located immediately adjacent to bone with underlying scalloping, irregular bone resorption, and little reactive change. The talus is the most common site of this rare variety of osteoid osteoma.

Osteoid osteomas commonly occur in the spine, especially the posterior elements. The patient can develop a painful scoliosis, with the lesion being formed at the concave margin of the apex of the curve. There is no rotatory component to this scoliosis. Because of the sclerotic reaction to the underlying nidus, an osteoid osteoma in the posterior elements of the spine can be mistaken for a blastic metastasis or sclerosis related to abnormal stress, particularly in a patient with contralateral spondylolysis.

Osteoid osteomas have a typical clinical presentation of aching pain, which is worse at night and relieved with aspirin. This presentation is not unique, but is suggestive of the diagnosis. These symptoms are dramatically relieved by complete excision of the lesion. The radiologist plays a key role in the treatment of these lesions, because precise localization of the very small nidus without interruption of the surrounding bone is required. The localization is usually provided by CT scan. To aid a surgeon intent on operative resection,

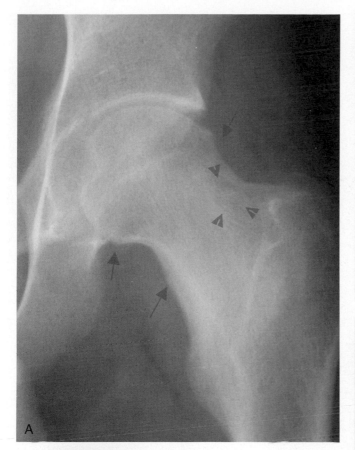

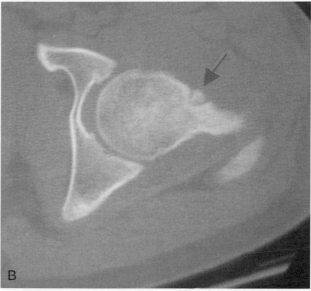

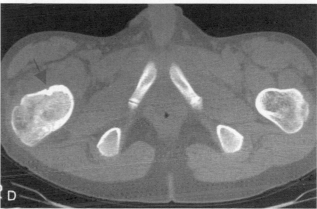

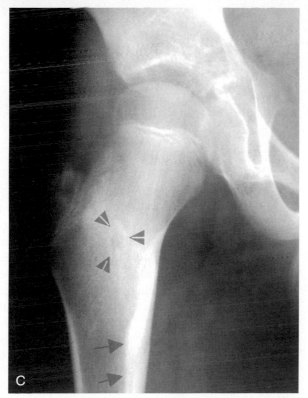

Fig. 1-12   Intracapsular osteoid osteoma. **A,** An AP radiograph of the hip in a 17-year-old male which demonstrates reactive change in the form of femoral head osteophytes and calcar buttressing (*short arrows*). The nidus of the osteoid osteoma is found in the femoral neck (*arrowheads*) which is within the capsule in this joint. **B,** CT localizes the nidus of the osteoid osteoma to the anterior cortex (*arrow*). **C,** An intracapsular osteoid osteoma with resultant growth deformities in a 10-year-old male. This AP radiograph of the hip shows dense and distant cortical reactive bone formation (*arrows*), a wide and valgus femoral neck, and the faintly seen nidus of the osteoid osteoma (*arrowheads*). **D,** The nidus is localized with CT (*arrow*). (Reprinted with permission from the ACR learning file.)

injection of a drop of methylene blue dye into the periosteum overlying the lesion allows precise localization (see Fig. 1-11). Such localization allows the surgeon to minimize the amount of cortical bone destroyed in the resection, decreasing the risk of postoperative fracture. Radiologists may themselves treat the lesion, either with core needle excision or radiofrequency ablations, using CT as a control.

MRI generally is not used in diagnosing or localizing osteoid osteomas. If the MRI slices are small enough to show the nidus, the nidus will appear with low signal intensity on T1 imaging and with variably low to high signal intensity on T2, usually enhancing intensely if contrast is given. The adjacent marrow may show either edema or sclerosis, with the attendant expected signal intensities. If the nidus is not noted, the appearance in the region of host reaction may mislead one toward a diagnosis of a larger, more aggressive lesion.

Osteoblastoma

Osteoblastoma is a rare benign bone-forming tumor that may be difficult to differentiate from osteoid osteoma histologically, but is quite distinct radiographically. Osteoblastoma may be characterized by its common location in the posterior elements of the spine (42%); the remainder of the lesions are found in long bones. Osteoblastomas are usually geographic, causing expansion of the underlying bone, with a narrow zone of transition and sclerotic margin. Although these are bone forming tumors, they have a wide range of density, from lucent through a mixed pattern, to a completely blastic appearance (Fig. 1-13). Because of this range of mineralization, the signal intensities seen on both T1 and T2 imaging can be highly variable. Generally, the lesions appear nonaggressive, with only occasional cortical breakthrough. Unlike osteoid osteomas, they may rarely undergo malignant transformation. Treatment is with curettage or marginal excision, and recurrence is rare. Because of the usual location in the posterior elements of the spine, differential diagnosis may include aneurysmal bone cyst. Because of the

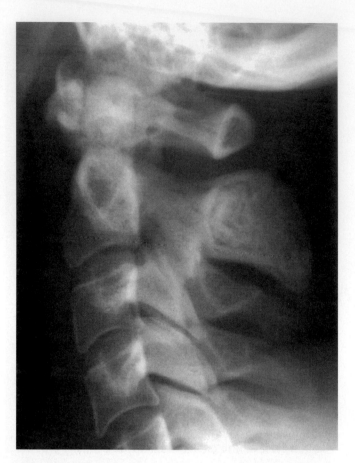

Fig. 1-13 Osteoblastoma. The expanded mixed lytic and blastic lesion located in the spinous process of C2 is a typical appearance of osteoblastoma in this 36-year-old female.

occasional finding of osteoid matrix, these lesions can be mistaken for osteosarcoma.

Ossifying Fibroma

Ossifying fibroma (also called osteofibrous dysplasia) is an extremely rare, benign lesion found almost exclusively in the proximal tibia. It most often appears in the first through third decades of life and appears as a cortically based geographic, oval lesion. It is associated with cortical bowing and generally causes local expansion of bone. It has a sclerotic rim and may be entirely lucent or may contain osteoid. This is an interesting lesion, as it can be similar, both histologically and radiographically, to cortically based fibrous dysplasia, or to an adamantinoma. These three lesions are believed, by some, to represent a spectrum of lesions although there are subtle histologic differentiating characteristics. Therefore, as there are no other radiographic distinguishing features, the radiologist should consider ossifying fibroma as well as cortically based fibrous dysplasia and

---

Key Concepts	Osteoblastoma

- The lesion is expansile and usually nonaggressive.
- The most common location is posterior elements of the spine.
- There is variable osteoid formation, resulting in appearance ranging from lytic (most common) to densely sclerotic.

adamantinoma whenever the location and appearance such as this dictates (Fig. 1-14).

Liposclerosing Myxofibrous Tumor

Liposclerosing myxofibrous tumor (LSMFT) is a fibrous benign lesion of bone that usually occurs in the fourth through sixth decades, and is most specifically characterized by its location. The vast majority (over 90%) of these lesions occur in the central metadiaphysis of the proximal femur. The lesion does not appear aggressive; it usually appears as a lytic or ground glass geographic lesion with a narrow zone of transition and often markedly sclerotic border (Fig. 1-15). Mineralized matrix is present in the majority of lesions.[12] The matrix appears globular and irregular. Because of the presence of matrix, MRI appearance is heterogeneous on T2 imaging, with decreased signal intensity in the regions of matrix and the stroma appearing to have higher signal intensity. T1-weighted images are more homogeneous, and isointese to muscle.

Although included in this section of benign bone forming tumors, the lesion actually contains a complex mixture of fatty, fibrous, xanthomatous, and myxoid elements. Ischemic ossification may be found within altered fat. Some feel that LSMFT may relate to osteofibrous dysplasia or ancient intraosseous lipoma. An important feature of this lesion is the fact that approximately 10% are reported to show malignant transformation, despite the initial nonaggressive appearance.[12] The lesion may present either with pain or may be incidental, but in any event must be monitored closely. Location in the intertrochanteric region of the femur is the key element to consideration of this lesion.

BONE-FORMING TUMORS: MALIGNANT (OSTEOSARCOMA)

Osteosarcoma is the most common primary malignant bone tumor in adolescents. Among all ages, it is second only to myeloma in frequency of primary bone malignancy (15%–20%). Several types of osteosarcoma are described and, because of their varying prognosis, treatment, and imaging features, we will consider them individually.

High-Grade Intramedullary (Conventional) Osteosarcoma

Conventional osteosarcoma comprises 75% of all osteosarcomas. Most arise in children between 10 and 25 years of age. Most osteosarcomas (90%) are metaphyseal in origin, but can be diaphyseal. Despite the metaphyseal origin, the tumor frequently crosses the physeal plate to

Key Concepts   Conventional Osteosarcoma

- This is the most common primary bone sarcoma in the adolescent age group.
- It is a highly aggressive lesion with permeative change, cortical breakthrough, and soft-tissue mass.
- The majority show osteoid matrix.
- It is frequently located about the knee, originating in the metaphasis and often extending across the physeal plate to the epiphysis.

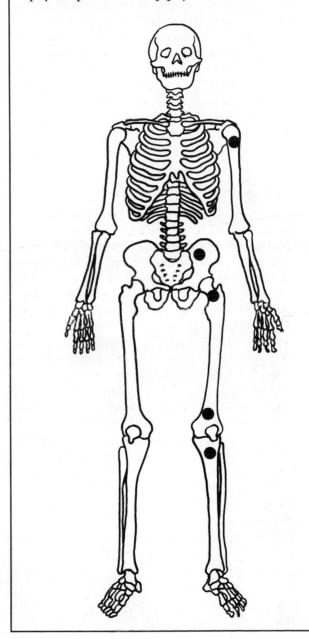

involve the epiphysis. Such epiphyseal involvement is found in 75% of cases and, although infrequently detected by radiography, can be easily seen on coronal or sagittal MRI images. Epiphyseal spread of tumor must be sought as there are significant therapeutic implications (the pre-

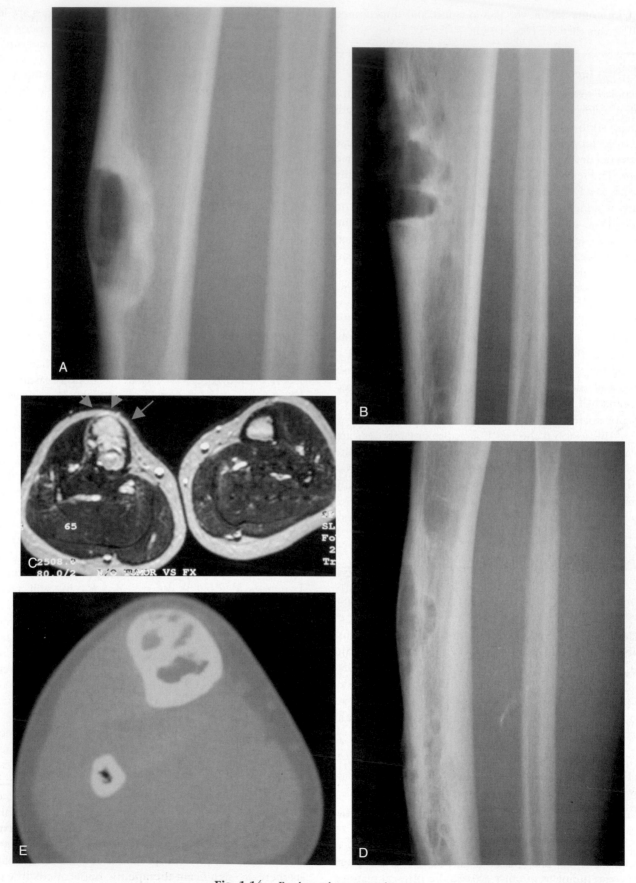

Fig. 1-14   For legend see opposite page

Fig. 1-14   Spectrum of osteofibrous dysplasia, cortical fibrous dysplasia, and adamantinoma. **A,** An AP radiograph of a cortically based lytic lesion in the proximal tibia of a 12-year-old female. This is typical of osteofibrous dysplasia (also known as ossifying fibroma). However, it is not always radiographically distinguishable from a cortically based fibrous dysplasia or adamantinoma. **B,** A lytic cortically based lesion in the anterior tibia of a 12-year-old female. This lesion has adjacent daughter lesions and at biopsy was found to be fibrous dysplasia. **C,** The T2-weighted axial MR image (2500/80), confirming the cortically based location of the lesion (*arrow*). **D,** Also shows cortically based lytic lesions in the anterior tibia, this time in a 10-year-old male, which proved to be adamantinoma. **E,** The CT confirms the cortical nature of this lesion. Note that there are no radiographically distinguishing features among these three lesions.

---

ferred allograft cannot be used; rather, osteoarticular graft or a prosthesis must be placed).

Conventional osteosarcoma occurs most frequently in the long bones, with the distal femur outnumbering the proximal tibia, which in turn is more frequently involved

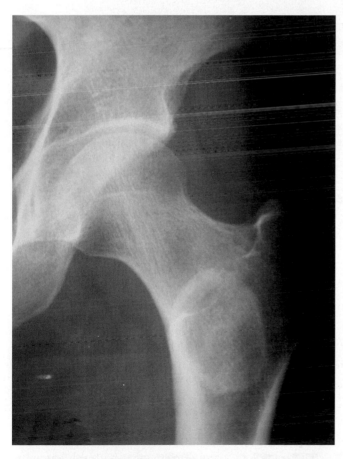

Fig. 1-15   LSMFT. This AP radiograph shows a well marginated, mixed lytic and sclerotic central lesion in the intertrochanteric region of the femur. This appearance and location is typical of liposclerosing myxofibrous tumor (LSMFT).

than the proximal humerus. Although flat bones are less frequently involved than long bones, osteosarcoma of the iliac wing deserves mention.

Osteosarcomas have a very rapid doubling rate and frequently are large when first noticed. They are highly aggressive in appearance, with a permeative pattern and wide zone of transition without margination (Fig. 1-16). Cortical breakthrough is usually seen, often with a large soft-tissue mass. Periosteal reaction is usually present and often appears aggressive, with a sunburst or Codman's triangle pattern.

Ninety percent of osteosarcomas produce osteoid matrix, which is visible on radiography or CT images. The amount of matrix, however, varies so that the radiographic appearance may range from densely blastic to nearly completely lytic (Figs. 1-16 to 1-18 and see 1-1B and C). The matrix most often appears amorphous or cloudlike, being less dense than normal bone, and without any organized trabecular pattern. It should be noted that, although 90% of osteosarcomas produce tumor bone matrix, which is visible radiographically, the lesions have different histologic terminology based on the fact that 50% produce enough osteoid to be termed "osteoblastic," whereas 25% produce predominately cartilage (chondroblastic) and 25% produce predominately spindle cells (fibroblastic). The radiographic appearance often corresponds to these histologic findings, with the matrix calcification in the cartilage and spindle cell variety being more subtle relative to that of the osteoblastic variety. It should also be noted that the matrix appears denser in the bone than in the soft tissue mass, as that in the bone is superimposed on the density of the remaining bone.

The MRI appearance of conventional osteosarcoma varies, according to the degree of mineralization of the matrix. If the matrix is quite dense, that portion of the tumor will appear to have low signal intensity on all sequences. If it is less dense, T1 weighting will have a nonspecific low signal intensity whereas T2 sequences will have inhomogeneous high signal intensity. Please note that because so many of these lesions occur around the knee, coronal or sagittal imaging may be required to evaluate for joint involvement. In addition, careful attention must be paid to imaging the remainder of the involved bone to detect "skip" lesions, said to occur in 1%–10% of cases.

There is no differential if the lesion shows osteoid matrix in the soft tissue mass and is typical in location. The differential diagnosis for osteosarcoma can include Ewing's sarcoma. Although Ewing's sarcoma tends to be diaphyseal in location, it can be metadiaphyseal. Furthermore, Ewing's sarcoma can elicit an extensive reactive bone formation that can mimic osteoid matrix. However, the reactive bone formation is restricted to the involved bone and does not extend into the soft tissue mass in a Ewing's sarcoma. This usually helps differentiate the two.

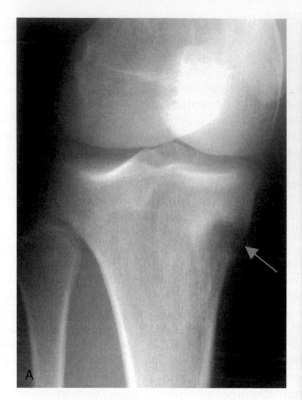
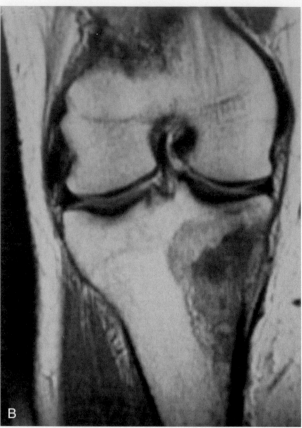

Fig. 1-16   Osteosarcoma. **A,** An oblique radiograph demonstrating a predominately lytic lesion in the metaphysis of the proximal tibia. There is a very small region of sclerosis within the bone which could represent either tumor matrix or reactive bone formation. Although the lesion appears small, it is aggressive, with cortical breakthrough (*arrow*) and is a predominately lytic osteosarcoma. **B,** The MR shows that the lesion is larger than might be expected by radiograph and that it is heterogenous, with both increased and decreased signal intensity on this proton density image (3000/20). The decreased signal intensity within the lesion represents osteoid matrix, which is not visible on the radiograph.

Any lesion that produces bone can be confused with osteosarcoma, including healing fractures and cortical desmoid. Cortical desmoid is an avulsive irregularity located posterior to the adductor tubercle in the distal femoral metaphysis. It may appear as a scalloped defect in the cortex, sometimes with a small soft tissue mass and periosteal elevation and occasionally even matrix calcification due to repair (see Fig. 1-60). Location is the key to diagnosis of a cortical desmoid; the cortical desmoid is always located on the posteromedial surface of the distal femoral metaphysis and, other than scalloping, does not affect the underlying bone. It is important to recognize a cortical desmoid to avoid biopsy, as tissue obtained during the active repair phase may be difficult to distinguish histologically from osteosarcoma.

Early myositis ossificans can be mistaken for a soft tissue or surface osteosarcoma (see Figs. 1-94, 1-95, and 1-96). The appearance of myositis ossificans is highly

dependent on time relative to the injury. After the first 4–8 weeks, amorphous calcification may develop in the soft tissue overlying bone, and periosteal reaction may be associated. This can be highly suggestive of osteosarcoma, although no underlying permeative change is found. Careful evaluation, including patient history, may mitigate a potentially confusing biopsy.

The metastatic potential of conventional osteosarcoma is high, with hematogenous spread to lungs or bones and lymphatic spread locally. Metastases are found in 10%–20% of patients at clinical presentation. Eighty percent of tumor relapses occur in the lung, and 20% in bone. Both local recurrence and systemic disease usually occur within two years after initial diagnosis.

The radiologic work-up begins with radiography, which usually establishes the diagnosis. Bone scan is used to assure that the lesion is monostotic, chest x-ray and CT to exclude metastatic disease to the lung, and MRI

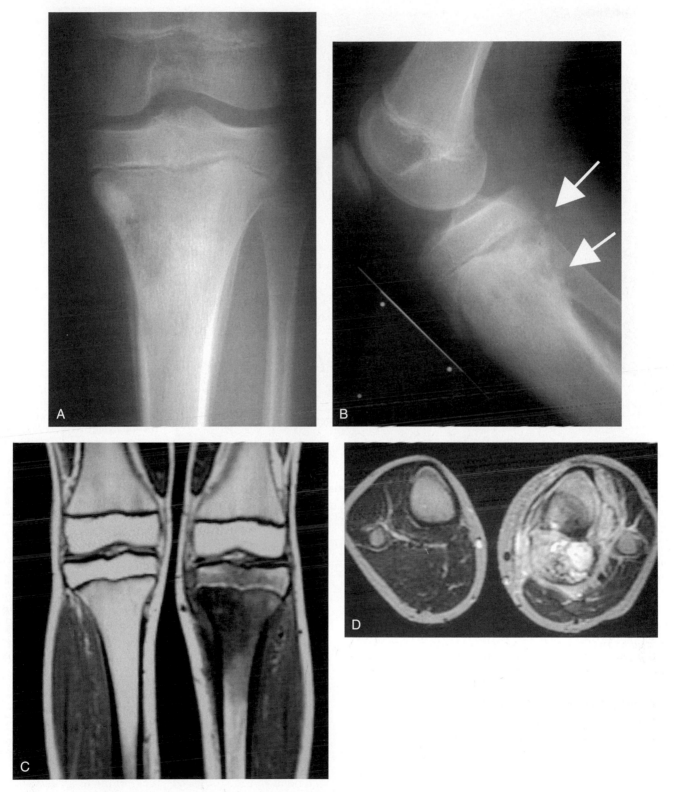

Fig. 1-17   Osteosarcoma. **A,** The AP and **B** lateral radiographs demonstrate a mixed lytic and sclerotic permeative lesion in the metadiaphysis of the tibia in this 14-year-old male. The lesion is highly aggressive, with abundant periosteal reaction and a tiny amount of tumor matrix seen in the posterior soft tissues (*arrow*). By radiographic criteria, this is the classic appearance of osteosarcoma. Also, by radiographic criteria, the epiphysis appears spared. **C,** However, the T1-weighted MR image (500/10) clearly shows extension of the lesion into the proximal epiphysis. **D,** The T2-weighted MRI (2030/80) demonstrates the large soft-tissue mass involving both the anterior and posterior compartments as well as the major neurovascular bundle.

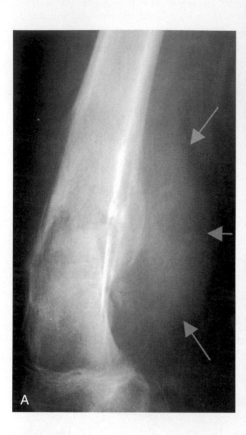

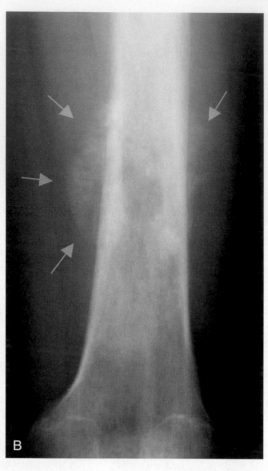

Fig. 1-18 Osteosarcoma. **A,** A lateral radiograph of a highly aggressive lesion involving the distal metaphysis of the femur in a 12-year-old female. Periosteal reaction is prominent. There is a large soft-tissue mass extending well beyond the periosteal reaction, and the mass contains very subtle amorphous tumor matrix (*arrows*). **B,** An AP radiograph of an osteosarcoma in a different patient that shows much more obvious osteoid matrix formation in the soft tissue mass (*arrows*). The range of density of osteoid can be wide.

to evaluate the local extent of the lesion, plan the biopsy, and plan definitive therapy. Treatment begins with induction chemotherapy, which helps to control the development of micrometastases, and to shrink the primary tumor, which would allow easier excision. Following the chemotherapy regimen, the tumor is re-staged with MRI. Pathologic assessment of the chemotherapy regimen judges percent of tumor necrosis at the time of surgery for limb salvage. Wide excision is required, and limb salvage is preferred if possible. The patient concludes therapy with adjuvant multidrug chemotherapy.

Telangiectatic Osteosarcoma

Telangiectatic osteosarcoma is a rare variant that has the hallmark of being difficult to diagnose as it is entirely lytic and appears much less aggressive than the conventional osteosarcoma. Telangiectatic osteosarcoma occurs in the same age range and location as conventional osteosarcoma but it differs in radiographic appearance, being primarily geographic rather than permeative. Although geographic in large part (Fig. 1-19), there may be a wide zone of transition in portions of the lesion and cortical breakthrough with soft-tissue mass. The lesion is highly vascular and contains necrotic

tissue and large pools of blood with tumor located only at the periphery and along septations. The tumor may show subtle osteoid matrix and also enhances in most cases.[13]

As described above, the plain radiograph can appear misleadingly nonaggressive, although there is usually some suggestion to alert the radiologist that the lesion is not completely nonaggressive (see Fig. 1-1D). The MRI may have prominent fluid-fluid levels, with hemorrhage frequently observed as areas with high signal intensity. With careful observation, the peripheral tumor can be seen to appear nodular in some areas, and irregular in others. Careful observation is required to avoid misdiagnosing telangiectatic osteosarcoma as the less aggressive aneurysmal bone cyst or even giant cell tumor.

The metastatic potential, work-up, prognosis, and therapy are identical to that of conventional osteosarcoma.

Parosteal Osteosarcoma

Parosteal osteosarcoma is a surface lesion that represents the second most common variety of osteosarcoma. Although there is a wide age range, including adolescents, more than 80% occur between the age of 20

Key Concepts   Parosteal Osteosarcoma

- The median age is older than for conventional sarcoma.
- Prognosis is better than conventional sarcoma.
- It is metaphysial surface lesion, most commonly found in the posterior aspect of the distal femur.
- Produces more mature osteoid than does conventional osteosarcoma.
- As it enlarges, it gives the appearance of wrapping around the underlying bone.

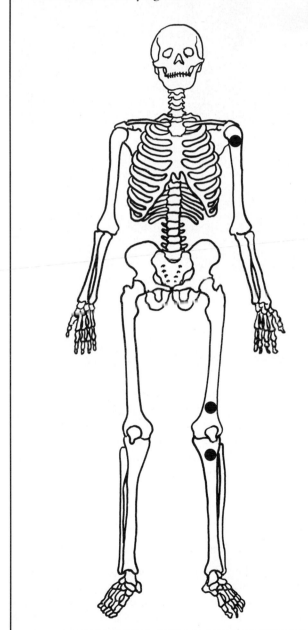

and 50, giving an older median age than is found with conventional osteosarcoma. The lesion also tends to be of lower grade and is better differentiated than conventional osteosarcoma, resulting in a substantially better prognosis.

This surface osteosarcoma is found most frequently at the posterior distal femoral metaphysis, with other common locations being the proximal tibia and proximal humerus. The lesion arises from the surface of the bone at the site of origin but is otherwise located nearly entirely in the soft tissues, wrapping around the underlying bone in a lobulated fashion as it enlarges (Figs. 1-20 and see 1-3C). This results in a cleavage plane between much of the lesion and the underlying bone. There is local invasion of the underlying bone in approximately 50% of cases. This is usually not seen by plain film, but confirmed on MRI examination (Fig. 1-21).[14]

Parosteal osteosarcoma is often large by the time of discovery. The tumor matrix is usually densely sclerotic mature osteoid, quite different in appearance from the immature osteoid of conventional osteosarcoma. Parosteal osteosarcomas show greater maturity of the tumor matrix centrally, while peripherally the matrix may be less mature or even nonossified (Fig. 1-22). This zoning pattern distinguishes the lesion from myositis ossificans, in which the more mature bone is found peripherally. CT can demonstrate this zoning phenomenon, as may MRI. The MRI appearance is variable, depending on the degree of matrix ossification. If it is not cellular and contains little cartilage there will be low signal on all sequences. However, there is often more cellularity present, as well as cartilaginous regions and soft-tissue mass, which give an inhomogeneous appearance. The extent of marrow involvement should be carefully assessed, as should regions that are more cellular, which might suggest a higher grade or dedifferentiation.[14]

Parosteal osteosarcomas tend to be very slow growing and low grade, but with inadequate excision may recur in a more aggressive form. With multiple recurrences they may dedifferentiate. These lesions can be ideal for limb salvage techniques of wide marginal resection. Because of the low-grade nature of the lesion, chemotherapy is generally not necessary. Metastases to the lung in parosteal osteosarcoma occur both later and with considerably less frequency compared with metastases in conventional osteosarcoma.

Parosteal osteosarcoma is generally not a difficult diagnosis to make. In its earliest stages, it could be mistaken for myositis ossificans, though the zoning of the mature bone differentiates the two both radiographically and histologically. Parosteal osteosarcoma is easily distinguished from an osteochondroma; the latter should show a cortex and marrow, each of which has continuity with its counterpart in the underlying bone.

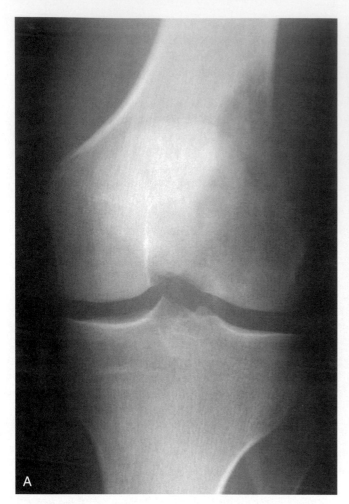

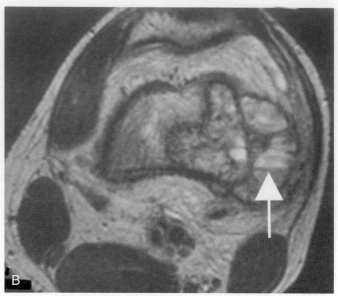

Fig. 1-19   Telangiectatic osteosarcoma. **A,** AP radiograph demonstrates a fairly geographic lytic lesion in the distal femoral metaphysis, extending to the subchondral region. The lesion is largely nonaggressive in appearance, particularly when compared with the highly aggressive osteosarcomas seen in Figures 1-16, 1-17, and 1-18. Telangiectatic osteosarcomas are often misjudged as being nonaggressive lesions. **B,** The T2-weighted MRI (2400/100) demonstrates the large extraosseous soft-tissue mass that contains fluid levels (*arrows*). Fluid levels are typically seen in telangiectatic osteosarcomas, but are seen in other lesions as well.

Periosteal Osteosarcoma

Periosteal osteosarcoma is a rare surface osteosarcoma. It has a distinct radiographic appearance compared with parosteal or conventional osteosarcomas. As it is a surface lesion, it usually causes scalloping of the underlying cortex, although occasionally cortical thickening is seen (Fig. 1-23). The soft-tissue mass extends from the surface of the lesion, usually with spicules of bone seen emanating in a sunburst pattern (see Fig. 1-2E and F). Periosteal reaction is common, often in the form of Codman's triangles. MRI demonstrates the extent of the soft-tissue mass and usually shows no intermedullary extension of the lesion, although the rare intramedullary extension of lesion should be sought as this will affect limb salvage plans. The MRI signal is nonspecific, being low intensity on T1-weighted images and high signal intensity on T2-weighted images. The perpendicular reactive bone formation may be seen as low signal linear rays on all sequences.[13]

Periosteal osteosarcomas are usually located in a more diaphyseal position than either conventional or parosteal osteosarcomas. The femur and the tibia are the most common locations for periosteal osteosarcoma. Periosteal osteosarcomas generally arise in the second or third decade, similar to or slightly later than conventional osteosarcomas. Treatment is by wide excision. Their prognosis is better than conventional osteosarcomas, although not as good as parosteal osteosarcomas.

The major differential diagnosis is of juxtacortical chondroma, another surface lesion that can have a very similar appearance (see Fig. 1-27). The rare high-grade surface osteosarcoma can be difficult to differentiate as well.

High-Grade Surface Osteosarcoma

High-grade surface osteosarcoma is rare. Like periosteal osteosarcomas, they tend to involve the diaphysis of long bones. They are similar in appearance to periosteal osteosarcomas although intramedullary involvement is more frequent in the high-grade surface lesions. High-grade surface osteosarcomas have a prognosis identical to that of conventional osteosarcoma.

Low-Grade Intraosseous Osteosarcoma

Low-grade intraosseous osteosarcoma is a rare variant that is entirely intraosseous. Its appearance ranges from

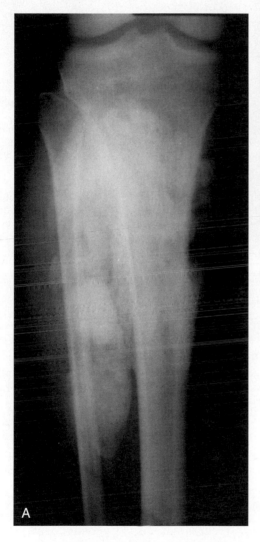

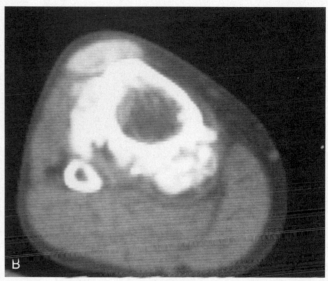

Fig. 1-20   Parosteal osteosarcoma. **A,** AP radiograph shows a dense well-defined osteoid matrix forming this tumor, which appears to "wrap around" the proximal tibial metadiaphysis in this 41-year-old male. **B,** The appearance of the tumor being a surface lesion, wrapping around the underlying bone is confirmed on CT. This is a large parosteal osteosarcoma in a typical location with characteristic mature osteoid formation.

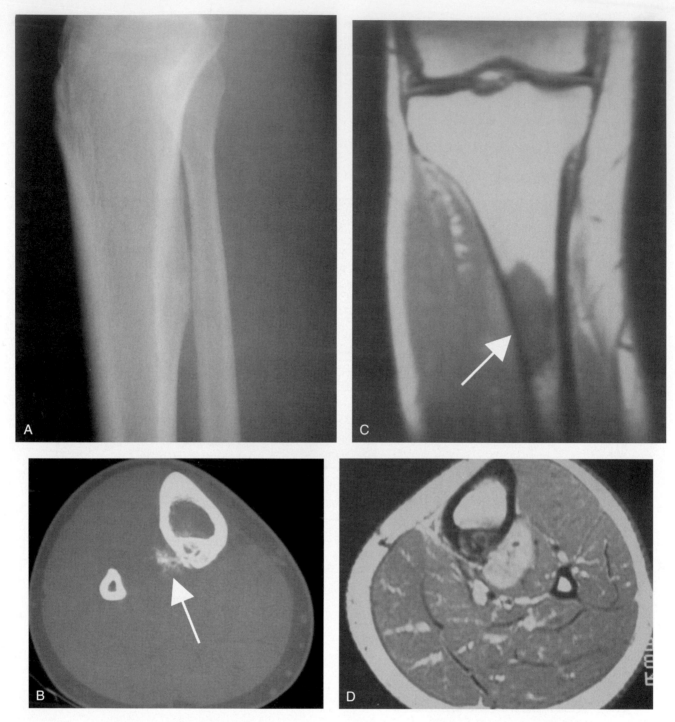

Fig. 1-21 Parosteal osteosarcoma. **A,** Lateral radiograph shows prominent focal cortical bone formation in the posterior tibial metadiaphysis, a location that is typical for a stress fracture in this active 28-year-old male. **B,** However, CT demonstrates a small amount of dense tumor bone formation in the soft tissues (*arrow*). The dense cortical bone formation is also demonstrated. The CT confirms the diagnosis of an early parosteal osteosarcoma. **C,** T1-weighted MRI (800/20) demonstrates that the surface parosteal osteosarcoma has invaded the underlying marrow (*arrow*). Fifty percent of parosteal osteosarcomas show focal marrow invasion. **D,** The T2-weighted image (2400/30) shows the soft tissue mass and, more subtly, the marrow extension of this parosteal osteosarcoma.

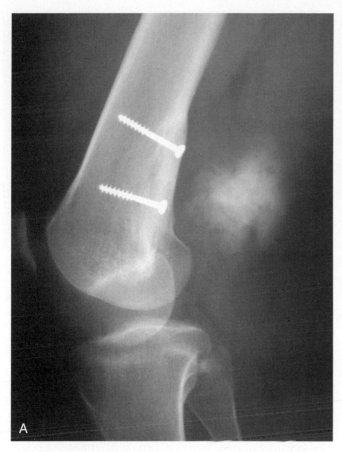

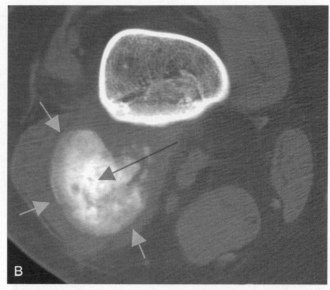

Fig. 1-22   Recurrent parosteal osteosarcoma. **A,** A lateral radiograph demonstrating a previously resected parosteal osteosarcoma with bone graft secured with screws at the posterior cortex, now incorporated. The recurrent tumor is in the soft tissues and demonstrates the zoning phenomenon typical of parosteal osteosarcoma, with the more mature bone formation located centrally in the mass and the periphery showing less mature osteoid formation. **B,** The zoning phenomenon is emphasized on the CT where the dense center (*long arrow*) is surrounded by less mature peripheral osteoid formation (*short arrows*).

being well circumscribed and very nonaggressive to a more permeative pattern. The lesion is diaphyseal or metadiaphyseal in the long bones. It can range from being entirely lytic to quite sclerotic. The median age is slightly older than for conventional osteosarcoma.

If the lesion is not highly aggressive in appearance, it may be mistaken for fibrous dysplasia or a cartilage lesion. If it is more aggressive in appearance, it may be mistaken for Ewing's sarcoma, lymphoma, or malignant fibrous histiocytoma.

If the lesion is recognized initially and completely resected, the survival is excellent. With recurrence, a higher grade lesion may be found.

Soft Tissue Osteosarcoma

This is a rare extraosseous osteosarcoma, generally occurring later in life (40–70 years). It is found most frequently in the thigh, with less frequent occurrence in the upper extremity and retroperitoneum. The soft-tissue mass has variable amounts of mineralized osteoid. Treatment is with wide resection and adjuvant chemotherapy or radiation therapy and prognosis is poor, being worse than that for conventional osteosarcoma.

Osteosarcomatosis (Multicentric Osteosarcoma)

Osteosarcomatosis is a rare process, with the synchronous appearance of osteosarcoma at multiple sites, often bilaterally symmetric. The lesions are nearly always osteoblastic and are rapidly progressive. Although this was originally described as truly synchronous development of multicentric osteosarcomas, some researchers believe that osteosarcomatosis represents rapidly progressive metastatic disease. The latter theory is based upon the fact that in many of the cases there is a dominant lesion and pulmonary metastases at the time of diagnosis.[15]

Although the origin of osteosarcomatosis may be controversial, the results unfortunately are not, with all of these patients having an extremely poor prognosis.

Osteosarcoma in the Older Age Group

Osteosarcomas arising in patients older than 60 years often do not have the classic appearance of conventional osteosarcoma. Their location tends to be different (27% in the axial skeleton, 13% in the cranial/facial bones, and

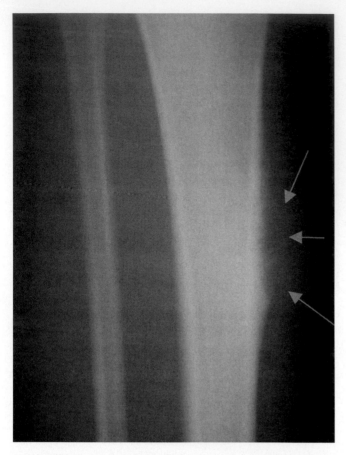

Fig. 1-23   Periosteal osteosarcoma. AP radiograph demonstrates the surface periosteal osteosarcoma in a 12-year-old female, with the typical tumor osteoid arising from the surface of the lesion and a faint scalloping of the cortex (*arrows*). For another example of periosteal osteosarcoma, see Figure 1-2E and F.

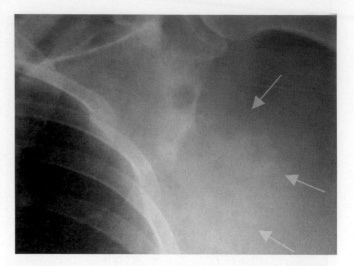

Fig. 1-24   Secondary osteosarcoma. AP radiograph of the shoulder demonstrates frank destruction of the scapula, along with a large soft tissue mass containing tumor osteoid in the axilla (*arrows*). This 66-year-old female had axillary radiation for breast carcinoma and 12 years later developed a radiation-induced osteosarcoma.

11% in the soft tissues).[16] Eighty percent of these lesions present as purely lytic without tumor bone formation and all appear aggressive. Although some are primary osteosarcomas, 56% arise in pre-existing lesions. Common pre-existing lesions for secondary osteosarcoma include Paget's disease, previously radiated bone, and dedifferentiated chondrosarcoma. It is likely that no more than 1% of patients with Paget's disease are at risk for developing osteosarcoma; in such cases there is generally long-standing and severe Paget's disease. Postradiation osteosarcomas (Fig. 1-24; see also Fig. 1-7b) have locations that parallel that of commonly irradiated areas (shoulder girdle for breast carcinoma, pelvis for genitourinary tumors). Irradiated bone can degenerate to osteosarcoma (50%), fibrosarcoma, chondrosarcoma, or undifferentiated sarcoma, with the interval between radiation and diagnosis ranging from 3 to 40 years but averaging 14 years.

Up to 10% of well-differentiated chondrosarcomas can dedifferentiate into osteosarcoma or other high-grade sarcoma. Radiographically, there is often a sharp transition between the well-differentiated chondrosarcoma and the highly aggressive dedifferentiated tumor. This tumor may contain elements of fibrosarcoma, malignant fibrous histiocytoma, high-grade chondrosarcoma, as well as osteosarcoma. Osteosarcoma may also rarely arise from benign conditions, including osteochondroma, chronic osteomylitis, osteoblastoma, bone infarct, and fibrous dysplasia.

Treatment is with radical excision and chemotherapy. However, survival is poor, averaging 37% at 5 years in primary osteosarcomas in the older patient and 7.5% in osteosarcoma arising in a pre-existing lesion.

CARTILAGE FORMING TUMORS: BENIGN

Chondroblastoma

Chondroblastoma is a rare benign cartilaginous tumor found almost exclusively in the epiphysis in skeletally immature patients. This is one of the few lesions found in the epiphysis.

Chondroblastoma tends to be eccentrically located within the epiphysis. If there is partial epiphyseal plate closure, the lesion may extend into the metaphysis. The most common site of involvement is the proximal humerus, followed by the proximal femur, distal femur, and proximal tibia. The bones of the hindfoot may also be involved.

The lesion is geographic with sclerotic margins. It is predominately lytic, although 50% show some amount of chondroid matrix. This may be very subtle, seen only by CT. Note, even though the lesion is nonaggressive in

Key Concepts | Chondroblastoma

- Epiphyseal location predominates.
- Found in skeletally immature patients.
- Proximal humerus is the most common location.
- Cartilage matrix present only 50% of the time.
- It may elicit prominent periosteal reaction in the metaphysis.

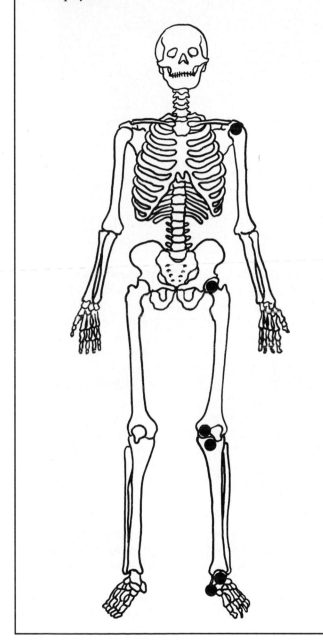

appearance, most chondroblastomas elicit a thick periosteal reaction along the metaphysis, a location remote from the lesion (Fig. 1-25).

MRI shows isointense signal intensity with muscle on T1-weighted images and intermediate heterogeneous to high signal intensity on T2-weighted images, often in a lobulated pattern. Lobulated MRI margins are typical of cartilaginous lesions. MRI shows not only the prominent periosteal reaction in the metaphysial region, but also reaction demonstrated by bone marrow and adjacent soft tissue edema. MRI therefore simulates a more aggressive lesion than is demonstrated by plain film.

Diagnosis is made by radiography, and CT can be helpful in confirming matrix calcification. MRI is generally not necessary but can help establish the relationship of the chondroblastoma to the adjacent joint. Treatment is by curettage and bone graft. Recurrence rate is 15% and metastatic potential is almost negligible, with only isolated case reports of malignant chondroblastoma. The major differential diagnoses in the adolescent or young adult include giant cell tumor crossing into the epiphysis, articular lesions with large cysts (such as pigmented villonodular synovitis), and clear cell chondrosarcoma. In the pediatric age group, the differential diagnoses include eosinophilic granuloma and epiphyseal osteomyelitis.

Chondromyxoid Fibroma

Chondromyxoid fibroma is a very rare benign cartilaginous lesion, which also contains fibrous and myxoid tissue. Although the age range is wide, it is most frequently seen in the second and third decades. The lesion is geographic, often lobulated, and usually occurs eccentrically in the metaphysis. One-third of the lesions are found in the proximal tibia with the others distributed in the proximal and distal femur, flat bones, tarsals, and other small bones of the hand or foot. Chondromyxoid fibroma usually has a thick sclerotic margin and may cause mild cortical expansion (Figs. 1-26 and see 1-2B). Although this is a cartilaginous lesion, it is rare to find tumor matrix within it. The overall appearance is nonaggressive. The MRI appearance is nonspecific, with low signal intensity on T1 and high signal intensity on T2, which is often inhomogenous. The lesion follows a benign course with malignant transformation only rarely reported. Treatment is with curettage with bone grafting. There is a high recurrence rate (approximately 25%) following curettage, perhaps due to incomplete removal of this lobulated lesion.

Juxtacortical (Periosteal) Chondroma

Juxtacortical chondroma is a benign cartilaginous lesion originating at the periosteal surface (Fig. 1-27). The lesion produces a soft tissue mass and cortical pressure erosion that can be difficult to differentiate from that seen in periosteal osteosarcoma. Furthermore, calcification is produced in the soft-tissue mass in 50% of juxtacortical chondromas. This makes differentiation from periosteal osteosarcoma even more difficult.

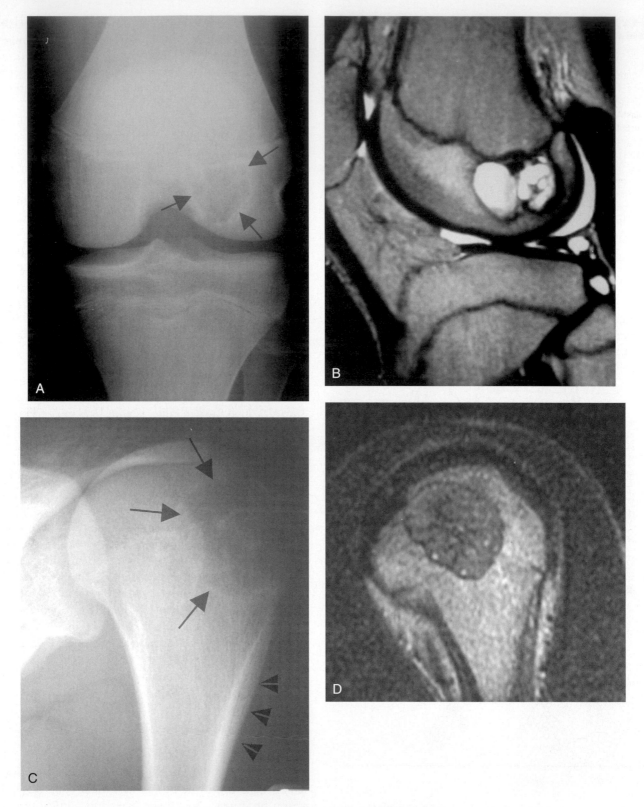

Fig. 1-25   For legend see opposite page

Fig. 1-25, cont'd   Chondroblastoma. **A,** An AP radiograph of the knee in a 14-year-old male. It gives the typical appearance of chondroblastoma, a lytic well-marginated lesion located in the epiphysis of a skeletally immature patient (*arrows*). **B,** The fast spin echo (FSE) T2-weighted MR in a sagittal plane demonstrates the epiphyseal location, as well as the largely homogenous high signal appearance that can be typical of cartilage lesions. **C,** An AP radiograph of a chondroblastoma in a different patient, an 18-year-old male. In this case, the lytic lesion is again located predominately in the epiphysis and has a narrow zone of transition (*arrows*). The margin is not quite as sclerotic as on the previous example, but there is a very dense and regular periosteal reaction seen in the metaphyseal region of the bone (*arrowheads*). Both the location of the lesion in the humerus and the dense periosteal reaction are typical of chondroblastoma. **D,** A sagittal T2-weighted MRI (2000/70) showing several areas of low signal intensity within the lesion. This represents matrix which was not discernable on the radiograph.

Juxtacortical chondromas occur in a wide age range and are seen in both large and small tubular bones. Periosteal reaction can be striking, falsely leading one to believe the lesion to be aggressive. MRI appearance is nonspecific. However, the soft tissue mass adjacent to the bone destruction may make the lesion appear more aggressive by MRI than by radiograph. The behavior, however is benign. The lesion is treated with enbloc excision, whenever possible, to preclude recurrence.

The major differential diagnosis, as noted above, is periosteal osteosarcoma. Giant cell tumor of the tendon sheath can cause cortical saucerization with a soft-tissue mass which appears to be a surface lesion.

Enchondroma

Enchondromas (occasionally termed chondromas) are common benign cartilaginous neoplasms, which are thought to arise in the medullary canal owing to continued growth of residual benign cartilaginous rests that are displaced from the growth plate. Enchondromas are most frequently discovered incidentally, as they are usually asymptomatic in the absence of pathologic fracture or malignant transformation. Enchondromas are common, representing from 3%–17% of primary bone tumors in biopsy series and found in 1.7% of individuals at autopsy series.[17]

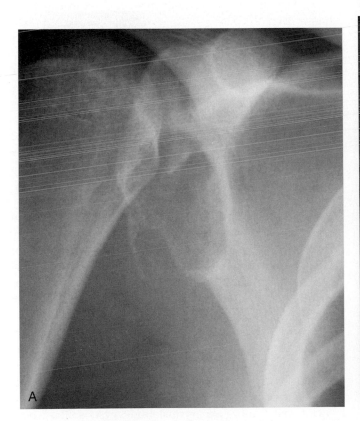
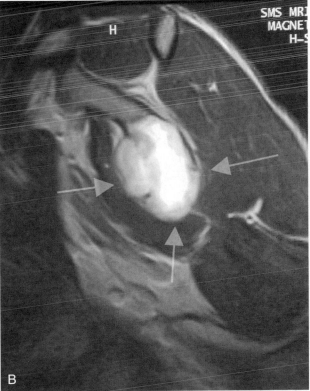

Fig. 1-26   Chondromyxoid fibroma. **A,** AP radiograph of the shoulder in a 31-year-old male demonstrates an expanded lytic lesion in a metaphyseal equivalent of the scapula. There is no matrix present. This is a typical appearance of chondromyxoid fibroma, but it should be remembered that the lesion is quite rare and that this is an unusual location for it. A more typical location is the proximal tibia, as seen in Figure 1-2B. **B,** The homogenous high signal intensity of the chondromyxoid fibroma (*arrows*) is seen in this sagittal T2-weighted MRI (4000/96).

Key Concepts	Enchondroma

- It is a common benign cartilaginous neoplasm.
- It is often discovered incidentally.
- It has a central, metaphyseal location.
- Fifty percent occur in the tubular bones of the hands or feet.
- Fifty percent are found in the metaphyseal regions of the long tubular bones.
- Most have chondroid matrix, although they may be entirely lytic (especially in the hand or foot).
- It is geographic, although often without a sclerotic margin.
- MRI shows lobulated bright signal on T2-weighted images, with low signal calcification.

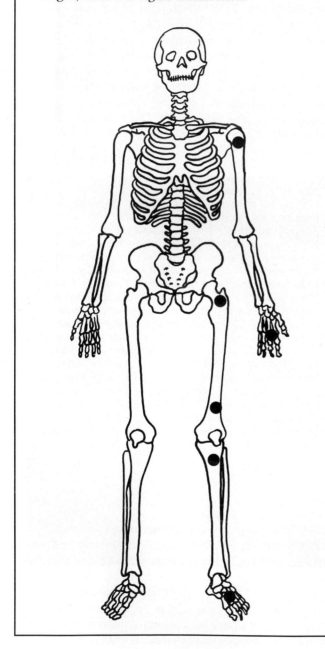

Enchondromas are especially common in the tubular bones of the hands or feet, which comprise up to 50% of all enchondromas. They are also commonly distributed among metaphyseal regions of the long tubular bones, especially the humerus, femur, and tibia, yet they are rarely seen in the pelvis, shoulder girdle, and axial skeleton.

The most common appearance of an enchondroma is that of a geographic lesion, which may mildly expand bony margins, causing cortical thinning. The zone of transition is usually narrow, although the lesion may be lobulated. The geographic nature of the lesion is often defined by a fine sclerotic margin in enchondromas of the hands or feet. There is often no definite sclerotic margin seen in the metaphyseal lesions of the larger tubular bones. Enchondromas usually contain typical cartilaginous matrix, which may be stippled or have the "arcs and rings" architecture, generally appearing denser than normal bone (Fig. 1-28). However, enchondromas can also appear completely lytic and be discovered only incidentally by MRI examination or by thinning or endosteal erosion (Fig. 1-28C). There is no cortical break, soft tissue mass, or host response in the absence of pathologic fracture. Overall, the appearance of an enchondroma is non-aggressive.

Enchondromas are usually monostotic. They may, however, be multiple when found in the hands or feet (Fig. 1-29). Patients with multiple enchondromatosis (Ollier's disease; see later discussion) have more than one enchondroma in locations other than the hands or feet.

An enchondroma has a typical MRI appearance of a cartilaginous neoplasm, but the appearance is not specific for enchondroma. Cartilaginous neoplasms show low signal intensity on T1-weighted images and very high signal intensity on T2-weighted images with lobular margins, occasional internal septations, and punctate signal voids representing matrix calcifications. The very high signal intensity is due to the high water content of the mucopolysaccharide extracellular matrix of the tumor, and combined with the lobular pattern makes the characteristic appearance of a cartilage neoplasm. On the other hand, the appearance on MRI rarely allows one to distinguish between cartilage tumor types.

The differential diagnosis of an enchondroma in the hands or feet is different from that of an enchondroma in the more proximal tubular bones. In the hands or feet, if the lesion shows no matrix calcification, one might also consider a diagnosis of epidermoid inclusion cyst, giant cell tumor, aneurysmal bone cyst, solitary bone cyst, or fibrous dysplasia. Enchondromas in the hands or feet almost always behave in a benign manner, even if the radiology and histology appears aggressive (Fig. 1-29). They are generally treated with curettage and bone grafting.

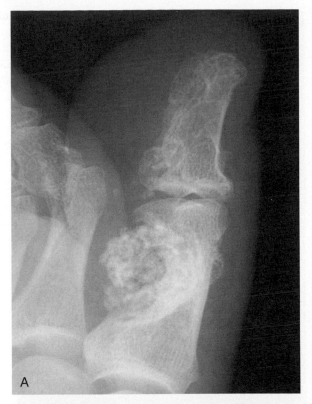

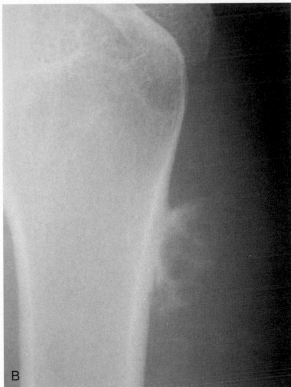

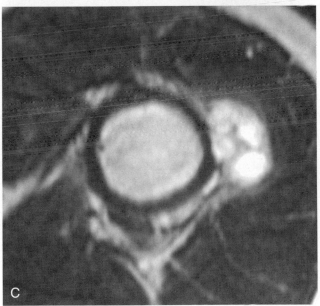

Fig. 1-27 Juxtacortical chondroma. **A,** A lateral radiograph of the great toe in a 50-year-old female. It demonstrates a lesion in both the proximal and distal phalanx, with each showing scalloping of the underlying bone and a densely calcified matrix. These findings are of a surface lesion, and each is a typical example of a juxtacortical chondroma. It is somewhat unusual to see two adjacent lesions. **B,** Another example with a somewhat different appearance is seen in an AP radiograph of the proximal humerus in an 18-year-old female. Again, a surface lesion is demonstrated, this time without scalloping and with prominent matrix extending into the soft tissues. **C,** The axial T2-weighted MRI (36000/92) shows some low signal intensity matrix within otherwise high signal intensity surface mass, which is typical of, although not an exclusive appearance for, cartilage. Although this proved at biopsy to be a juxtacortical chondroma, a diagnosis of parosteal osteosarcoma would be reasonable based on the imaging characteristics.

In sites other than the hands or feet, enchondroma may occasionally be confused with bone infarct; the serpiginous pattern of calcification found in a bone infarct usually allows clear differentiation. One might also consider a diagnosis of chondromyxoid fibroma because of the chondroid matrix. However, the rarity of chondromyxoid fibroma, its usual lack of chondroid matrix, its sclerotic margin, and its preference for the proximal tibia usually allows differentiation from enchondroma.

The major diagnostic dilemma, which occurs fairly frequently because of considerable histologic and radiographic overlap, is the differentiation between enchondroma and low-grade chondrosarcoma. In sites other than the hands and feet, malignant transformation of enchondroma to chondrosarcoma is not uncommon. Large and proximal lesions have the highest incidence of malignant change. The difficulty lies in the fact that early malignant change may not be detectable radiographically. Even with

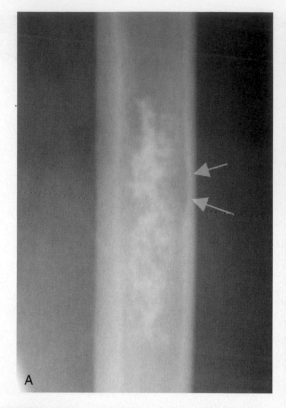

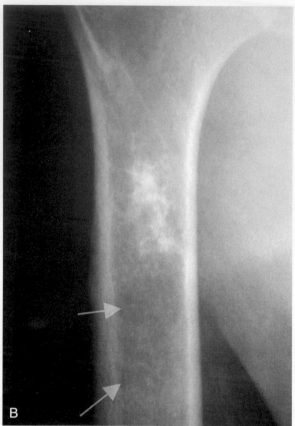

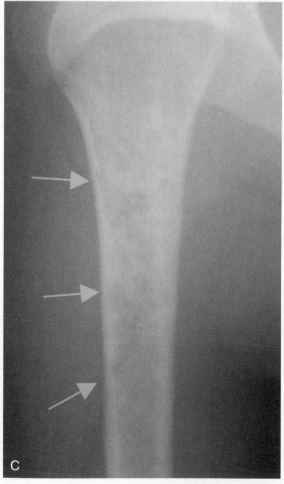

Fig. 1-28   Enchondroma. **A,** An AP radiograph of a metadiaphyseal lesion in the proximal humerus of a 47-year-old female. The appearance is typical of enchondroma, with dense matrix, some of which has the "rings and arcs" appearance of cartilage matrix. There is mild scalloping of the endosteal bone (*arrows*). Other than the matrix, which gives a geographic appearance, the lesion itself is not defined by a margin. **B,** An AP radiograph of the proximal humerus in a 58-year-old male. In this case, the matrix again has the typical appearance of cartilage matrix and the lesion is an enchondroma. However, the character of the lesion in its distal aspect is very different from that in its proximal aspect. In the more distal portion of the lesion, the matrix is more scattered, less distinct, and there are destructive permeative changes in the bone (*arrows*). This more distal portion of the enchondroma has transformed to a chondrosarcoma. **C,** An AP radiograph of the proximal humerus in a 31-year-old female (*arrows*). In this case, there is no calcified matrix present. However, the lesion shows mild scalloping of the endosteal cortex and the lesion is located in the proximal metadiaphysis of the humerus. This lesion was not painful and had shown no radiographic change over the period of one year, and represents an enchondroma, despite the absence of calcified matrix. This is an uncommon appearance of a common lesion (Fig. 1-28C reprinted with permission from the ACR learning file.)

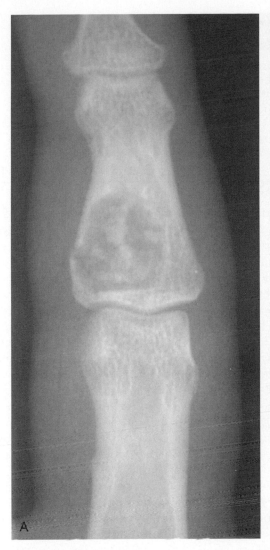

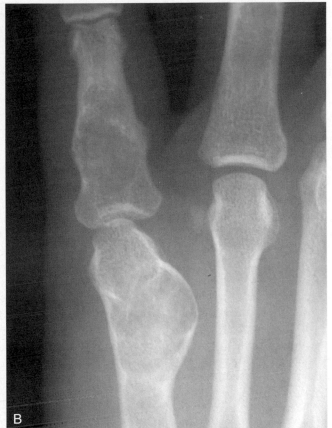

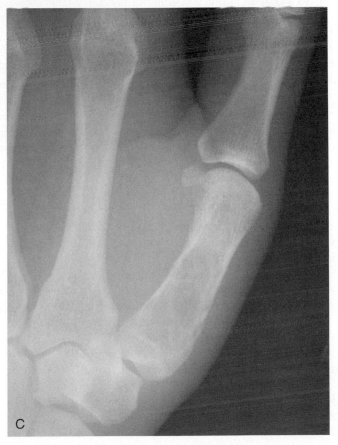

Fig. 1-29   Enchondroma. Fifty percent of enchondromas arise in the hands or feet. **A,** An AP radiograph of a typical enchondroma in the middle phalanx of a finger in a 35-year-old male. In this case there is a geographic lesion with densely spiculated matrix and pathologic fracture. This is a pathognomonic appearance of an enchondroma. **B,** An AP radiograph of two fingers in a different patient, a 23-year-old male. In this case the matrix is much less dense and the lesions are more expanded. Nonetheless, they are typical for an enchondroma. It should be noted that a patient can have several enchondromas in the hand or foot, which can behave simply as a typical enchondroma, without implying the diagnosis of multiple enchondromatosis. **C,** An AP radiograph of the thumb in yet a different patient, showing a completely lytic central lesion. Although this could represent a solitary bone cyst, aneurysmal bone cyst, or giant cell tumor, enchondroma is still statistically the most likely diagnosis. Note the wide variety of appearance of cartilaginous matrix in these cases.

serial radiographs, bone scans, CT, and MRI, no interval change may be shown with early transformation. The diagnosis of malignant transformation of an enchondroma, therefore, is often suspected solely on the basis of local pain. The difficulty in diagnosis is compounded by the fact that biopsy in early malignant transformation most commonly shows either a low grade (grade 1/2) chondrosarcoma or "atypical" enchondroma. The pathologist needs a very large sample size to determine whether or not the lesion is malignant. Sampling representative of the entire lesion is generally not obtained by percutaneous biopsy, but requires curettage of the entire lesion.

Because differentiating between enchondroma and low-grade chondrosarcoma is a relatively common problem in assessing musculoskeletal neoplasms, several researchers have endeavored to find distinguishing characteristics. For many years it was felt that the most helpful radiographic features favoring chondrosarcoma were location in the axial skeleton and larger size.[18] One group suggested that if abnormal peritumoral marrow and soft tissue signal on short tau inversion recovery (STIR) images is demonstrated, chondrosarcoma is a more likely diagnosis than enchondroma.[19] Another group is studying the possibility of differentiating enchondroma and low-grade chondrosarcoma using fast, contrast enhanced MR imaging. The work is encouraging, but not yet conclusive, with differentiation of malignant or benign having a sensitivity of only 61% but a specificity of 95%.[20] The largest and most comprehensive study using more traditional MR imaging is from the AFIP.[17] This study concurs with the generally accepted notion that enchondromas more frequently occur distally and chondrosarcomas more proximally. It is interesting to note that, although epiphyseal location of these lesions is uncommon, when epiphyseal rather than metaphyseal lesions do occur, with the appearance of enchondroma/low grade chondrosarcoma, histologic analysis most often proves them to be low-grade chondrosarcoma. The AFIP confirms that the presence or absence and type of matrix mineralization is not statistically different between enchondroma and chondrosarcoma. They also confirm that the homogeneity or heterogeneity of the nonmineralized component as seen on MRI is not statistically different and that lobulated margins are common in both enchondromas and chondrosarcomas. Furthermore, the degree of enhancement on MRI does not differentiate between malignant and benign lesions. As all would agree, if cortical destruction or soft tissue extension is seen, malignancy is indicated. One interesting parameter, which this group noted, was that, although endosteal scalloping can be seen in both enchondroma and low grade chondrosarcoma on radiography, CT, or MRI, deeper (greater than two-thirds the cortical width) and more extensive (along more than two-thirds of the lesion) endosteal scalloping suggests chondrosarcoma rather than enchondroma.

Key Concepts — Enchondroma vs. Chondrosarcoma

The following observations favor the diagnosis of chondrosarcoma over enchondroma:
- Axial location
- Epiphysial location
- Lesional pain
- Larger size
- Any destructive change
- Significant depth and length of cortical scalloping

The presence of pain relating to these confusing lesions has long felt to be a clinical indicator suggesting transformation to chondrosarcoma. Although one study[18] did not find a statistically significant correlation between clinical symptoms and the benign or malignant histology of these neoplasms, the larger AFIP study[17] confirms that 95% of patients with chondrosarcoma experience pain, and that the symptom favors the diagnosis of malignancy 4.7 times more often than enchondroma. However, they note that enchondromas are commonly painful as well. In considering pain as an indicator for suggesting a malignant rather than benign nature of such a lesion, it is important to differentiate between joint and other sources of pain commonly found in the older patient age group. This differentiation can be made on the basis of physical examination, conservative therapy, or even intra-articular injection of lidocaine.

Because the distinction between enchondroma and low-grade chondrosarcoma can be so difficult if such a lesion is asymptomatic, it may be reasonable to elect watchful waiting as a treatment. If the lesion is painful and there are any radiographic features suggesting malignant transformation, the surgeon faces the choice of curettage and bone grafting or complete excision. Curettage of these low-grade lesions may succeed without recurrence, but a limb salvage procedure more assuredly represents a curative resection, although carrying greater morbidity. The decision is usually made on the basis of the patient's age and condition.

Multiple Enchondromatosis (Ollier's Disease)

Multiple enchondromatosis is a rare developmental abnormality characterized by the presence of enchondromas in the metaphyses and diaphyses of multiple bones. The disease appears in early childhood and is neither hereditary nor familial. It tends to be unilateral and localized to one extremity. The lesions may look like typical enchondromas or may be much larger and even appear grotesque, especially in the fingers. The lesions in the metaphases of the long bones frequently do not have a typical appearance of enchondroma, but rather appear striated, with vertical lucencies and densities. Most have some chondroid matrix (Fig. 1-30). The involved limb usually is short and demonstrates epiphyseal deformities. The risk of malignant degeneration (usually chondrosarcoma) falls in the range of 10% to 25%. Maffucci's syndrome falls in the spectrum of multiple enchondromatosis, demonstrating enchondromatosis in combination with soft tissue and visceral hemangiomas. Phleboliths may be present, which, in addition to the features of enchondromatosis, make the radiographic diagnosis (Fig. 1-31). Maffucci's syndrome is believed to have a much higher malignant potential than enchondromatosis alone.

Osteochondroma (Exostosis)

Exostoses are one of the most common benign neoplasms, seen in approximately 3% of the population.[21] Exostoses arise from growth plate cartilage, which is displaced to the metaphyseal region. They are characterized by having completely normal underlying osseous structures, with the lesion arising as an excrescence from the underlying metaphyseal bone. There is continuity of the normal cortex into the cortex of the exostosis as well as continuity of the periosteum and marrow. The exostosis is covered by a cartilaginous cap, which is its source of growth. An exostosis can be pedunculated (cauliflower-like) (Fig. 1-32) or a broad-based sessile type (Fig. 1-33).

The radiographic appearance of an exostosis is distinct, with no sclerotic margin as the normal bone extends from the host bone to the exostotic bone. There is no host response, although remodeling of adjacent normal bone occasionally occurs from mechanical erosion. There may be cartilaginous matrix seen within the cartilaginous cap, but otherwise the appearance is that of normal bone. The size may range from small to very

Key Concepts   Exostosis

- It is a very common benign neoplasm.
- Metaphyseal: exostosis usually points away from the adjacent joint.
- The knee is the most common location, but can occur anywhere.
- Ninety-five percent are found in the extremities.
- It has a distinct appearance, with normal marrow, cortex, and periosteum extending from the underlying bone into the exostosis, and a cartilage cap, which may or may not show chondroid matrix.
- The majority are solitary.
- Growth ceases at skeletal maturity.
- Mechanical complications are common.
- Pain or continued growth after skeletal maturity warrants exclusion of sarcomatous transformation.

large and although soft tissues are displaced by the bony mass, there is no soft tissue extension from the mass.

Exostoses are metaphyseal lesions, with the exostosis usually pointing away from the adjacent joint. Ninety-five percent occur in the extremities and 36% are found around the knee. Ninety percent are solitary. Exostoses are distinctive in that growth normally ceases at skeletal maturity. Growth of an exostosis after maturity suggests malignant transformation. Such transformation occurs in fewer than 1% of solitary exostoses.

The MRI appearance of an exostosis is characteristic, with continuity of normal appearing host bone marrow and cortex extending into the lesion. The overlying hyaline cartilage is high signal on T2-weighted MR image, typical of cartilage, and is expected to be thin (generally less than 1 cm thick) (compare Figs. 1-32 and 1-34).

Diagnosis of an exostosis is generally not difficult. The pedunculated or cauliflower variety of exostosis should be differentiated from a parosteal osteosarcoma by the type of matrix and the lack of continuity of the cortex and marrow with host bone seen in the osteosarcoma. Occasionally, myositis ossificans that is adjacent to cortex may be confused with an exostosis, but careful examination demonstrates no cortical or marrow continuity with myositis ossificans. CT may be helpful in cases where differentiation is difficult. The broad-based sessile type of exostosis (Figs. 1-34, 1-35) may be confused with a metaphyseal dysplasia or the occasional cortically based fibrous dysplasia.

It may be difficult to determine early malignant transformation in an exostosis. Fewer than 1% of solitary exostoses undergo malignant degeneration. If destructive changes at the neck or base of the exostosis, or new mineral deposition beyond the previously documented contours is seen, then the diagnosis of chondrosarcoma is secure. More frequently, there is no early radiographic change but the patient complains of pain or growth of the exostosis after skeletal maturity. In the absence of mechanical reasons for pain or the formation of a bursa simulating the growth of the exostosis, such clinical symptoms indicate malignant transformation until proven otherwise. If malignant degeneration is suspected, a chondrosarcoma work-up is done, which requires MRI examination. MRI of a degenerating exostosis may demonstrate a thicker cartilage cap, a soft-tissue mass, and osseous destruction (Fig. 1-34). Bone scan usually shows mildly increased uptake in osteochondromas and variable uptake in chondrosarcomas. Although serial scans may be helpful in distinguishing an osteochondroma from transformation to chondrosarcoma, a single bone scan may not be specific for diagnosis.

Although pain and growth after skeletal maturity are hallmarks of malignant transformation in exostoses, they can each be mimicked by mechanical complications of an exostosis.[21] Exostoses can cause limitation of motion

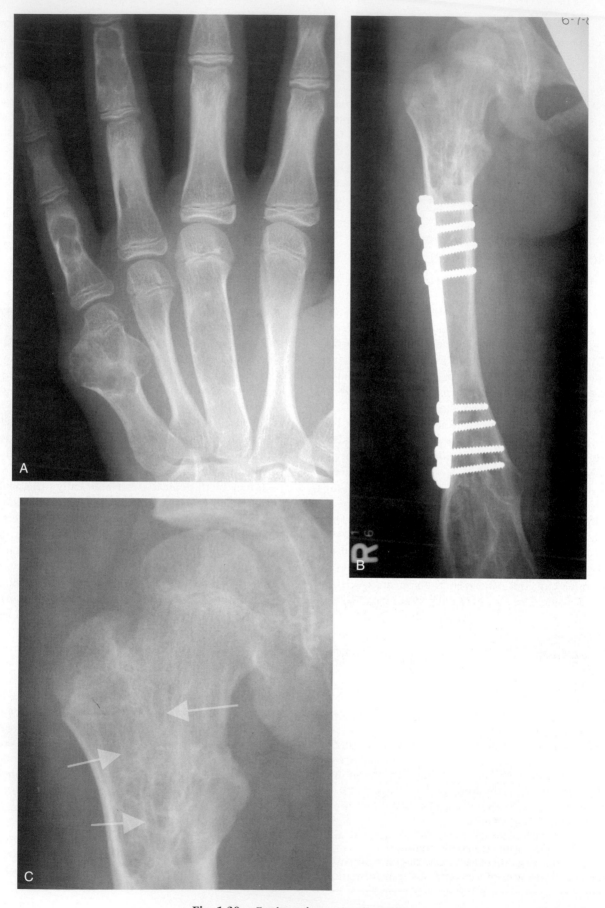

Fig. 1-30   For legend see opposite page

Fig. 1-30, cont'd   Multiple enchondromatosis (Ollier's disease). **A,** The AP radiograph of the hand (30A) in a 13-year-old male shows several enchondromas, in the third through fifth metacarpals, fourth and fifth proximal phalanges, and fourth middle phalanx. Several of these show cartilaginous matrix typical of enchondromas. Although one of the enchondromas in this case is significantly expanded, in Ollier's disease the expansion can be much more significant, to the point of being grotesque. **B,** An AP radiograph of the femur in a 9-year-old patient with Ollier's disease. Note that the dysplasia involves the metaphyses and epiphyses but not the diaphyses. In this case, the patient has undergone limb lengthening, which is the reason for the lateral plating. **C,** The vertical striations which can be seen in multiple enchondromatosis are shown (*arrows*). Notice that the appearance of the dysplasia in multiple enchondromatosis can be very different from that of a routine enchondroma (for example, Fig. 1-28). Chondroid matrix need not be seen in multiple enchondromatosis. (Fig. 1-30B and C printed with permission from the ACR learning file).

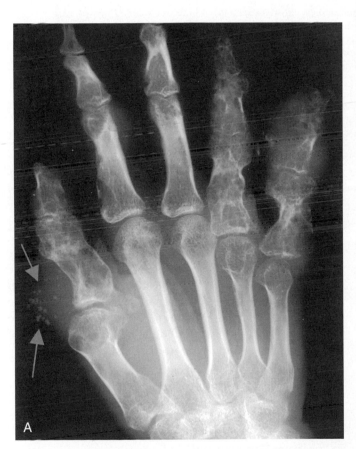
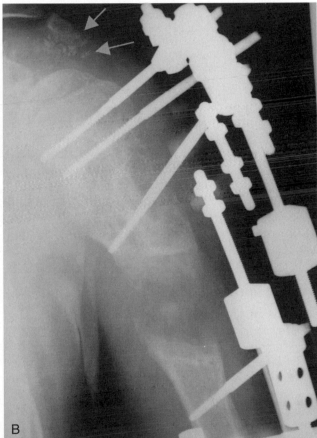

Fig. 1-31   Maffucci's Syndrome. **A,** An AP radiograph of the hand in a 31-year-old patient with Maffucci's syndrome. Note the multiple, fairly typical appearing enchondromas that are accompanied by soft tissue hemangiomas. The most prominent of these is seen at the proximal phalanx of the thumb (*arrows*), where phleboliths are seen in the soft tissue mass. **B,** An AP radiograph of the proximal humerus in a different patient, an 11-year-old female, with Maffucci's syndrome. Note the dysplastic appearance of the proximal humerus, which would be typical of either Ollier's disease or Maffucci's disease. However, the soft tissue hemangioma in the shoulder (*arrows*) leads to the diagnosis of Maffucci's. This patient is undergoing limb lengthening. This dysplasia routinely results in severely shortened limbs.

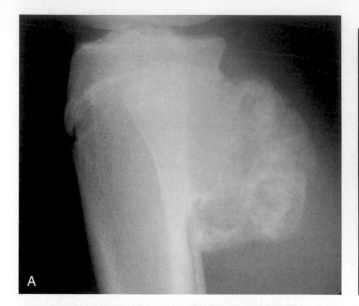 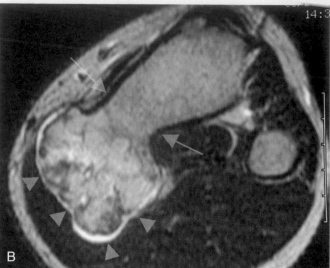

Fig. 1-32   Exostosis. **A,** A lateral radiograph of a typical exostosis seen in a 15-year-old male. The lesion arises from the metaphysis, with continuity of the cortex and the marrow extending from the underlying bone into the exostosis. **B,** This continuity is demonstrated well on the axial T2-weighted (3000/80) MR. The marrow and cortex extend into the exostosis (*arrows*). The cartilaginous cap (high signal, *arrowheads*) is uniform and thin.

and mechanical erosions of adjacent bone. The exostosis itself can fracture, causing pain. Bursa formation can both be painful and cause an apparent enlargement. Nerve impingement and pseudoaneurysm formation can occasionally occur, especially in the region of the popliteal fossa. All of these findings are demonstrated with MR imaging and can help differentiate the painful or "growing" exostosis from malignant degeneration to chondrosarcoma.

Multiple Hereditary Exostoses

This is an uncommon autosomal dominant disorder that also may arise sporadically. Patients present with multiple exostoses and short stature. Although some of the exostoses are cauliflower-like, most are broad-based sessile lesions. These sessile exostoses result in a greater circumference of the metaphases (Fig. 1-35), and the radiographic appearance may simulate a dysplasia. The lesions first appear in childhood as lumps adjacent to joints. The multiple exostoses result in limb shortening and frequent deformities. There is a higher incidence of sarcomatous degeneration (approximately 10%) than in individuals with isolated exostoses, especially in the more proximal lesions. Transformation to chondrosarcoma occurs earlier in life than it does for patients with solitary exostoses. Treatment depends on circumstances, with local resections as necessary for mechanical problems. The patients are observed for sarcomatous transformation.

Dysplasia Epiphysealis Hemimelica (Trevor-Fairbank Disease)

Trevor-Fairbank disease is multiple intra-articular epiphyseal osteochondromas (Fig. 1-36). The lesions may occur in single or multiple joints, though generally they occur only in one extremity. The knee and ankle are the most common sites of occurrence. Histologically, the lesions are identical to exostoses. Radiographically, they give the appearance of a lobulated mass arising from the epiphysis which is usually well mineralized. MRI can help define the extent of the lesion and its relationship to the joint surfaces. Not surprisingly, Trevor-Fairbanks disease causes joint deformity, pain, and limited range of motion. It is treated by local resection.

CARTILAGE FORMING TUMORS: MALIGNANT

Chondrosarcoma

Chondrosarcoma is a cartilage producing sarcoma. This is the third most common primary malignant bone tumor, following osteosarcoma and multiple myeloma. These sarcomas are often asymptomatic, resulting in large tumors at presentation. Errors in diagnosis are also common, leading to delay in appropriate treatment. Chondrosarcomas are classified into central (medullary) and peripheral (exostotic) varieties.

Key Concepts   Chondrosarcoma

- They are a common primary malignant bone tumor.
- They usually but not invariably demonstrate chondroid tumor matrix.
- They are usually low grade.
- They often appear radiographically nonaggressive.
- Central metaphyseal lesions with a minimally aggressive appearance should suggest the diagnosis.
- Endosteal thickening in a minimally aggressive central lesion should suggest the diagnosis.
- Increasing pain or lesion growth in an adult exostosis should suggest the diagnosis.
- Cartilage cap thickness of greater than 1 cm suggests the diagnosis.

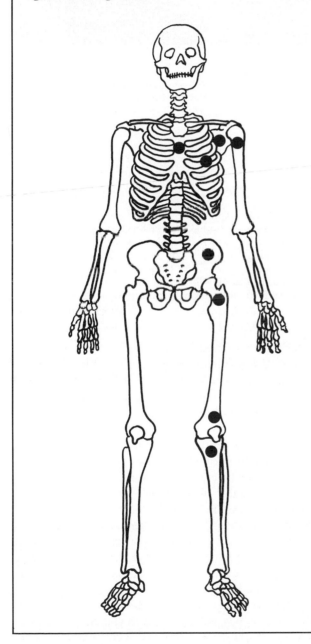

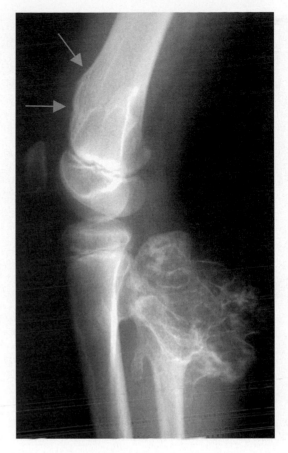

Fig. 1-33 Sessile exostosis. This lateral radiograph of the knee in a 7-year-old female demonstrates not only the large cauliflower-like exostosis of the proximal fibula, but the widened metaphysis of the distal femur and the undulating character of sessile exostoses (*arrows*). These sessile exostoses occasionally are mistaken for a metaphyseal dysplasia, leading to a missed diagnosis of multiple hereditary exostoses.

Central chondrosarcoma may be either primary or secondary, that is, arising de novo or from transformation. These lesions are usually central and metaphyseal in location, and are particularly common in the proximal long bones and the pelvis and shoulder girdle. They most frequently occur in the fourth through sixth decades.

Ninety percent of central chondrosarcomas are low-grade lesions. Although they are generally large (greater than 5 cm) they tend to be geographic in appearance. They may show mild cortical expansion and/or endosteal scalloping. They often have a narrow zone of transition, but there is usually no sclerotic margin. The presence of chondroid tumor matrix is variable, ranging from completely lytic lesions to lytic with only a few flecks of calcification, to dense aggregates of annular calcification (Fig. 1-37). There often is no soft-tissue mass, although high-grade lesions may extend to soft tissues. Because there may be no cortical breakthrough, periosteal reaction is variable; there may be none, or the endosteum may be significantly thickened (Fig. 1-38). This latter

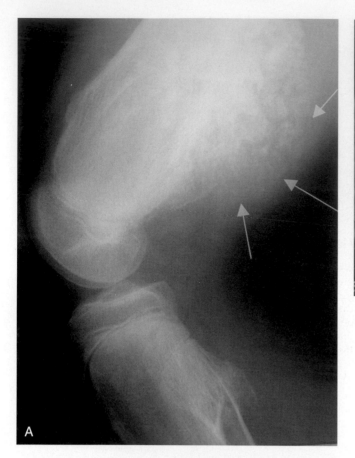

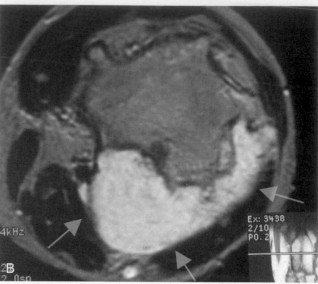

Fig. 1-34 Malignant degeneration of an exostosis. **A,** A lateral radiograph of the knee in a 13-year-old male who has multiple hereditary exostoses. Note the posterior lesion in the distal femur. It shows a soft tissue mass and a "snowstorm" effect of the chondroid matrix (*arrows*). This indicates transformation of an exostosis to a chondrosarcoma. Radiographs do not always demonstrate a transformation so clearly. However, MR will show an enlarged and very abnormal cartilage cap, confirming chondrosarcoma. This is seen in **B,** an axial MR in the same patient, showing the multiple small exostoses along with the large posterior exostosis and its thick and irregular cartilage cap (high signal intensity, *arrows*), (T2-weighting 2400/90).

feature of endosteal thickening, when present, may suggest the diagnosis. It is only seen in a few other aggressive lesions in patients of this age group, including primary lymphoma of bone (Ewing's Sarcoma in a younger age group) and osteomyelitis. It is very important to be aware that chondrosarcomas are common malignant tumors of bone, and usually are not aggressive in radiographic appearance. Therefore, if a central lesion in the correct age group appears slightly to moderately aggressive, with a possible small zone of permeative pattern or questionable zone of transition, subtle calcification should be sought and the diagnosis of chondrosarcoma should be offered, whether or not cartilaginous calcification is found. Note the variety of appearances central chondrosarcoma can show in Figures 1-37 and 1-38. This lesion is very commonly underdiagnosed as it so often appears nonaggressive. Underdiagnosis results in undertreatment, which puts the patient at risk for recurrence or metastatic disease.

A well-differentiated chondrosarcoma may show the lobulated T2-bright features of hyaline cartilage typical of benign cartilage lesions. Higher-grade lesions will appear nonspecific and have inhomogeneous high signal intensity on T2-weighted imaging. Mineralized matrix will be seen as low signal intensity on all sequences.

The major differential diagnosis of a central chondrosarcoma is enchondroma. If the lesion appears more aggressive and calcification is present, it can be confused with a bone infarct degenerating to malignant fibrous histiocytoma (see Fig. 1-64). If there is no chondroid matrix present, the differential diagnosis includes metastasis, plasmacytoma, malignant fibrous histiocytoma, fibrosarcoma, and lymphoma. If the lesion is less aggressive in appearance and without matrix, giant cell tumor might be considered.

Peripheral (exostotic) chondrosarcomas may be either primary or may secondarily arise from malignant transformation of an exostosis. They are seen most frequently

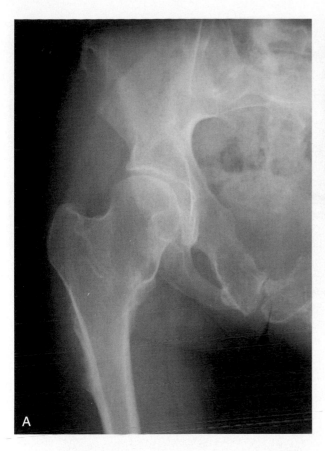

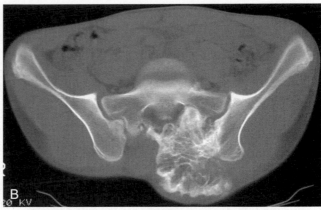

Fig. 1-35   Multiple exostoses. **A,** An AP radiograph of the hip in a 39-year-old female. This demonstrates the wide femoral neck, wide superior pubic ramus, and small irregular excrescences along the metaphyses, which are typical of multiple sessile exostoses. Not surprisingly, these are sometimes misinterpreted as a metaphyseal dysplasia. **B,** A different patient, a 10-year-old male with multiple hereditary exostoses. This axial CT demonstrates one large cauliflower-like exostosis as well as the small sessile exostoses arising from the anterior portion of the iliac wings.

in the third, fourth, and fifth decades. They are large extraosseous lesions, arising from the metaphyses of long bones as well as the pelvis, shoulder girdle, sternum, and ribs (Figs. 1-34 and 1-39). They most frequently show normal appearing underlying host bone extending into

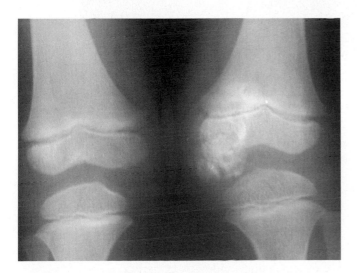

Fig. 1-36   Trevor Fairbank disease. This AP radiograph of the knees of a 9-year-old male is typical for Trevor Fairbank, demonstrating exostosis-like lesions arising from the epiphysis. This intraarticular process is usually unilateral. (Printed with permission from the ACR learning file.)

an exostosis but with a large cartilaginous cap (greater than 1 cm in thickness). Changes over time in the appearance of chondroid calcification in an exostosis may help to diagnose transformation to a chondrosarcoma, but MRI may frequently be necessary to evaluate the cartilaginous cap thickness. Higher-grade lesions may show destruction of the stalk as well as soft tissue mass beyond that of the cartilaginous cap. As described in the earlier section on exostoses, degeneration to chondrosarcoma may produce no distinct radiographic signs. Therefore clinical signs of new onset nonmechanical pain and increased size after epiphysial closure should be considered of primary importance in suggesting the diagnosis of peripheral chondrosarcoma.

Ninety percent of chondrosarcomas, either central or peripheral, are low-grade lesions. Therefore local recurrence is more common than is metastatic disease. Prognosis is worse for proximal and axial than distal lesions. Five-year survival is approximately 75%, and this can be improved by both a more prompt radiologic diagnosis and meticulous surgical technique. It must be remembered that chondrosarcoma can be readily implanted in soft tissues as it does not need a blood supply to survive. Therefore recurrences may be due to tumor spill at the time of biopsy or resection. Wide excision is the therapy of choice. Generally radiation and chemotherapy do not improve survival or decrease local recurrence rates.

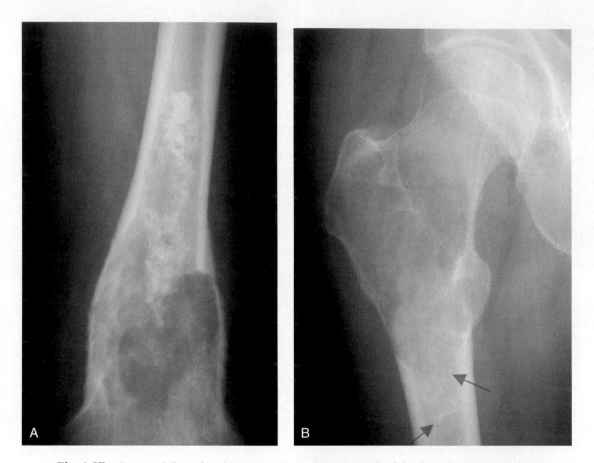

Fig. 1-37   Intramedullary chondrosarcoma. **A,** An AP radiograph of the distal femur in a 79-year-old male. This demonstrates the typical matrix of an enchondroma in its proximal portion, extending into a highly destructive lesion more distally. This is a chondrosarcoma arising in an enchondroma (see also Fig. 1-28B). **B,** An AP radiograph of a moderately destructive lesion in the hip of a 52-year-old male. There is a tiny bit of speckled chondroid matrix seen in the distal portion of the lesion (*arrows*). With this matrix and the location, as well as the moderately destructive lytic portion of the lesion, the diagnosis can only be chondrosarcoma. Note the spectrum of chondroid matrix one might expect to see in chondrosarcoma.

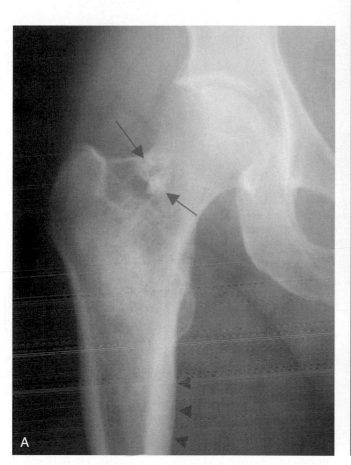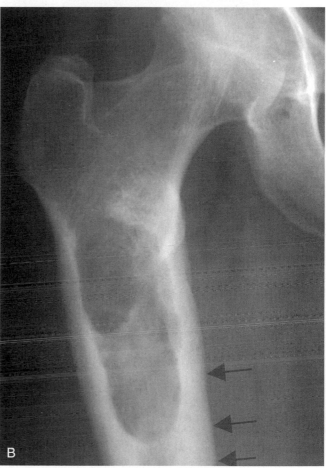

Fig. 1-38   Intramedullary chondrosarcoma. **A,** An AP radiograph of the proximal femur in a 38-year-old male. There is chondroid matrix present, particularly in the proximal portion of the lesion (*arrows*) and the lesion shows a destructive pattern with a wide zone of transition. These features alone make it a chondrosarcoma. Additionally, there is prominent thickening of the cortex (*arrowheads*). This is also a feature which may be seen in intramedullary chondrosarcoma. **B,** An AP radiograph of the hip in a 51-year-old female, also an intramedullary chondrosarcoma. In this case, there is no chondroid matrix present. The lesion is only moderately aggressive in appearance. However, there is prominent periosteal thickening (*arrows*). The location, age of the patient, and periosteal thickening lead to a diagnosis of chondrosarcoma despite the absence of chondroid matrix.

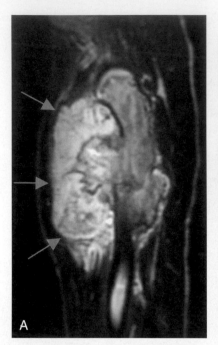
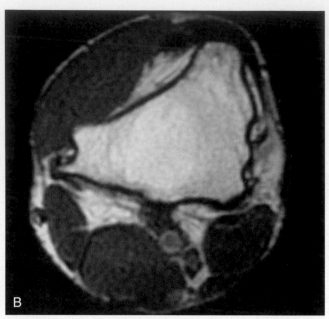

Fig. 1-39   Exostotic chondrosarcoma. **A,** A coronal T2-weighted image (3000/102) of the proximal femur in a 20-year-old male. There are multiple sessile exostoses present, but one large cauliflower-like exostosis arising from the medial aspect of the proximal femur. The very large cartilage cap (*arrows*) allows for a diagnosis of chondrosarcoma. Another example of this large cartilage cap indicative of chondrosarcoma is seen in Fig. 1-34. **B,** An axial T1-weighted image (500/16) of the distal femur in the same patient. In this case, the multiple sessile exostoses have normal cortex surrounding them and normal marrow extending into them, without a prominent cartilage cap.

Clear Cell Chondrosarcoma

Clear cell chondrosarcoma is a very rare lesion that is most often mistaken for a chondroblastoma because it is nonaggressive in appearance and arises in the epiphyses, especially of the proximal femur and humerus. Clear cell chondrosarcoma occurs in older patients than does chondroblastoma, peaking in the third decade. It is usually geographic in appearance with a rather narrow zone of transition and sharp sclerotic margin. Periosteal reaction and cortical breakthrough are rare. Chondroid matrix is usually absent.

This description is very similar to that of chondroblastoma, except the occurrence in a slightly older age group in patients with clear cell chondrosarcoma. The age of the patient may be the only hint of the true diagnosis. After growing slowly for a number of years, however, clear cell chondrosarcoma may become much more aggressive. Treatment is wide excision; curettage alone can result in an aggressive recurrence.

Dedifferentiated Chondrosarcoma

A portion of a low grade chondrosarcomas may devolve into a highly aggressive lesion. This dedifferentia-tion results in a neoplasm that may have several elements, including fibrosarcoma, malignant fibrous histiocytoma, high-grade chondrosarcoma, and osteosarcoma. As many as 10% of chondrosarcomas dedifferentiate.

The radiographic appearance of dedifferentiated chondrosarcoma usually shows areas with features of low-grade chondrosarcoma, with other areas appearing highly aggressive with clear destructive elements. It is important to choose a biopsy site that includes the more aggressive portion of the lesion (Fig. 1-40).

Prognosis of dedifferentiated chondrosarcoma is poor with only a 20% five-year survival. Metastases to the lung are common. Treatment is radical excision and chemotherapy.

Mesenchymal Chondrosarcoma

This is an exceedingly rare, high grade chondrosarcoma.[22] The age group for mesenchymal chondrosarcoma is younger than standard chondrosarcoma (first through fourth decades). The site is unusual, with one-third arising in the soft tissues. In the skeleton, rib and jaw lesions are common, whereas long bone lesions are unusual. Chondroid calcification is usually present, which in the radiographically aggressive lesion may suggest the diagnosis.

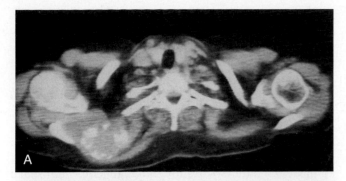

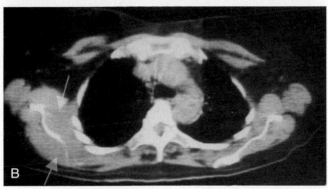

Fig. 1-40 Dedifferentiated chondrosarcoma. **A,** A CT of the scapula in a 62-year-old female that demonstrates chondroid matrix in a mass arising from the supraspinous fossa of the right scapula. This gives the appearance of a typical chondrosarcoma. **B,** However, more distally the character of the lesion is different, with a large soft tissue mass surrounding and destroying the scapula (*arrows*) but no matrix present. Because of the different features in this lesion, one should suspect a dedifferentiated chondrosarcoma and should biopsy the region with no matrix, which will show the more aggressive nature of this tumor. (Printed with permission from the ACR learning file.)

OTHER MUSCULOSKELETAL TUMORS

GIANT CELL TUMOR

Giant cell tumor is a common, benign neoplasm constituting 5% of primary bone tumors. It consists of multinucleated giant cells in a fibroid stroma, distinct from many other lesions that may contain reactive giant cells. Giant cell tumor has a typical radiographic appearance, but it is not unusual for variants of that appearance to be seen. In addition, it can have unusual variants in behavior, which are not clearly related to radiographic appearance.

Giant cell tumors nearly always occur after epiphyseal fusion; 70% of them occur between the third and fifth decades. Radiographically, it appears as a geographic expanding lesion. Most of the lesions have the unusual distinction of a narrow zone of transition *without* a sclerotic margin. There is generally little host response in the absence of fracture. Cortical breakthrough and soft-

| Key Concepts | Giant Cell Tumor |

- They are lytic, with a narrow zone of transition but no sclerotic margin.
- Commonly occur at the knee and distal radius.
- In the spine, the sacrum or body of vertebra is the preferred location.
- The site of origin is metaphysis; usually extends to the subarticular region.
- They almost always occur after epiphyseal fusion, most commonly between 20 and 40 years of age.
- Most are benign, but may have a more aggressive radiographic appearance.

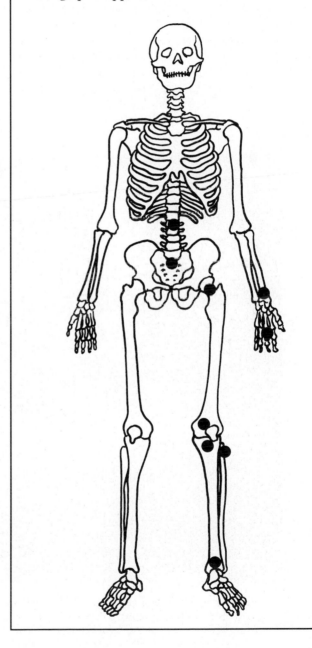

tissue mass are infrequently seen. The above description is typical (Fig. 1-41). However, it should be noted that occasionally the lesion appears less aggressive, with a sclerotic margin. The lesion can also appear more aggressive, with cortical breakthrough and soft-tissue mass in up to 24% (Fig. 1-42).

Location is an important feature in diagnosing giant cell tumors. The lesion is most frequently found about the knee (distal femur and proximal tibia) or wrist (distal radius or ulna), with these cases comprising 65% of all cases. Location in another sense is important. The lesion arises eccentrically in the metaphysis and it extends to the subarticular end of the bone. Because of this eventual subarticular extension of most giant cell tumors, it is sometimes mistakenly believed that these are epiphyseal lesions. However, early lesions are located in the metaphysis (Fig. 1-43). Giant cell tumors also occur in the spine, where they most often involve the sacrum or body of a

vertebra (Fig. 1-44). It only rarely arises in the posterior elements.

Giant cell tumors are generally monostotic. They may be rarely multicentric, especially in the skull and facial bones that are affected by Paget's disease. Multicentric giant cell tumors may be difficult to differentiate from metastatic giant cell tumor; fortunately, both are rare.

The MRI appearance typically is that of a solid lesion with nonspecific low signal intensity on T1 imaging. There is no calcified matrix in these lesions. Forty percent of giant cell tumors will show homogeneous high signal intensity on T2 imaging. However, 60% will have T2 imaging demonstrating high signal intensity with low signal intensity regions that may be nodular, zonal, whorled, or diffuse. The low signal intensity regions may occupy 20%–25% of tumor volume and relate to hemosiderin and collagen content.[23] Fluid levels are occasionally seen on MR imaging of giant cell tumors.

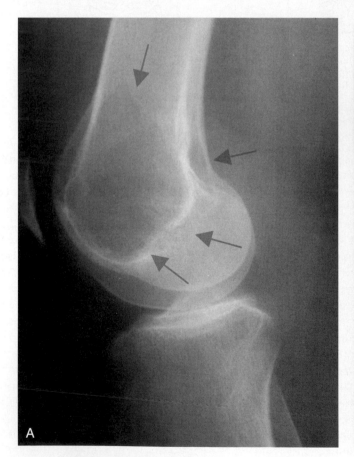
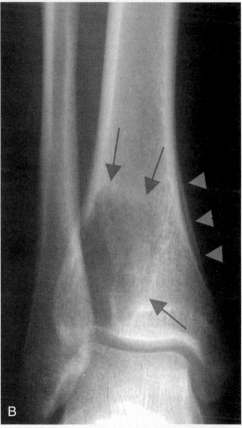

Fig. 1-41 Giant cell tumor. **A,** A lateral radiograph showing a large lytic lesion located in the distal femoral metaphysis (*arrows*), extending to the subchondral bone at the anterior portion of the femoral condyle. There is no matrix, and the zone of transition is narrow despite the lack of a sclerotic margin. This is a typical appearance of giant cell tumor, seen in a 31-year-old female. **B,** A giant cell tumor seen in the distal tibia of a 16-year-old male (*arrows*), again demonstrating the eccentric metaphyseal location of these lesions and the narrow zone of transition without sclerotic margin. Arrowheads outline the periosteal reaction, which can be associated with giant cell tumor.

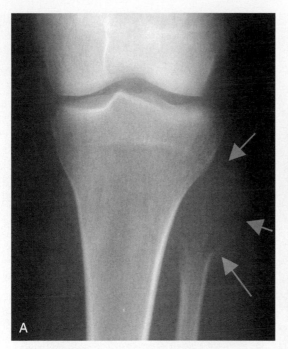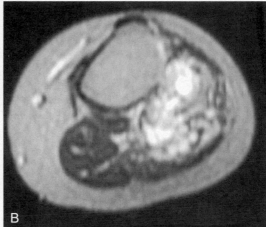

Fig. 1-42   Aggressive giant cell tumor. **A,** This AP radiograph demonstrates a lytic lesion in the proximal fibula (*arrows*) which is expanded and has a somewhat wide zone of transition. **B,** The MRI shows the lesion to be even more aggressive than it appeared on plain film, with a large soft-tissue mass involving the anterior, lateral, and posterior compartments (T2-weighted, 2500/80). This proved to be an aggressive giant cell tumor in this 29-year-old female.

Giant cell tumor is generally not a difficult diagnosis to make. In the long bones, one might consider a diagnosis of chondroblastoma because of the subarticular nature of the lesion. However, chondroblastomas are generally found in skeletally immature patients and also have typical sclerotic margins. Brown tumor of hyperparathyroidism may also have an appearance similar to giant cell tumor. However, these patients have appropriate clinical history and will manifest typical radiographic features of hyperparathyroidism. Nonossifying fibroma is a cortically based metaphyseal lesion. Its slightly different location as well as sclerotic border should differentiate this lesion from giant cell tumor. Rarely, a low-grade chondrosarcoma, if it lacks matrix, or plasmacytoma could be confused with giant cell tumor. In the spine, giant cell tumor could be confused most frequently with cordoma or chondrosarcoma as the location in the body of the sacrum or vertebra is similar. Differential diagnosis also includes plasmacytoma and metastasis. Aneurysmal bone cyst and osteoblastoma, also lesions found in the spine, should not be confused with giant cell tumor as they are most frequently found in the posterior spinal elements.

The biologic behavior of giant cell tumor may be confusing. The vast majority are benign with low histologic grade. However, 5% are malignant, and can metastasize to the lungs. Of those that metastasize, the prognosis may be good with surgical resection of the lung metastases. The difficulty lies in the fact that one cannot reliably differentiate benign from malignant giant cell tumors radiologically, even by detecting lung metastases, as benign giant cell tumors can also metastasize. The histologic features are not predictive of the tumor's ultimate behavior either. However, a higher grade giant cell tumor that has recurred does increase the likelihood of developing metastatic disease.[24] Treatment of giant cell tumors is problematic. Curative treatment would be to regard the lesion as a low-grade malignant neoplasm and to treat it with wide resection. With such therapy, the recurrence rate is only 10%. However, for wide resection, the subarticular location of the lesion requires resection of the joint and fusion, placement of an osteoarticular graft, or placement of a long-stem custom prosthesis. In a young patient, such a prosthesis might require multiple revisions throughout life, causing considerable morbidity. To avoid this morbidity, curettage and bone grafting or methacrylate injection may be chosen as the initial treatment. The recurrence rate following this treatment ranges from 10% to 50%. If cryosurgery is added, recurrence rates may be lower. In following these patients for recurrence, a thin halo of resorption of bone graft at the margins of the lesion might be expected. However, nonsymmetric lytic regions that are progressive in the tumor bed indicate recurrence (Fig. 1-45).

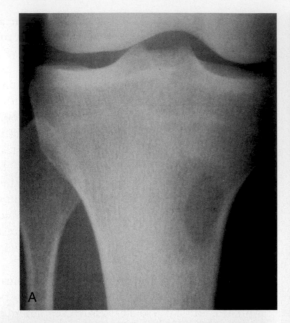

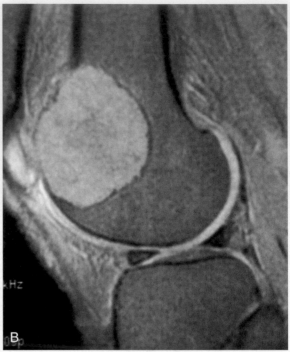

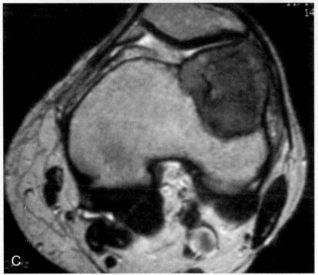

Fig. 1-43   Metaphyseal giant cell tumor. **A,** An AP radiograph of the proximal tibia in a 22-year-old female. It demonstrates a lytic lesion arising eccentrically in the metaphysis having a narrow zone of transition but no sclerotic margin. This is a typical appearance for a giant cell tumor, but some might have a difficult time arriving at the diagnosis because the lesion does not extend all the way to the subchondral bone. It should be remembered that giant cell tumors arise in the metaphysis and may only reach the subchondral bone when they are moderately large. **B,** A sagittal fat saturated T1-weighted MR (600/15) image of a metaphyseal giant cell tumor in a 63-year-old male. **C,** The T2-weighted (5000/98) axial image demonstrates significant low signal intensity, which may be a feature of giant cell tumors. (Figure 1-43A reprinted with permission from the ACR learning file.)

MARROW TUMORS

Ewing's Sarcoma

Ewing's sarcoma is a highly malignant round cell tumor found primarily in children. It is the most common primary malignant bone tumor found in children in the first decade of life. In the second decade, it is second to osteosarcoma. Ninety-five percent occur between the ages of 4 and 25, with the most frequent occurrence between 5 and 14. Ewing's sarcoma is a central lesion, most commonly within the diaphysis or metadiaphysis. Seventy-five percent of cases involve the pelvis or long tubular bones. Other sites of involvement include the shoulder girdle, rib, and vertebral body. The expected location relates to the age at presentation; Ewing's sarcoma tends to involve the tubular bones in children under the age of 10 and the axial skeleton, pelvis, and shoulder girdle in patients older than the first decade. The lesion is generally diffuse and permeative. The zone of transition is wide, with no sclerotic margin (Fig. 1-46). There is invariably cortical permeation with a large soft tissue mass. No calcified tumor matrix is produced, but sclerotic reactive bone may be seen within the permeative tumor. Sixty-two percent of Ewing's sarcomas are completely lytic, 23% have minimal reactive bone, and 15% have marked sclerotic reactive bone (Fig. 1-47). The presence of this sclerotic reactive bone might suggest osteosarcoma as a diagnosis. However, it should be noted that this reactive bone in Ewing's sarcoma is found only within the osseous structures and is not produced within the soft-tissue component of the mass. This feature helps to differ-

Key Concepts | Ewing's Sarcoma

- It is the most common primary malignant bone neoplasm in the first decade of life.
- It is one of the "small round cell" lesions, having a differential diagnosis and similar radiographic appearance to some cases of osteomyelitis, Langerhan's histiocytosis, metastatic neuroblastoma, primative neuroectodermal tumor (PNET), lymphoma, leukemia.
- It is highly aggressive, with a permeative pattern and large soft-tissue mass and prominent host reaction.
- Tubular bones are more frequently involved in the younger age group and flat bones and the axial skeleton more frequently involved in adolescents and young adults.
- It is central and either diaphyseal or metadiaphyseal.
- Systemic symptoms are frequent.
- Bone and lung metastases are common.

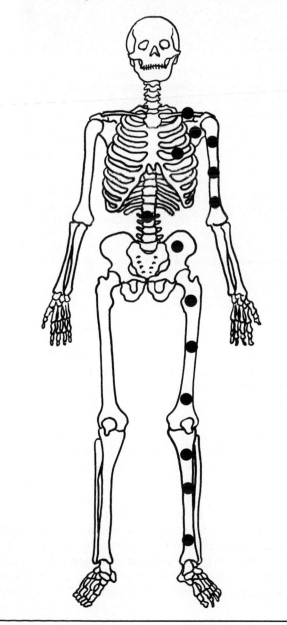

entiate a sclerotic Ewing's sarcoma from an osteosarcoma, which most frequently shows tumor matrix formation in both the permeative osseous lesion and its soft tissue mass.

Aggressive periosteal reaction is a prominent feature found in Ewing's sarcoma. Occasionally, thick reactive endosteal bone formation is seen. Systemic reaction may be prominent as well, as one-third of the patients present with fever, leukocytosis, and elevated erythrocyte sedimentation rate (ESR). This clinical presentation simulates infection. Unfortunately, the radiographic appearance as an aggressive permeative lesion with periosteal change also suggests infection. Clinical findings therefore may be misleading. Another interesting clinical feature is that Ewing's sarcoma is extremely rare in black patients.

The MRI appearance of Ewing's sarcoma is nonspecific, with low signal intensity on T1 and high signal intensity on T2. The soft-tissue component of the mass is typically large and may contain central necrosis.

Ewing's sarcoma is initially monostotic, but metastases to bone are common so that the lesion may present initially as a polyostotic disease. This can contribute to difficulty in diagnosis. The differential diagnosis is primarily that of the other "small round cell" lesions, including osteomyelitis, Langerhan's histiocytosis, neuroblastoma metastases, lymphoma, and leukemia. Although benign and highly malignant lesions are included in this same differential diagnosis, each of these lesions mentioned above can have a highly aggressive permeative appearance similar to Ewing's sarcoma. The duration of symptoms may be helpful in differentiating among these round cell lesions. Langerhan's histiocytosis may be one of the most locally aggressive, with the shortest time course of osseous destruction (1 to 2 weeks). Osteomyelitis also has a relatively short course of osseous destruction (2 to 4 weeks). Ewing's sarcoma, although highly aggressive, has a somewhat slower course with destructive changes seen at 6–12 weeks.

The 5 year survival of patients with Ewing's sarcoma is relatively low, at 50%. Fifteen percent to 30% have metastases at the time of diagnosis, with these metastases affecting lung and bone with equal frequency. Of all the primary bone sarcomas, Ewing's sarcoma most frequently metastasizes to other bones. It should be noted that more central and larger lesions have a worse prognosis than more distal smaller lesions.

Treatment includes combined radiation and chemotherapy. When surgically and functionally possible, wide resection following treatment is frequently done.

Primary Lymphoma of Bone

Primary lymphoma of bone is an uncommon presentation of lymphoma. Although the age range is wide,

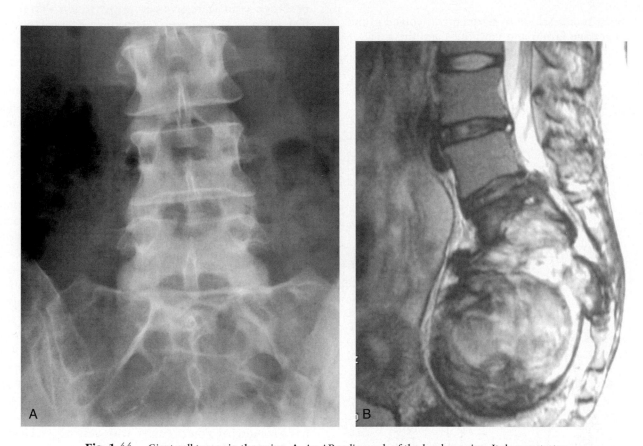

Fig. 1-44   Giant cell tumor in the spine. **A,** An AP radiograph of the lumbar spine. It demonstrates an expanded lytic lesion occupying the entire sacrum. The extent of the lesion is seen better with MR imaging. **B,** A sagittal T2-weighted (3200/102) image that demonstrates a very large mass extending anteriorly from the sacrum. It is inhomogeneous, with mixed high and low signal intensity. The spine, and particularly the sacrum, are favorite locations for giant cell tumor in the axial skeleton.

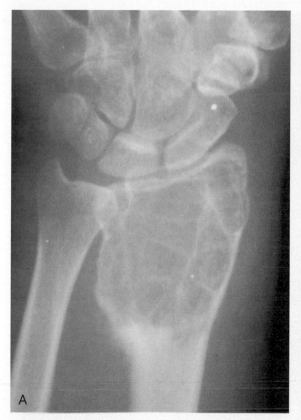

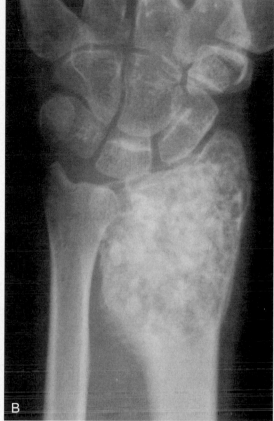

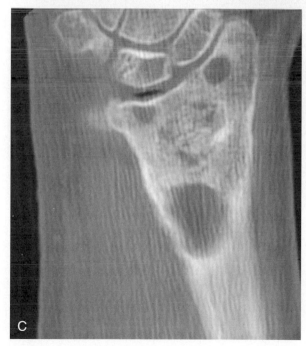

Fig. 1-45   Recurrent giant cell tumor. **A,** The initial AP radiograph of a giant cell tumor in this 25-year-old female. The wrist is a common location for giant cell tumor, and this case is atypical only in the degree of pseudotrabeculation seen. **B,** The lesion was treated with curettage and grafting, as shown in the radiograph. **C,** One year later, a direct coronal CT demonstrates that although much of the bone graft has incorporated and matured, there are three separate sites of recurrence within the distal radius. Recurrence is a common complication of giant cell tumor.

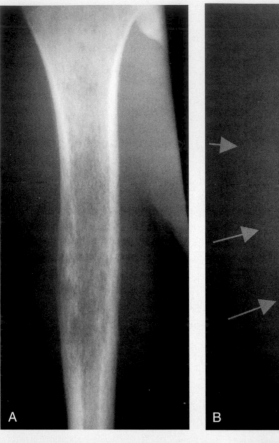

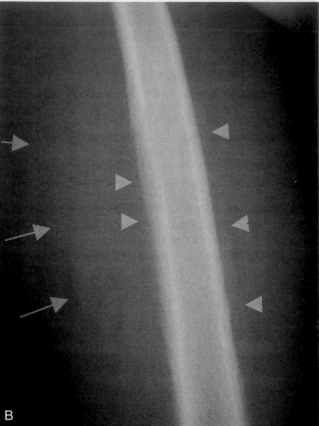

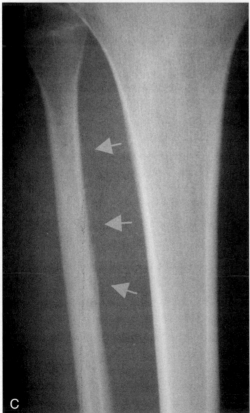

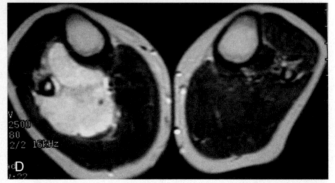

Fig. 1-46   Ewing's sarcoma. **A,** An AP radiograph of the humerus in a 14-year-old female. This highly permeative diaphyseal lesion is a very typical appearance for Ewing's sarcoma. **B,** However, permeative change is not always this obvious. The latter is a sagittal radiograph of the mid-diaphysis of the femur in a 10-year-old female. The permeative change in the bone is almost impossible to see, but there is very prominent and aggressive appearing periosteal reaction (*arrowheads*) as well as a large soft tissue mass (*arrows*). This is also a typical radiographic appearance of Ewing's sarcoma. **C,** An even more subtle case of Ewing's sarcoma is seen in an AP radiograph of the proximal fibula in a 23-year-old female. The fibula only appears slightly irregular, but there is permeative change with subtle periosteal reaction (*arrows*). **D,** The MR of this lesion T2-weighted (2500/80) shows what a large soft tissue mass can be seen in Ewing's sarcoma.

- It is permeative and aggressive, usually diaphyseal in location.
- It has enormous soft-tissue mass with relative preservation of cortex.
- Sequestra.
- Most common age range is 30 to 60 years.
- Large tubular bones, pelvis, and scapula are most common sites of origin.

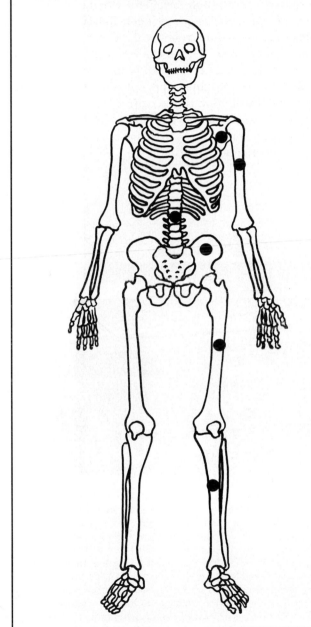

the most common range is 30–60 years. The lesion most frequently is permeative and lytic (Fig. 1-48) but it can appear to be of mixed density because of reactive bone formation and prominent endosteal thickening. The lesion tends to arise in appendicular central diaphy-seal sites, particularly the femur, tibia, and humerus but also can occur in the pelvis, scapula, and spine.

This lesion can enlarge very rapidly, giving rise to two features that can be suggestive of the diagnosis, seen on radiography, CT, or MRI. One of these features is a very large soft-tissue mass without extensive cortical destruction. In addition, sequestra have been reported in 16% of the AFIP series. It is felt that the sequestra result from rapid growth of tumor overwhelming blood supply to residual bone.[25] The MRI appearance is nonspecific.

The major differential diagnosis relates to other aggressive lesions occurring in this age range. Therefore the differential includes malignant fibrous histiocytoma/fibrosarcoma, osteomyelitis, Ewing's sarcoma, and lytic chondrosarcoma.

Primary lymphoma can metastasize to lymph nodes and bone. Lung metastases are uncommon, but when present may increase in size and number quickly. Treatment is whole bone radiation, with chemotherapy reserved for disseminated disease.

Hodgkin's Disease

Hodgkin's disease in bone is almost always metastatic in etiology. Twenty percent of patients with Hodgkin's disease have radiographic evidence of bone involvement, but it is extremely rare as a primary bone tumor. Metastatic Hodgkin's disease can involve bone either by hematogenous dissemination or by contiguous spread from adjacent nodes. The sternum is a common site of contiguous tumor involvement.

Hodgkin's disease of bone is seen most frequently in the second through fourth decades of life. The lesion most frequently is found in the axial skeleton, especially the vertebral bodies. The lesion may be lytic, but most frequently is either blastic or mixed lytic and blastic. The ivory vertebrae (Fig. 1-49) is a classic manifestation of Hodgkin's disease, although it is also seen in metastatic disease and Paget's disease. Two thirds of cases are polyostotic. The lesions may be moderately aggressive in appearance and may show a soft-tissue mass.

Multiple Myeloma

This neoplastic proliferation of plasma cells is the most common primary bone tumor, seen either in its solitary form (plasmacytoma) or as the more common multiple myeloma. Ninety-five percent of patients are over 40 years of age.

Plasmacytomas are lytic expansile geographic lesions (Fig. 1-50). They have a relatively narrow zone of transition without sclerotic margins. There is no matrix calcification present. The most common sites of occurrence for plasmacytoma are the vertebral bodies, pelvis, femur, and humerus. The differential diagnosis of plasmacytoma

Key Concepts	Multiple Myeloma

- Most common appearance is multiple punched out lytic lesions.
- May present as diffuse osteopenia, without focal lytic lesion.
- Occasionally presents as a focal lytic expansile lesion (plasmacytoma).
- Bone scan and skeletal survey are complementary studies, as each misses a significant number of myeloma lesions.
- MR may be used as a survey.

depends on its degree of aggressiveness. Other lesions, which best fit the description above, include metastasis, intramedullary chondrosarcoma, giant cell tumor, and brown tumor of hyperparathyroidism.

Seventy percent of patients with a plasma cell neoplasia have multifocal myeloma, which most often presents with numerous focal (punched out) lytic lesions. These lesions are generally less than 5 cm in size, and often are less than 1 cm in size (Fig. 1-51). The zone of transition is narrow in these punched out lesions. Less commonly, multiple myeloma presents as generalized osteopenia (Fig. 1-52), showing no focal lesions. Such a generalized osteopenia, perhaps with a compression fracture, in a middle aged male should suggest the diagnosis of multiple myeloma in the absence of other predisposing factors for osteoporosis. Multiple myeloma, whether it presents as focal punched out lesions or as generalized osteopenia, originates in the red marrow but then progresses to cortex and other areas. The skull, vertebral bodies, ribs, and pelvis are the most frequently involved structures, followed by the proximal appendicular skeleton. This reflects the distribution of red marrow in the adult. The major differential diagnosis for multiple myeloma is metastatic disease, and the less frequent multiple brown tumors of hyperparathyroidism.

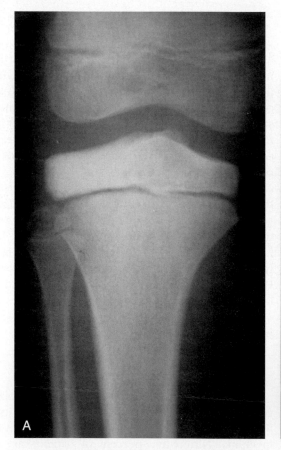
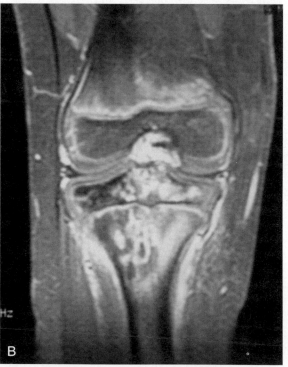

Fig. 1-47 Sclerotic Ewing's sarcoma. **A,** An AP radiograph of the knee in a 9-year-old male. The proximal epiphysis of the tibia stands out as being sclerotic, but no definite destructive change is seen. It is worth remembering that Ewing's sarcoma can elicit such dense reactive bone formation that the permeative change can be disguised by the reactive bone. **B,** The T1-weighted MRI (733/10) obtained in a coronal plane following contrast administration shows that the lesion involves not only the proximal tibial epiphysis, but extends well into the metaphysis as well. There is a soft-tissue mass, although it is not as large as was seen in an earlier case (Fig. 1-46D).

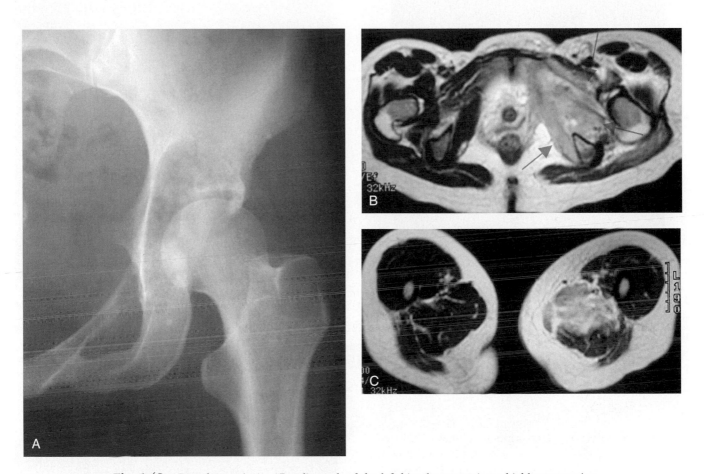

Fig. 1-48   Lymphoma. **A,** An AP radiograph of the left hip, demonstrating a highly permeative lesion involving the acetabulum and extending into the superior pubic ramus. Lymphoma is certainly a strong consideration for this aggressive lesion in a 31-year-old female. **B** and **C,** The T2-weighted MRI (2700/104) demonstrates an unusually extensive soft-tissue mass associated with this lesion. In its proximal portion, the soft-tissue mass involves both the obturator internus and externus (*arrows*), and the mass is seen to extend well down into the proximal half of the thigh, involving the adductor musculature. This extensive and infiltrative soft-tissue mass is typical of lymphoma.

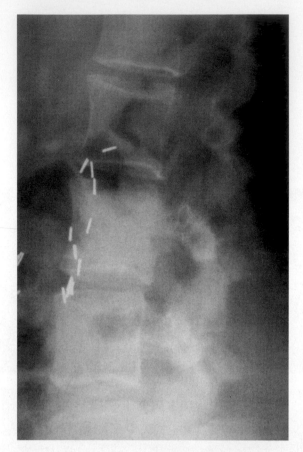

Fig. 1-49   Hodgkin's Disease. This lateral radiograph of the spine demonstrates an ivory vertebra at L3. Although ivory vertebra can be seen in other disease processes, the periaortic lymph node dissection suggested by the position of the clips helps to make the diagnosis of Hodgkin's disease in this case. (Reprinted with permission from the ACR learning file.)

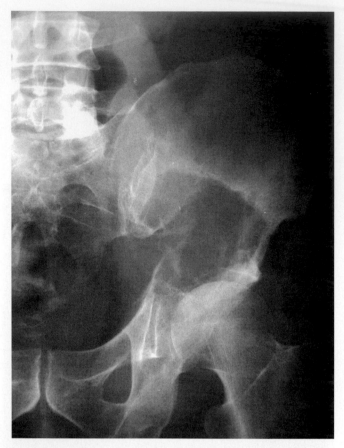

Fig. 1-50   Myeloma. A solitary large lytic lesion of the iliac wing is seen, which is fairly well marginated, but shows medial cortical breakthrough. This is a typical appearance of plasmacytoma in this 53-year-old male.

Some manifestations of multiple myeloma are unusual. Ten percent to 15% of cases of multiple myeloma are associated with amyloidosis. When amyloid is deposited in the synovium, the radiographic picture may simulate rheumatoid arthritis. Rarely, multiple myeloma may have a sclerotic pattern, with either a sclerotic margin around the lytic lesion or else entirely sclerotic round lesions. Sclerosing myeloma (Fig. 1-53) is associated with the POEMS syndrome. This acronym stands for the syndrome of polyneuropathy (P), organomegally (O), endocrinopathy (E), myeloma (M), and skin (S) changes.

The radiographic work-up for multiple myeloma is somewhat controversial, as no single study appears to demonstrate all lesions. It seems that skeletal surveys and bone scans are complementary studies for multiple myeloma. Technetium radionuclide bone scanning is positive in only 25%–40% of myeloma lesions. Therefore it is thought to be less reliable than a skeletal survey in a lesions search. However, it is worthwhile to

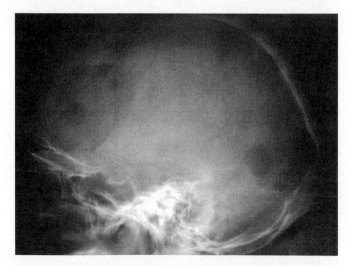

Fig. 1-51   Myeloma. Multiple "punched out" lesions of the skull. These non-marginated lesions are classically seen with multiple myeloma, proven in this 60-year-old male.

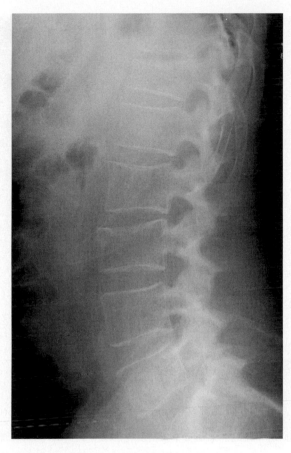

Fig. 1-52   Myeloma. A more difficult case, where one sees only diffuse osteopenia and compression fractures of the superior end plates of T12 and L3. However, this radiograph is taken in a 32-year-old male who has no known metabolic disease or use of steroids. When severe generalized osteopenia is seen in a patient whose age and gender does not suggest senile osteoporosis, multiple myeloma should be strongly considered.

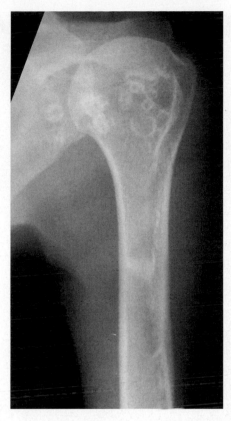

Fig. 1-53   Sclerosing myeloma. Multiple myeloma need not show only focal lytic lesions. Another manifestation of multiple myeloma is seen in this case, where the lesions are either entirely sclerotic or show a sclerotic rim. Sclerosing myeloma is rare and is part of the POEMS syndrome.

remember that although plain film is more sensitive than technetium in 38% of lesions, bone scanning is more sensitive than radiographs in 18% of lesions. An additional option for determining tumor burden may be MR imaging, which is sensitive and may be helpful in resolving a discrepancy between bone scan and radiographic results. The MR imaging appearance of both the plasmacytoma and multiple myeloma is non-specific. T1 demonstrates either a diffuse or mottled decrease in signal intensity whereas there is generalized increased signal intensity on T2 imaging. Screening MR is used in some centers to evaluate tumor burden in cases of multiple myeloma.

Most cases of plasmacytoma go on to multi-focal or generalized disease, though a few remain localized. Multiple myeloma has a relatively low 5-year survival rate. Treatment consists of chemotherapy, bone marrow transplant, and palliative radiation therapy, with occasional ablative surgery for plasmacytomas. Serial filming is used to follow tumor burden as well as to identify lesions

at risk for pathologic fracture (large lesions, or those involving greater than 50% of cortical width).

VASCULAR TUMORS

Vascular Tumors: Benign

Hemangiomas are vascular malformations. They may arise anywhere, and may be either osseous or soft tissue in origin. Although the lesions are found most frequently in the fourth and fifth decades, the age range is wide.

The majority (75%) of osseous hemangiomas are found in the vertebral bodies, skull, and facial bones. In the vertebral bodies, the vertical trabecular pattern becomes coarsened, usually without collapse. This gives a vertical striated appearance on plain film and a "polka dot" appearance on axial CT. There may be mild expansion in the vertebral body lesions (Fig. 1-54) and occasionally a soft-tissue mass, which may lead to neurologic symptoms. The expansion is often much more prominent in skull lesions, where the outer table rather than the inner table expands. In the skull lesions, there are also coarsened

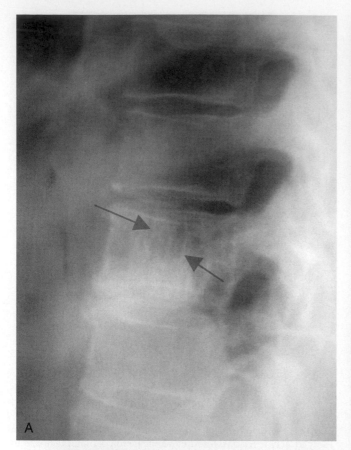

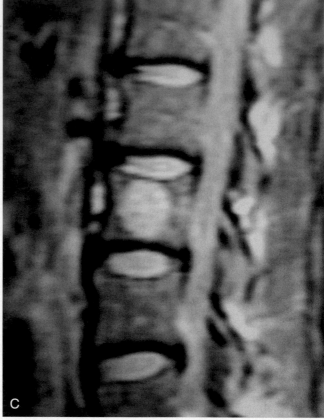

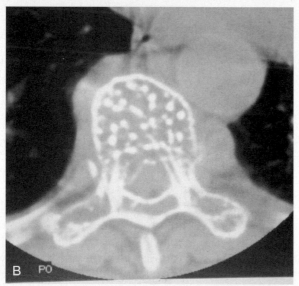

Fig. 1-54   Vertebral body hemangioma **A,** A lateral radiograph of a lower thoracic vertebral body showing the vertical striations (*arrows*) that are typical for hemangioma. **B,** CT shows the thickened vertical trabeculae as a "polka-dot" pattern. MR most typically shows a stroma that follows the signal intensity of fat on all sequences. **C,** The sagittal MR shows the vertebral body hemangioma with fatty signal in this proton density sequence (2200/35). (Reprinted with permission from the ACR learning file.)

trabeculae but their pattern is to radiate in a sunburst pattern toward the expanded outer table. This is a pathognomonic appearance. The much less frequent appearance of hemangiomas in other bones generally shows a geographic lytic pattern, sometimes with a radiating or spoke-wheel pattern of ossification.

The MRI appearance of osseous hemangioma is quite characteristic owing to the fact that there is a variable amount of fatty stroma within the lesion. This fatty stroma leads to an increased signal intensity on both T1- and T2-weighted imaging.

Soft tissue hemangiomas are characterized by a mass, often containing phleboliths (Fig. 1-55). Although the vessels of a hemangioma are generally not demonstrated in osseous lesions, they are seen, both on contrast enhanced CT and on MRI (Fig. 1-56) as a characteristic "can of worms" within the underlying stroma. As with the osseous lesions, the stroma contains areas of fat that yield high signal intensity on both T1 and T2 imaging. On MRI, the tortuous vessels are seen either

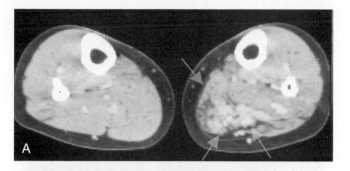

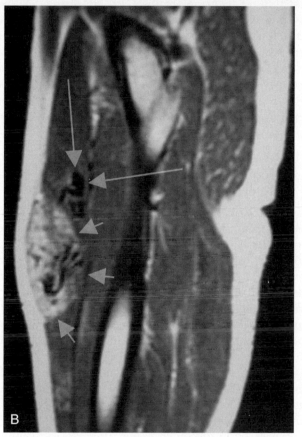

Fig. 1-56   Soft tissue hemangioma. **A,** A CT of a patient in which a hemangioma is seen in the posterior compartment of the leg (*arrows*). This CT is obtained after administration of IV contrast, and shows the tortuous vascular structure that has been given the term "can of worms." **B,** A different patient with a soft tissue hemangioma. In this sagittal T1-weighted MRI (630/30), we see an anteriorly located intramuscular hemangioma that has fatty stroma surrounding vessels showing a flow void (*short arrows*). A large feeding vessel is seen proximal to the mass, again with flow void, low signal characteristics (*long arrow*).

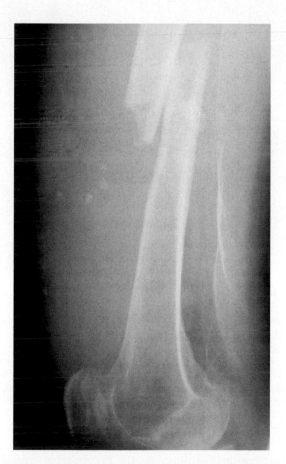

Fig. 1-55   Soft tissue hemangioma. A lateral radiograph showing a large soft-tissue mass that contains multiple phleboliths. The phleboliths are diagnostic of hemangioma. In this case, the hemangioma caused extrinsic scalloping and thinning of the anterior femoral cortex, which resulted in pathologic fracture.

as high signal or flow void, depending on the rate of flow. Soft tissue hemangiomas are usually intramuscular and may scallop or extend into adjacent bone. If a hemangioma occurs in a skeletally immature patient, it may cause focal bone overgrowth due to chronic hyperemia. Finally, the rare synovial hemangioma may cause repetitive bleeding into the joint and an appearance similar to hemophilia. The knee and elbow are favored sites for synovial hemangioma; this site preference also makes it difficult to differentiate from the appearance of hemophilia.

Other benign vascular tumors are rare, including the extremely uncommon osseous lymphangioma and the somewhat more common soft tissue lymphangioma. Cystic angiomatosis is a rare benign multicentric manifestation of hemangiomatosis or lymphangiomatosis, often with severe visceral involvement. The multiple lytic lesions of bone are nonspecific in appearance unless calcified phleboliths are present in the soft tissues. Another variant is Gorham's disease, or massive osteolysis. This is a disease of multicentric angiomatosis with regional dissolution of bone, which is rapid and severely destructive, spreading contiguously across joints.

Vascular Lesions Intermediate or Indeterminate for Malignancy

Hemangiopericytoma and hemangioendothelioma fit within this category. These are vascular lesions seen in soft tissues which may erode bone, and may rarely originate within bone. They are benign or low-grade malignant lesions, which can be difficult to differentiate histologically from angiosarcoma. Hemangiopericytoma and hemangioendothelioma are not radiographically distinguishable. Their soft tissue mass is nonspecific and their osseous involvement may range from a nonaggressive to a moderately aggressive appearance. The MRI appearance of each is nonspecific, although vascular channels are occasionally seen. There is no underlying fatty stroma as might be seen in hemangioma. These vascular tumors of intermediate aggressiveness may be multicentric. Interestingly, when they are multicentric they tend to involve several bones of a single extremity, often the feet. The lesions which are multicentric tend to have a better prognosis than the solitary lesions.

Malignant Vascular Tumors: Angiosarcoma

Angiosarcoma is a rare malignant vascular tumor (Fig. 1-57), which may be difficult to differentiate histologically from the less aggressive hemangioendothelioma. Angiosarcoma is seen most frequently in the fourth and fifth decades, but can be seen in younger patients if it is multifocal. Osseous angiosarcomas are extremely rare and are permeative, aggressive appearing lesions without matrix. The most common location is metaphyseal, in the femur, tibia, humerus, and pelvis. Thirty-eight percent of angiosarcomas are polyostotic. If they are polyostotic, the lesions tend to be regional

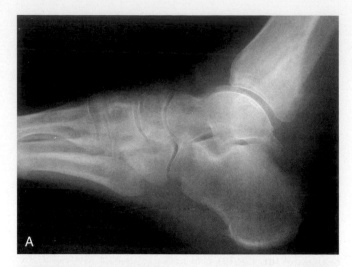

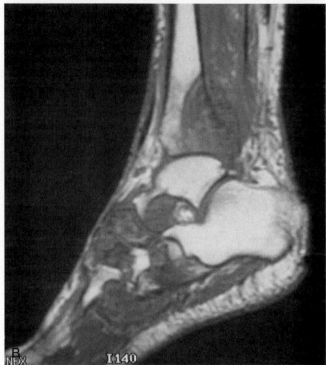

Fig. 1-57 Angiosarcoma. **A,** A lateral radiograph of the foot in a 67-year-old male. There is an ill-defined destructive lesion involving the posterior aspect of the distal tibia. One might consider that the lucencies seen throughout the bones of the hindfoot and midfoot represents disuse osteopenia. **B,** However, the T1-weighted MRI (700/16) demonstrates the low signal intensity lesions involving the distal tibia, distal talus, navicular, cuboid, cuneiforms, and several of the metatarsals. Multiple lesions involving the lower extremities frequently prove to be vascular tumors. In this case, the diagnosis is angiosarcoma.

in distribution. Furthermore, the prognosis is somewhat improved if the lesions are multifocal. Five-year survival is poor for the solitary lesions, with metastases spreading to the lungs or skeleton. Treatment is wide resection.

OTHER CONNECTIVE TISSUE TUMORS: FIBROUS ORIGIN

Fibromatoses

The fibromatoses are a heterogeneous group of tumors that have been described with a variety of terms and classifications, though histologically all the lesions are similar. The vast majority arise in soft tissue. As a group, soft-tissue fibromatoses tend to be large, locally infiltrative, and occasionally multicentric. Tumor often infiltrates through compartmental barriers and has no visible capsule either at surgery or with imaging. This aggressive appearance may lead to a misdiagnosis of a malignant lesion. However, MRI signal characteristics can be helpful in making the correct diagnosis. In up to 80% of cases, the signal intensity is low on both T1 and T2 imaging because of the hypocellularity of the lesion. In the remaining 20% of cases, the nonspecific low signal intensity on T1 and high signal intensity on T2 sequences make the diagnosis more difficult.

Soft tissue fibromatoses tend to be grouped according to the age and location of occurrence. *Congenital generalized fibromatosis* is a variant that develops in utero, with disseminating fibromatoses involving much of the musculature and viscera. This is usually fatal within a few months. Another category is *infantile dermal fibromatosis*. In this case, the lesion infiltrates the extensor surface of the digits, presenting as firm nodules attached to the skin, tendon, fascia, and periosteum. Bony erosion may occasionally occur. The lesion is usually seen in children 1-2 years of age and recurrence after excision is frequent. *Juvenile aponeurotic fibroma* is seen in children and adolescents as a slowly infiltrating lesion arising in the aponeurotic tissue of the hands (usually the volar portion), wrist, and feet (usually the plantar region). This lesion may calcify, especially in the interosseous membrane of the distal forearm (Fig. 1-58). It may be locally aggressive, with recurrence commonly following resection.

The most common of the soft tissue fibromatoses is the *desmoid tumor,* which is also commonly called *aggressive fibromatosis,* desmoid fibromatosis, or fibrosarcoma grade I desmoid type. This is a fairly common lesion, comprising 7% of benign soft-tissue tumors.[8] Aggressive fibromatosis presents as a painless infiltrative soft-tissue mass, which originates in abdominal or extra-abdominal muscle. The lesion is often large by the time it is detected, and shows aggressive local infiltration of adjacent muscle, vessels, nerves, and tendons (Fig. 1-59). Bone involvement is rare (6% of cases) and arises from extrinsic invasion (Fig. 1-59D). However, when bone is affected by aggressive fibromatosis, it may have a spectacular appearance with huge frondlike excrescences arising

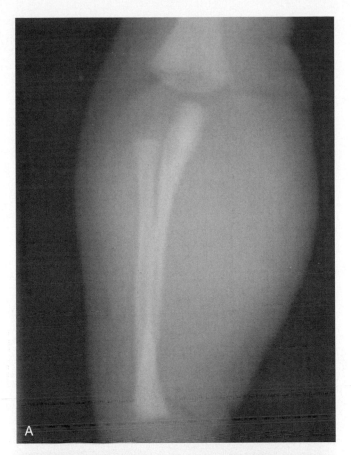

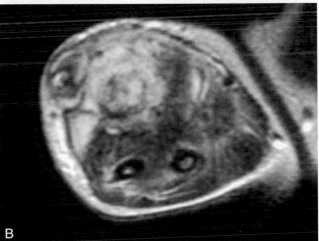

Fig. 1-58 Juvenile aponeurotic fibromatosis. **A,** An AP radiograph of the forearm in a 6-day-old infant. It demonstrates a large soft-tissue mass, along with scalloping and deformity of the forearm bones. **B,** On the T2-weighted MRI (3933/100), the mass is shown to be volar in location and both heterogeneous and infiltrative. Despite the aggressive appearance on MRI, the deformity of the bones, age of the patient, and prevalence of the disease suggests this is a congenital form of fibromatosis.

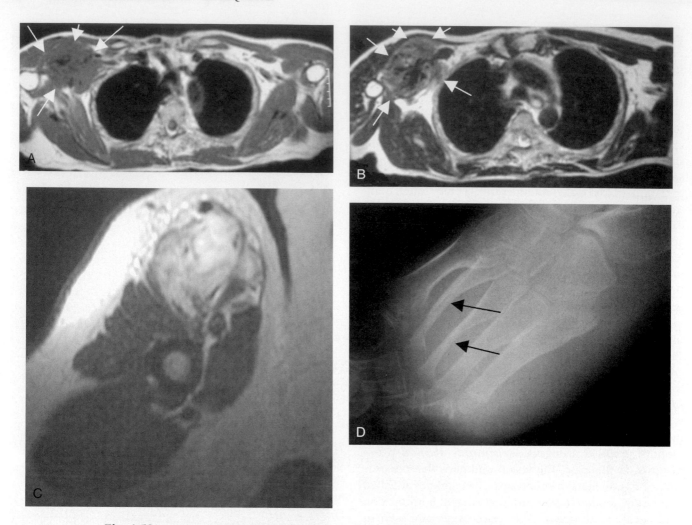

Fig. 1-59 Aggressive fibromatosis. **A,** A T1-weighted axial MRI (549/10) showing a low signal intensity infiltrative lesion involving the anterior chest wall (*arrows*) in a 61-year-old male. **B,** The T2-weighted MRI shows the mass to remain mostly low signal intensity (*arrows*). The MRI signal characteristics, in combination with the invasiveness of the lesion and location on the chest wall make the diagnosis of aggressive fibromatosis extremely likely in this case. However, aggressive fibromatosis does not always show low signal characteristics on T2-weighted imaging, as shown in **C,** an axial T2-weighted MR image (2000/80) showing an invasive high signal intensity mass lesion in the proximal humerus in a 42-year-old male. This proved at biopsy to also be an example of aggressive fibromatosis. **D,** An oblique radiograph of a foot in a 12-year-old male, showing the osseous deformity (*arrows*) that can occur in cases of aggressive fibromatosis.

from a stimulated periosteum, with spicules of bone radiating into the adjacent soft-tissue mass. Aggressive fibromatosis often presents in children and young adults and may be indolent for long periods of time. However, it may also act in a highly aggressive fashion, with a postresection recurrence rate of 65%–75%. As margins can be difficult to assess with imaging studies or by direct palpation at surgery, a wide margin beyond the apparent defined tumor limit should be obtained at surgery.

Desmoplastic fibroma is the rare form of fibromatosis in bone. The majority of these lesions present in the second decade of life and have a geographic pattern with cortical expansion and endosteal erosion. The lesions are located centrally in the metaphysis, most frequently in

the long bones but also the pelvis and mandible. The zone of transition is variable and can simulate a more aggressive lesion. There is no tumor matrix and generally no significant host response. Because these can be radiographically aggressive, they can be difficult to differentiate radiographically as well as histologically from a well differentiated fibrosarcoma. Their behavior is not malignant, but recurrence is very common.

Cortical "Desmoid" (periosteal desmoid) is not a neoplasm, but fibroblastic proliferation probably secondary to trauma at the insertion of the adductor magnus muscle or medial head of the gastrocnemius. Cortical desmoid is sometimes considered a normal variant that is better termed "avulsive cortical irregularity" or "medial supracondylar defect.'' Because cortical desmoid causes erosion of the cortex as well as an exuberant periostitis, it may be misdiagnosed both radiographically and histologically as an osteosarcoma (Fig. 1-60). The location of the lesion is the hallmark that leads to the correct diagnosis: it is always found on the posterio-medial cortex on the distal metaphysis of the femur, adjacent to the medial femoral condyle. If at all possible, the diagnosis should be made on radiographs as MRI may further confuse the issue, with low signal intensity on T1 and high signal intensity on T2. There is occasionally a low signal rim, but this is not always present.

Nonossifying Fibroma/Benign Fibrous Cortical Defect (Fibroxanthoma)

Nonossifying fibroma and benign fibrous cortical defect are histologically identical, cortically based lesions that in fact are not neoplasms but may arise secondary

Key Concepts	NOF/BFCD

- It is a cortical metadiaphyseal lesion.
- It is common in children.
- It is radiographically nonaggressive.
- Its typical appearance does not require further work-up.
- The most common natural evolution of the lesion is to heal in with a smooth sclerosis.

to epiphyseal plate defects that migrate away from the plate with growth. It is estimated that benign fibrous cortical defect occurs in 30%–40% of children over the age of two. They are seen infrequently in adults, as they convert to normal bone spontaneously. Occasionally benign fibrous cortical defect may enlarge, forming a nonossifying fibroma. These lesions are asymptomatic in the absence of pathologic fracture and are so radiographically

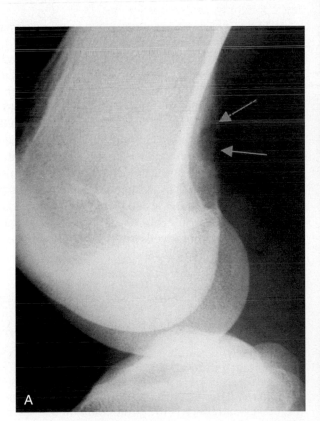 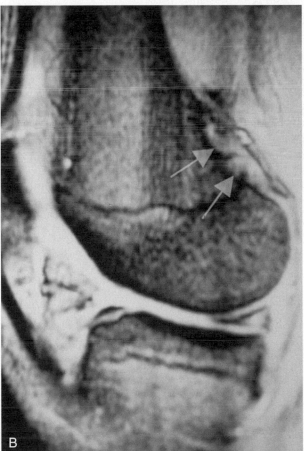

Fig. 1-60   Cortical desmoid. **A,** A lateral radiograph of the knee in a 17-year-old male. The posteromedial cortex of the distal femoral metaphysis is scalloped, with elevated periosteum (*arrows*). Although this might have the appearance of an aggressive lesion, its location should allow for the appropriate diagnosis. **B,** MRI (gradient echo imaging) shows the elevated periosteum and interruption of the cortex with scalloping, but no soft tissue mass (*arrows*). Also shown is the torn posterior horn of the medial meniscus, the source of the patient's pain. (Reprinted with permission from ACR learning file.)

specific that they fall among the "leave me alone" lesions that should be ignored unless symptomatic. There is no real significance in the popular distinction made between nonossifying fibromas and benign cortical defects; nonossifying fibromas are occasionally large enough to present some diagnostic difficulty by radiograph.

Eighty percent of these lesions occur in the diametaphyses of the long bones of the lower extremity. They are cortically based. Although nonossifying fibroma arises in the cortex, it may enlarge to involve the intramedullary region and even appear central when found in very small bones such as the fibula or ulna (see Fig. 1-2G). These lesions have a narrow zone of transition, sclerotic margin, and no matrix calcification (Fig. 1-61). There is no periosteal reaction. However, during the spontaneous healing process they may demonstrate homogeneous sclerotic bone formation (Fig. 1-2G). Not surprisingly, MRI shows low signal intensity on T1-weighted images and a variable signal intensity on T2-weighted images, depending on the extent of hypercellular fibrous tissue and hemosiderin versus healing bone that is present.

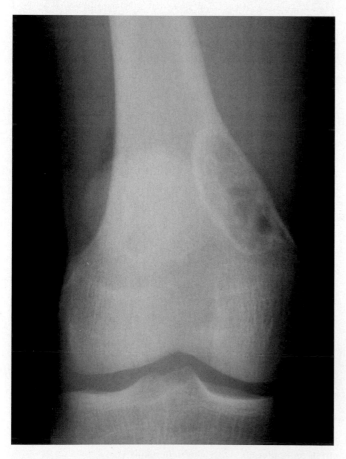

Fig. 1-61 Nonossifying fibroma. This AP radiograph shows a cortically based metaphyseal lesion that has a sclerotic rim and narrow zone of transition, in a 19-year-old male. This is a typical nonossifying fibroma.

Benign Fibrous Histiocytoma

Benign fibrous histiocytoma is a rare osseous lesion that has a histologic appearance very similar to that of nonossifying fibroma but demonstrates different radiographic features, being geographic and arising centrally in the metaphyseal region of long bones. CT and MRI features are nonspecific. Unlike nonossifying fibromas, benign fibrous histiocytoma has a tendency to recur after curettage and may be symptomatic. Benign fibrous histiocytoma may also originate in soft tissue.

Malignant Fibrous Histiocytoma/ Fibrosarcoma

Malignant fibrous histiocytoma (MFH) is a pleomorphic sarcoma that contains both fibroblastic and histiocytic elements in varying proportions. Fibrosarcoma is distinguishable histologically, having a more regular appearance of fibroblastic cells. The lesions are not distinguishable radiographically and will be discussed together in this section. Both malignant fibrous histiocytoma and fibrosarcoma may originate either in the soft tissues or, less commonly, as osseous lesions.

MFH is the most frequent soft-tissue sarcoma in adults, found to represent 24% of the cases in a large series.[9] Soft tissue MFH occurs in a wide age range (10–90 years of age), with most patients between 30 and 60 years old. Soft tissue MFH is usually located in the extremities, with 50% of all cases found in the lower extremity.[26] Soft tissue MFH is usually not detected by plain film, but is worked up with MRI for local staging. The MRI appearance is generally nonspecific, with T1-weighted images appearing isointense with muscle, and T2-weighted images showing inhomogeneous high signal intensity. These lesions may appear to have a reactive pseudocapsule, but must be regarded as aggressive lesions with tumor cells invariably infiltrating locally

Key Concepts	Malignant Fibrous Histiocytoma

- It is the most common soft tissue sarcoma in adults.
- Relatively common osseous sarcoma, especially in the fourth through seventh decades.
- The osseous MFH may be either primary or secondary.
- Lower extremity is the most common site for both the soft tissue and osseous MFH.
- Dystrophic calcification is seen in 15% (particularly in lesions secondary to bone infarct degeneration).
- Both soft tissue and osseous lesions are highly aggressive clinically.

usually appears as an aggressive geographic lytic lesion (Fig. 1-63). They generally appear permeative or moth-eaten, with a wide zone of transition seen in at least part of the lesion. The lesion is lytic, although dystrophic calcification may be seen in as many as 15% of cases. MR imaging is nonspecific, with low signal intensity T1 and a heterogeneous high signal intensity T2 appearance, with occasional low signal intensity regions relating to dystrophic calcification.

Although most osseous MFH arise as primary lesions, up to 20% arise in areas of abnormal bone.[27] Underlying lesions include Paget's disease, previously radiated bone, dedifferentiated chondrosarcoma, nonossifying fibroma, fibrous dysplasia, enchondroma, chronic osteomyelitis, and bone infarct (osteonecrosis). With these secondary forms of MFH, an aggressive lesion will be found in contiguity with the benign counterpart from which it arises. For example, MFH arising in bone infarct may demonstrate the nonaggressive serpiginous pattern of calcifica-

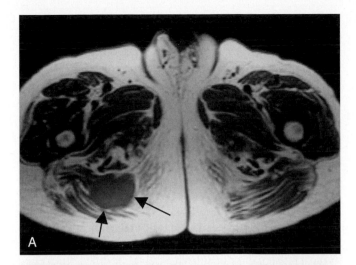
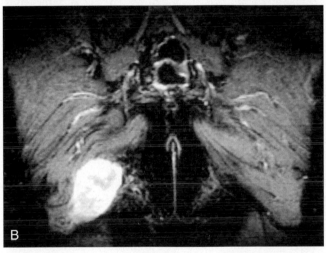

Fig. 1-62   Soft-tissue malignant fibrous histiocytoma (MFH). **A,** An axial T1-weighted MRI (486/15) showing an intramuscular soft tissue mass that is isointense with muscle (*arrows*). **B,** The coronal T2-weighted image (1500/20) shows a slightly inhomogeneous high signal intensity mass lesion. This is a nonspecific appearance, but given the age of the patient and prevalence of the lesion, MFH is a reasonable diagnostic choice.

at the margins (Fig. 1-62). When the soft tissue mass is adjacent to a long bone, it may cause a smooth cortical pressure erosion. Dystrophic calcification occasionally occurs, usually in the periphery in either a curvilinear or punctate pattern.[26] There is a myxoid variety of MFH that demonstrates low signal intensity central portions on T1 and T2 imaging, with nodular peripheral enhancement.

Osseous MFH and fibrosarcoma may arise either primarily or secondarily. MFH comprises 5% of all primary malignant bone tumors. As with soft-tissue MFH, the age range is wide but the peak prevalence is in the 30–60 year age range.

Most osseous MFH lesions occur in the long tubular bones, usually centrally in the metaphysis. Primary MFH

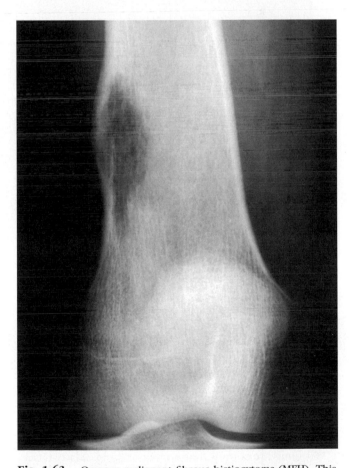

Fig. 1-63   Osseous malignant fibrous histiocytoma (MFH). This is an AP radiograph of a moderately aggressive appearing lesion in the distal metadiaphysis of the femur in a 22-year-old male. The zone of transition is wide and there is no calcific matrix. This is a nonspecific appearance, but a moderately aggressive lytic lesion in an adult should include MFH as diagnostic consideration.

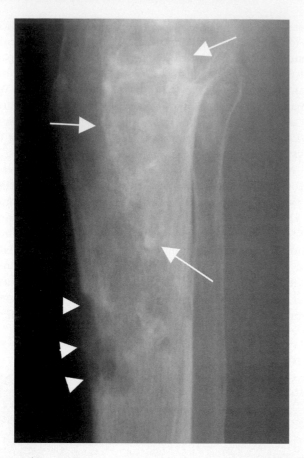

Fig. 1-64   Secondary osseous MFH. This is a lateral radiograph of the proximal tibia in a 66-year-old female that demonstrates dystrophic calcific matrix in a serpiginous pattern typical of bone infarct (*arrows*). However, there is a more destructive lesion found in contiguity but slightly distal to the bone infarct (*arrowheads*). This aggressive lesion arising from a bone infarct represents a secondary osseous MFH. (Reprinted with permission from the ACR learning file.)

tion commonly seen in bone infarct, immediately contiguous with a highly destructive pattern (Fig. 1-64).

Most MFHs are high-grade, with a 5-year survival of 25%. Metastases involve lung, bone, lymph nodes, and liver. Local recurrence after resection is common. Treatment consists of aggressive surgical excision, chemotherapy, often supplemented by radiation therapy.

OTHER CONNECTIVE TISSUE TUMORS: FATTY TISSUE

Lipoma

Lipomas are common tumors consisting of fatty tissue, most commonly found in soft tissues but rarely arising as an intraosseous lesion. Lipoma and lipoma variants constitute 16% of benign soft-tissue tumors.[8] Fully 80% of lipomas are found in the subcutaneous tissues. Others are inter or intramuscular. They may extensively infiltrate fascial planes and muscle compartments. Lipomas present as an asymptomatic, soft, compressible, mobile mass (Fig. 1-65). If they are large enough on radiographs they may appear as radiolucent (fat tissue density) masses. They show fat attenuation on CT. MRI is highly characteristic, showing a sharply bordered lesion with high signal intensity matching that of subcutaneous fat on both T1 and T2 imaging, which suppresses with fat saturation. Lipomas do not enhance. They may rarely contain metaplastic cartilage and bone calcification. The only true difficulty with lipomas is detecting the rare atypical lipoma or low grade, well-differentiated liposarcoma. Atypical lipomas are well-differentiated lipomas that recur locally but do not metastasize. MR image should be carefully scrutinized to detect any site within a lipoma where typical fat signal is not shown, such as nodules, thickened margin, or areas of enhancement, that may raise concern for atypical lipoma or low-grade liposarcoma.

There are other variants of lipoma that are of interest. *Lipomatosis* is a congenital abnormality with multiple lipomas distributed either randomly or symmetrically over the body. *Macrodystrophia lipomatosa* is a more localized form, which results in overgrowth of the soft tissues and bone, usually in the hand or foot (Fig. 1-66). Macrodystrophia lipomatosa falls into the differential for localized giantism. Included in this differential are neurofibromatosis and vascular lesions.

Lipoblastoma is a benign embryonal fatty tumor seen in young children. It simulates liposarcoma histologically.

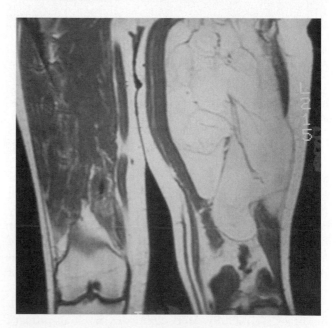

Fig. 1-65   Lipoma. This coronal T1-(750/20) weighted MRI demonstrates an extensive lipoma infiltrating the muscle of the left thigh in a 77-year-old male. Note that the signal of the tumor is identical with that of the subcutaneous fat. This would hold true on all sequences, and it would suppress with fat suppression techniques.

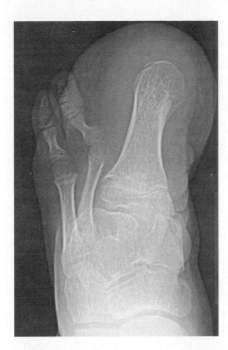

Fig. 1-66   Macrodystropia lipomatosa. This AP radiograph shows a massively overgrown midfoot and first metatarsal. The second and third rays have been resected, as have been the phalanges of the great toe, in this 13-year-old male, in order for his foot to accommodate a shoe. This is one form of focal giantism.

This is a confusing lesion as CT or MRI characteristically will show nonadipose tissue in the periphery of the lesion. Although recurrence after surgery is common, it is important not to mistake this lesion for liposarcoma. Age at onset is the major factor differentiating lipoblastoma from liposarcoma; the latter occurs almost exclusively in adults.

Other lipomas have characteristic appearances according to their location. *Osseous lipoma* is a rare fatty lesion of bone. This is generally asymptomatic and presents as a lytic lesion with a geographic sclerotic margin and no matrix or host reaction. It is usually fat density on CT and fat signal intensity on MRI. It may be distinguished by having a central nidus of dystrophic calcification. Osseous lipomas are found in the metaphyses of long bones and the calcaneus (Fig. 1-67). In the calcaneus, it occurs in the triangular region between the major trabecular arcs (Fig. 1-68). Occasionally a lipoma is located in a *parosteal* position. This position may elicit intense periosteal reaction that may take the form of hyperostosis or may produce large bony spicules radiating from the periosteum into the lesion (Fig. 1-69).

Lipoma arborescens is a rare monoarticular process, usually found in the knee.[21] MR features are characteristic, with hypertrophic synovial villi distended with fat protruding into a large joint effusion. This synovial mass has a signal intensity of fat on all sequences, including those

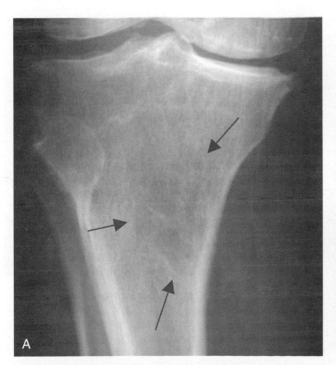
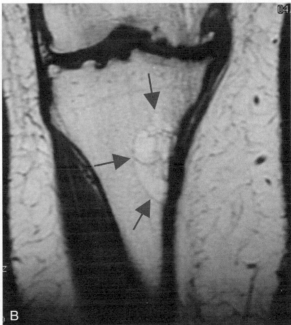

Fig. 1-67   Osseous lipoma. **A,** An AP radiograph of the proximal tibia in a 60-year-old male. There is an ill-defined lytic lesion in the tibial metaphysis (*arrows*), which does not have an aggressive appearance but is otherwise nonspecific. **B,** The MRI allows definitive diagnosis. This coronal T1-weighted image (750/11) shows the lesion (*arrows*) to have the same signal intensity and appearance as nearby subcutaneous fat.

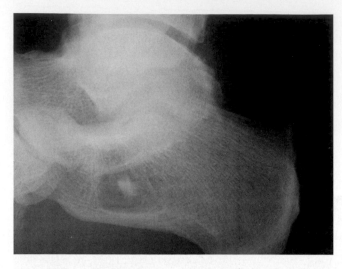

Fig. 1-68   Calcaneal lipoma. A lytic lesion seen on the sagittal radiograph of the mid-calcaneus often represents a lipoma, with the diagnosis approaching certainty when there is central calcific density as in this case.

with chemical fat suppression. Although most cases demonstrate a frondlike appearance, it may occasionally appear as masslike subsynovial fat deposits. Occasional contiguous osseous erosions are seen.[27]

Liposarcoma

Osseous liposarcoma is extremely rare. It is an aggressive neoplasm biologically and at imaging. On the other hand, soft tissue liposarcomas are common, and represent 14% of all malignant soft tissue tumors, second only to malignant fibrous histiocytoma.[9] Soft tissue liposarcoma may range from a well differentiated to a high-grade lesion. The most common age range is 30–60 years, and most arise in the buttock, thigh, leg, and retroperitoneum.

Liposarcoma may have a widely variable appearance on imaging studies, depending on the grade and histology of the lesion. A low grade, well-differentiated lesion may show fat density at radiography and CT, and fat signal intensity on MR imaging. Such well-differentiated liposarcomas can be difficult to differentiate from benign lipomas or atypical lipomas. Differentiating factors include nodularity, usually found at the margins of the tumor, or thick and enhancing septa within the fatty tissue. Although benign lipomas can contain septalike structures, they are generally thin, nonenhancing, and few in number.[28] Unlike low-grade liposarcomas, which show fat density or signal, high-grade liposarcomas may be so cellular that no fat is detectable at imaging. Thus,

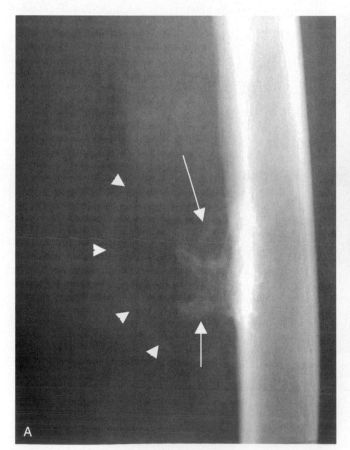

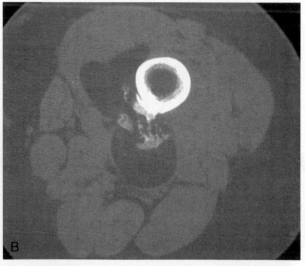

Fig. 1-69   Parosteal lipoma. **A,** A lateral radiograph of the mid-thigh in a 63-year-old male. This is an interesting lesion, showing fat density in the soft tissues (*arrowheads*) and exuberant osseous reaction (*arrow*). Both this radiograph and the CT **B,** which mirrors the findings of the osseous reaction and lipomatous lesion, make the diagnosis of parosteal lipoma.

a high-grade liposarcoma may be completely nonspecific at MR imaging, having a low signal intensity T1 and high inhomogeneous signal intensity at T2 imaging (Fig. 1-70). Other appearances of liposarcoma may relate to the occasional well-differentiated liposarcoma dedifferentiating into a high-grade sarcoma, giving the appearance of a juxtaposed predominately fatty tumor and more highly cellular tumor. Finally, myxoid liposarcoma can also be potentially confusing in appearance, as it shows amorphous fatty areas within an otherwise nonspecific soft tissue mass that may contain cystic areas of myxoid material. The fatty regions may be inconspicuous.

High-grade liposarcomas are aggressive and require wide excision, chemotherapy, often combined with radiation therapy.

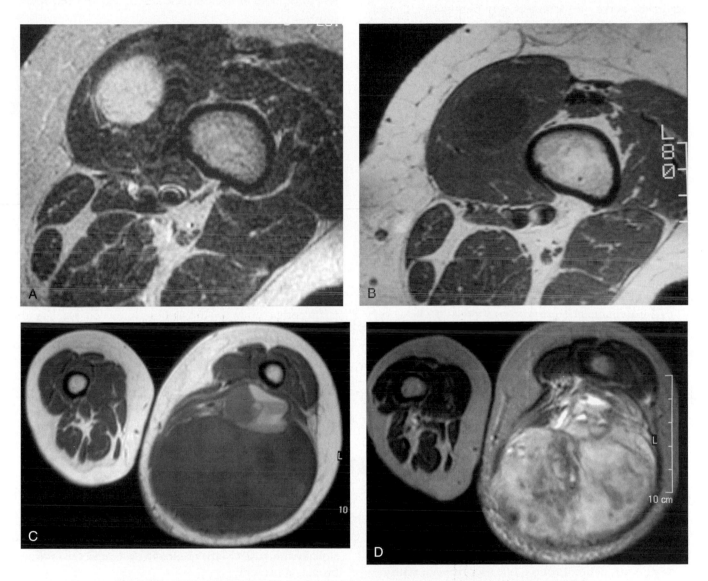

Fig. 1-70   Liposarcoma. **A,** A T2-weighted axial image (2000/70) of a lesion in the vastus medialis. One clinician was tempted to call this a lipoma because it appears so round and is of a similar signal intensity to subcutaneous fat. **B,** However, the T1-weighted image (700/20) shows the lesion to be of low signal intensity, completely different from that of the subcutaneous fat. Even though this does not give the appearance of an aggressive lesion, it is a high-grade liposarcoma. **C,** A very large lesion in the left thigh of a 46-year-old female. This T1-weighted image (815/15) shows that the majority of the lesion is low signal intensity, but that there is high signal intensity adjacent to the femur. This was misinterpreted as representing a hematoma. **D,** The T2-weighted image (2934/80) shows the majority of the lesion to be inhomogeneous, high signal, and aggressive in appearance. This is a high-grade liposarcoma. Although the specific variety of sarcoma cannot be diagnosed from the MRI, it is important to remember that large sarcomas can have intratumoral necrosis and bleeding, and these must not be mistaken for hematoma.

OTHER CONNECTIVE TISSUE TUMORS

Peripheral Nerve Sheath Tumors (PNST)

Peripheral nerve sheath tumors, whether benign or malignant, are most frequently distinguished by their fusiform pattern, with the mass tapering at either end to accommodate the nerve entering and exiting the tumor. Together, neurofibromas and schwannomas represent 10% of all benign soft tissue tumors.[8] Both types of benign peripheral nerve sheath tumors most frequently affect patients in the 20–30 age range. Both show initial slow growth and small size; larger tumors can be exquisitely painful.

Neurofibromas may be localized, plexiform, or diffuse. Ninety percent of neurofibromas are solitary, and are not associated with neurofibromatosis (NF1). These most often affect the superficial cutaneous nerves. Although fusiform enlargement may not be seen in superficial cutaneous neurofibromas, it is indeed a feature of deeper lesions. Neurofibromas invade the nerve fascicles, which become separated and intimately involved with tumor. This feature is not always discernable on MRI. MR shows low signal intensity T1-weighted images and heterogeneously increased signal intensity on T2-weighted images. The "target sign" has been described as being nearly pathognomonic for neurofibroma. This sign is seen on T2-weighted MR images and consists of low signal intensity centrally with a ring of higher signal intensity peripherally (Fig. 1-71). The experienced observers at the AFIP, however, note that the target sign can be seen in schwannomas as well as neurofibromas, and even occasionally in malignant peripheral nerve sheath tumors.[29] The other MR feature that the AFIP group specifies as typical of the lower grade peripheral nerve sheath tumors is the fascicular sign, an image obtained with the involved nerve in cross section, consisting of multiple small ringlike structures corresponding to fascicular bundles.

Key Concepts | **Peripheral Nerve Sheath Tumors**

- They have fusiform shape.
- Entering and exiting nerve.
- Target sign on MRI is said to be more frequently seen with neurofibromas, but may be seen with schwannoma and malignant PNST.
- Neurofibromas are usually found in cutaneous nerves, with the fascicles separated and intimately involved with tumor.
- Schwannomas most frequently involve the ulnar and peroneal nerves, with the tumor lying on the surface of the nerve.
- Malignant PNSTs are more frequently associated with NF1.

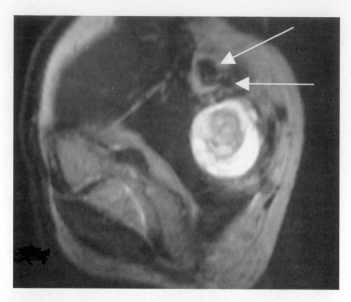

Fig. 1-71 Neurofibroma. This axial T2-weighted image (2600/80) located at the elbow of a 52-year-old male demonstrates a lesion immediately adjacent to and involved with the neurovascular bundle (*arrows* pointing to neurovascuar bundle) on the volar aspect of the arm. The lesion is high signal intensity, with central low signal, an appearance described as a "target sign." The target sign is frequently seen in neurofibroma but can also be seen in other peripheral nerve sheath tumors.

Schwannomas, also known as neurilemoma, neurinoma, perineural fibroblastoma, and peripheral glioma, is the other common benign peripheral nerve sheath tumor. Besides the spinal and sympathetic nerve roots, schwannomas affect nerves in the flexor surfaces of the upper and lower extremities, particularly the ulnar and peroneal nerves. Like neurofibromas, schwannomas are usually solitary. If there are multiple schwannomas, they generally occur in a cutaneous distribution, with a very small proportion of these associated with neurofibromatosis (NF1).

Like neurofibromas, schwannomas are fusiform in shape. However, the nerve lies on the surface of the neoplasm. Because of this characteristic, the tumor can be peeled away from the adjacent nerve at surgical excision. Other than the fusiform shape, and association with a nerve, the MRI appearance is usually nonspecific. Occasionally the target sign, originally described for neurofibroma, is present.

Malignant peripheral nerve sheath tumors (PNST, also called neurofibrosarcoma or malignant schwannoma) comprise 5%–10% of all soft tissue sarcomas. They are generally seen in patients in the 20–50 year age range. Unlike the benign PNST, malignant PNST are much more frequently associated with NF1 (25%–70% of cases).[29] Malignant PNSTs are usually deep lesions, involving the major nerve trunks, such as sciatic nerve, brachial plexus, and sacral plexus (Fig. 1-72). These lesions may be fusi-

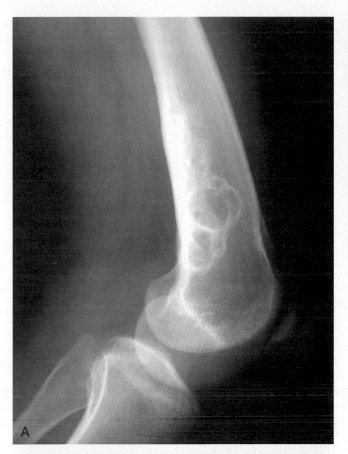

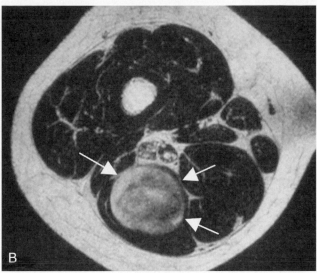

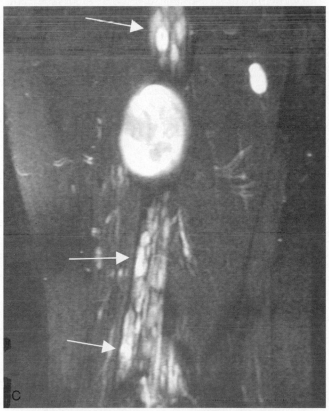

Fig. 1-72   Neurofibromatosis. **A,** A lateral radiograph of the knee in a 21-year-old female that demonstrates a cortically based well-marginated lytic lesion typical of a nonossifying fibroma. **B,** This patient had a palpable mass located more proximally in the thigh, shown on the axial T2-weighted MRI (3200/119). This mass is inhomogenously high signal intensity on T1, with a semi-target sign (*arrows*). **C,** The fat saturated T2 coronal MR image (5000/96) re-demonstrates the mass, which at biopsy was a malignant peripheral nerve sheath tumor, but also demonstrates the multiple smaller neurofibromas arising from the tibial and common peroneal nerves of the thigh (*arrows*).

form in shape and intimately associated with a large nerve, suggesting the diagnosis. Although their generally large size may suggest malignancy, signal characteristics, margination, and inhomogeneity on MRI are not distinctive features. Malignant PNSTs are aggressive lesions, requiring wide surgical excision, chemotherapy, and often radiation therapy. Local recurrence is common (40%), as are distant metastases (60%).[29]

Morton Neuroma

A Morton neuroma is not a tumor, rather it consists of perineural fibrosis and nerve degeneration occurring in the interdigital space. The etiology is likely to be trauma, with the digital nerve rubbing the intermetatarsal ligament between two metatarsal heads. The association with high heeled shoes and repetitive trauma is suggested by the gender frequency (18:1, female to male). The lesions are most frequently found between the third and fourth or second and third metatarsal heads. The diagnosis can be made clinically and may be confused with other lesions such as stress fractures, intermetatarsal bursitis, and Morton's neuromas in unexpected locations. MR is helpful to the clinicians in differentiating among these possibilities. If MRI is used, the lesions are usually identified as low signal, round lesions in the appropriate location seen on small field of view T1-weighted imaging as a teardrop shaped mass along the planter interspace between the metatarsal heads and necks. The lesion is

often obscured on T2-weighted imaging. Contrast enhanced imaging with fat suppression may be used if the diagnosis from T1 imaging is uncertain because the lesions intensely enhance. Ultrasound of these lesions has also been described, but small lesions can be missed. Power Doppler ultrasound may show increased vacularity around the lesion.[29]

Fibrolipomatous Hamartoma (Neural Fibrolipoma)

This lesion is a tumorlike lipomatous process in which fatty tissue is interposed among thickened nerve bundles. The lesion is usually seen in children or young adults and there is a marked predilection for the median nerve. The MRI appearance is pathognomonic, with lipomatous high signal surrounding longitudinally oriented fasicular low signal thickened nerve bundles (Fig. 1-73). This lesion may be associated with macrodactyly.

Giant Cell Tumor of the Tendon Sheath

Giant cell tumor (GCT) of the tendon sheath is generally a painless, slow growing lesion in the tendon sheath, usually of the finger and is considered a form of pigmented villonodular synovitis (PVNS) arising in a tendon sheath. Like PVNS, the etiology may be reactive rather than neoplastic. Histologically, GCT tendon sheath is identical to intraarticular pigmented villonodular synovi-

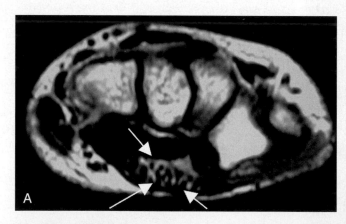
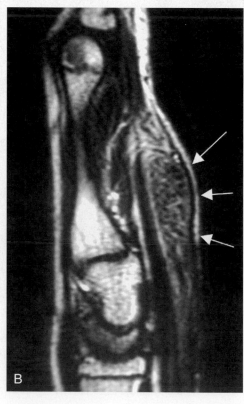

Fig. 1-73 Fibrolipomatous hamartoma. **A,** The axial T1-weighted image (700/10) of the wrist in this 13-year-old female demonstrates multiple nerve fascicles within the carpal tunnel, surrounded by lipomatous signal (*arrows*). **B,** The sagittal T2-weighted MRI (5200/96) re-demonstrates both the fatty stroma and the thickened wavy nerve bundles (*arrows*).

tis. The patient's complaint is of a soft-tissue mass and radiographically, a localized soft-tissue mass is seen. This mass is usually not centered around a joint and may have an associated bony erosion (10% of cases) (Fig. 1-74). Diagnosis may be made by clinical and radiographic features. However, if MRI is done, the lesion is hypointense to muscle on T1, and like PVNS, is variably hypo to hyper intense on T2, depending on the amount of hemosiderin present.[30]

Synovial Cell Sarcoma

This is a soft-tissue sarcoma of cells similar histologically to synovial cells, representing 5% of malignant soft-tissue sarcomas. Synovial sarcoma is often distinguished from the other common soft tissue sarcomas by its being found in younger adult patients (15–35 years of age). Although the name of the lesion suggests an articular process, it should be noted that synovial cell sarcomas are usually not associated with joints, though they are often found nearby. Fewer than 10% of synovial

Key Concepts	Synovial Cell Sarcoma

- They are a common soft tissue sarcoma in young adults.
- They most frequently occur around the knee but are not intra-articular.
- Dystrophic calcification is relatively common.
- MRI appearance is deceptively nonaggressive.

cell sarcomas occur in a joint capsule. Synovial sarcomas are characteristically found in the lower extremity, especially about the knee. Synovial cell sarcomas have a higher prevalence of dystrophic calcification than do the other soft tissue sarcomas (20%–30%). Thus, the age, location, and calcification, if present, can suggest this tumor (Fig. 1-75). The MRI appearance is nonspecific and even sometimes misleadingly nonaggressive. T1 is usually isointense with muscle and T2 shows inhomogeneous high signal intensity, often with areas

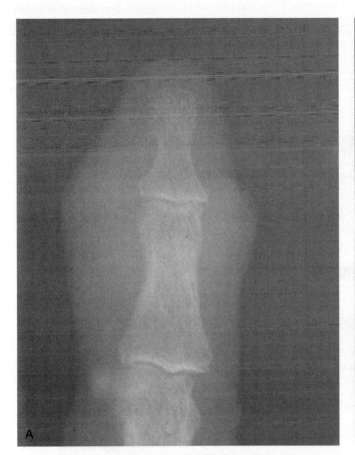
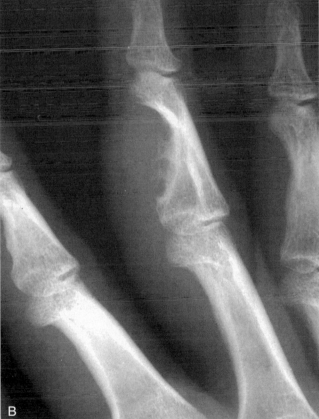

Fig. 1-74 Giant cell tumor of the tendon sheath. **A,** An AP radiograph of the finger in a 52-year-old female, demonstrating a nodular soft-tissue mass with normal underlying bone. This is the most typical appearance for giant cell tumor of the tendon sheath. However, these lesions occasionally cause scalloping of the underlying bone, resulting in an appearance such as that seen in **B,** a finger in a 20-year-old male patient.

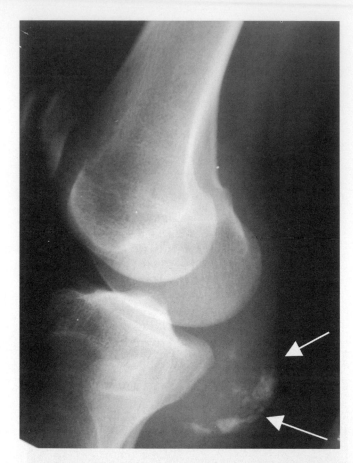

Fig. 1-75 Synovial cell sarcoma. This is an oblique radiograph of the knee in an 18-year-old male, demonstrating a soft-tissue mass adjacent to the joint, with the mass containing dystrophic calcification (*arrows*). The location, calcification, age of the patient, and prevalence information should yield a strong suspicion of synovial cell sarcoma in this case (Reprinted with permission from the ACR learning file.)

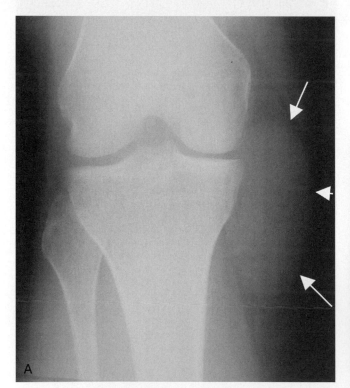

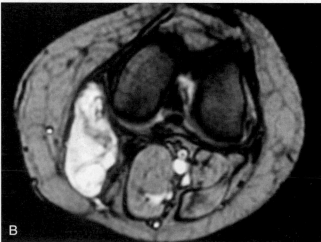

Fig. 1-76 Synovial cell sarcoma. **A,** An AP radiograph of the knee in a 17-year-old female that demonstrates a soft tissue mass adjacent to, but not within the knee joint (*arrows*). **B,** The axial gradient echo image of the lesion, demonstrated here to be extra-articular. Despite the lack of calcification and the encapsulated appearance of this lesion, the age of the patient, location, and prevalence of the lesion lead one to suspect the diagnosis is synovial cell sarcoma, which was proven at biopsy.

of hemorrhage and occasional fluid-fluid levels. Most synovial sarcomas appear "encapsulated" or clearly delineated from surrounding tissues (Fig. 1-76).[31] It is important not to be misled by this appearance of a pseudocapsule, as tumor cells are invariably found peripheral to the lesion. Synovial cell sarcomas are aggressive lesions, metastasizing to the lung. They are treated with wide excision, often with adjuvant chemotherapy and occasional radiation therapy.

CHORDOMA

Chordoma is a low-grade malignant neoplasm that arises from notocord remnants. Because of this cell of origin, it is specifically restricted in location to the sa-

Key Concepts Chordoma

- Generally found in the sacrum, clivus, spine (posterior body, not posterior elements).
- Locally aggressive, with soft-tissue mass.
- May metastasize, but local morbidity may be of greater concern.

crum, clivus, and spine. The greatest number (50%) arise in the sacrum, and chordomas represent 40% of all sacral tumors. Chordomas are next most frequently found in the clivus (35%), and 15% are found in the spine, most frequently the lumbar region (Fig. 1-77).

Chordomas arise in adults, with a wide age range (fourth through seventh decades). They begin in the

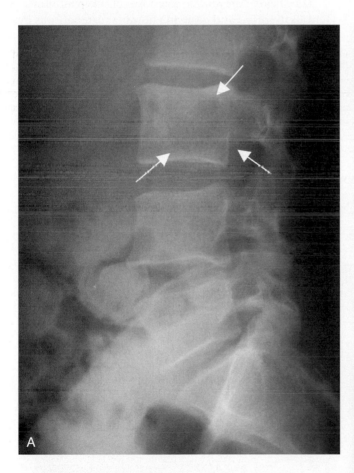
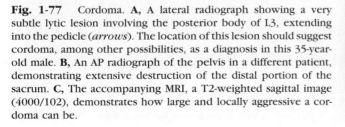
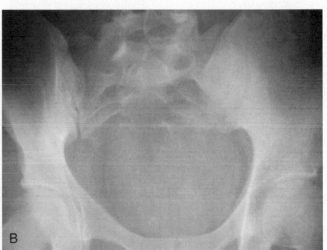
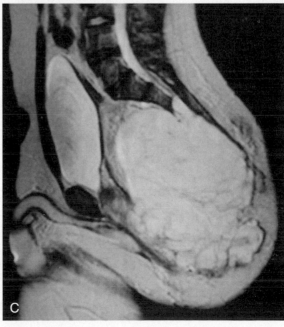

Fig. 1-77 Cordoma. **A,** A lateral radiograph showing a very subtle lytic lesion involving the posterior body of L3, extending into the pedicle (*arrows*). The location of this lesion should suggest cordoma, among other possibilities, as a diagnosis in this 35-year-old male. **B,** An AP radiograph of the pelvis in a different patient, demonstrating extensive destruction of the distal portion of the sacrum. **C,** The accompanying MRI, a T2-weighted sagittal image (4000/102), demonstrates how large and locally aggressive a cordoma can be.

body rather than the posterior elements of the spine but may extend into the posterior elements. Extensive local bone destruction is also seen, with soft-tissue mass (see Fig. 1-77) extending either in an epidural pattern or anteriorly. However, the time course of growth of the chordoma is often so slow that the lesion acquires a sclerotic rim and has a narrow zone of transition, giving it radiographic characteristics of a moderately aggressive lesion despite its size and soft-tissue mass.

In the sacrum, the major differential diagnosis is giant cell tumor, followed by chondrosarcoma and plasmacytoma. In the vertebral body, metastatic disease, multiple myeloma, giant cell tumor, and lymphoma belong in the differential diagnosis.

Twenty-five percent of chordomas have distant metastases to the lung, but these often occur very late. Greater difficulty usually arises with the morbidity and mortality associated with local recurrence and associated complications. Treatment is early wide resection, if possible, with radiation often used for recurrence. Five-year survival is 50%.

ADAMANTINOMA

Adamantinoma is a rare epithelioid lesion of unknown pathogenesis, containing elements of squamous, alveolar, and vascular tissue (Fig. 1-78). Adamantinoma is considered a low-grade and sometimes multicentric malignant neoplasm. The most frequent location of adamantinoma is in the tibial diaphysis (90%), usually eccentric or cortically based. This may be the most distinctive feature of adamantinoma. The early pattern of bone destruction is geographic, but may appear more aggressive with more advanced disease. There is generally a sclerotic margin, but soft-tissue mass and periosteal reaction may occur as the lesion becomes larger. Although the lesion is monostotic, it may have satellite foci adjacent to the initial lesion in the tibia or even in the adjacent fibula.

The major differential diagnosis of adamantinoma is fibrous dysplasia and ossifying fibroma (osteofibrous dysplasia). In fact, many investigators believe there is a spectrum of all three of these disease processes. All may be cortically based and located in the tibia and appear

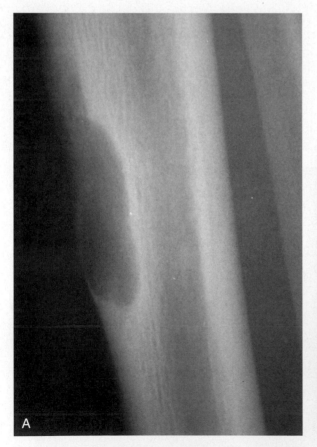

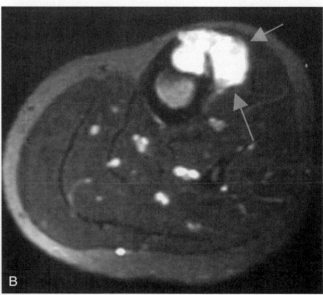

Fig. 1-78 Adamantinoma. **A,** AP radiograph demonstrates a cortically based lytic lesion in the tibia in a 17-year-old female. **B,** T2-weighted MR image confirms the cortical location of this lesion, as well as extension of a soft-tissue mass (*arrows*), which indicates a more aggressive lesion than might be expected from the radiograph.

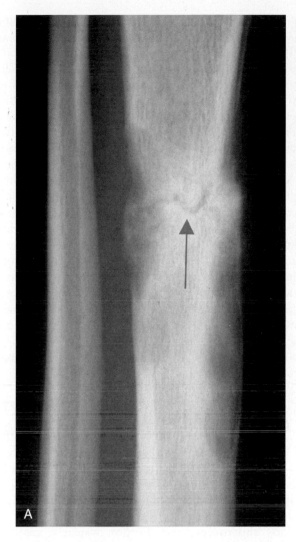

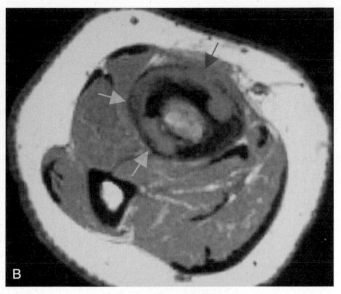

Fig. 1-79   Adamantinoma. **A,** AP radiograph of the tibia in a 17-year-old female demonstrates what appears to be multiple cortically based lytic lesions with a pathologic fracture (arrow). **B,** T1-weighted MRI (600/15) demonstrates that in fact this is a single cortically based lesion that wraps around the cortex (*arrows*). Although this cortically based tibial lesion is typical of an adamantinoma, it cannot be radiographically distinguished from osteofibrous dysplasia or cortically based fibrous dysplasia (see Fig. 1-14).

somewhat aggressive (Fig. 1-79). Histologic distinctions are subtle.[32]

Adamantinoma is a malignant lesion in that 20% metastasize to the lung, lymph nodes, or even skeleton. However, it is generally locally nonaggressive so that the lesion may be present for several years before developing metastatic lesions. Recurrence is common after surgery. Five-year survival is 60%. The ideal treatment is wide excision. However, because the lesion is often mistaken as nonaggressive, the initial treatment is often an inadequate curettage.

TUMORLIKE LESIONS

SOLITARY BONE CYST (SBC)

Solitary bone cyst, also termed simple or unicameral bone cyst, is a very common nonneoplastic lesion of childhood. It is often found incidentally, or as a pathologic fracture.

Solitary bone cyst is most frequently discovered in the first and second decades but uncommonly has been seen in adults. It is characterized by its location, with the proximal humerus and proximal femur being the most common sites (50% and 20% respectively). Solitary bone cyst is a central lesion, which initially is metaphyseal in location, abutting the epiphyseal plate. However, with advancing skeletal maturation and the cessation of lesion growth, a solitary bone cyst "migrates" into the diaphysis. This "migration" actually represents growth of normal bone away from the cyst (Figs. 1-80 and see 1-2A). Although the above described location is typical in a child, the rare solitary bone cyst in an adult tends to be found in unusual locations, such as the iliac wing or calcaneus (Fig. 1-81).

Solitary bone cyst is a mildly expansile lesion, which thins the cortex and has a narrow zone of transition with a fine sclerotic rim. There is no tumor matrix, but in fracture one might see a "fallen fragment," which represents a fracture fragment that settles inferiorly in the dependent portion of fluid filled cyst (Fig. 1-80A). There is generally no host response to a solitary bone cyst, with periosteal reaction seen only following a pathologic fracture. Thus, the

Key Concepts	Solitary Bone Cyst

- They are common in first and second decades.
- Location is a key to diagnosis, with a central metaphyseal or metadiaphyseal proximal humeral location being most common.
- It is an expansile, geographic, nonaggressive lesion.
- "Fallen fragment" sign is nearly pathognomonic if present.
- It has a high recurrence rate following curettage.

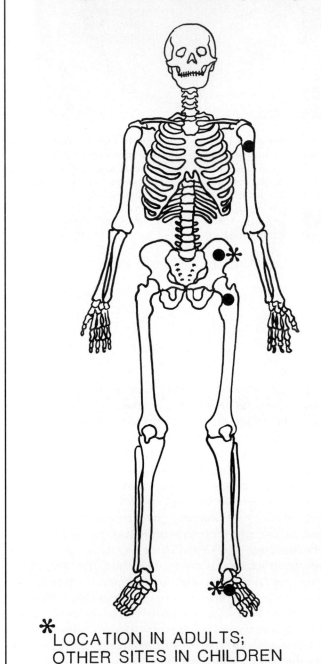

*LOCATION IN ADULTS;
OTHER SITES IN CHILDREN

total appearance is of a nonaggressive monostotic lesion. The major differential diagnosis includes fibrous dysplasia (if there is no matrix present to give the typical "ground glass" appearance), and Langerhans' cell histiocytosis (eosinophilic granuloma). Aneurysmal bone cyst (ABC) is usually not part of this differential diagnosis because ABC is eccentrically located. In the adult calcaneal lesion, the location of a solitary bone cyst is identical to that of intraosseous lipoma and pseudocyst, which is seen as a relative lucency between areas of primary trabeculae.

MRI is rarely required for solitary bone cyst. However, the MRI appearance is typical of a cyst with low signal T1 and high signal T2 and occasional fluid levels.

Solitary bone cyst is treated with curettage and bone grafting or steroid injection into the cyst. The lesion occasionally may heal spontaneously following fracture. Complications of treatment include either acceleration or arrest of limb growth following curettage of a lesion adjacent to the epiphyseal plate. There is a high recurrence rate (35%–50%). The likelihood of recurrence relates predominately to patient age, with younger patients (those under the age of 10) having a much higher likelihood of recurrence.

ANEURYSMAL BONE CYST

Aneurysmal bone cyst (ABC) is an expansile, eccentric bone lesion consisting of blood-filled cystic cavities. It is an interesting lesion in that there are two associations: (1) trauma-related expansion of bone and (2) occurrence in pre-existing osseous tumors (most frequently chondroblastoma, fibrous dysplasia, giant cell tumor, osteoblastoma, and nonossifying fibroma). These associations may be found in 30%–50% of cases. One theory of the pathogenesis of ABC is that it is a vascular anomaly induced by interference with venous drainage, either by trauma or a precursor lesion. It has been hypothesized that an ABC obliterates the precursor lesion in some cases. These observations underline the need for careful evaluation of ABCs so as not miss the

Key Concepts	Aneurysmal Bone Cyst

- It is expansile and eccentric.
- It is metaphyseal in long bones and also found in posterior elements in the spine.
- It is lytic with a narrow zone of transition.
- Generally found in those under 30 years of age.
- CT and MRI demonstrate fluid levels in most cases.
- Occasionally it is rapidly progressive, simulating a more aggressive lesion.
- It may be associated with neoplasms or trauma.
- Fluid-filled level differential: giant cell tumor, osteoblastoma, telangiectatic osteosarcoma.

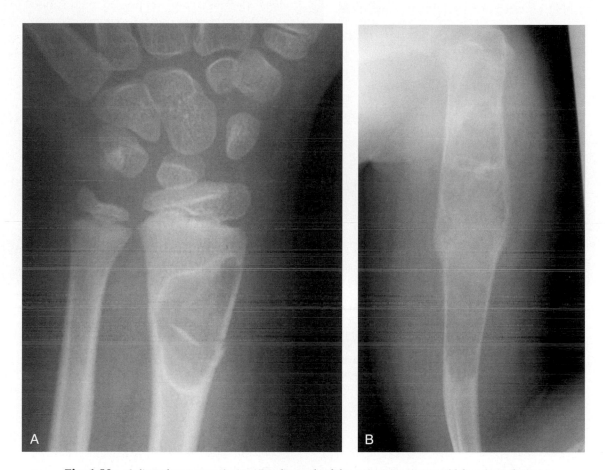

Fig. 1-80   Solitary bone cyst. **A,** An AP radiograph of the wrist in an 8-year-old female. It demonstrates a central lytic lesion, located in the metaphysis near the epiphyseal plate. It has thinned the cortex, has no matrix, but has developed a pathologic fracture resulting in a "fallen fragment" seen centrally within the lesion. This is the classic appearance of a solitary bone cyst. Another solitary bone cyst can be seen in Figure 1-2A. **B,** A lateral radiograph of the humerus in a 14-year-old male, demonstrates a more mature solitary bone cyst, which has "migrated away" from the metaphysis, and demonstrates a healing mid-diaphyseal fracture.

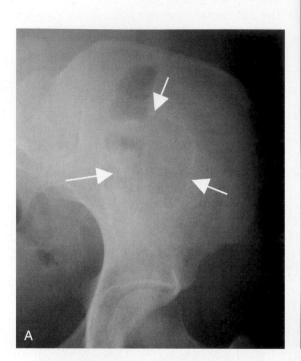
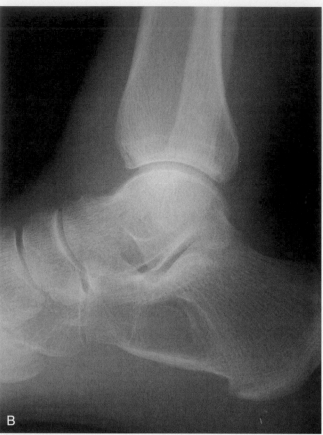

Fig. 1-81   Adult solitary bone cyst. **A,** An AP radiograph of the iliac wing in a 32-year-old female, demonstrating a well-marginated lytic lesion (*arrows*). There are not many nonaggressive lesions that occur in the pelvis in this age group, and solitary bone cyst might be considered, although it is unusual for a patient of this age. **B,** A lateral radiograph of the calcaneus in a 43-year-old male, demonstrating a lytic lesion in the anterior portion of the calcaneus. This is a typical location for either solitary bone cyst or intraosseous lipoma. Biopsy in this case demonstrated solitary bone cyst.

presence of an underlying tumor or incompletely sample a lesion during biopsy (Fig. 1-82).

Aneurysmal bone cyst is found most frequently in the first through third decades, with 70% occurring between 5 and 20 years of age. It is usually a geographic lesion, often large, with a narrow zone of transition and fine sclerotic rim. This sclerotic rim may not be seen on radiographs, but is more completely seen with CT. There is no tumor matrix. The lesion is monostotic and occurs in the metaphyses of long bones, where it is eccentrically located (Fig. 1-83). Aneurysmal bone cysts also occur in posterior elements of the spine (Fig. 1-83) and occasionally the pelvis.

The lesion is nonaggressive in appearance, but may occasionally enlarge rapidly and elicit a periosteal reaction, in which case it may be mistaken for a more aggressive lesion.

The major differential diagnosis of aneurysmal bone cyst includes nonossifying fibroma and fibrous dysplasia in the long bones. As it occurs in the posterior elements of the spine, osteoblastoma belongs in the differential diagnosis for that site.

Aneurysmal bone cyst is a benign lesion. However, as it may appear more aggressive or may be associated with an underlying tumor (Fig. 1-84), MR imaging generally helps further define the lesion. MRI usually shows fluid-fluid levels, but it should be noted that such levels are not specific for aneurysmal bone cyst; they also have been described in solitary bone cyst, giant cell tumor, telangiectatic osteosarcoma, osteoblastoma, and rarely in other lesions. It should also be noted that occasionally there is a solid variety of ABC (5%) that does not show fluid levels. Associated lesions may be suggested by a thick rind, thick septations, or peripheral nodules.

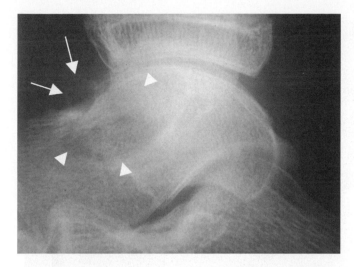

Fig. 1-82   ABC arising in underlying lesion. This is a lateral radiograph of the talus in a 12-year-old male. It demonstrates a typical appearing chondroblastoma (*arrowheads*), associated with a blisterlike lytic lesion on the dorsum (*arrow*). This small, different appearing portion of the lesion is an aneurysmal bone cyst arising in the underlying chondroblastoma. (Reprinted with permission from the ACR learning file.)

Treatment consists of curettage, often with cryosurgery as there is a 20%–50% recurrence rate. Low dose radiation may be used for surgically inaccessible lesions.

LANGERHANS' CELL HISTIOCYTOSIS (HISTIOCYTOSIS X)

Langerhans' cell histiocytosis represents a spectrum of diseases, all with histiocytic infiltration of various tissues and aggressive bone lesions. The most common and mildest form was formerly termed eosinophilic granuloma (EG).

Langerhans' cell histiocytosis has a peak incidence in the age range of 5–10 years, but the disease process can be seen through the third decade. Although the process is most commonly monostotic, 10%–20% develop polyostotic disease within 6 months of developing the first lesion. Those who present with a lesion at a young age are more likely to develop polyostotic disease.

At first presentation, the pattern usually appears motheaten or permeative. However, as it evolves it may become more geographic in appearance (Fig. 1-85). Thus, the zone of transition can range from wide to narrow. Skull lesions, in particular, have a narrow zone of transition with nonuniform involvement of the inner and outer skull tables, giving a beveled-edge appearance. The lesions tend not to have a sclerotic margin. There is no tumor matrix, but, rarely, a fragment of bone may be left centrally, resembling a sequestrum. Periosteal reaction is common, and there may be a soft-tissue mass (Fig. 1-86).

Key Concepts   **Langerhans' Cell Histiocytosis**

- This is a common lesion of childhood.
- They may develop and enlarge extremely rapidly.
- They may appear aggressive, with a permeative pattern and soft tissue mass.
- The differential diagnosis includes Ewing's sarcoma, osteomyleitis, and metastatic neuroblastoma.
- Ten percent to 20% are polyostotic.
- They have a distinctive vertebra plana appearance in spine.
- Common sites include skull, spine, pelvis, femur.

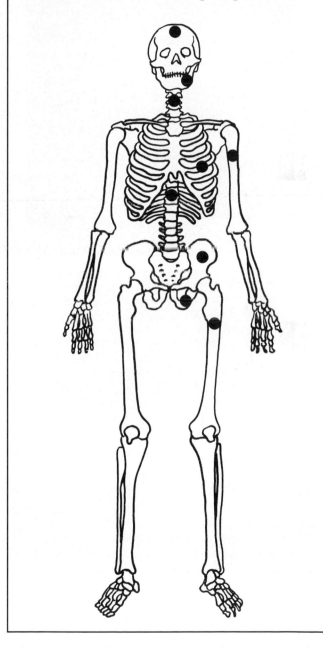

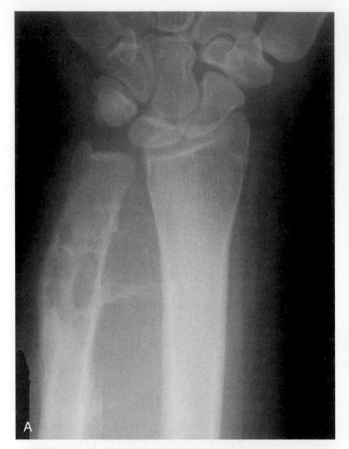

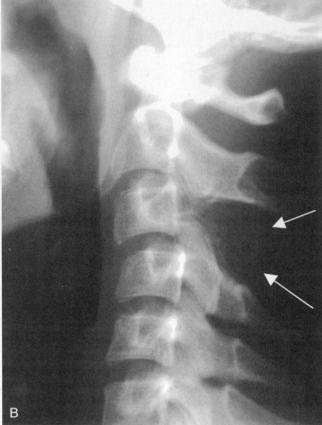

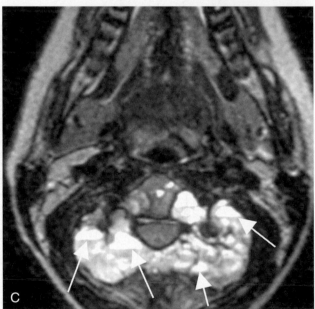

Fig. 1-83   ABC. **A,** An AP radiograph of the distal forearm in a 16-year-old male, demonstrating an eccentrically located metaphyseal expansile lesion. This is a large but nonaggressive lesion, typical for aneurysmal bone cyst. **B,** A lateral radiograph of the cervical spine in a different patient, demonstrating expansion and near complete destruction of the spinous process of C3 (*arrows*). **C,** The T2-weighted MRI (5000/95) shows that the lesion is indeed large, involving all of the posterior elements, but containing fluid levels throughout (*arrows*). The age of the patient, along with the location of the lesion in the posterior elements of the spine and the presence of multiple fluid levels, makes the diagnosis of ABC.

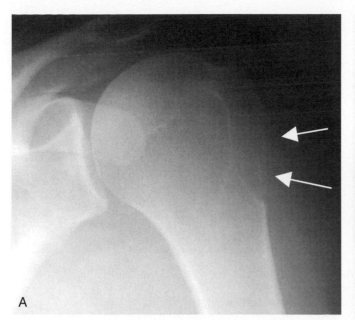

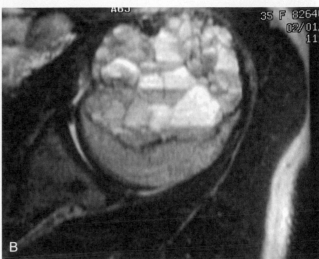

Fig. 1-84   ABC. **A,** An AP radiograph of the proximal humerus in a 19-year-old male that gives the appearance of a permeative, aggressive lesion with cortical breakthrough laterally (*arrows*). **B,** The lesion appears less aggressive by MRI (axial image, T2-weighted, 2416/85). Multiple fluid levels are noted throughout the lesion, making one consider the diagnosis of aneurysmal bone cyst. However, given the lack of margination of the lesion as seen on the radiograph, other diagnoses such as telangiectatic osteosarcoma must be considered. At biopsy this proved to be an ABC.

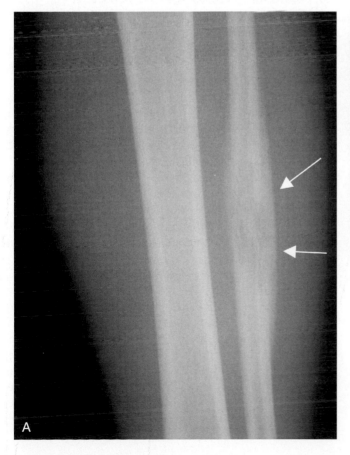

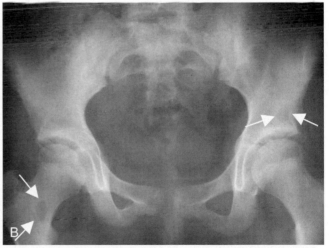

Fig. 1-85   Langerhans' cell histiocytosis. **A,** An AP radiograph showing an aggressive permeative lesion (*arrows*) involving the mid-diaphysis of the fibula in a 3-year-old female. There is periosteal reaction and a wide zone of transition. Although this very aggressive lesion is suggestive of Ewing's sarcoma, Langerhans' cell histiocytosis (also termed eosinophilic granuloma, EG) must also be considered. This proved to be the diagnosis at biopsy. **B,** A less aggressive manifestation of Langerhans' cell histiocytosis in a different patient, a 12-year-old female. In this case, the disease is polyostotic and the lesions appear well-defined (*arrows*). Langerhans' cell histiocytosis can appear either highly aggressive or completely nonaggressive.

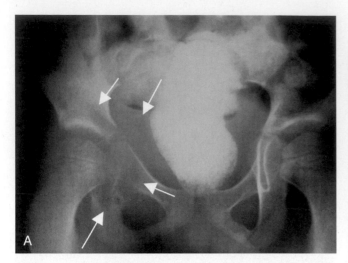 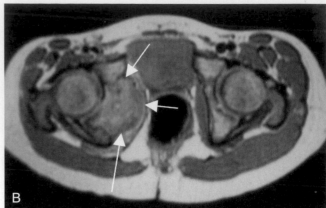

Fig. 1-86 Langerhans' cell histiocytosis. **A,** An AP pelvis radiograph in a 6-year-old male, demonstrating a highly aggressive lesion involving the right acetabulum, with a soft tissue mass (*arrows*). Note that the radiographic teardrop in the right hip has been destroyed, compared with the left side. **B,** The presence of a large soft-tissue mass (axial PD, 2000/20) (*arrows*) is confirmed. With this severe osseous destruction and soft-tissue mass in a patient of this age, Ewing's sarcoma should be most strongly considered, but it should be remembered that Langerhans' cell histiocytosis can be an aggressive, although benign, lesion. This was proven to be Langerhans' cell histiocytosis at biopsy. (Reprinted with permission from the ACR learning file.)

Langerhans' cell histiocytosis is commonly seen in the calvarium (50%). Twenty percent of lesions are found in the long tubular bones, with the femur being most common. Within the tubular bones, the lesions are usually central and metadiaphyseal. Finally, the axial skeleton represents another common location. Pelvic lesions are frequently seen, and Langerhans' cell histiocytosis can also involve the vertebral body. The vertebral body involvement has a classic radiographic appearance of a compressed vertebral body (vertebra plana), with intact posterior elements and disks (Fig. 1-87).

Because Langerhans' cell histiocytosis can be highly aggressive in its radiographic appearance as well as its rapid evolution, it has a place in the differential diagnosis of Ewing's sarcoma, lymphoma, osteomyelitis, and aggressive bone metastases. Although Langerhans' cell histiocytosis can have a soft tissue mass and an aggressive appearance, it is a benign lesion. Radiography may suggest the diagnosis, particularly when the lesion is polyostotic, but biopsy may be required for definitive histologic diagnosis.

Many therapeutic regimens have been used, with the healing rate being similar whether there is curettage, wide excision, low dose radiation, intralesional steroid injection, or no therapy at all. As each of these methods of treatment leads to the same rate of recurrence or reconstitution, therapy is often reserved for painful lesions or widespread disease.

FIBROUS DYSPLASIA

Fibrous dysplasia is a hamartomatous fibro-osseous metaplasia consisting of a fibrous stroma with islands of osteoid and woven bone. The lesion is relatively common. Although there is a wide age range of occurrence, it is most often first seen in the second and third decade. Fibrous dysplasia is often polyostotic (30%), and this form has a more aggressive appearing lesion and usually occurs before the age of 10. Interestingly, in 90% of polyostotic cases, the lesions are unilateral.

Fibrous dysplasia can be found in any bone, but vertebral localization is uncommon. The most common areas of involvement include the tubular bones, in which the lesions are usually central and metadiaphyseal, ribs, pelvis, and skull (particularly the base of skull and facial bones). The lesions tend to have a specific appearance, depending on whether they reside in the skull, pelvis, or tubular bones.

There is no distinct matrix pattern in fibrous dysplasia. The lesions range from being completely lucent, through a more opaque (termed "ground glass") density, to densely sclerotic lesions. The density depends on the amount of woven bone present within the fibrous stroma. In general, lesions in the base of the skull tend to be sclerotic (Fig. 1-88). Calvarial lesions range from lytic to dense and show a nonaggressive expansion of bone.

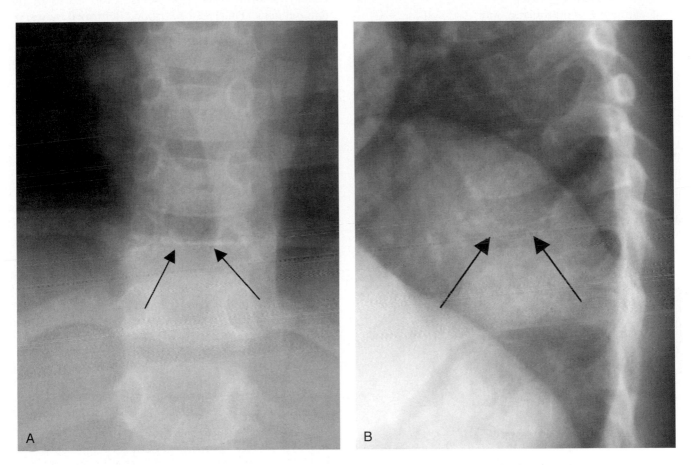

Fig. 1-87   Langerhans' cell histiocytosis. **A,** An AP radiograph of the thoracolumbar spine in a 10-year-old patient, demonstrating complete flattening of the body of T10 (*arrows*), although the posterior elements remain intact as do the adjacent vertebral bodies. **B,** This complete flattening of the vertebral body is confirmed on the lateral view (arrows). This appearance of "vertebra plana" is typical for EG, a variety of Langerhans' cell histiocytosis.

Key Concepts   **Fibrous Dysplasia**

- Thirty percent are polyostotic, usually unilateral.
- The lesions are typically expansile and nonaggressive.
- Lesions in the skull involve the calvarium and base, and may be densely sclerotic.
- Rib and long bone lesions often have a "ground glass" appearance and may have bowing deformities.
- Pelvic lesions may be either lytic and bubbly, often large, or mildly expansile.
- Treatment is symptomatic only.

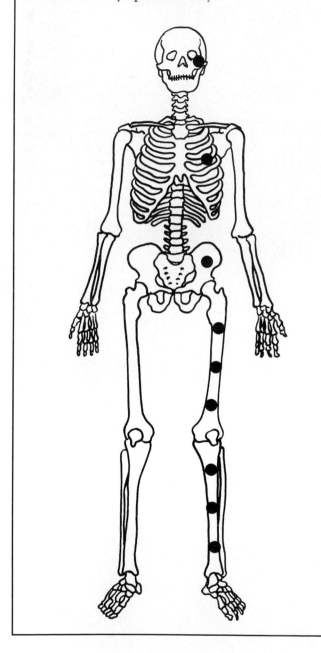

Fibrous dysplasia in the ribs and tubular bones tend to have "ground glass" density (Fig. 1-89). On the other hand, the typical pelvic lesion may be quite bubbly and expansile (Fig. 1-90).

Similar to the other sites, the ribs and tubular bones show expansion when involved with fibrous dysplasia, often with cortical thinning (Fig. 1-91). The thin expanded bones, with weight bearing, often result in bowing and angulation. In the femur, the physical deformity that is typical of fibrous dysplasia is called a "Shepherd's Crook" deformity and represents severe varus of the femoral neck (Fig. 1-92). Expanded deformed bones, often with a ground glass density, lacking trabecular definition, and often polyostotic, make a very distinctive radiographic appearance. Although the lesions in the long bones are usually central, fibrous dysplasia can also be cortically based. When this occurs in the tibia, it falls within the spectrum of appearance of osteofibrous dysplasia (ossifying fibroma) and adamantanoma (Figs. 1-2C, D, and 1-14B, C). MR imaging of fibrous dysplasia is nonspecific, with low signal on T1-weighted and variable signal on T2-weighted sequences.

Fibrous dysplasia is usually easily diagnosed. Most lesions remain quiescent throughout life, neither improving nor resolving. Only 5% continue to enlarge after skeletal maturity. Malignant transformation, usually to fibrosarcoma or osteosarcoma, is a rare occurrence. In consideration of these observations, treatment is generally reserved for symptomatic lesions only, such as fractures or deformities. Limb length discrepancy, angular deformity, and pseudoarthrosis seen in the tibia of young children with fibrous dysplasia may require osteotomy, bone grafting, and immobilization. However, resection or curettage of a nonsymptomatic site of fibrous dysplasia is usually both futile and unnecessary.

BROWN TUMOR OF HYPERPARATHYROIDISM

Brown tumors are localized accumulations of osteoclasts that produce expanded lytic lesions in patients with hyperparathyroidism. Radiographically and pathologically a brown tumor may be difficult to differentiate from a giant cell tumor. However, other manifestations of hyperparathyroidism are usually present as well, making possible the diagnosis (Fig. 1-93). Following treatment of hyperparathyroidism, a brown tumor may hyperossify.

MYOSITIS OSSIFICANS

Myositis ossificans represents heterotopic formation of nonneoplastic bone and cartilage in soft tissue, usually muscle. The etiology is usually traumatic, although the episode of trauma may be minor. Myositis ossificans can

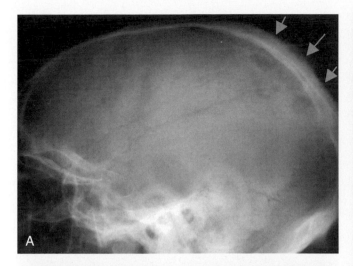

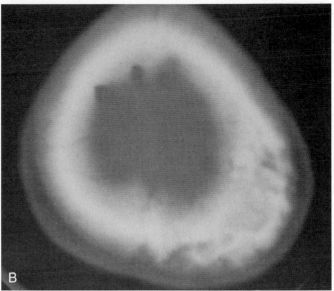

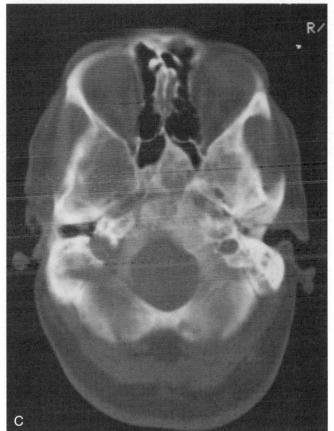

Fig. 1-88   Fibrous dysplasia, skull. **A,** Lateral radiograph of the skull demonstrates lytic lesions in the cranium and widened diploic space (*arrows*). There is also increased density in the skull base. **B,** Axial CT reveals prominent widening of the diploic space in this 44-year-old male with fibrous dysplasia. **C,** CT of the skull base shows mild enlargement and sclerosis of the left skull base compared with the right. The enlargement and sclerosis is typical of fibrous dysplasia in the skull.

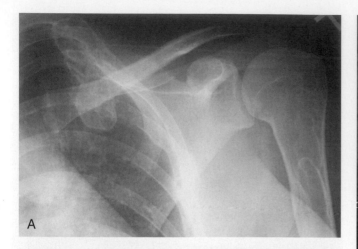

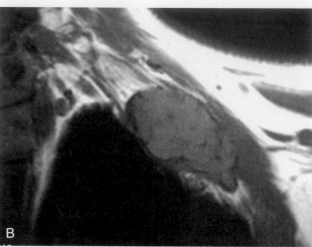

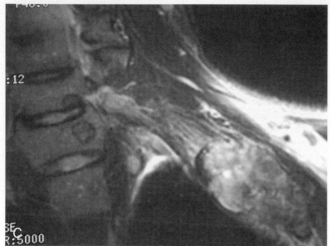

Fig. 1-89   Fibrous dysplasia of a rib. This 24-year-old female had a brachial plexopathy. **A,** AP radiograph demonstrates an expanded first rib (*arrows*), as well as lesions in the proximal humerus. **B,** T1-weighted coronal MRI (500/14) shows an expanded mass in the first rib, which is isointense with muscle and which shows mixed high and low signal intensity on T2 imaging **C,** (5000/90). This mass is seen to compress the brachial plexus. Note additional lesions in the adjacent vertebrae. Ribs are a common location for fibrous dysplasia.

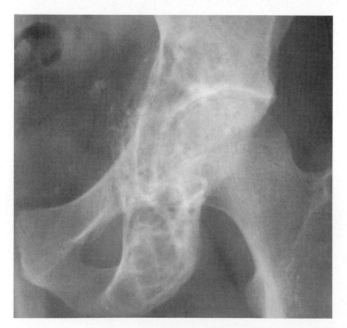

Fig. 1-90   Fibrous dysplasia. Fibrous dysplasia of the pelvis most frequently appears as a bubbly and expanded lesion, as is seen in this 29-year-old male. The lesion does not have an aggressive appearance.

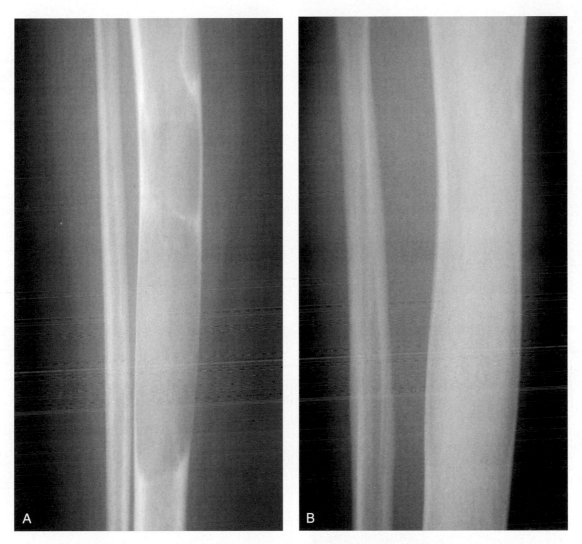

Fig. 1-91   Fibrous dysplasia of the tubular bones. **A,** An AP radiograph of the tibia in a 10-year-old female which demonstrates mild expansion and a mostly lytic appearance of multiple lesions. This is a typical appearance of fibrous dysplasia in the long bones. **B,** A more dense "ground glass" appearance, again with mild expansion of the tibia is seen in a different patient. The juxtaposition of these two cases demonstrates the spectrum of the "ground glass" appearance of fibrous dysplasia. Remember that although most cases of fibrous dysplasia are central medullary lesions, fibrous dysplasia can occasionally be cortically based. These cortically based lesions can be significantly different in appearance. For examples, please see Fig. 1-2C and D as well as Fig. 1-14B and C.

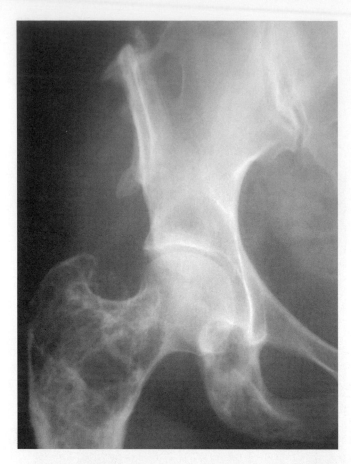

Fig. 1-92   Fibrous dysplasia. The AP radiograph shows a bubbly lesion in the ischium, as well as a rather bubbly appearing lesion in the proximal femur. The femoral neck is in a varus configuration, which has been termed a "shepherds crook" deformity and is typical of fibrous dysplasia. What is unusual about this case is that this 45-year-old female has undergone curettage and bone grafting of the femoral neck lesion, with the bone graft obtained from the right iliac wing, leaving a defect at that spot. Generally, bone grafting and other surgery is reserved for only complications of fibrous dysplasia.

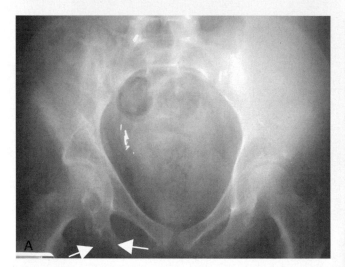

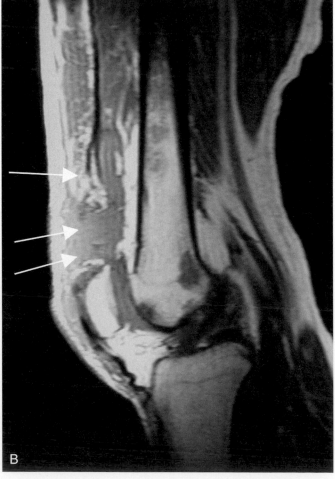

Fig. 1-93   Brown tumor of hyperparathyroidism. A, An AP radiograph of the pelvis in a 21-year-old female. There is a lytic lesion in the right ischium (*arrows*). Clips in the pelvis and a soft-tissue mass in the left iliac fossa suggests that the patient has had a renal transplant and gives the underlying diagnosis of brown tumor due to renal osteodystrophy. B, A sagittal T1-weighted (650/15) MRI of the knee in a 45-year-old male. This demonstrates multiple low signal intensity lesions in the distal femur. Additionally, the patient has a rupture of the patellar tendon (*arrow*). Patellar tendon ruptures are uncommon, so when seen in conjunction with multiple lytic lesions, the diagnosis of brown tumor of hyperparathyroidism can be assumed.

occur anywhere, but is most commonly found in the areas prone to trauma such as thigh and elbow. Myositis ossificans also can be associated with burns and neurologic disorders, with greater than one-third of paraplegics showing extensive myositis ossificans.

The histologic evolution of myositis ossificans parallels the radiographic evolution and MRI appearance. Histologically, during the first 4 weeks of evolution, myositis ossificans has a pseudosarcomatous appearance in its central zone, which may suggest malignant neoplasm. During weeks 4 through 8, histology shows a centrifugal pattern of maturation, where the periphery of the lesion is demarcated by immature osteoid formation that gradually organizes into mature bone surrounding a cellular center. The radiographic evolution parallels this. In the first 2 weeks, there is only a soft tissue mass present, which clinically may be painful, warm, and doughy. Weeks 3 to 4 begin to show amorphous density within the mass, often with periosteal reaction in the underlying

bone. At this stage myositis may be mistaken for an early osteosarcoma as the calcification has the appearance of tumor osteoid. Over weeks 6 through 8, the amorphous osteoid matures into compact bone that surrounds a lacy pattern of less mature bone (Fig. 1-94). Maturation proceeds centrifugally, as is seen histologically. Over ensuing months, the osseous mass reaches full maturity, often with reduction in size. Thus, the history and timing are crucial in supporting the early diagnosis of myositis ossificans and avoiding a potentially disastrous diagnosis of osteosarcoma.

The MRI appearance of myositis ossificans relates to the age of the lesion, similar to the radiograph. Early lesions show a mass that is isointense to muscle on T1-weighted and high signal with inhomogeneity on T2-weighted imaging (Fig. 1-95). Surrounding edema is prominent. Periosteal reaction and bone marrow edema may be seen if the myositis is located near bone. More mature lesions (over 8 weeks) are better defined. The

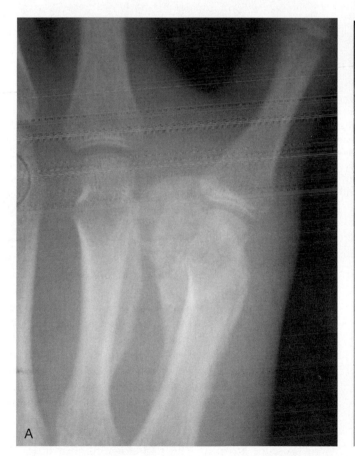 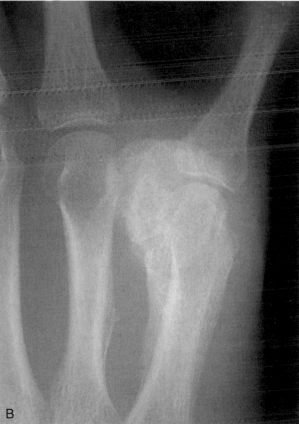

Fig. 1-94 Myositis ossificans. **A,** An AP radiograph of the hand in an 18-year-old male taken 7 weeks after crush injury. It demonstrates an immature myositis ossificans involving both the fourth and fifth metacarpals. The matrix is clearly osteoid, but it does not yet show the mature periphery. **B,** An AP radiograph of the same region taken 5 months postinjury. At this time, the myositis involving both the fourth and fifth metacarpals has evolved to a more mature phase, having decreased in size on the fourth and showing a defined rim on the fifth. This represents a mature myositis ossificans. (Reprinted with permission from the ACR learning file.)

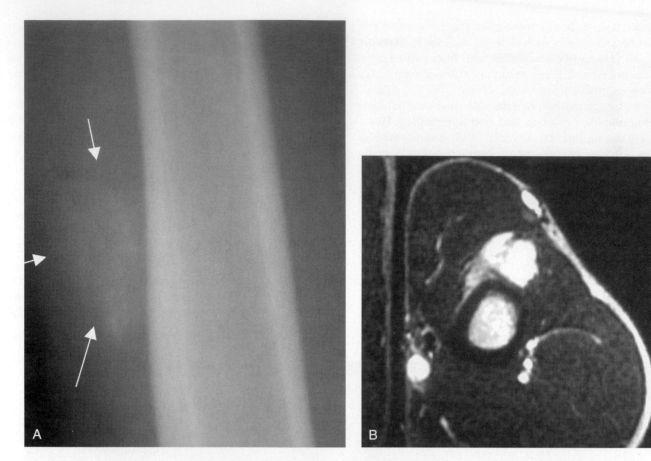

Fig. 1-95   Myositis ossificans. **A,** An AP radiograph of the mid-portion of the arm in a 17-year-old male. It demonstrates amorphous bone formation, which is typical of immature myositis ossificans (*arrows*). The T1-weighted MR (not shown) showed a lesion isointense with muscle, although the T2-weighted image **B,** (2200/80) demonstrates a high signal lesion adjacent to the humerus. This is a nonspecific MR appearance, but is certainly consistent with the diagnosis of myositis ossificans made on the radiograph. (Reprinted with permission of the ACR learning file.)

center remains inhomogeneous, but may be rimmed by a halo of decreased signal on all sequences.[33] Thus, the zoning seen on radiographs and histology is mirrored on MRI imaging (Fig. 1-96).

The differential diagnosis of myositis ossificans includes parosteal osteosarcoma. However, the latter is attached to the underlying bone and usually shows marrow extension of the tumor, as well as a reversed zonal phenomenon with more heavily calcified central tumor and a less densely calcified periphery. Periosteal osteosarcoma might also be found in the differential diagnosis of myositis ossificans; periosteal osteosarcoma usually appears more aggressive, often scalloping the underlying cortex. Juxtacortical chondroma also often presents with scalloped underlying cortex and juxtacortical calcific densities. An early myositis ossificans could possibly mimic this appearance. An exostosis should not be confused with myositis, as it arises from the underlying bone, with continuation of cortical and medullary bone into

the lesion. Tumoral calcinosis presents as periarticular calcified soft-tissue masses, usually around the hip, shoulder, and elbows. The masses are usually separate from the underlying bone and could, at some stage, appear similar to myositis ossificans.

Myositis ossificans progressiva is a hereditary mesodermal disorder characterized by progressive ossification of striated muscles, tendons, and ligaments. It has an autosomal dominant mode of inheritance with a wide range of expressivity though may appear as a spontaneous mutation. The target tissue in this disease is thought to be the interstitial tissues, with muscle involvement secondary to pressure atrophy. The pathologic abnormalities are similar to those of myositis ossificans. The most frequent presenting symptom and location is acute torticollis, with a painful mass seen in the sternocleidomastoid muscle. The process then progresses to the shoulder girdle, upper arms, spine, and pelvis. The heterotopic bone often bridges between adjacent bones of the skeleton (Fig.

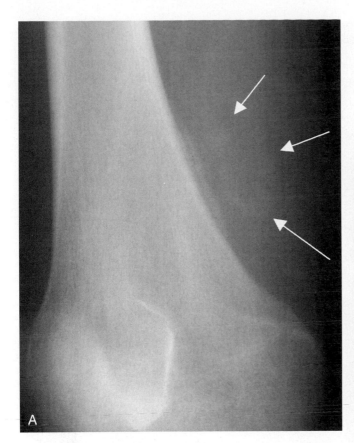
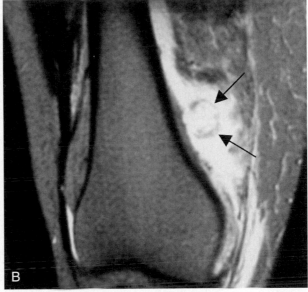

Fig. 1-96   Myositis ossificans. **A,** An oblique radiograph of the distal thigh in a 15-year-old female with a painful mass. The radiograph demonstrates faintly seen osteoid within a mass (*arrows*), as well as periosteal reaction along the femoral shaft. This is a nonspecific appearance and could represent either myositis ossificans or an early surface osteosarcoma. **B,** The MRI is extremely helpful with the T2 coronal images (2300/90) showing extensive soft tissue edema surrounding a low signal intensity rim, which itself surrounds high signal intensity material. This "halo" (*arrows*), when seen on MR in this circumstance, represents the zoning phenomenon of myositis ossificans.

1-97) and eventually causes a severe restriction of motion.

METASTATIC DISEASE OF BONE

Osseous metastasis occurs in 20%–35% of extraskeletal as well as skeletal malignancies. Metastases to bone are significantly more common (in a ratio of 25 : 1) than are primary bone tumors. About (80%) of bone metastases arise from primary tumors of the breast, prostate, lung, or kidney. Other common primaries metastasizing to bone include gastrointestinal, thyroid, and round cell malignancies.

Metastases are most frequently identified by radiographs or bone scans. Bone scans are highly sensitive compared with radiographs in that 10% to 40% of metastatic lesions may be abnormal on bone scan but normal radiographically. On the other hand, fewer than 5% of metastatic lesions are normal on bone scan but detected by radiograph. However, bone scan specificity is very

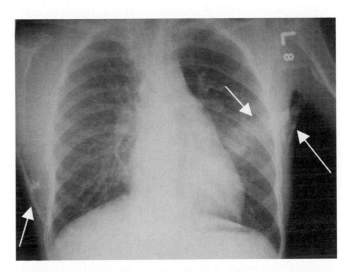

Fig. 1-97   Myositis ossificans progressiva. This AP radiograph of the chest demonstrates ossific masses forming in the latissimus dorsi and pectoralis muscles, showing early bridging between the humeri and the thorax in this 6-year-old patient (*arrows*). Progressive ossification will occur.

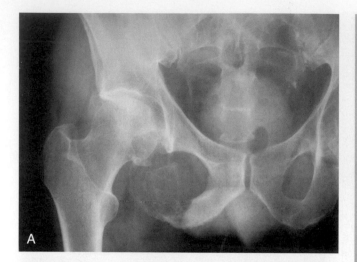

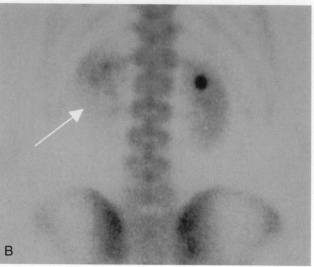

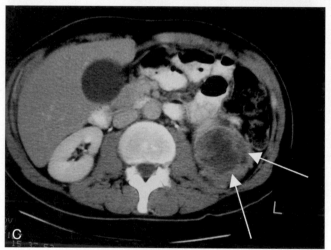

Fig. 1-98   Metastasis. **A,** An AP radiograph of the pelvis in a 50-year-old male that demonstrates an expanded ''bubbly'' lesion in the right ischium. This was a solitary lesion. **B,** Radionuclide bone scan performed to evaluate for polyostotic lesions, demonstrated the osseous lesion to be solitary but also showed a defect in the left kidney (posterior image, *arrow*). This combination is highly suspicious for renal cell carcinoma, and CT (**C**) demonstrates the tumor (*arrows*).

poor. Therefore radiographs are used in a complementary fashion with bone scans, helping to improve specificity. Furthermore, radiographs should be evaluated for signs of impending pathologic fracture that would warrant prophylactic fixation. These signs include lesions that are 2.5 cm or larger, and those showing 50% or greater cortical width destruction.

Metastases usually have a moth-eaten pattern with an ill-defined zone of transition, no sclerotic margin, and often little periosteal reaction or soft tissue mass. Occasionally, a metastatic site may present as a geographic, bubbly, expansile mass (Fig. 1-98). These may be solitary and in this case the primary site of tumor is usually kidney or thyroid. The density of metastases is variable. Purely lytic metastases are most frequently lung, but are also seen with kidney, breast, thyroid, gastrointestinal (GI), and neuroblastoma. Blastic metastases include prostate, breast, bladder, GI (adenocarcinoma and carcinoid), lung (usually small cell), and medulloblastoma. Mixed lytic and blastic metastases can be seen in breast, lung, prostate, bladder, and neuroblastoma metastases. With therapy or

radiation necrosis, one may see changing patterns of density.

Most metastases occur where red bone marrow is found; 80% of metastases are located in the axial skeleton (ribs, pelvis, vertebrae, skull), and proximal humerus and proximal femur (Fig. 1-99). Lesions distal to the elbows or knees are usually due to primary lung cancers. Although most metastases are central lesions found within the distribution of bone marrow, occasionally a cortically based metastasis can occur, most often due to pulmonary or breast origin (Fig. 1-100). Metastases are frequently found in the spine, where they may appear as nonspecific compression fractures. However, it is more frequent to detect vertebral metastases through focal destruction of a pedicle. Pedicle involvement is often stated to be the hallmark of vertebral metastases. However, the origin of the metastasis is usually in the posterior vertebral body, due to the distribution of the vertebral vascular supply. Pedicle involvement is secondary, but is more easily visualized on radiographs than is early destructive change in the posterior vertebral body. About 50% of a vertebral

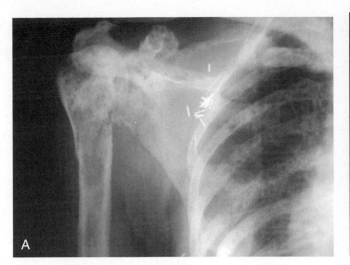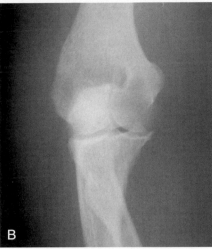

Fig. 1-99   Metastasis. **A,** Multiple lytic destructive lesions involving the rib cage as well as proximal appendicular skeleton are seen in this 45-year-old female with widespread metastatic breast carcinoma. Interestingly, the elbow and distal tubular bones **(B)** show normal mineralization and no evidence of metastatic disease. This case typifies the distribution of the metastases within the hematopoietic portions of the bone marrow.

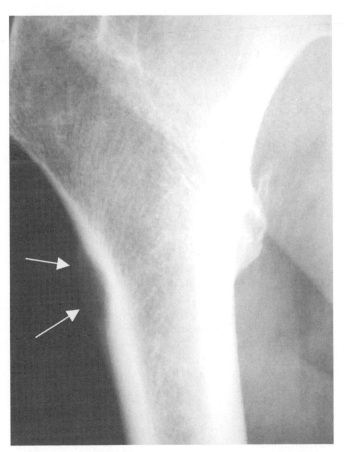

Fig. 1-100   Metastatic lung carcinoma. AP radiograph of the proximal femur in this 65-year-old male demonstrates a cortically based lytic lesion (*arrows*). Cortical metastases are uncommon, but when they occur are most likely due to pulmonary or breast tumors.

body must be destroyed before it can be detected radiographically.

Two specific sites are worthy of mention with respect to metastatic disease. First, lesser trochanter fractures in the adult should be considered pathologic until proven otherwise. Secondly, in patients with known breast cancer, a solitary sternal lesion is rare, but if present, has an 80% probability of being due to metastatic disease. Finally, in general, the presence of a transverse fracture in a long bone, without a significant episode of trauma, should alert the radiologist to the possibility of its being a pathologic fracture.

REFERENCES

1. Enneking WF: Staging of musculoskeletal neoplasms. *Skeletal Radiology* 13:183-194, 1985.
2. Griffith LK, Dehdashti F, McGuire A et al: PET evaluation of soft tissue masses with FDG. *Radiology* 182 (1):185-194, 1992.
3. Nieweg O, Pruins J, Von Ginkel R et al: FDG. PET imaging of soft tissue sarcoma. *J Nuclear Medicine* 37 (2):257-261, 1996.
4. Kormaz M, Kim F, Wong F et al: FDG and Methionine PET in differentiation of recurrent or residual musculoskeletal sarcomas from post-therapy changes. *J Nuclear Medicine* 34 (5):33 p (abst), 1993.
5. DeSchepper AM, Ed: *Imaging of soft tissue tumors.* Berlin, 1997, Springer.
6. DeSchepper A, Ramon F, Degryseh P: Statistical analysis of MRI parameters predicting malignancy in 141 soft tissue masses. *Fortschr Roentgenstr* 156:587-591, 1992.
7. Moulton J, Blebea J, Dunco D, Braley S, Bisset G, Emory K: MR imaging of soft tissue masses: Diagnostic efficacy and value of distinguishing between benign and malignant lesions. *Am J Roentgenol* 164:1191-1199, 1995.
8. Kransdorf M: Benign soft tissue tumors in a large referral population: Distribution of specific diagnosis by age, sex, and location. *Am J Roentgenol* 164:395-402, 1995.
9. Kransdorf M: Malignant soft tissue tumors in a large referral population: distribution of specific diagnosis by age, sex, and location. *Am J Roentgenol* 164:129-134, 1995.
10. Kransdorf M, Murphey M: *Imaging of soft tissue tumors.* Philadelphia, 1997, WB Saunders.
11. Manaster BJ, Dalinka M, Alazraki N et al: Follow-up examinations for bone tumors, soft tissue tumors, and suspected metastasis post therapy. American College of Radiology ACR Appropriateness Criteria, Supplement to Radiology 215(s):379–387, 2000.
12. Kransdorf M, Murphey M, Sweet D: Liposclerosing myxofibrous tumor: A radiologic/pathologic distinct fibroosseous lesion of bone with a marked predelection for the intertrochanteric region of the femur. *Radiology* 212:693-698, 1999.
13. Murphey M, Robbin M, McRae G, Flemming D, Temple H, Kransdorf M: The many faces of osteosarcoma. *Radiographics* 17:1205-1231, 1997.
14. Jelinek J, Murphey M, Kransdorf M, Shmookler B, Malawer M, Hur R: Parosteal osteosarcoma: Value of MR imaging and CT in the prediction of histologic grade. *Radiology* 201:837-842, 1996.
15. Hopper K, Moser R, Haseman D, Sweet D, Madewell J, Kransdorf M: Osteosarcomatosis. *Radiology* 175:233-239, 1990.
16. Huvos A: Osteogenic sarcoma of bones in soft tissues of older persons. *Cancer* 57:1442-1449, 1986.
17. Murphey M, Flemming D, Boyea S, Bojescul J, Sweet D, Temple H: Enchondroma vs chondrosarcoma in the appendicular skeleton: Differentiating features. *RadioGraphics* 18:1213-1237, 1998.
18. Geirnaerdt M, Hermans J, Bloem J et al: Usefulness of radiography in differentiating enchondroma from central grade one chondrosarcoma. *AJR* 169:1097-1104, 1997.
19. Janzen L, Logan P, O'Connell J, Connell D, Munk P: Intramedullary chondroid tumors of bone: correlation of abnormal peritumoral marrow and soft tissue MRI signal with tumor type. *Skeletal Radiology* 26:100-106, 1997.
20. Geirnaerdt M, Hogendoorn P, Bloem J, Taminiau A, Van Der Woude H: Cartilaginous tumors: fast contrast enhanced MR imaging. *Radiology* 214:539-546, 2000.
21. Methta M, White L, Knapp T, Kandel R, Wunder J, Bell R: MR imaging of symptomatic osteochondromas with pathological correlation. *Skeletal Radiology* 27:427-433, 1998.
22. Shapeero L, Vanel D, Couanet D, Contesso G, Ackerman C: Extra skeletal mesenchymal chondrosarcoma. *Radiology* 186:819-826, 1993.
23. Aoki J, Tanikawa H, Ishii K et al: MR findings indicative of hemosiderin in giant cell tumor of bone: frequency, cause, and diagnostic significance. *AJR* 166:145-148, 1996.
24. Manaster B, Doyle A: Giant cell tumor of the bone. *Radiolog Clin North Am* 31:299-323, 1993.
25. Mulligan M, McRae G, Murphey M: Imaging features of primary lymphoma of bone. *AJR* 173:1691-1697, 1993.
26. Murphey M, Gross T, Rosenthal H: Musculoskeletal malignant fibrous histiocytoma: radiologic pathologic correlation. *RadioGraphics* 14:807-826, 1994.
27. Ryu K, Jaovisidha S, Schweitzer M, Motta A, Resnick D: MR imaging of lipoma arborescens of the knee joint. *AJR* 167:1229-1232, 1996.
28. Hosono M, Kobayashi H, Fujimoto R et al: Septum like structures in lipoma and liposarcoma: MR imaging and pathologic correlation. *Skeletal Radiology* 26:150-154, 1997.
29. Murphey M, Smith W, Smith S, Kransdorf M, Temple H: Imaging of musculoskeletal neurogenic tumors: Radiologic pathologic correlation. *RadioGraphics* 19:1253-1280, 1999.
30. Jelinek J, Kransdorf M, Shmookler B, Aboulafia A, Malawer M: Giant cell tumor of the tendon sheath: MR findings in nine cases. *AJR* 162:919-922, 1994.
31. Jones B, Sundaram M, Kransdorf M. Synovial sarcoma: MR imaging findings in 34 patients. *AJR* 161:827-830, 1993.
32. Springfield D, Rosenberg A, Mankin H: Relationship between osteofibrous displasia and adamantinoma. *Clinical Orthopaedics* 309:234-244, 1994.
33. Kransdorf M, Meis J, Jelinek J: Myositis ossificans: MR appearance with radiologic pathologic correlation. *AJR* 157:1243-1248, 1991.

CHAPTER 2

Arthritis

B.J. MANASTER M.D., Ph.D.

INTRODUCTION

Classic cases of arthritis are generally seen in their chronic stages, which makes them relatively easy to distinguish radiographically. However, early arthritic processes may be much more subtle and the radiologist needs to be able to distinguish among similar appearing joint processes. There is a wide range of parameters that, when used in combination, will usually lead to correct diagnosis. These considerations include clinical evaluation, age and gender of the patient, laboratory values, distribution of the joints involved, joint deformities, and the general appearance of inflammatory erosive versus productive bony change. Of all these parameters, the radiologist is generally provided only with the age and gender of the patient and must rely on the location of involvement and the general appearance of the arthritic process to render a diagnosis. Almost all arthritic processes have a preferential distribution, including specific joints, as well as specific locations within a joint. As with both real estate and tumor evaluation, "location" is of prime importance in distinguishing among the arthritides. Throughout this chapter, you will find "location" is stressed as a vital piece of information.

The other important parameter in evaluation of an arthritic process is the determination of whether it is primarily erosive, productive of bone, or mixed. In general, erosive arthropathies have an initial inflammatory stage that produces pannus (inflammatory granulation tissue). The pannus destroys cartilage and bone by means of lytic enzymes and by direct interference with movement of nutrients across the joint surface. Rheumatoid arthritis is the most purely erosive arthritic process. Osteoarthritis (degenerative joint disease) stands at the other end of the spectrum, with productive rather than erosive manifestations. Although osteoarthritis also involves cartilaginous and subchondral bone destruction, abnormal mechanical forces combine with host reactive processes to produce changes, such as osteophyte formation, subchondral sclerosis, and cortical buttressing. As you will note, most of the other arthropathies generally fall between the erosive and productive ends of the spectrum, often demonstrating both erosive and productive changes.

Radiographs are the imaging modality of choice for the diagnosis of arthritis. However, radiographs often do not reflect the most subtle alterations that might be useful in evaluating efficacy of therapy. Although currently only used in therapeutic trials, MR imaging with intravenous contrast can be used to follow synovial enhancement and has been shown to be useful in judging treatment efficacy in small studies. On a more routine basis, MR imaging is sensitive to early arthritic changes, but is generally nonspecific. Effusion and synovial proliferation can be seen with MR imaging. With specialized MR imaging techniques, cartilaginous defects can be seen. Physical properties of cartilage relating to degeneration may be measurable by MR spectroscopy.

RHEUMATOID ARTHRITIS (RA)

Rheumatoid arthritis (RA) is the most common purely erosive inflammatory arthropathy. The synovial inflammation and articular destruction found in this disease is invariably polyarticular, involving the axial as well as appendicular skeleton, the upper and lower extremities, and the large and small joints. RA can first develop in either young or middle aged adults. There is a distinct gender preference, with females affected more frequently than males in a 2:1 or 3:1 ratio.

Clinical symptoms may be continous or episodic. These symptoms include early morning stiffness, pain, boggy synovial swelling, tendon contractures and ruptures, and result in several characteristic deformities. Rheumatoid factor (RF) is not entirely specific; it may be negative early in the disease process, but does eventually become positive in 90%–95% of cases. RF may, however, be falsely positive in older individuals. Patients with RA may have extra-articular manifestations, including nodules in tendon sheaths or subcutaneous locations, tenosynovitis or bursitis, pleural effusion, rheumatoid pulmonary nodules, and diffuse interstitial pneumonitis.

Radiographic characteristics of a joint involved with RA include fusiform swelling secondary to effusion and synovitis. There is usually osteoporosis resulting from a combination of hyperemia and disuse. The osteoporosis may be juxta-articular early in the disease but later becomes generalized. Cartilage destruction is uniform within a joint. The earliest hint of erosive change may be a "dot dash" pattern of the articular cortex within a joint. True bone destruction initially is marginal, at the bare areas of bone that are within the joint capsule but not protected by overlying cartilage.

Following cartilaginous destruction, subchondral erosions occur, along with subchondral cysts (Fig. 2-1). It is important to note that productive bone of any type is extremely unusual; specifically, periositis and enthesopathy do not occur in RA. Ankylosis of a joint is extraordinarily rare and limited to carpal and tarsal bones. Osteophytes are not seen in the absence of secondary degenerative joint disease. The exception to this rule is found in the distal ulna, where bone formation may be seen in a minority of RA patients who have long-term

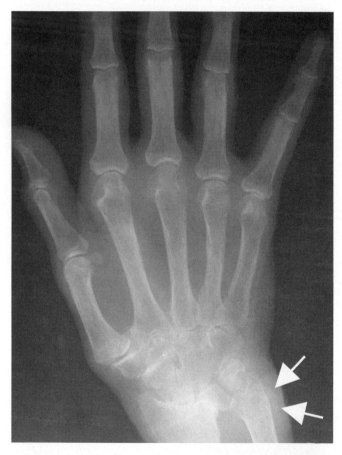

Fig. 2-1 Rheumatoid arthritis. PA view of the hand demonstrates the typical findings of RA, with diffuse osteopenia, soft tissue swelling at the MCPs, loss of cartilage width at the radiocarpal joint, erosions at the distal radioulnar joint and ulnar styloid, and carpal instability with ulnar translocation of the entire carpus. Note the only productive change is around the ulna, termed "ulnar capping" (*arrows*).

disease. This productive change is termed "ulnar capping."

RA is remarkable for its symmetry. Although most joints in the body can be affected by RA, survey films for the disease should include postero-anterior (PA) and ball catcher's views of the hand, AP and lateral views of the feet, and a lateral cervical spine.

Rheumatoid Arthritis: Hand and Wrist

Proximal disease is the hallmark of RA of the hand and wrist, and the wrist demonstrates some of the earliest findings in RA. Early erosions are found in the distal radioulnar joint, ulnar styloid, radial styloid, and waist of the scaphoid (Fig. 2-2). Early erosions in the triquetrum and pisiform are best seen on the ball catcher's view (Fig. 2-3). Thus, although rheumatoid arthritis eventually involves the mid-carpal row and the carpal-metacarpal joints, its initial involvement in the hand and wrist is in the distal radioulnar joint and radiocarpal joint. In addition to the erosive change, ligamentous rupture can result in instability patterns and deformities (Fig. 2-4), including

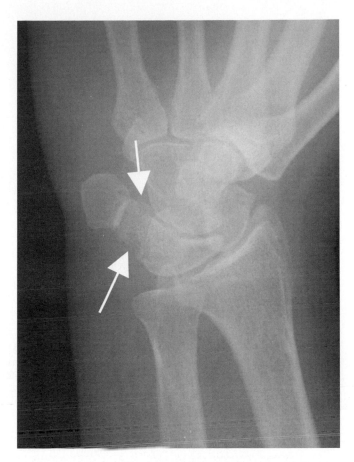

Fig. 2-3 Rheumatoid arthritis, wrist. Ball catcher's or Norgard view of the wrist demonstrates an erosion in the triquetrum (*arrows*), which was not demonstrated on the PA view. There were no other abnormalities on this patient's hand, but this single erosion in this typical location allows for a diagnosis of RA. (Reprinted with permission of the ACR learning file.)

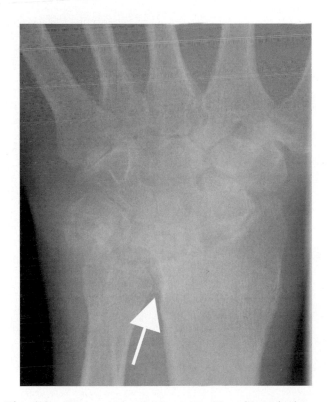

Fig. 2-2 Rheumatoid arthritis, wrist. PA radiograph demonstrates osteopenia, complete loss of cartilage width in the radiocarpal as well as intercarpal joints, soft tissue swelling, and typical erosions of the distal radioulnar joint (*arrow*), ulnar styloid, radiocarpal structures, and intercarpals. Note also that the entire carpus is slightly translocated in the ulnar direction.

ulnar translocation in which the entire carpus translates in an ulnar direction, scapholunate dissociation, distal radioulnar dissociation, and dorsal as well as volar flexion carpal instability patterns. More distally, the early erosive pattern is seen in the metacarpal-phalangeal joints (MCP). Although MCP erosions can be seen on the usual PA view, they sometimes are better seen on the ball catcher's view (Fig. 2-5). MCP involvement is usually followed by proximal interphalangeal (PIP) involvement (Fig. 2-6). Distal interphalangeal joints (DIPs) are spared early in the disease but may be involved once the disease becomes diffuse. As in the wrist, tendon ruptures are frequent, resulting in characteristic deformities. At the MCPs, ulnar deviation and volar subluxations or dislocations are frequent, often with associated pressure erosions (Fig. 2-4). Swan neck deformities (PIP hyperextension and DIP hyperflexion) as well as boutonnière deformities (PIP hyperflexion and DIP hyperextension) are frequent. Hitchhiker's thumb (MCP flexion and IP extension) is seen frequently as well.

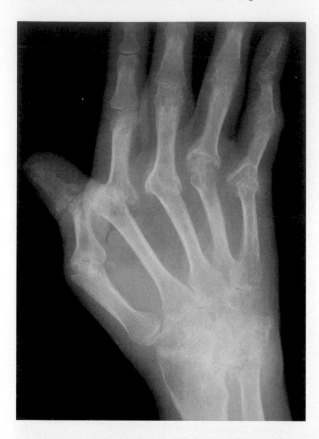

Fig. 2-4   Rheumatoid arthritis, instability. PA view demonstrates the instability that can be seen in late RA, with ulnar translocation of the carpus, a "hitchhiker's thumb," volar subluxation, ulnar deviation of the MCPs, and a boutonniere deformity of the fifth finger. A lateral view (not shown) might show dorsi or volar flexion instability patterns of the carpus. (Reprinted with permission of the ACR learning file.)

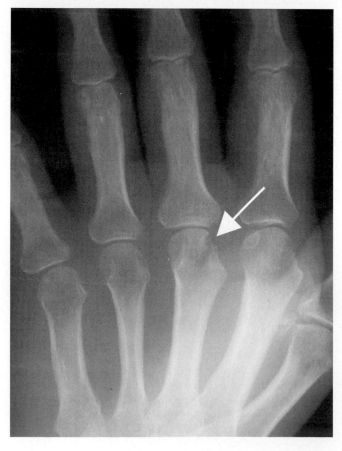

Fig. 2-5   Rheumatoid arthritis, MCPs. Ball catcher's view demonstrates periarticular osteopenia, soft tissue swelling at the MCPs, and a solitary erosion at the head of the third metacarpal (*arrow*). This was the only erosion seen in this patient, and the only view in which it was discernible. (Reprinted with permission of the ACR learning file.)

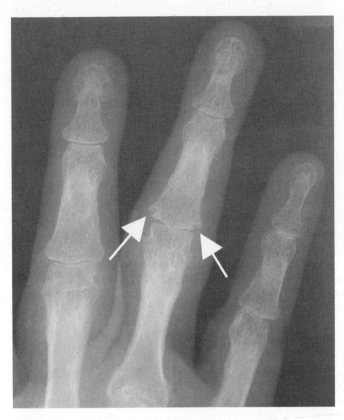

Fig. 2-6   Rheumatoid arthritis, IP marginal erosions. Cartilage narrowing is seen in all of the IP joints pictured on this AP radiograph. The fourth PIP shows marginal erosions (*arrows*), occasionally likened to "mouse-ears" (Reprinted with permission of the ACR learning file.)

Rheumatoid Arthritis: Elbow

The elbow is frequently involved in RA. The entire articulation is involved, with a positive fat pad sign indicating effusion, and prominent erosions of the distal humerus, radial head and neck, and coranoid process (Fig. 2-7). Olecranon bursitis may be seen as a "mass" at the olecranon bursa, without joint involvement necessarily being associated.

Rheumatoid Arthritis: Shoulder Girdle

The acromiclavicular joint is frequently involved with RA, with early changes seen as lysis of the distal clavicle and erosion of the coracoclavicular ligament insertion (Fig. 2-8). Although the sternomanubrial and sternoclavicular joints frequently have erosions, they are infrequently imaged. Marginal erosions can be found at the humeral head adjacent to the greater tuberosity, at the capsular insertion on the anatomic neck of the humerus. As with other joints, tendons are frequently disrupted. In the case of the shoulder, the rotator cuff is frequently torn. These tears of course can be diagnosed on MRI or at arthrogra-

phy. However, the chronicity of the rotator cuff tear is so prominent in RA patients that they often develop the elevated humeral head and mechanical erosion at the undersurface of the acromion, which make the diagnosis obvious by radiograph (Fig. 2-9). With the elevation of the humeral head due to rotator cuff tear, mechanical erosion of the medial surgical neck of the humerus by the inferior glenoid can occur, occasionally resulting in a pathologic surgical neck fracture.

Rheumatoid Arthritis: Feet

The metatarsal-phalangeal (MTP) joints commonly show early erosive changes, particularly at the fifth digit (Fig. 2-10). Interphalangeal and intertarsal erosions occur later in the disease. Associated deformities in the digits include lateral deviation at the MTPs, hammer toe deformities (flexion of the PIPs and DIPs), and cock-up deformities (hyperextended MTPs). Lateral foot films may demonstrate a retrocalcaneal bursitis, which may obliterate the normal pre-Achilles fat triangle, occasionally associated with erosive change at the posterior calcaneus (Fig. 2-11). This posterior calcaneal inflammatory and erosive change is also seen in psoriatic arthritis and Reiter's disease.

Rheumatoid Arthritis: Knee

The knee is very frequently involved in rheumatoid arthritis, with joint effusion and popliteal synovial cysts seen early in the disease (Fig. 2-12). The latter may present as a large mass lesion. Once erosive change begins, all three compartments of the knee demonstrate uniform cartilage loss, erosions, and subchondral cyst formation. Valgus deformity most often occurs. Patellar tendon ruptures occasionally occur and the distal femoral shaft can develop anterior mechanical erosion from patellar pressure.

Rheumatoid Arthritis: Hip

Rheumatoid involvement in the hip results in a concentric decrease in joint space with resultant protrusio deformity (medial displacement of the femoral head such that the medial femoral head cortex lies medial to the ilioischial line) (Fig. 2-13). These two characteristics should make the entity distinct from osteoarthritis of the hip, which shows preferential decrease in joint space width at the weight-bearing region, usually with superolateral subluxation. However, up to 20% of cases of osteoarthritis show protrusio. Even with protrusio, osteoarthritis shows osteophytes and normal bone density whereas RA shows erosions and osteoporosis; these findings serve to differentiate the two.

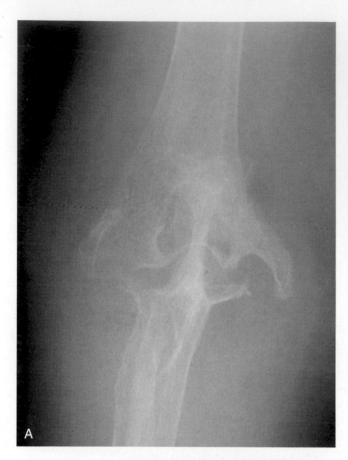

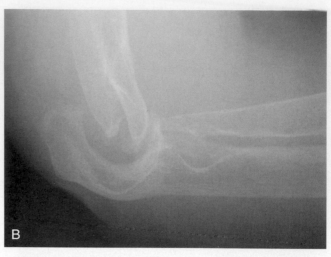

Fig. 2-7   Rheumatoid arthritis, elbow. **A,** AP and **B,** lateral radiographs of the elbow in a patient with advanced RA demonstrates the diffuse and uniform erosive change that can be seen in this disease process.

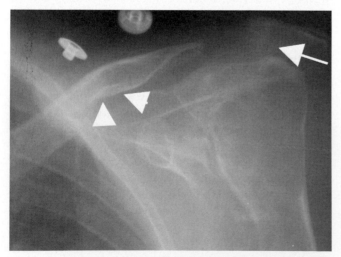

Fig. 2-8   Rheumatoid arthritis, acromioclavicular joint. AP radiograph of the AC joint demonstrates the elevation of the humeral head associated with the patient's chronic rotator cuff tear, as well as erosions involving both the distal end of the clavicle (*arrow*) and the site of insertion of the coracoclavicular ligament (*arrowheads*).

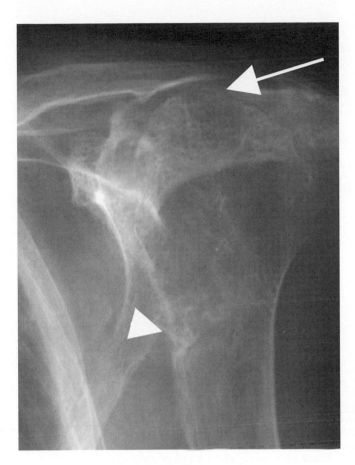

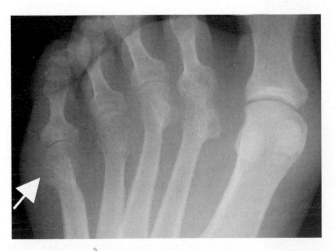

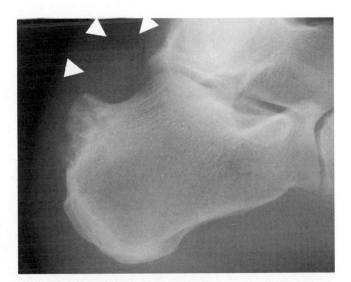

Fig. 2-9   Rheumatoid arthritis, shoulder. This AP radiograph shows severe osteopenia and elevation of the humeral head. Note that with the chronic rotator cuff tear, the humeral head now articulates with the undersurface of the acromion (*arrow*). The patient also has developed a mechanical erosion at the surgical neck of the humerus (*arrowheads*) related to its rubbing against the inferior glenoid. This is at risk for fracture.

Fig. 2-10   RA, MTPs. AP radiograph of the foot demonstrates soft tissue swelling at the MTPs and prominent erosions at the second, third, and fifth (*arrow*). Erosions at the MTPs are a frequent finding in RA. (Reprinted with permission of the ACR learning file.)

Fig. 2-11   Rheumatoid arthritis, calcaneus. Lateral radiograph of the calcaneus demonstrates both erosive change at the posterior calcaneus, and inflammatory change obliterating the pre-Achilles fat triangle (*arrowheads*). Most radiologists think of Reifer's disease when they see this appearance, but it should be remembered that the inflammatory erosive changes of RA can affect the posterior calcaneus as well. (Reprinted with permission of the ACR learning file.)

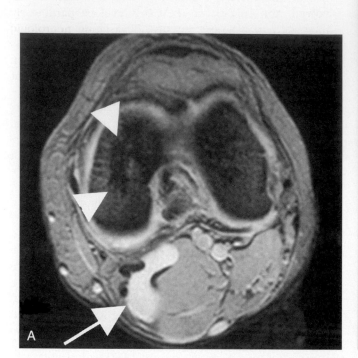

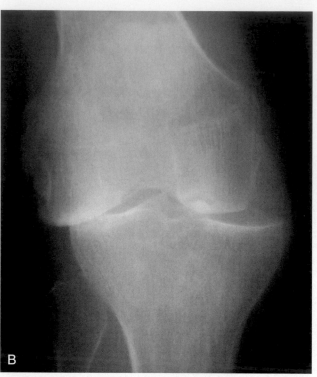

Fig. 2-12   Rheumatoid arthritis, knee. **A,** An axial gradient echo MR image of the knee in a 29-year-old female with RA. The popliteal cyst, arising in the typical location in the semimembranosus gastrocnemius bursa is seen (*arrow*), along with low signal in the femoral condyles (*arrowheads*), a site of osteonecrosis in this patient who has been taking steroids for her disease. **B,** An AP radiograph of a different patient with RA, showing diffuse osteopenia, uniform loss of cartilage width in the medial and lateral compartments, and medial subluxation of the tibia with apex valgus angulation. This is a typical alignment and appearance of RA involving the knee. (Figure 2-12B reprinted with permission of the ACR learning file.)

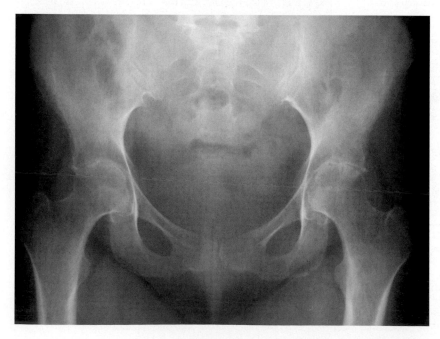

Fig. 2-13   Rheumatoid arthritis, hip. AP radiograph of the pelvis demonstrates diffuse osteopenia, symmetric loss of cartilage width, early erosive change, and early protrusio of both hips. The appearance is typical of RA. (Reprinted with permission of the ACR learning file.)

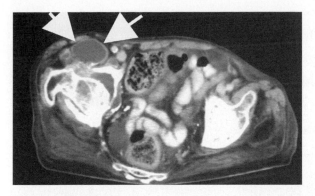

Fig. 2-14   Rheumatoid arthritis, hip. Axial CT demonstrates a water density mass located in the right iliopsoas bursa (*arrows*), deviating the neurovascular bundle medially. Note that the hip shows severe protrusio and erosive disease. The combination of the erosive disease in the hip with this mass makes the diagnosis of RA with decompression of synovial fluid into the iliopsoas bursa a straightforward process. (Reprinted with permission of the ACR learning file.)

Soft-tissue abnormalities may occur around hips in patients with RA. A soft-tissue mass may develop anterior to the hip joint; in a patient with RA this almost invariably represents decompression of a large synovial effusion into the iliopsoas bursa. This is seen as a fluid collection elevating the neurovascular bundle on CT (Fig. 2-14) as well as MRI (Fig. 2-15). Tendon ruptures occasionally occur around the hip. These are best diagnosed with MRI (Fig. 2-15).

Rheumatoid Arthritis: Spine

Involvement of the thoracic spine, lumbar spine, and sacroiliac joints by RA is usually mild and infrequently noted. The cervical region, however, is commonly involved. Abnormalities at the C1-2 level are particularly important to diagnose because devastating neurologic deficits can result. The most frequently noted complication of RA in the C1-2 region is atlantoaxial subluxation. In this process, there is transverse atlantoaxial ligament laxity or disruption, resulting in the atlantoaxial distance measuring greater than 2.5 mm. Atlantoaxial subluxation often increases in flexion and reduces in extension (Fig. 2-16). Furthermore, pannus formation anterior and posterior to the odontoid process can decrease canal width; this can be diagnosed by MRI. Although atlantoaxial subluxation is diagnosed with an atlantoaxial measurement of greater than 2.5 mm, it is often not symptomatic until subluxation approaches 9 mm.

Another important complication of RA at C1-2 is atlantoaxial impaction. This impaction is due to C1-2 facet erosion and subsequent collapse of the facets. With the facet collapse, the odontoid process protrudes into the foramen magnum. As the odontoid itself can be difficult to observe in patients with RA owing to superimposed mastoids and generalized osteopenia, atlantoaxial impaction is perhaps best detected by observation of the relationship of the anterior arch of the atlas with the odontoid process. On the lateral film, the atlas usually is aligned with the cranial portion of the odontoid. With impaction, the anterior arch of the atlas aligns with the body of C2 (Fig. 2-17). This relationship is important to detect, as neurologic symptoms are more often associated with atlantoaxial impaction than subluxation.

Other abnormalities of RA involving the cervical spine include odontoid erosion, unilateral facet erosion that may result in torticollis, erosions at the facets and joints of Lushka, mechanical erosion of the spinal processes, and the appearance of "discitis" at several levels. Discitis

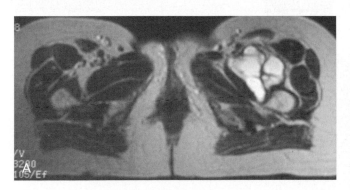

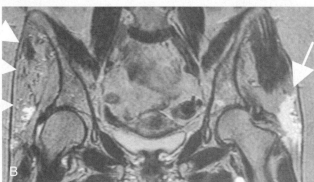

Fig. 2-15   Rheumatoid arthritis, hip. **A,** An axial T2 weighted (3200/105) MR image of the hips in a 35-year-old female with RA. It demonstrates a multi-loculated appearing mass, which is located within the iliopsoas bursa. Like the mass seen in Figure 2-14, this represents decompression of synovial fluid from the hip into the iliopsoas bursa through the relatively weak anterior hip capsule. **B,** A coronal T2-weighted image in the same patient (3750/108), demonstrating bilateral gluteal tendon ruptures. On the left, we see high signal intensity at the site of the rupture (*arrow*). The left rupture is relatively recent, as the musculature remains. On the right side, the gluteal musculature shows complete fatty atrophy, indicating a longer term tendon rupture (*arrowheads*).

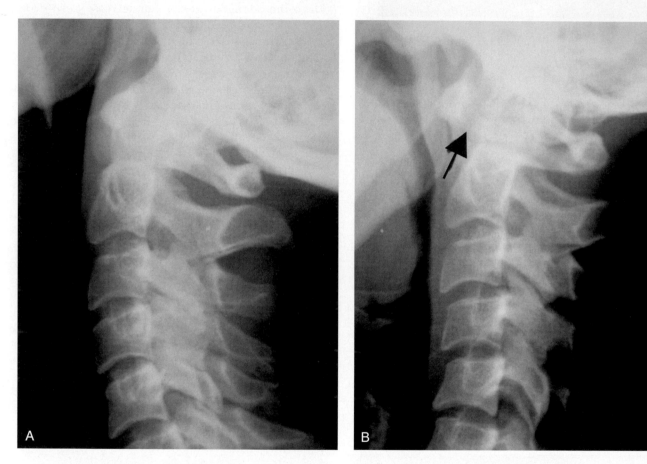

Fig. 2-16   Rheumatoid arthritis, cervical spine. Atlantoaxial subluxation can be prominently seen, especially in flexion of the cervical spine. Note that in this case with extension **A,** there is no evidence of atlantoaxial subluxation. However, in flexion **B,** atlantoaxial subluxation of 8 mm is seen (*arrow*). Even if it is difficult to see the odontoid process through the mastoids, the disruption of the spinal laminar line at C1–2 indicates atlantoaxial subluxation. The other finding of RA in this patient is the lack of cortical distinctness of the facets of C3, 4, and 5.

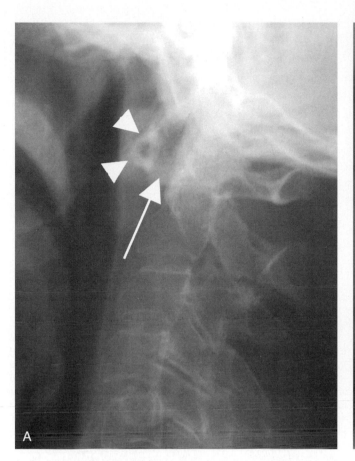 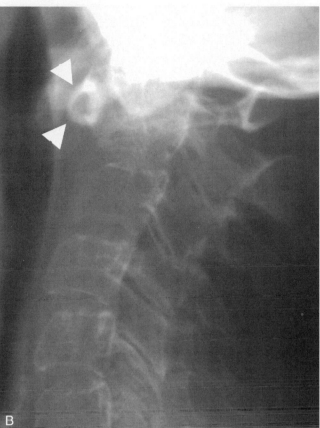

Fig. 2-17   Rheumatoid arthritis, cervical spine. **A,** A lateral radiograph demonstrating atlantoaxial subluxation (*arrow*) and osteopenia. Note that the anterior arch of the atlas (*arrowheads*) is located at the level of the odontoid process and that at this point there is no evidence of atlantoaxial impaction. However, a film taken 2 years later **B,** demonstrates that severe atlantoaxial impaction has occurred, with the anterior arch of the atlas (*arrowheads*) now located opposite the inferior portion of the body of C2. Although you cannot actually see the odontoid process, it must be presumed to have impacted into the foramen magnum. Note the severe constriction of the spinal canal between the posterior aspect of the body of C2 and the anterior aspect of the spinous process of C1. Atlantoaxial impaction can be even more devastating to the patient's neurologic status than atlantoaxial subluxation. (Reprinted with permission of the ACR learning file.)

is thought to be due to a combination of osteoporosis and posterior ligament laxity that results in decreased disk height, irregularity of the endplates, and a "stair-step" deformity is seen on the lateral film.

Rheumatoid Arthritis: Robust Rheumatoid Arthritis

Robust RA is a type of RA featuring large subchondral cysts and normal bone density. The distribution of abnormalities is identical to that of RA and the abnormality seems predominantly erosive, without productive change. It is generally seen in men who maintain normal activity, thus retaining their normal bone density and forcing decompression of synovial fluid into enlarging subchondral cysts (Fig. 2-18).

Rheumatoid Arthritis: Adult Still's Disease

Adult Still's disease is clinically similar to the systemic form of juvenile chronic arthritis, with intermittent fever, skin rash, pleuritis, pericarditis, lymphadenopathy, and hepatosplenomegaly. Radiographically, carpal disease predominates. Pericapitate erosions and fusions are seen more frequently than radiocarpal disease (Fig. 2-19).

Rheumatoid Arthritis: Differential Diagnosis

The distribution of abnormalities and pure erosive character of RA usually serves to distinguish it from other arthritides. Occasionally, psoriatic arthritis may appear

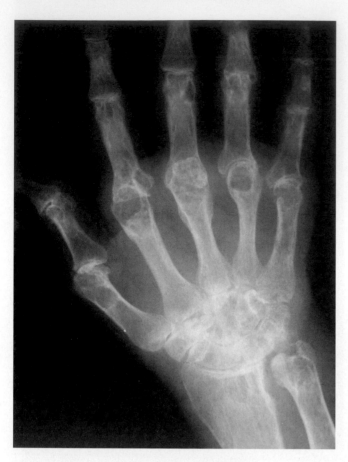

Fig. 2-18   Robust rheumatoid arthritis. PA radiograph of the hand in this 47-year-old male demonstrates tremendous subchondral cyst formation as well as erosive change in the distribution of rheumatoid arthritis. The bone density is decreased, but not as much as one might expect for the severity of disease. This is a carpenter who has continued working in his profession despite his severe rheumatoid arthritis, leading to these changes of robust RA. (Reprinted with permission of the ACR learning file.)

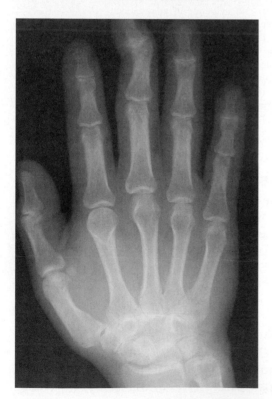

Fig. 2-19   Adult Still's disease. PA radiograph demonstrates carpal and DIP disease. The pericapitate distribution of the carpal disease is typical for adult Still's disease. (Reprinted with permission of the ACR learning file.)

Key Concepts | **Rheumatoid Arthritis**

- It is purely an erosive arthropathy.
- Exhibits synovitis with osteoporosis.
- There is uniform cartilage destruction.
- There is no productive change (absent osteo-phytes, fusion, or periostitis).
- It is bilaterally symmetric.
- There is wrist involvement at the radiocarpal joint, distal radioulnar joint.
- There is hand involvement at the MCPs and PIPs.
- There is foot involvement at the MTPs and retrocal-caneal bursa.
- Exhibits rotator cuff tears.
- Exhibits valgus deformity of the knee.
- Exhibits protusio of hips.
- Upper cervical spine pathology (facet erosions, at-lantoaxial impaction, atlantoaxial subluxation).

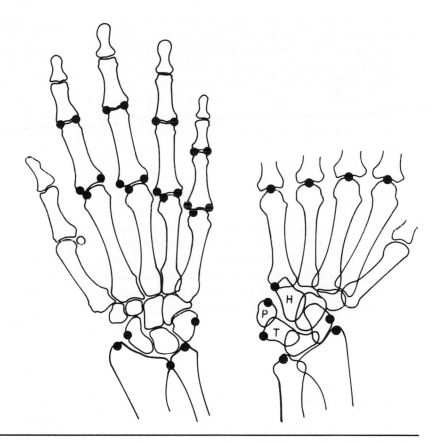

similar in the hand or foot but the DIP distribution of psoriatic arthritis tends to predominate. The retrocalcaneal bursitis and erosive change may appear identical in RA and Reiter's disease, but Reiter's may have superimposed enthesophyte productive change and often has characteristic additional joint distribution (sacroiliac joints; foot findings predominating over those of the hand). The deformities seen so frequently in RA are mimicked with systemic lupus erythematosis (SLE), but the latter disease process is rarely erosive. Finally, spondyloarthropathy of hemodialysis may have similar discovertebral junction abnormalities as those found in the cervical spine in RA. However, C1-2 and the facet joints are usually normal in spondyloarthropathy of hemodialysis, in which disc and endplate changes predominate, distinguishing this from RA.

JUVENILE CHRONIC ARTHRITIS (INCLUDING JUVENILE RHEUMATOID ARTHRITIS: JRA)

Juvenile chronic arthritis is a group of related diseases of unknown etiology arising in childhood with symptom complexes that have been divided into the following categories.

1. Still's Disease. Twenty percent of patients with JRA have Still's disease, which presents as an acute systemic process occurring in children under 5 years of age. Patients with Still's disease present with high fever, anemia, polymorphonuclear leukocytosis, hepatosplenomegaly, lymphadenopathy, and polyarthritis. They do not have iridocyclitis. Radiographic findings are often mild and may not show erosions, but 25% of patients with Still's disease have chronic and destructive arthritis.

Key Concepts | **JRA**

- Periostitis may be seen in children.
- Knee, elbow, hip are most common locations.
- Exhibits metaphyseal/epiphyseal "ballooning" due to hyperemia.
- Exhibits early growth plate closure due to hyperemia.
- Exhibits asymmetric maturation of ossification centers due to hyperemia.
- Cartilage destruction and erosions occur later than in RA.
- Exhibits distinctive fusion and growth abnormalities in the cervical spine.
- Exhibits facet and carpal ankylosis.

---

2. Pauciarticular Disease. This is the most common type of JRA, seen in 40% of the patients. One fourth of such patients have chronic iridocyclitis. They are RF negative. This type is most frequently seen in young girls. Inflammation is typically seen in one to three joints (usually large joints such as the knee, ankle, or elbow) and is rarely severe.

3. Seronegative Polyarticular Disease. Twenty-five percent of patients with JRA have seronegative polyarticular disease. There is a female preponderance and the disease may occur at any age but the patient remains RF negative. These patients show synovitis with the adult type of symmetric and wide-spread distribution involving both large and small joints.

4. Seropositive Polyarticular Disease (juvenile onset adult RA). This comprises only 5% of patients with JRA. These patients show polyarticular changes typical of RA with severe erosive changes, similar distribution to RA, and most become RA positive. These disease generally starts in the second decade.

5. Juvenile ankylosing spondylitis (AS). Juvenile AS is an inflammatory arthropathy with a strong male predominance (7 : 1) and strong HLA B27 positivity. These patients usually present with extra-axial arthritis and only rarely present with the classical signs and symptoms of sacroiliitis and spondylitis, which are more typical of the adult form of AS. Radiographically, sacroiliac joint abnormalities in these patients may be underdiagnosed because adolescent sacroiliac joints are normally wide, with indistinct cortices. Symptoms of pain at the symphysis pubis, ischial tuberosities, and costochondral junction are uncommon but strongly support the diagnosis. It should be remembered that juvenile AS is often misdiagnosed as JRA because the abnormalities are not typical of those of adult AS and the sacroiliac joint abnormalities are particularly difficult to detect in adolescents.

Whatever the clinical symptom complex may be, the radiographic changes of the arthropathy of JRA are similar among the various categories, particularly Still's and pauciarticular disease. It should be noted that patients with JRA have a distinct radiologic appearance from that of adult RA. The joints are usully osteoporotic, but cartilage destruction and erosive change occur as late manifestations. Subchondral cysts are rarely present. Periosteal reaction may be seen in early JRA (Fig. 2-20), and fusion is more common in JRA than adult RA. Joint contractures are common. One very distinctive feature of JRA is growth abnormalities. With hyperemia in the skeletally immature patient, there is overgrowth of the involved epiphyses. This leads to "ballooning" of joints clinically, and radiographically demonstrates advanced skeletal maturation and premature fusion in those joints that are

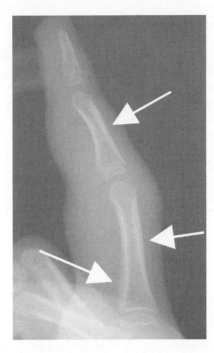

Fig. 2-20   JRA. Lateral radiograph of the index finger in a 6-year-old female demonstrates soft tissue swelling and dense periosteal reaction (*arrows*). Although these changes are not pathognomonic for JRA (they could be seen in a bone infarct in a young patient with sickle cell disease, or infection), they are typical as the first manifestation of JRA.

involved. Therefore asymmetry in epiphyseal size and maturation may suggest JRA as a diagnosis (Fig. 2-21). With premature fusion, one may find shortened limb on the affected side.

The distribution of joint involvement in JRA can be similar to that of adult RA. However, there is generally a predilection for large joints rather than small joints. Thus, the knee and the elbow are commonly and distinctively involved. The knee shows an effusion, widened intercondylar notch, metaphyseal and epiphyseal flaring, and overgrowth relating to the hyperemia, and uniform cartilage and destructive change (Fig. 2-22). The elbow also shows effusion, enlargement of the trochlear notch, radial head enlargement due to overgrowth from hyperemia, and uniform cartilage loss and destructive change (Fig. 2-23). The hip also shows common distinctive involvement, with femoral head enlargement, a short neck with valgus, and significant protusio acetabuli (Fig. 2-24). The iliac wings are often hypoplastic and the femoral shaft can be gracile. The small bones combined with the coxa valga abnormality can make joint replacement difficult.

The hand and wrist in JRA shows MCP and PIP involvement similar to adult RA. However, in the wrist the radiocarpal joint may be spared and the mid-carpal joint involved, particularly in the pericapitate region. This may distinguish JRA from adult RA. Adult Still's disease is similar to JRA in this aspect. Ankylosis is very common in the hand and wrist in JRA (Fig. 2-25).

As in adult RA, the cervical spine is commonly affected in JRA. Atlantoaxial subluxation and odontoid erosions are prominent findings. Facet erosions are seen as well. However, with JRA, cervical spine ankylosis is common and this ankylosis is thought to protect these patients from developing the discovertebral junction abnormalities seen so often in adult RA. If ankylosis of cervical

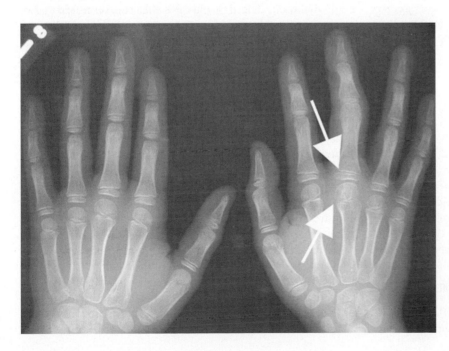

Fig. 2-21   JRA. PA radiograph of both hands in this 8-year-old female demonstrates soft tissue swelling of the right third digit, and asymmetrically large epiphyses at the right third metacarpal head and base of its proximal phalanx (*arrows,* compared with the opposite normal left side). This focal advancement and skeletal maturation results from chronic hyperemia at this site with pauciarticular JRA.

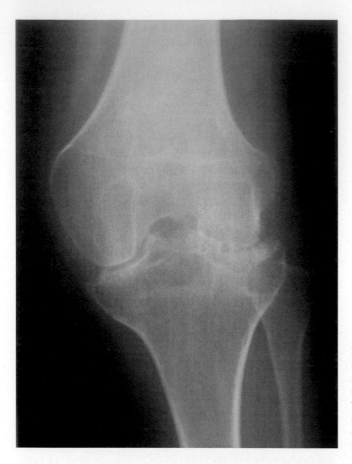

Fig. 2-22 JRA, knee. AP radiograph of the knee in this 23-year-old patient demonstrates typical findings of JRA, with epiphyses and metaphyses that are overgrown or enlarged relative to the diaphyses, a wide intercondylar notch, and erosive change with cartilage loss. The relative enlargement of the bones at the joint compared with the diaphyses is seen in JRA because of the chronic hyperemia occurring during skeletal growth. (Reprinted with permission of the ACR learning file.)

bodies occurs before skeletal maturation, there is vertebral body hypoplasia both in height and in AP dimension, resulting in the appearance of "waisting" of the bodies (Fig. 2-26). This is a very distinctive appearance for JRA.

ANKYLOSING SPONDYLITIS (AS) AND SPONDYLITIS OF INFLAMMATORY BOWEL DISEASE (IBD)

Ankylosing spondylitis (AS) is the most common of the seronegative spondyloarthropathies. It is of unknown etiology, and is characterized by being a mixed erosive and osseous productive disease, which involves predominately the axial skeleton and large proximal joints.

AS has a strikingly higher incidence in males than females, with a male-to-female ratio of between 4:1 and 10:1. The onset occurs either in adolescence or young adulthood, ranging between 15 and 35 years of age. Clinical signs are of low back pain and limited chest expansion. As the disease progresses, stiffness of the spine can progress to distinct postural changes, with prominent thoracic kyphosis and limited lumbar lordosis. Laboratory testing can be helpful in the diagnosis; more than 90% of patients with ankylosing spondylitis are HLA B27 positive. This is not a specific finding, as between 6% and

8% of the normal population show HLA B27 positivity and between 50% and 80% of patients with Reiter's disease and psoriatic arthritis are positive as well.

A key feature of AS remains its distribution of disease. The sacroiliac joints are classically the site of initial involvement. The first changes that can be noted radiographically are the loss of cortical definition, followed by erosions and joint widening (Fig. 2-27). These findings may be most prominent on the iliac side of the joint as the cartilage is normally thinner on that side; both sides are eventually involved. Later in the disease process sclerosis and fusion of the synovial portion of the sacroiliac joints develop. Although the abnormalities may initially be asymmetric, they eventually become bilaterally symmetric in the disease process. Thus, the hallmark of late disease is bilateral sacroiliac joint fusion, which can be easily identified on a radiograph (Fig. 2-28). Very early disease may be suspected radiographically, but may require cross-sectional imaging for confirmation. It should be remembered that only the synovial portion of the "sacroiliac joint" is involved in the erosive disease; the synovial portion is the anterior-inferior aspect of the joint. The posterosuperior portions of the sacroiliac regions are syndesmoses without cartilage, synovium, or capsule. They are joined together by interosseous ligaments that may ossify in some disorders without representing a true

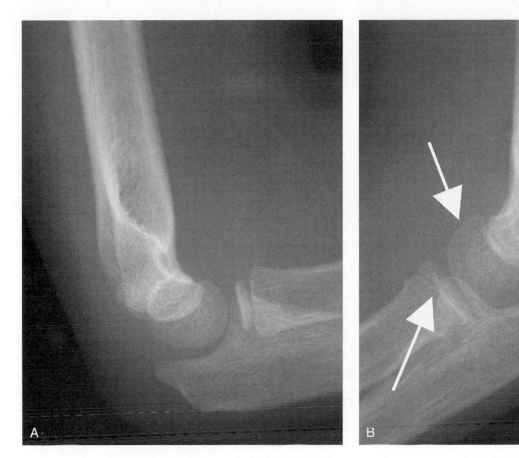

Fig. 2-23   JRA, elbow. **A,** Normal left and **B,** abnormal right elbow lateral radiographs in this patient with JRA demonstrate relative overgrowth of the capitellum and radial head on the right side (*arrows*). Additionally, the right elbow shows ossification of the olecranon apophysis and an AP radiograph (not shown) demonstrates asymmetric ossification of the lateral epicondyle on the right compared with ossification of that structure not yet occurring on the left. This advancement of skeletal maturation is typical in a joint affected by JRA. The adult elbow will show relative enlargement compared with the left, particularly of the radial head.

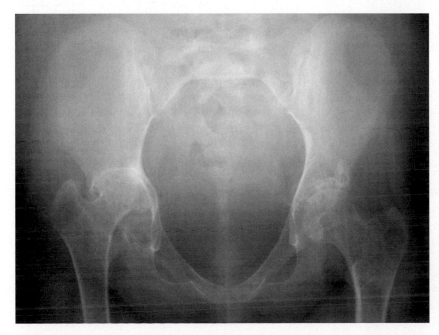

Fig. 2-24   JRA, pelvis. AP radiograph of the pelvis of a 20-year-old female with JRA demonstrates the small stature and gracile diaphyses typically seen in these patients. It also shows severe erosive change involving both hips with protrusio particularly on the right side. This particular case does not show the valgus deformity that can occur in the femoral necks. (Reprinted with permission of the ACR learning file.)

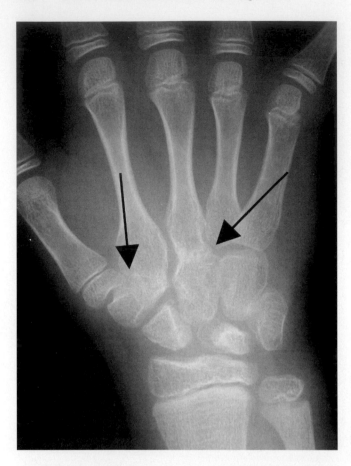

Fig. 2-25 JRA, hand. PA radiograph in this 11-year-old female demonstrates little loss of cartilage width in the wrist or MCPs, but abnormal fusion between the capitate and third metacarpal, as well as between the trapezium and second metacarpal and trapezoid (*arrows*). Early fusion in the absence of substantial erosive change or loss of cartilage is typical finding in JRA.

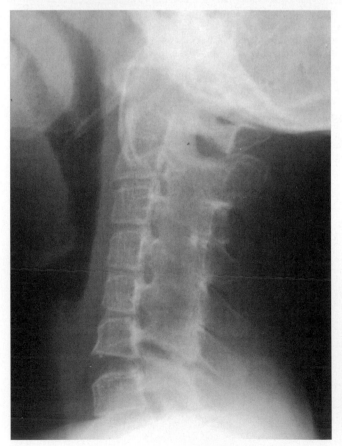

Fig. 2-26 JRA, cervical spine. Lateral radiograph of the cervical spine demonstrates complete fusion of the facets of C2 though C6. This fusion protects the endplates and disk spaces from the deterioration that is seen in advanced adult RA. Fusion at an early age also results in restriction of growth of the vertebral bodies in an AP dimension (note how much smaller the bodies of C3, 4, and 5 are than C2, 6, and 7 in the AP diameter). This appearance has been termed "waisting" of the cervical bodies. (Reprinted with permission of the ACR learning file.)

Key Concepts Ankylosing Spondylitis

- It is the most common spondyloarthropathy.
- Develops most frequently in the adolescent or young adult male, but may occur in females.
- It is a mixed erosive and osseous productive arthropathy.
- It involves the axial skeleton and large proximal appendicular joints.
- Sacroiliitis shows erosive changes and early symmetric widening of the SI joints, followed by ankylosis.
- Thin vertical syndesmophytes in the spine may result in a "bamboo" appearance late in the disease.
- Spine fracture may occur after mild trauma, most common at cervicothoracic and thoracolumbar junctions.

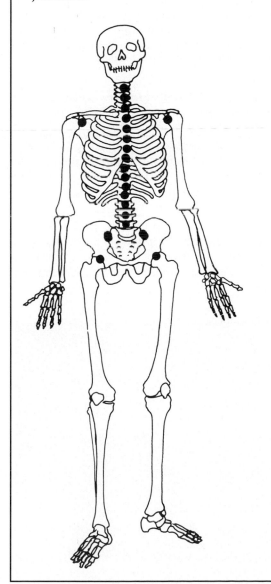

sacroiliitis. Thus, nonsynovial SI joint bridging enthesophytes as is seen in DISH (diffuse idiopathic skeletal hyperostosis) should not be confused with fusion of the true SI joints in AS.

In AS, involvement of the thoracolumbar spine classically follows SI abnormalities. It usually begins at the thoracolumbar and lumbosacral junctions and extends contiguously without skip areas. Again, it should be noted that skips and asymmetry may be seen, but are far less common in AS than in Reiter's disease or psoriatic arthropathy. Vertebral involvement in anklyosing spondylitis begins with osteitis, related to erosive enthesitis at the peripheral corners of the vertebral bodies. Reactive sclerosis at the sites of osteitis may result in the "shiny corner" sign. The osteitis in turn leads to loss of the normal concavity of the anterior vertebral body, giving it a characteristic "squaring" (Fig. 2-29). Eventually, syndesmophytes form in the anulus fibrosis at the discovertebral junction, seen as thin vertical ossifications. These are distinct in appearance from the bulky horizontal nonmarginal osteophytes that arise from the vertebral body itself, seen in Reiter's syndrome and psoriatic arthropathy. By the end stage of the process, several segments will show ankylosis as a "bamboo" spine (Fig. 2-30), with undulating fusion of the vertebral bodies as well as fusion of the apophyseal joints. Although, initially, bone density is normal in patients with AS, after fusion disuse osteoporosis ensues. This can be very significant late in the disease, leaving the fused osteoporotic spine vulnerable to fracture from minor trauma. Such extremely subtle fractures may not be initially detected yet must be sought because of the instability that accompanies those fractures. They occur most frequently at the cervicothoracic and thoracolumbar junctions. The fracture usually extends through the disk space and the posterior elements (Fig. 2-31). As subtle as these may appear, traumatically induced fractures of this sort may result in sudden death or severe neurologic sequelae. MRI is often useful in evaluating cord injury, disk herniation, or epidural hematoma in such cases. If the fracture itself goes undetected, motion across this segment of osteoporotic bone results in osseous breakdown with an appearance similar to neuropathic arthropathy.

The hip is the most common appendicular joint involved in AS, with abnormalities seen in up to 50% of patients. The hip usually shows a combination of erosive and productive change, with concentric joint narrowing, mild erosions, protrusio acetabuli, and later, ring osteophytes (Fig. 2-32). In any young adult such incongruent radiographic appearances alone should suggest a diagnosis of ankylosing spondylitis and lead to careful scrutiny of the SI joints, as the SI joints are the earliest site of involvement in AS. As with the SI joints, involvement of the hips is often bilateral but may be asymmetric.

After the hip, the glenohumeral joint is the next most commonly involved appendicular joint in AS. The sym-

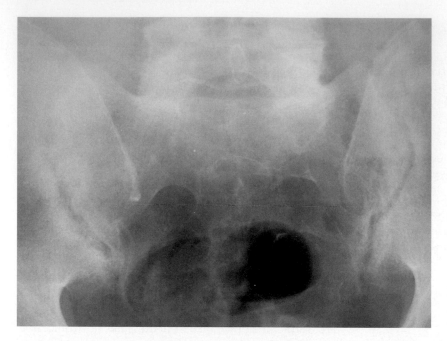

Fig. 2-27 Ankylosing spondylitis, SI joints. This AP radiograph of the SI joints demonstrates very early changes that can be found in the spondyloarthropathy of ankylosing spondylitis. The cortices of the SI joints lack the normal distinctness. No specific erosion or fusion is seen at this time. This loss of cortical distinctness is the earliest change that will be seen on radiography, and in this case is a symmetric finding.

physis pubis, sternomanubrial, and costochondral joints are commonly involved, with eventual anklyosis. The knees, ankles, hands, and feet are much less commonly involved than the large proximal joints.

Subchondral cysts, periostitis, and ligament disruption are not common features in AS. Enthesopathy, however, is usually seen, especially in the pelvis, calcaneus, and patella.

Although AS is less common in women, the diagnosis should not be excluded based on female gender. The radiographic findings tend to be neither as severe nor as typical in distribution as in male patients. The disease also can present later in females and skip levels in the spine.

The arthropathy of inflammatory bowel disease (IBD) can be seen in two forms. One group of disease processes occurs as a result of *Salmonella, Shigella,* or *Yersinia* infections. These diseases may produce a self-limited polyarthritis, usually without radiographic findings but occasionally with SI joint clinical symptoms. A more pronounced spondyloarthropathy may occur with ulcerative colitis, Crohn disease, and Whipple disease. As many as 10%–15% of these patients develop chronic arthropathy. The majority of these are peripheral with mild clinical manifestations, but one-third may develop a sacroiliitis identical clinically and radiographically to that of ankylosing spondylitis.

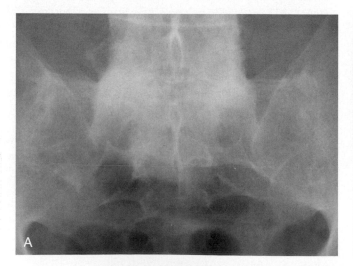 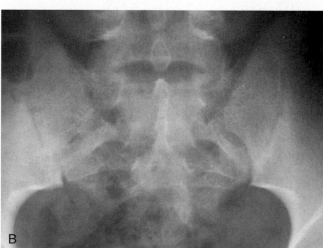

Fig. 2-28 Ankylosing spondylitis, SI joints. **A,** This AP radiograph shows SI joints that are completely fused bilaterally. This is a later finding in this case of ankylosing spondylitis than that demonstrated in Figure 2-27. **B,** demonstrates an intermediate phase of sacroiliitis and ankylosing spondylitis, with slight widening of the SI joints, sclerosis, and erosive change.

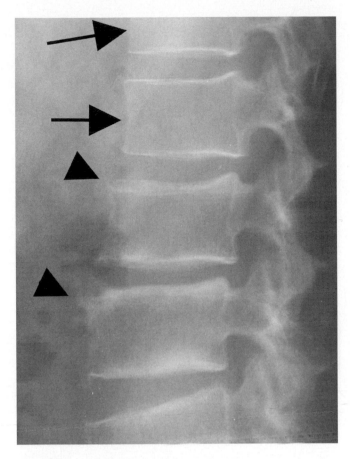

Fig. 2-29   Ankylosing spondylitis, spine. This lateral radiograph in a patient with ankylosing spondylitis demonstrates the squaring of some of the vertebral bodies (*arrows*) as well as the irregular osteitis at the corner of others (*arrowheads*). A single vertical syndesmophyte is beginning to form at the inferior endplate of the lower body seen on this film. The osteitis and resultant squaring are the first vertebral body abnormalities seen in ankylosing spondylitis, followed by formation of the syndesmophytes.

PSORIATIC ARTHRITIS

Psoriatic arthritis occurs in from 0.5% to 25% of patients with psoriasis. Five distinct manifestations have been described, including polyarthritis (predominately distal interphalangeal joints), arthritis mutilans (deforming type), symmetric type (resembling RA), oligoarthritis, and spondyloarthropathy. Of the patients with psoriatic arthritis, 30%–50% will develop a spondyloarthropathy.

Patients who develop psoriatic arthritis are generally young adults. Unlike AS, psoriatic arthritis affects males and females with equal prevalence. Although skin disease is usually present before the arthropathy, arthritis may predate skin findings in up to 20% of cases. This can obscure the clinical diagnosis.

Clinically, the patients present with soft tissue swelling, particularly in the small joints of the hands and feet. The swelling may involve the entire digit and be so extreme as to be termed a "sausage digit." There is pain and reduced range of motion. Patients may complain of low back pain. Nail changes, including thickening, pitting, or discoloration, are common and highly correlated with the severity of the arthropathy. These patients' serum is negative for RF and shows HLA B27 positivity in 25%–60% of the cases, usually in the patients with spondyloarthropathy.

The characteristic distribution of psoriatic arthritis involves the small joints of the hands and feet, with or without a spondyloarthropathy. In the hand, tuft resorption and DIP erosive disease are usually seen early and involvement tends to be more severe in the DIPs than in the PIP or MCP joints. This pattern helps to differentiate psoriatic arthritis from RA. In addition, asymmetric involvement is far more common in psoriatic than in RA.

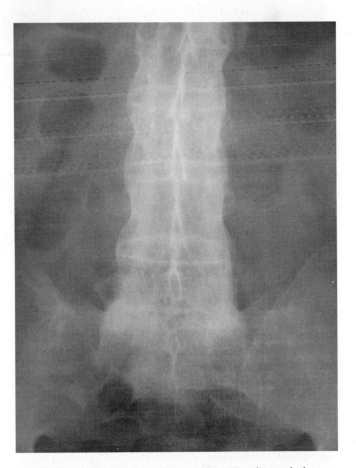

Fig. 2-30   Ankylosing spondylitis, spine. AP radiograph demonstrates advanced ankylosing spondylitis, with complete fusion of the SI joints as well as fusion of the lumbar vertebral bodies. The thin vertical syndesmophytes seen at all levels of the lumbar spine outline the relatively dense endplates, giving the spine its "bamboo" appearance.

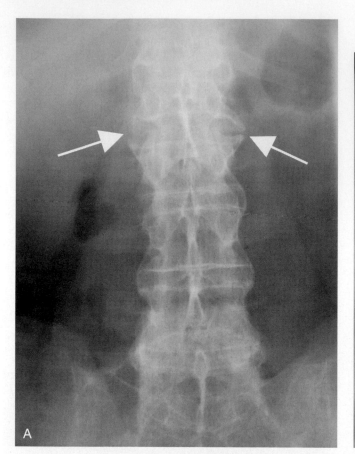

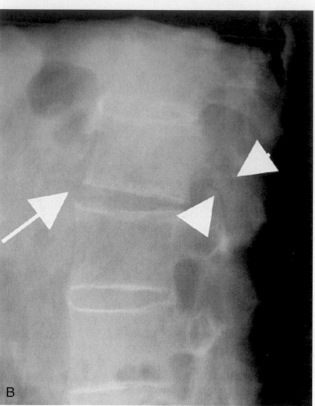

Fig. 2-31   Ankylosing spondylitis, pseudarthrosis. **A,** An AP radiograph of the lumbar spine in a patient with ankylosing spondylitis, showing the advanced disease with fused SI joints and the "bamboo" appearance of the spine. However, there is interruption in the bamboo spine at the level of L1–2, with fractures of the syndesmophytes (*arrows*). **B,** The lateral view at the same level demonstrates the thin syndesmophytes at all levels except the L1–2 site (*arrow*), where there is gapping and instability. A very subtle fracture is seen through the pars intra-articularis (*arrowheads*), completing the fracture across this disk space level. Pseudarthroses such as this are seen typically at the cervicothoracic or thoracolumbar junctions, and may be very subtle to detect radiographically.

The erosions seen in these joints begin marginally, as in RA, but often progress to severe subchondral erosions, occasionally resulting in pencil-in-cup deformity (Fig. 2-33). Once severe erosive change has developed, the clinical "telescoping" of the joint can be observed. Although erosive changes predominate, bone productive changes are usually seen, frequently in the form of subtle bone excrescences at and around the joint. Unlike RA, subchondral cysts are not commonly seen.

Other features that serve to differentiate psoriatic arthritis from RA are the character of the soft tissue swelling, which in psoriatic arthritis may be either fusiform around a joint or may involve the entire digit (sausage digit). In addition, periosteal reaction is often seen in the phalanges (Fig. 2-34). Such periostitis is not seen in patients with RA, except in the very youngest patients with JRA. Ankylosis is common in the hands and feet

of patients with psoriatic arthritis, a feature that also differentiates this disease from RA. In addition, the bone density is generally normal in psoriatic arthritis and the joint distribution in the hands is distal and asymmetric.

The wrists are not as frequently involved in psoriatic arthritis as in RA; if there is wrist involvement, any compartment may be abnormal and, as with the hands, symmetry is far less common in psoriatic than in RA. In the foot, IP and MTP erosive disease is common. A retrocalcaneal bursitis with erosions at the site of the Achilles tendon may be seen, indistinguishable from that in RA or Reiter's disease. Large joint involvement (ankle, knee, hip, shoulder) is much less common, but does occur. If large joints are affected, the distal small joints are almost invariably involved as well.

When present, the character of the sacroiliitis seen in these patients follows the same pattern as that seen in

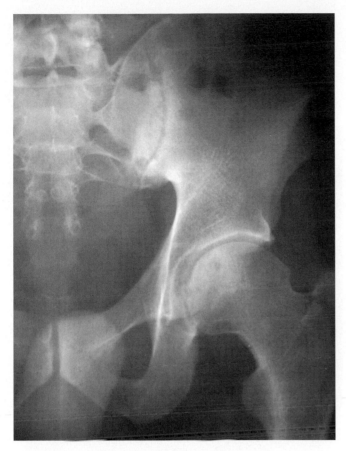

Fig. 2-32   Ankylosing spondylitis, hip. Large joint involvement is typical in the appendicular skeleton with ankylosing spondylitis. This 25-year-old man has degenerative type changes of the right hip, with osteophytes and subchondral cyst formation in the femoral head. Such degenerative change is distinctly unusual in a 25-year-old, but a glance at the SI joint demonstrates erosive change with sclerosis, confirming the diagnosis of ankylosing spondylitis.

AS, with cortical indistinctness, erosions, widening, sclerosis, and eventually, fusion. However, involvement of the SI joints is usually asymmetric (Fig. 2-35). Although sacroiliitis is usually adequately assessed with radiographs, occasionally cross-section imaging is used. One study showed the combination of T1- and T2-weighted MR images to be more accurate than CT[1] in the detection of early joint inflammation, whereas another showed gadolinium enhancement to be particularly helpful in demonstrating abnormalities in patients with clinically inflamed joints who had normal radiographic and precontrast MR imaging.[2]

The thoracolumbar spine involvement in psoriatic arthritis usually appears quite distinct from that of AS, with bulky asymmetric osteophytes rather than delicate syndesmophytes (Fig. 2-35). These generally start in the thoracolumbar junction region, usually skip levels, and show asymmetry in the size of osteophyte formation. The axial involvement seen in psoriatic arthritis is indistinguishable from Reiter's disease.

Key Concepts	**Psoriatic Arthritis**

- It is an asymmetric erosive arthropathy, with superimposed bone productive changes.
- The DIP joints are most commonly involved, followed by PIP and MCPs.
- Erosions may be spectacularly destructive, resulting in a pencil-in-cup deformity.
- Periostitis and "sausage digit" may help distinguish psoriatic from RA.
- Bone density is generally normal.
- Distal phalanges may show either tuft resorption or reactive sclerosis (ivory phalanx).
- Sacroiliitis may be bilateral but is usually asymmetric.
- Bulky asymmetric osteophytes in spine usually starting at the thoracolumbar junction and noncontiguous.
- Arthropathy may antedate skin changes.

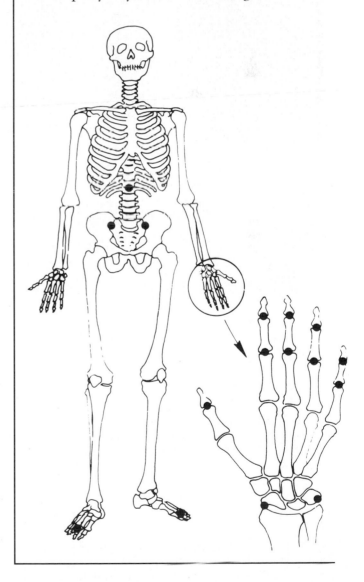

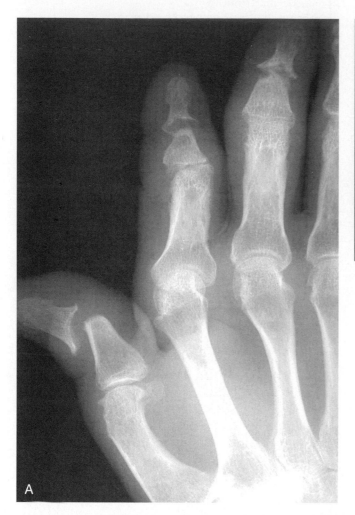

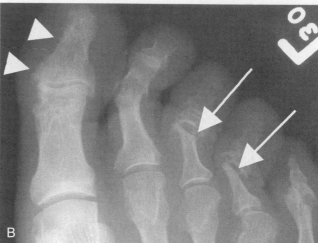

Fig. 2-33   Psoriatic arthritis. **A,** An AP radiograph of the hand showing advanced psoriatic arthritis changes, with so much destruction at the DIP joints of digits 1, 2, and 3 that they have developed a "pencil-in-cup" appearance. This appearance is mimicked in a second patient **B** showing not only the "pencil-in-cup" appearance of the third and fourth PIP joints (*arrows*), but also the periostitis at the distal phalanx of the great toe (*arrowheads*). (Figure 2-33A reprinted with permission of the ACR learning file.)

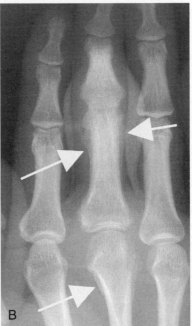

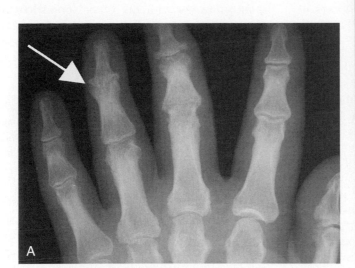

Fig. 2-34   Psoriatic arthritis. **A,** A PA view of the hand demonstrating predominantely DIP disease, with fusion at the fourth DIP (*arrow*). Note also the subtle periostitis at the base of the proximal phalanx of the third and fourth digits. Fusion and periostitis are hallmarks of psoriatic arthritis. (Figure 2-34A reprinted with permission of the ACR learning file.) **B,** A PA radiograph of the hand in a different patient with psoriatic arthritis, demonstrating the swelling in the form of a "sausage digit" in the third ray, with prominent periostitis along the metacarpal and proximal phalanx of the third ray (*arrows*).

The diagnosis of psoriatic arthritis can occasionally be difficult. Early psoriatic arthritis is occasionally indistinguishable from RA, but the involvement of DIP joints in psoriatic arthritis usually leads to the correct diagnosis. Any periostitis serves to differentiate the two. Adult Still's disease, with its DIP distribution, may be indistinguishable from psoriatic arthritis. Erosive osteoarthritis is potentially confusing with psoriatic arthritis because of the DIP erosions. However, erosive osteoarthritis usually has abnormalities in the first carpal-metacarpal joint or the scaphoid-trapezium-trapazoid joints; the carpal distribution is a reliable distinguishing factor between erosive

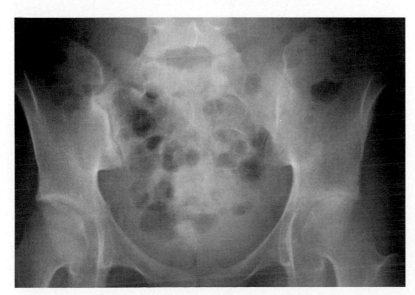

Fig. 2-35   Psoriatic arthritis. AP radiograph of the pelvis in this 17-year-old female demonstrates an erosive process involving the left hip and unilateral sacroiliitis, with prominent sclerosis seen in the right SI joint. Note that the spondyloarthropathy seen in psoriatic arthritis tends to have unilateral, or at least asymmetric, involvement of the SI joints. (Reprinted with permission of the ACR learning file.)

osteoarthritis and psoriatic arthritis. Finally, the spondyloarthropathy of psoriatic arthritis is indistinguishable from that of Reiter's disease. In these cases, the peripheral distribution must be relied upon, with foot disease being found more prominently in Reiter's and hand disease in psoriatic. The asymmetry of the SI joint disease in psoriatic and Reiter's usually distinguishes them from AS/IBD. The spine disease is more clearly different, as is the small joint distribution.

SAPHO (synovitis, acne, pustulosis, hyperostosis, osteitis) is likely an uncommon form of spondyloarthropathy in which patients can have various osteoarticular manifestations, the most common being osteitis of the anterior chest wall. This is seen as hyperostosis and soft tissue ossification between the medial clavicle, anterior portion of the upper ribs, and manubrium. In addition to the anterior chest wall, the axial skeleton may be involved and, rarely, extra-axial tumor-simulating bone lesions are seen. Pustulosis, psoriatic lesions, and spondyloarthropathy may also be seen. The variety of manifestations exhibited by psoriatic arthritis leads to confusion resulting in several other names being applied to this process.

REITER'S DISEASE

Reiter's disease is a syndrome consisting of the triad of arthritis, urethritis (cervicitis in females), and conjunctivitis. Reiter's disease is usually seen in young adults. Males are affected much more commonly than females. Clinical signs of the arthropathy include low back pain and polyarticular arthritis, particularly with heel pain predominating. As with the other spondyloarthropathies, patients with Reiter's disease are rheumatoid factor negative and have a high positivity rate of HLA B27 (80%). Reiter's disease is far less common than either AS or psoriatic spondyloarthropathy.

The spondyloarthropathy seen in Reiter's disease is identical to that seen in psoriatic arthritis (Fig. 2-36). This consists of sacroiliitis, which may be unilateral, but if bilateral is asymmetric in appearance. Bulky asymmetric osteophytes are seen in the thorocolumbar spine, often with skip areas, and are better seen on AP than on lateral radiographs.

Although the spondyloarthropathy of Reiter's is indistinguishable from that of psoriatic arthritis, the distribution of acral disease is the distinguishing feature. In Reiter's disease the distribution predominates in the distal lower extremity, particularly the MTP joints, calcaneus, ankle, and knee (Fig. 2-37). Although the distribution of acral arthropathy is different than that of psoriatic, the radiographic appearance is similar. Soft-tissue swelling may be fusiform about the involved joint, but may also give the appearance of a sausage digit. Involved digits may show periostitis. Erosive changes predominate, but

---

Key Concepts **Reiter's Disease**

- It is the least common spondyloarthropathy.
- Males are far more frequently affected than females.
- Spondyloarthropathy identical to that of psoriatic arthritis but with acral involvement usually in the lower extremity.
- Calcaneal erosive disease and spur formation are prominent features.
- Usually exhibits bilaterally asymmetric sacroiliitis.
- Bulky asymmetric syndesmophytes in the thorocolumbar spine, with skip areas.

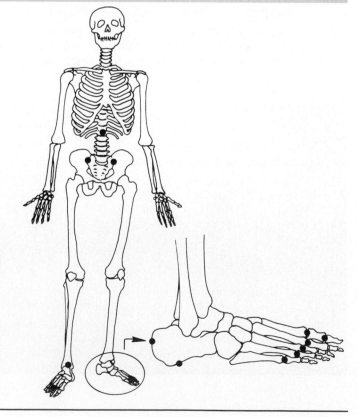

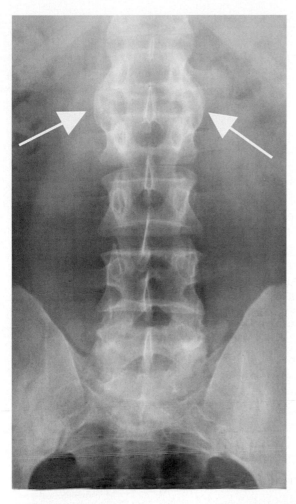

Fig. 2-36   Reiter's disease. AP radiograph of the lumbar spine demonstrates bilateral but somewhat asymmetric sacroiliitis, along with bulky syndesmophytes involving only the L1 - 2 level (*arrows*). This patient also had calcaneal erosive disease. Reiter's and psoriatic arthritis have an identical appearing spondyloarthropathy, with asymmetric sacroiliitis and bulky asymmetric syndesmophytes.

may be seen in conjunction with mild productive bony changes. Retrocalcaneal bursitis is particularly common, along with prominent enthesitis at the Achilles tendon and plantar aponeurosis origin.

CONNECTIVE TISSUE DISORDERS

Systemic Lupus Erythematosus (SLE)

SLE is an immunologic abnormality that produces severe and widely varied tissue injury. The musculoskeletal system is most commonly involved with a polyarthritis that is generally nonerosive but often deforming. Surprisingly, despite the destructive processes seen radiographically, the clinical musculoskeletal symptoms are mild.

Key Concepts	**SLE**

- It is a nonerosive but deforming arthropathy.
- The hands and wrists are commonly involved.
- Avascular necrosis, particularly in unusual sites, is common.
- There is occasional soft tissue calcification, particularly in the lower extremity.

There is a distinct gender distribution, with females more commonly affected than males (5 : 1 - 10 : 1). In addition, African-American patients are more commonly affected than Caucasians. The disease is usually manifested in young adults.

The patients present clinically with a typical skin rash, myositis, various neurologic abnormalities, pulmonary vasculitis, pulmonary fibrosis, pleural effusions, pericarditis, cardiomyopathy, and nephritis. The lupus erythematosus cell prep is positive, antinuclear antibody (ANA) is positive, and rheumatoid factor may be falsely positive.

The joints most frequently affected are those of the hand and wrist, although the foot may show similar abnormalities. These joints show classic deformities of ligamentous laxity, including reducible ulnar subluxation of the MCPs and of the first carpal-metacarpal joint, and variable flexion or extension deformities of the IP joints. A prominent feature of these deformities is their reducibility. Because of this feature, the deformities are more prominent when the hands are unsupported by the film cassette while being radiographed; this results in the deformities appearing much more severe on the oblique ball catcher's view than on the PA view (Fig. 2-38). The disease is usually nonerosive. This feature helps to distinguish RA from SLE, as the deformities are similar in appearance.

Subcutaneous calcifications are seen in approximately 10% of patients with SLE, usually in the lower extremities. This incidence is much less frequent than in dermatomyositis, but can lead to some diagnostic confusion.

Another radiographic feature of SLE is the remarkably high incidence of osteonecrosis. Up to one third of patients with SLE may show avascular necrosis (AVN) by MR imaging, although only 8% are symptomatic.[3] Steroid therapy is felt to be the major etiologic factor, but the disease process itself also predisposes to AVN. The femoral head, humeral head, and knee are common sites (Fig. 2-39). AVN found in unusual sites such as the talus should suggest an underlying diagnosis of SLE.

Progressive Systemic Sclerosis (PSS): Scleroderma

Scleroderma is a condition of unknown etiology that causes small vessel disease and fibrosis in several organ

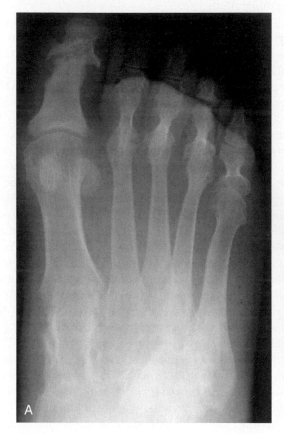

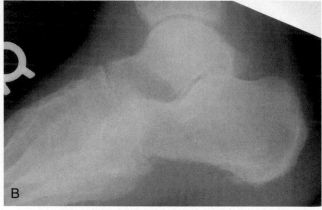

Fig. 2-37   Reiter's disease. **A,** An AP radiograph of the foot in a 50-year-old male. It demonstrates fusion of the intertarsal joints and tarsal metatarsal joints, fusion of MTPs 2–4, swelling of the great toe with periostitis and prominent erosive change at the IP joint. The lateral view **B,** demonstrates mild erosions at the posterior calcaneus and enthesopathy at the plantar aponeurosis. Acral disease in Reiter's tends to involve the foot and ankle.

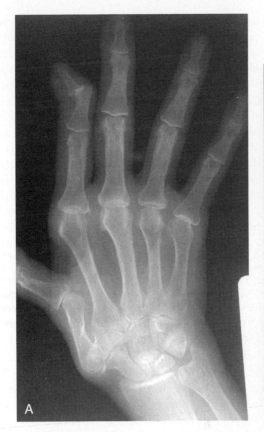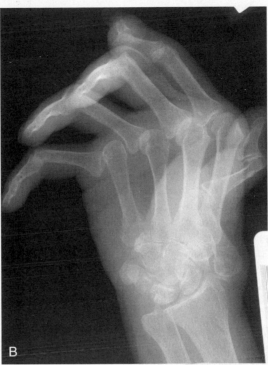

Fig. 2-38   SLE. **A,** PA and **B,** ball catcher's views in a patient with SLE demonstrate a patient with severe subluxation, which worsens when the hand is not supported on the cassette, as in the ball catcher's view. The process is predominately nonerosive. The findings are typical of the nonerosive but deforming arthropathy of SLE.

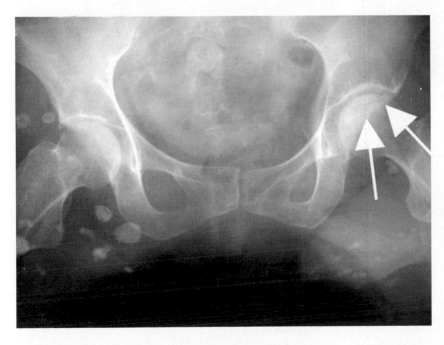

Fig. 2-39   SLE. The frog-leg pelvis radiograph demonstrates prominent soft tissue calcification, as well as a subchondral fracture and flattening indicating avascular necrosis of the left hip (*arrow*). This patient is known to have SLE, and it is not at all uncommon to develop avascular necrosis with this disease process and the associated steroid use. Soft tissue calcification is uncommon but well described in patients with SLE. (Reprinted with permission of the ACR learning file.)

Key Concepts Scleroderma

- It is a multisystem disease.
- There is acral soft tissue atrophy.
- There is acro-osteolysis.
- There is soft tissue calcification.
- Erosions occur, but arthritis is not a prominent feature.

systems, with scleroderma being the cutaneous manifestation of the disease. Scleroderma affects females more frequently than males, in a 3 : 1 ratio, and is most often diagnosed in the third to fifth decade of life. Laboratory tests are not specific, with an increased ESR and ANA in most patients but rheumatoid factor positive in up to 40%.

Patients with scleroderma may present with Raynaud's phenomenon, skin changes on the hands, feet, or face, distal joint pain and stiffness, dysphagia, and proximal myopathy. Esophageal atrophy and fibrosis lead to dismotility and reflux stricture, which may be noted as air

fluid levels within the esophagus on a chest film. The dismotility, as well as pseudosacculations of the colon, are seen with barium studies. The myopathy may be identified on MRI exam, although it is nonspecific.

Soft tissue abnormalities are extremely common, seen clinically at first as edema but eventually resulting in taut, shiny, and atrophic soft tissues with progressive distal phalangeal tapering. Radiographically, the acral (distal) tapering of the digits is seen both in the soft tissues and distal phalanges (Fig. 2-40). This acro-osteolysis may be seen in up to 80% of patients.[4] Acro-osteolysis is nonspecific, as it may be seen in several other disorders (Table 2-1). Resorption of bone, although most commonly seen in the phalangeal tufts, may also be severe at the first carpal-metacarpal joint, resulting in radial subluxation of the first metacarpal. This feature is thought to be distinctive for scleroderma. Resorption can also be seen at the angle of the mandible and at the posterior ribs, particularly rib number 3–6.

Other than acral resorption, the other distinctive radiographic feature in scleroderma is that of soft tissue calcification. Calcification is seen in 25% of cases,[4] and may be subcutaneous, extra-articular, intra-articular, or even in a punctate pattern within the terminal phalanx (Fig. 2-40). However, soft tissue calcification in conjunction with acro-osteolysis is not distinctive for scleroderma (See Tables 2-1 and 2-2, and Figs. 2-41 to 2-43).

Although acro-osteolysis and soft tissue calcification are the most frequent features of scleroderma, cartilage destruction and erosive changes are occasionally seen. It may be difficult to attribute erosive change only to

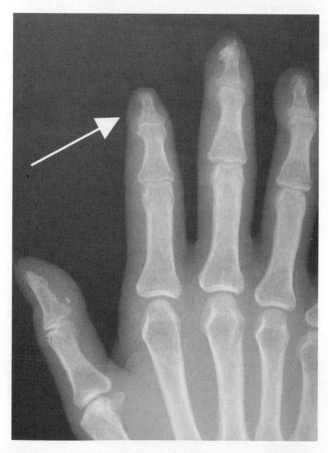

Fig. 2-40   Scleroderma. PA radiograph of the hand demonstrates the tapering of the fingers of digits 2 and 3, with acro-osteolysis seen at digit 2 (*arrow*). Soft-tissue calcification is seen both at the thumb and digit 3. This combination is typical for scleroderma. (Reprinted with permission of the ACR learning file.)

Table 2-1   Acro-osteolysis

1. Thermal injury
   a. burn: may have contracture and soft tissue calcifications (Fig. 2-41)
   b. frostbite: usually spares the thumb (Fig. 2-42)
2. Environmental: polyvinylchloride (PVC)
3. Metabolic
   a. hyperparathyroidism: tuft resorption, often accompanied by other signs of subperiosteal resorption, vascular calcification, or Brown tumors
   b. Lesch-Nyhan disease
4. Arthritis
   a. psoriatic: there should be associated DIP erosive disease
   b. neuroarthropathy, especially diabetic
5. Connective tissue disease
   a. scleroderma: often associated with soft tissue calcification
   b. other causes of vasculitis
6. Infection: leprosy, associated with linear calcifications of the digital nerve (Fig. 2-43)
7. Congenital
   a. pyknodysostosis: associated with dense bones and transverse fractures
   b. Hajdu-Cheney
   c. epidermolysis bullosa

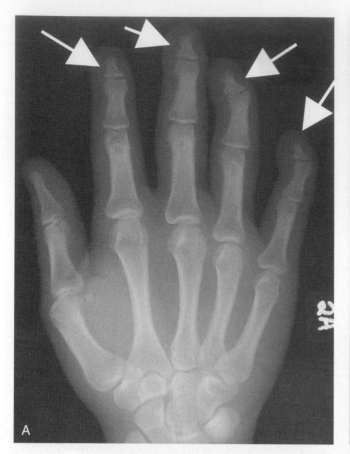 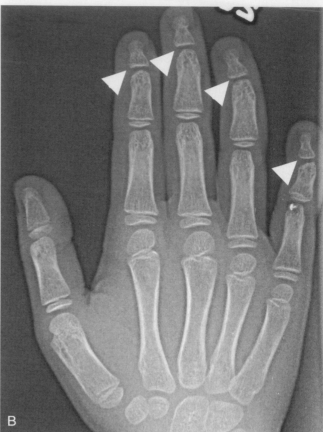

Fig. 2-42   Acro-osteolysis: frostbite. **A,** A PA radiograph of the hand in an adult who had frostbite. Note the short distal phalanges of digits 2 through 5 (*arrows*). The acro-osteolysis in this case results in shortening rather than tapering of the distal phalanges. Note also that the thumb is normal in size and morphology. This is typical of frostbite, since the thumb is usually protected by the cupped hand when one is cold. (Reprinted with permission of the ACR learning file.) **B,** A different patient, a 7-year-old child, who has suffered frostbite. Note that the growth centers of the distal phalanges of digits 2–5 are absent (*arrowheads*) whereas that at the thumb is normal. The growth centers are most at risk for thermal injury, and this patient's distal phalanges will not grow further.

with dermatomyositis a typical diffuse rash is an additional finding.

Polymyositis and dermatomyositis usually are noted in the third through fifth decades, and females are more frequently affected than males. Dermatomyositis may also be seen in children, associated with very severe systemic symptoms. Patients with this disease show muscle weakness and tenderness with eventual contracture and atrophy. The muscles involved are usually proximal girdle muscles. Early in the disease, the muscles develop edema, followed later by atrophy and calcification (Fig. 2-44). The early muscle disease may be identified on MR imaging with edema-like signal intensity in muscle, seen best with T2 fat saturated or inversion recovery sequences. The calcification of course may be seen on radiographs. The most common calcification pattern is a nonspecific subcutaneous calcification. "Sheetlike" calcification along fascial or muscle planes is less common but is thought to be pathognomonic for the disease. Classically, this

sheetlike calcification is seen in the proximal large muscles. Occasionally, periarticular calcification may also occur.

Although the hands, wrists, and knees are affected with arthralgias, radiographic abnormalities are rare. However, as these patients are treated with steroids, they may develop AVN as a complication of therapy.

AMYLOIDOSIS

Amyloidosis is a systemic deposition disease that may be either primary or secondary. The secondary form may be associated with multiple myeloma, long-term hemodialysis, RA, familial Mediterranean fever, chronic infection, spondyloarthropathy, and connective tissue disorders such as SLE, scleroderma, and dermatomyositis. Amyloid deposition can result in kidney disease, organomegally, pericardial and myocardial disease, pulmonary

Key Concepts **Amyloidosis**

- It may be primary or secondary (associated with multiple myeloma, long-term hemodialysis, rheumatoid arthritis).
- Exhibit bulky nodular synovitis.
- Shows well-marginated erosions.
- Wrist, elbow, and shoulder are most commonly involved.
- Cervical spine is involved in the spondyloarthropathy of hemodialysis.

septal infiltration, and GI tract involvement with submucosal thickening and decreased peristalsis. Five percent to 13% of patients with amyloidosis have bone or joint involvement, consisting of deposition in bone, synovium, and surrounding soft tissues. The soft-tissue deposition results in the formation of bulky nodules, seen particularly about the wrists, elbows, and shoulders. The "shoulder pad" sign has been attributed to amyloidosis, where bulky nodules are superimposed on atrophic musculature. MRI of the nodules shows a signal intensity intermediate between fibrocartilage and muscle on all sequences.[5] The MRI findings may help to distinguish amyloid deposits from cellular or water-containing processes such as inflammation or synovitis (Fig. 2-45).

Intra-articular amyloid deposits result in joint space widening due to infiltration, and later narrowing due to cartilage destruction. Erosions and subchondral cysts tend to be sharply marginated (Fig. 2-46). The joints most commonly involved are the wrists, elbow, and shoulder. Knees and hips are less commonly involved with amyloidosis. In patients on chronic hemodialysis, the spine, wrist, and hands are most commonly affected. In hemodialysis patients, spondyloarthropathy often occurs in the cervical spine with the appearance of disk space narrowing and end plate irregularity (Fig. 2-47), which can mimic vertebral disk space infection. The absence of a paravertebral soft-tissue mass and clinical signs of infection should help make the correct diagnosis.[6]

With the nodularity of the soft tissues and the erosive change particularly of the hands and wrist, amyloidosis is most frequently confused with RA. The presence of well-defined erosions and frequent preservation of joint space width in amyloidosis may help to differentiate the two. In addition, if the patient is known to have a predisposing factor such as multiple myeloma, the correct diagnosis is more frequently attained.

OSTEOARTHRITIS

Osteoarthritis (OA) is a degenerative joint disease of obscure etiology stimulated by either abnormal mechanical forces on the joint (joint deformity, obesity, occupational stresses), normal forces on abnormal cartilage (due to pre-existing arthritis such as RA, loose bodies, osteochondral fracture, or meniscal abnormalities), or collapse of subchondral bone (secondary to osteoporosis, AVN, or hyperparathyroidism). OA is the most common arthritis and affects males and females equally, with incidence increasing with age.

The clinical signs are of pain with weight bearing, limited range of motion, crepitus, and subluxation. The radiographic severity of disease does not always correlate with the amount of pain.

The radiographic manifestations include cartilage destruction in the weight bearing portions of the joint, lack of erosions, and bone productive change. Bone production consists of osteophyte formation, which may be marginated or central. Productive change is also seen as subchondral sclerosis and cortical buttressing, which is a response to abnormal mechanical forces and is seen particularly well on the medial and lateral aspects of the femoral neck. Bone density is normal in osteoarthritis. Subchondral cysts are common due to microfractures in the subchondral bone and synovial fluid pressure. The cysts tend to occur in weight bearing areas and generally have a sclerotic margin. Traction enthesophytes are an-

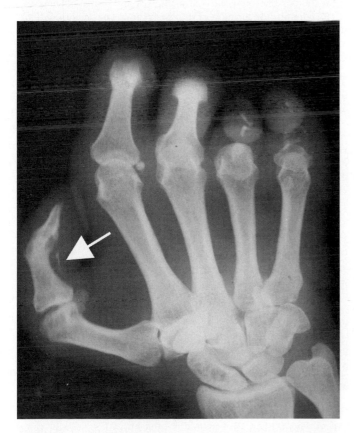

Fig. 2-43 Acro-osteolysis: leprosy. This patient has tremendous acro-osteolysis, involving all the digits, and has the added feature of a calcified digital nerve (*arrow*). This is a feature that is typical of leprosy.

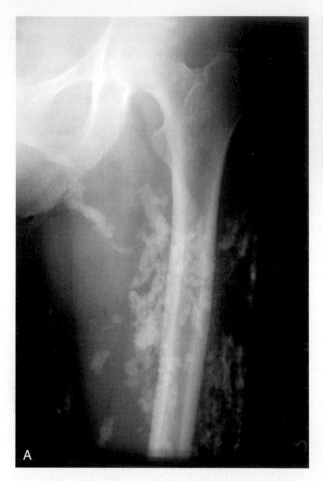

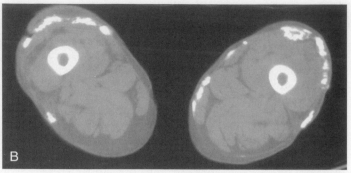

Fig. 2-44 Dermatomyositis. **A,** The AP radiograph demonstrates sheet-like calcifications in the soft tissues of the thigh of this 50-year-old female. The CT (**B**) confirms the location of the calcifications to be both within the muscle and fascial planes. Sheetlike calcifications are typically described with dermatomyositis, but the calcifications may assume other configurations. (Reprinted with permission of the ACR learning file.)

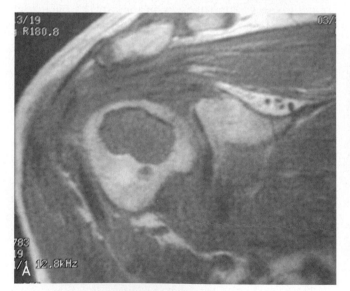

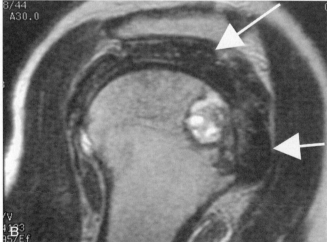

Fig. 2-45 Amyloid. **A,** A coronal T1-weighted (783/19) MR image of an amyloid deposit within the right humeral head. Its signal intensity is that of muscle. **B,** The T2-weighted sagittal image (4133/95) demonstrates the large erosion to have heterogeneous signal with areas of low signal intensity. In addition, note the thickened low signal supraspinatus and subscapularis tendons, which had amyloid deposits as well (*arrows*).

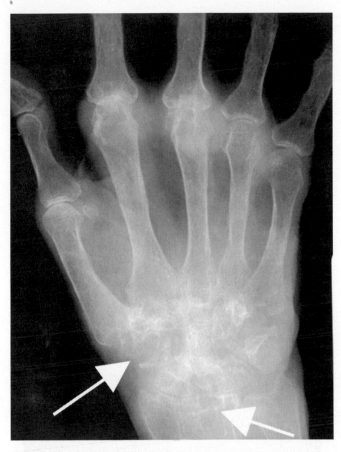

Fig. 2-46 Amyloid. PA radiograph of the hand demonstrates soft tissue swelling of the MCP joints and very prominent and well-defined erosions in the carpal bones (*arrows*). When bones are involved with amyloid, the erosions tend to be well defined. This is a patient who had multiple myeloma, with secondary amyloidosis.

other common productive process, relating to shifts in biomechanical loading, seen particularly on the anterior aspect of the patella and at the hip and pelvic apophyses. This enthesopathy is not distinguishable from that seen in AS and the other rheumatoid variants. Ankylosis is rare in the absence of trauma. Ligamentous abnormalities are commonly seen in OA. Focal cartilage loss leads to joint deformity, which in turn promotes ligamentous contractions and laxity. This ligamentous abnormality in turn promotes further arthropathy because of shifts in mechanical loading and further wear.

Primary OA most frequently involves the hand, wrist, acromioclavicular joint, hip, knee, foot, and spine. Within each of these, specific sites of involvement are expected for OA. Thus, location as well as the purely productive nature of the process helps to secure the diagnosis.

In the hand, several interphalangeal joints are often involved with uniform cartilage narrowing, subchondral sclerosis, and osteophyte formation. The MCPs are less commonly involved than the IPs, and virtually never are involved in the absence of findings of OA in the IP joints.

The diagnosis of OA in the hand can be substantiated by typical findings of sclerosis, osteophyte formation, and cartilage loss in the first carpometacarpal joint. The second most common site of involvement in the wrist is the scaphoid-trapezium-trapazoid complex (STT) (Fig. 2-48). Osteoarthritis involving the radiocarpal or distal radioulnar joint is extremely uncommon in the absence of trauma (as might be found, for example, in a patient with malunion of a scaphoid fracture or with ulnar plus variant resulting in ulnar impaction syndrome (Fig. 2-49).

The acromioclavicular joint frequently shows typical changes of OA. On the other hand, OA is unusual in the glenohumeral joint in the absence of previous trauma. When OA is present in the glenohumeral joint, the marginal osteophytes form around the glenoid and ring osteophytes form around the anatomic neck of the humerus, with the largest found inferiorly. Chronic rotator cuff tear and shoulder instability may predispose to OA of the glenohumeral joint.

The hip is an extremely common site of OA. Early signs include subchondral cyst formation in the acetabulum (termed Eggar's cyst) and calcar buttressing (Fig. 2-50).

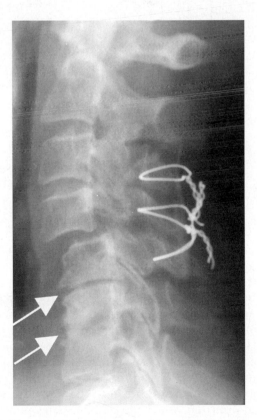

Fig. 2-47 Spondyloarthropathy of hemodialysis. This patient who was on hemodialysis developed neck pain and collapse, with the lateral radiograph demonstrating endplate and disk space abnormalities at both C5-6 and C5-7 (*arrows*). While disk space infection might be suspected in this patient, the circumstances also suggest the possibility of disk space deposition disease, often involving amyloid.

Key Concepts   Osteoarthritis

- Exhibits purely productive changes, including osteophyte formation, sclerosis, and normal bone density.
- Hip, knee (medial compartment), spine, and hand (DIP, first CMC, STT) are most common locations.
- EOA shows mixed productive and erosive changes of the IP joints, and is confirmed as the diagnosis if disease is seen at the CMC or STT joints.

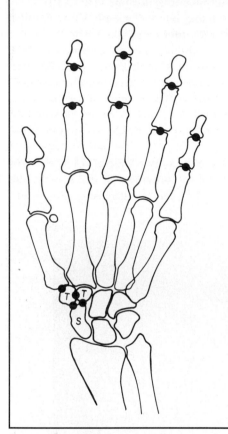

Later changes show typical signs of focal cartilage narrowing in the superior weight bearing portion, sclerosis, and osteophyte formation. Osteophytes are seen ringing the subcapital femoral neck, but can be particularly prominent medially. In 80% of patients, the hip migrates superolaterally (Fig. 2-51A). However, in 20% of patients with OA, the hip migrates in a medial direction. This may result in protrusio. RA also results in protrusion, and it is important not to confuse the two. OA is such a common disease, that it should not be surprising to find a hip in protrusio, which also demonstrates purely productive changes (Figure 2–51B). OA of the hip occasionally is reminiscent of other disease processes. If a late case of OA presents with particularly large inferomedial osteophytes at the femoral head, it may simulate superior flattening of the head and the appearance of avascular necrosis. As AVN itself can eventually develop degenera-

tive joint disease, the differentiation is not always possible. Other considerations in the differential diagnosis of OA of the hip include pseudogout or pigmented villonodular synovitis, particularly if large cysts are present. An early ring osteophyte in the subcapital position in OA may even be difficult to differentiate from an impacted subcapital fracture line. Finally, an unusual variant of OA in the hip is rapidly destructive hip disease (RDHD). This process is seen mostly in elderly females and results in atrophic destructive changes in the femoral head and acetabulum over a few months. The differential diagnosis includes infection and Charcot joint.[7]

The knee is a common site of involvement of OA. It may involve one, two, or all three compartments. If a patient has single compartment disease, it is likely to be the medial, although a patellar tracking abnormality can result in predominately patellofemoral compartment disease. With medial compartment predominance, one sees a typical varus deformity of the knee and lateral subluxation of the tibia. Single compartment disease should be specifically commented on in a report, as treatment may

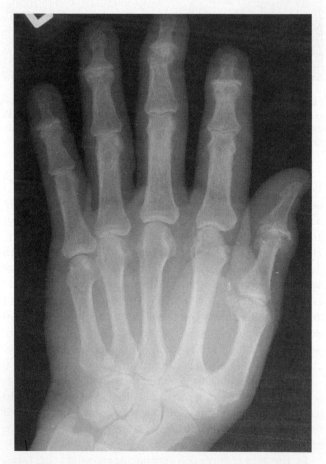

Fig. 2-48 Osteoarthritis: hands. The PA radiograph demonstrates the typical appearance of osteoarthritis, with normal bone density, and loss of cartilage width in the presence of osteophyte formation in the typical locations of the first carpal metacarpal joint and scaphotrapezium trapezoid joint, as well as the DIPs.

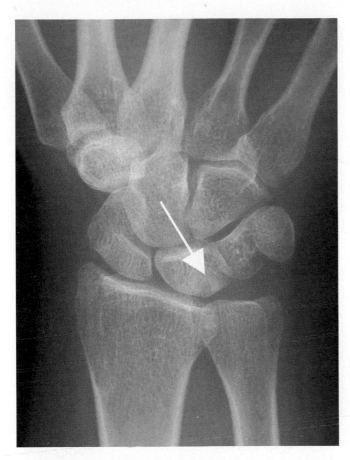

Fig. 2-49 Ulnar impaction syndrome. The PA view of the wrist demonstrates ulnar plus variance, with the lunate showing sclerosis and a subchondral cyst, indicating osteoarthritis secondary to the ulnar impaction.

be with a unicompartmental prosthesis or a high tibial osteotomy. The osteophyte formation in the knee tends to be marginal in all three compartments, as well as on the tibial spines. Enthesopathy is particularly prominent on the nonarticular surface of the patella at the quadriceps insertion. Differential diagnosis of OA of the knee includes pyrophosphate arthropathy or pigmented villonodular synovitis if subchondral cysts are especially prominent. Particularly if patellofemoral disease is prominent, one should consider pseudogout arthropathy and seek the presence of chondralcalcinosis for confirmation.

OA of the axial skeleton is extremely common. The SI joints manifest this disease with subchondral sclerosis and osteophytes, which are usually marginal in nature. Remember that only the inferior two-thirds of the SI joints are synovial and therefore vulnerable to OA. Large osteophytes bridge the joint anteriorly (Fig. 2-52). These bridging osteophytes may be misdiagnosed as focal osteoblastic metastases on a radiograph but should be properly identified as osteophytes based on location. If confirmation is needed, CT shows the bridging osteophytes. OA of the sacroiliac joint should be differentiated from the

early erosive and later sclerotic changes with fusion of ankylosing spondylitis. It also should not be confused with osteitis condensans ilii, which is a triangular sclerotic lesion found on the iliac side of the inferior SI joint, seen most often in multiparous women as a reactive change.

The spine shows several interdependent and coexistent signs of degeneration. These include degenerative disk disease, with decreased disk height and disk vacuum sign by radiograph, and disk herniation seen by CT or MRI. Degenerative disk disease often results in reactive sclerosis of the adjacent endplates, which is termed discogenic sclerosis or idiopathic segmental sclerosis. Discogenic sclerosis is a purely reactive process and the endplate remains intact, in contrast with disk infection, which destroys the adjacent endplates. In addition, the sclerosis of the superior endplate may be distinctive, being triangular shaped in the anterior portion of the vertebral body (Fig. 2-53). This distinctive shape may help distinguish discogenic sclerosis from a blastic metastatic tumor. It should be remembered that disk hernia-

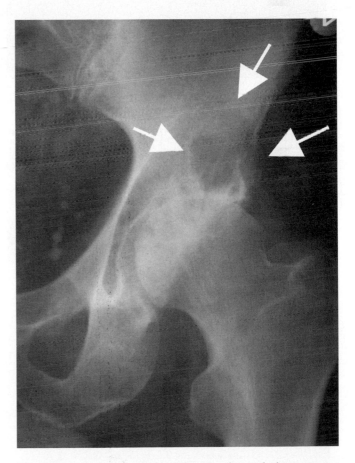

Fig. 2-50 Osteoarthritis: hip. The AP radiograph demonstrates typical OA with loss of cartilage width in the weight-bearing portion of the hip, osteophyte formation, and a large subchondral cyst located in the acetabulum. Cysts in this location have been termed Eggar's cysts (*arrows*).

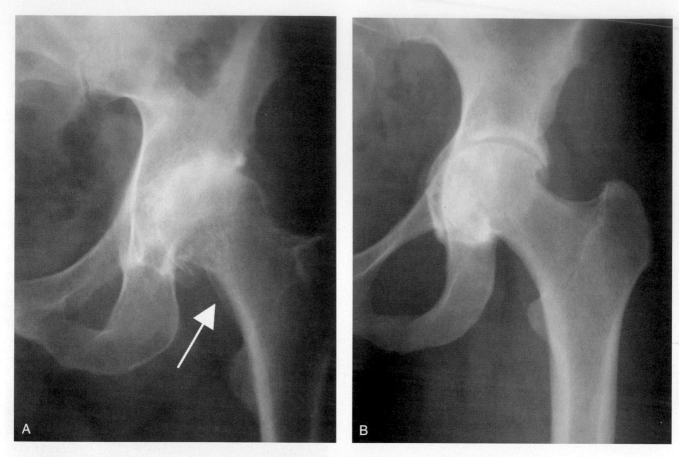

Fig. 2-51   Osteoarthritis: hip. **A,** An AP radiograph of classic appearing OA of the hip, with loss of cartilage width, osteophyte formation, mild superolateral subluxation of the femoral head, and buttressing along the femoral neck and calcar (*arrows*). **B,** An AP radiograph, in a different patient, also demonstrating OA as there are osteophytes present, but this time showing the hip to be moving into a protrusio position. Approximately 20% of patients with OA develop protrusio rather than the more common superolateral subluxation. (Reprinted with permission of the ACR learning file.)

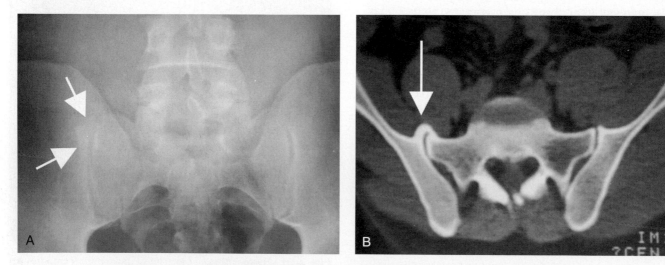

Fig. 2-52   Osteoarthritis: SI joint. **A,** The patchy sclerosis seen at the superior portion of the right SI joint (*arrows*) represents an osteophyte that is bridging over the top of the synovial part of the SI joint. It should not be mistaken for a blastic metastasis. If confirmation is necessary, CT **B,** will show the bridging osteophyte itself (*arrow*). (Reprinted with permission of the ACR learning file).

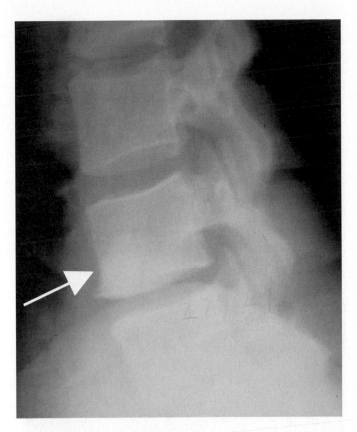

Fig. 2-53 Discogenic sclerosis. This patient shows disk space narrowing at L4–5, with a triangular-shaped sclerosis seen at the inferior endplate at L4 towards its anterior aspect (*arrows*). This appearance of the sclerosis of that seen as a reactive change to degenerative disk disease.

prominent, it can result in a spondylolisthesis of the body, without spondylolysis. This also contributes to foraminal and canal stenosis. OA also affects the cervical uncovertebral joints (also termed joints of Luschka). These joints are found only at C3–7, located posterolaterally at the vertebral bodies. In the cervical spine, these can contribute to neuroforaminal and central stenosis (Fig. 2-55).

Erosive (or inflammatory) osteoarthritis (EOA) is a variant of osteoarthritis. EOA is found primarily in middle aged women who experience distinct inflammatory episodes, similar to those of RA, with swollen, red IP joints. DIP and PIP joints are most frequently involved, with loss of cartilage, sclerosis, and combined erosive and productive bony changes. The erosions on the proximal side of the joint tend to be central and the osteophytes, marginal, which can give a distinctive "gull-wing" appearance (Fig. 2-56). The major differential diagnosis of EOA is psoriatic arthritis. In most cases of EOA, the first carpometacarpal joint and/or STT joints show typical OA changes. This location of carpal involvement is typical for OA and helpful in arriving at the correct diagnosis.

tion is most frequently posterior or posterolateral, but also can occur centrally into an adjacent vertebral body, seen as a Schmorl's node, or anteriorly, resulting in a limbus vertebra if it occurs before skeletal maturation. In a limbus vertebra, the anterior ring apophysis is separated from the underlying vertebral body by the disk herniation, resulting in a separate triangular ossicle, usually located at the anterosuperior border of the vertebral body as seen on the lateral film (Fig. 2-54). This is an incidental finding of no significance and should not be mistaken for fracture.

Another manifestation of degeneration of the spine is spondylosis deformans, resulting from bulging of the annulus fibrosis, stretching of Sharpey's fibers, and traction osteophyte formation on the anterior and lateral vertebral body. True OA involves the apophyseal (facet) joints of the spine. Apophyseal joint OA is seen most commonly at the C5–7, L4–5, and L5–S1 vertebrae. The severity of facet degenerative change is best judged by CT or MRI, with which direct observation of foraminal stenosis can also be made. If the OA of the facets is

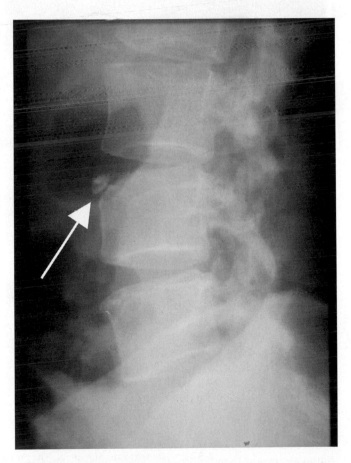

Fig. 2-54 Limbus vertebra. The normal variant limbus vertebra is seen, with a separated triangular fragment from the anterior superior endplate of L4 (*arrows*).

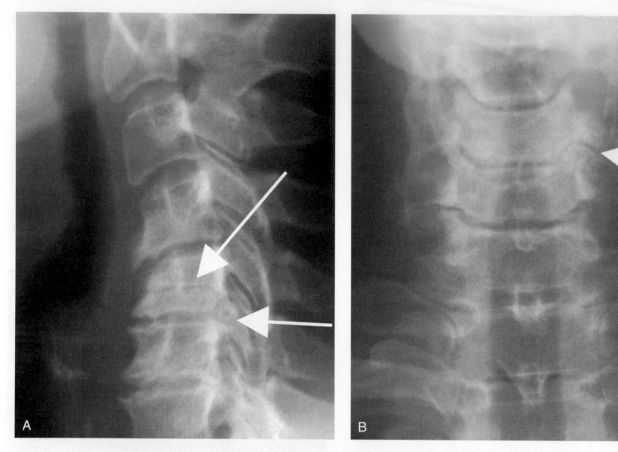

Fig. 2-55   Osteoarthritis: spine. OA is demonstrated in the spine by degenerative change of the facet joints. Spondylosis (anterior productive change at the vertebral bodies), is frequently seen as well. In the cervical spine, the uncovertebral joints also produce osteophytes. **A,** These are seen on the lateral view as posterolateral productive change at the vertebral bodies, and a lucency traversing the vertebral body (*arrows*). **B,** The AP view demonstrates the uncovertebral joints as prominent posterolateral structures which can cause neural foraminal encroachment (*arrows*).

NEUROPATHIC (CHARCOT) ARTHROPATHY

Neuropathic arthropathy is a severely destructive process, usually but not invariably monostotic, and related to one of several possible etiologies. Progression may be extremely rapid. Interestingly, the location of the neuropathic joint usually indicates its specific underlying etiology. The most common etiologies of neuropathic arthropathy are diabetes, tabes dorsalis, syringomyelia, and spinal cord injury. Less frequent etiologies include multiple sclerosis, Charcot-Marie-Tooth disease, alcoholism, amyloidosis, intra-articular steroids, congenital insensitivity to pain, congenital indifference to pain, and dysautonomia (Riley-Day Syndrome). The primary pathogenesis is uncertain, but most investigators agree that there is an initial alteration in sympathetic nerve control of osseous blood flow, which leads to hyperemia and active bone resorption. Secondarily, there seems to be a neurotrau-

Key Concepts | **Neuropathic Arthropathy**

- It is a severe destructive arthropathy.
- It may be hypertrophic or atrophic.
- It invariably has large effusions.
- Exhibits bony debris and fragmentation.
- Exhibits prominent cartilage destruction.
- Erosive and productive changes co-exist.
- Shows ligamentous laxity and joint subluxation or dislocation.
- Charcot feet are usually diabetic.
- Charcot knees may result from tabes dorsalis, diabetes, or congenital insensitivity/indifference to pain.
- Charcot shoulders result from syringomyelia.
- Charcot spines result from diabetes or instrumented spinal trauma in paraplegic patients.

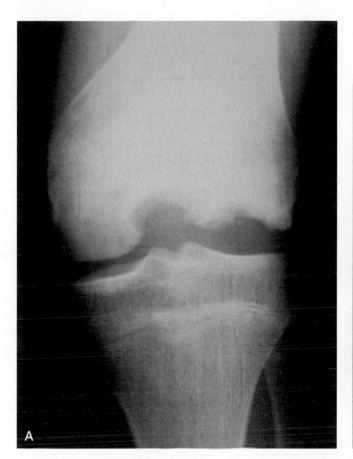
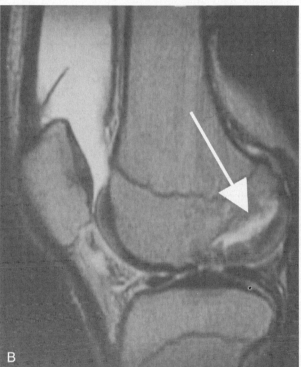

Fig. 2-59   Neuropathic knee. **A,** The AP radiograph shows fragmentation and destruction of the lateral femoral condyle in the knee of this 17-year-old male. There is normal bone density. **B,** The sagittal T2-weighted MRI (2500/80) demonstrates an enormous effusion and the fragmentation in the posterior aspect of the lateral femoral condyle (*arrows*). There is debris present. The constellation of findings are typical for a neuropathic joint. This particular patient had congenital insensitivity to pain.

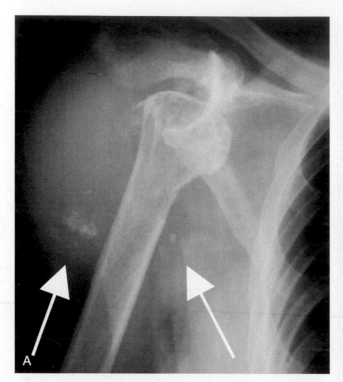

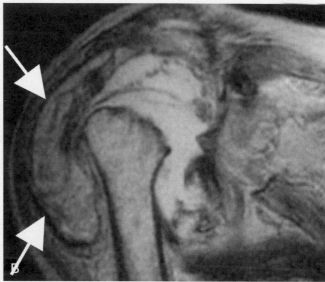

Fig. 2-60   Neuropathic shoulder. The diagnosis should be made on the radiograph in this case. **A,** demonstrates all the elements necessary to make the diagnosis of neuropathic shoulder. The glenohumeral joint is dislocated, there is an enormous effusion, and debris is seen floating in the effusion (*arrows*). If confirmation is needed, MRI demonstrates the entire abnormality, including the debris, to be intra-articular. **B,** A coronal T2-weighted MRI (2550/96) demonstrates the destroyed and dislocated humeral head surrounded by a large joint effusion, with more fluid and debris settling into the distended subdeltoid bursa (*arrows*). With this much destruction and a confirmed intra-articular process, the only logical diagnosis is neuropathic joint. Confirmation of the etiology of syringomyelia would be made with MRI of the cervical spine.

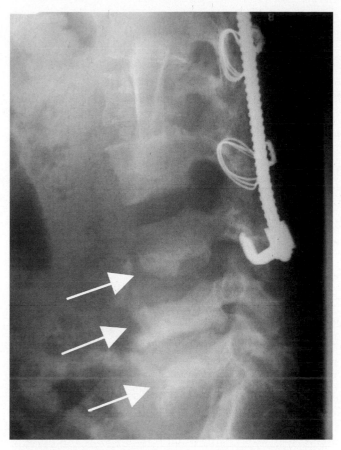

Fig. 2-61   Neuropathic spine. This patient had a burst fracture at the level of L1 and has had an anterior partial corpectomy with strut graft placement and posterior rodding from the levels of T10-L3. He remained paraplegic. Below the level of the solid rodding, the patient shows subluxation and destruction of the vertebral bodies and endplates (L3 inferior endplate, L4, and L5, *arrows*). With this much destruction in a paraplegic patient, neuropathic process must be considered.

BIOCHEMICAL ABNORMALITIES

Gout

Gout is a sodium urate crystal induced synovial inflammation that either may be limited to occasional acute attacks or may be a chronic arthropathy, with crystal deposition in capsular and synovial tissues, periarticular soft tissues, articular cartilage, and subchondral bone. This crystal deposition provokes very specific degenerative changes. Gout may be idiopathic or secondary to enzyme defects of purine metabolism. It also may be found secondary to chronic disease processes such as myeloproliferative disorders, renal disease, hyperparathyroidism, hypoparathyroidism, psoriasis, diuretic therapy, or chronic moonshine ingestion.

Gout typically occurs in middle aged or elderly males and in fact is extremely rare in premenopausal women

| Key Concepts | Gout |

- It is a sodium urate crystal induced arthropathy.
- Occurs usually in middle-aged to elderly males.
- Chronic disease processes may predispose to gout.
- Gouty tophus may show amorphus calcification on radiograph.
- Gouty tophus on MRI is low signal intensity on T1 and variably high or low signal intensity on T2, depending on the amount of calcification present.
- Shows normal bone density.
- Cartilage often is intact.
- Erosions are sharply marginated and may be intraarticular or para-articular.
- The "overhanging" edge of a para-articular erosion is virtually pathognomonic.
- First MTP, DIPs, PIPs, and patella are the most frequent joints involved.

unless there are other predisposing factors as outlined above. Caucasians are more commonly affected than African Americans. Gout is also seen relatively frequently in young Polynesian males. Gouty attacks may occur for several years before radiographic abnormalities appear. A monoarticular or oligoarticular arthropathy with the clinical appearance of red, swollen, extremely painful joints usually results in testing for hyperuricemia or sampling the synovial fluid for sodium urate crystals. Gouty tophi may be seen radiographically as eccentric soft tissue nodules either in a bursa or in the periarticular soft tissues. Gouty tophi often contain subtle amorphous calcification. The patient usually retains normal bone density, and the cartilage often remains intact, even late in the disease process, and even with adjacent erosions. This can be an important discriminating feature. Once erosions occur, they may be intra-articular (often marginal), or para-articular (nonmarginal, often beneath tophi). The para-articular erosions may be pathognomonic for gout and may show the additional feature of an "overhanging edge" (Fig. 2-62). The overhanging edge is a bony excrescence extending out toward the tophus, beyond the normal bony margin. The erosions tend to have a sclerotic margin and productive change may be seen in the form of secondary OA. Subchondral cysts are usually not present, but occasionally may be quite large (Fig. 2-63). Ligamentous laxity is not a common feature.

In general, the lower extremity is more commonly involved with gout than the upper extremity, and small joints more often than large joints. The first MTP is most frequently involved, but other MTPs and IPs as well as the mid and hindfoot may be involved as well. In the knee, the patellofemoral compartment is more frequently involved than either the medial or lateral compartments. The hand and wrist may show involvement in the DIPs, PIPs, and intercarpal joints, with the MCPs less frequently

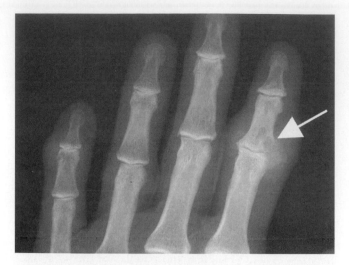

Fig. 2-62 Gout. PA view of the fingers demonstrates a classic appearance of gout, with dense soft-tissue swelling in the tophi seen at both the PIP of the second digit and the DIP of the fifth digit. In addition to the soft tissue tophus, there is a well-defined erosion with a "overhanging edge" at the base of the middle phalanx of the second digit (*arrow*). Overall bone density is normal.

involved. Gout is a relatively easy diagnosis to make when it follows all of the above rules, including being oligoarticular with tophi and discrete, nonmarginal erosions with overhanging edges. However, it may also present as a polyarticular disease, without obvious tophi but with

multiple well-marginated erosions. This appearance in an older male patient should always arouse suspicion for gout, but is often misdiagnosed as RA (Fig. 2-64). Finally, a younger patient with a gouty tophus may be clinically misdiagnosed with neoplasm. If MRI is done on these patients with atypical clinical and radiographic presentation (Fig. 2-65), the tophus demonstrates a low signal intensity on T1 but variably low to high signal itensity on T2, depending on the amount of amorphous calcification present in the tophus. It may even appear inhomogeneous and infiltrative. A gouty tophus usually enhances.[11] It is worthwhile to remember that gout can have a variety of appearances and is relatively common, so should always be kept in mind as a potential diagnosis. Definitive diagnosis is made by inspection of the synovial fluid.

Calcium Pyrophosphate Dihydrate (CPPD) Crystal Deposition Disease (Pyrophosphate Arthropathy)

CPPD crystal deposition disease is common. It is a disorder that results in intra-articular and para-articular crystal deposition, which leads to an associated arthropathy with radiographically distinctive features. The correct terminology for the arthropathy is pyrophosphate arthropathy. However, the clinical presentation of pyrophosphate arthropathy often resembles the intermittent

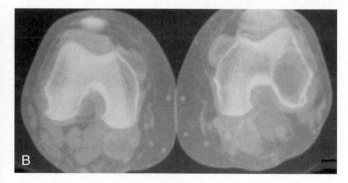

Fig. 2-63 Gout. **A,** An AP radiograph of the knee in a 45-year-old female. Both the radiographic findings and age and gender are unusual for the diagnosis of gout. However, when one sees a very large lytic lesion at a site which could be subchondral, an articular process should be considered. **B,** In this case, CT demonstrates that the patient has bilateral effusions. A bone scan (not shown) showed abnormal uptake in the great toe, a much more typical location for gout. Aspiration showed crystals that confirmed the diagnosis.

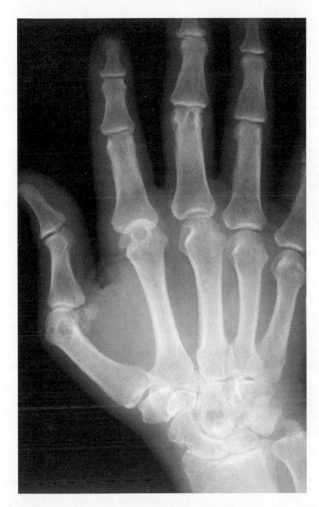

Fig. 2-64   Gout. Gout can occasionally have a pseudorheumatoid distribution. On the PA radiograph of the hand on this 50-year-old male, we see involvement of the radiocarpal joints, intercarpal joints, and MCPs of digits 1–3 as well as the PIP of digit 3. This distribution is characteristic of RA. However, the maintenance of normal bone density and the distinctness of the erosions makes one consider gout as a diagnosis, even in the absence of tophus formation. Aspiration proved gout in this case.

acute attacks of gout, and is more loosely termed "pseudogout." It is important to note that "pseudogout," "chondrocalcinosis," and "pyrophosphate arthropathy" are not synonomous terms. "Pseudogout" can only be used correctly to describe a type of clinical presentation. "Chondrocalcinosis" is the radiographic term for calcified mineral seen in the cartilage, and itself does not imply an arthritis. "Pyrophosphate arthropathy" is the form of arthritis resulting from pyrophosphate crystal deposition, and may or may not have either chondrocalcinosis or a goutlike clinical presentation.

Pyrophosphate arthropathy generally occurs among middle aged patients without gender predelection. It may clinically present as pseudogout (acute self-limited attacks simulating gout or infection), pseudo-RA (more continuous acute attacks simulating RA), pseudo-DJD

(chronic progressive arthropathy but with acute exacerbations), pseudo-DJD without acute exacerbations, pseudoneuropathic arthropathy (rapidly destructive form), or even as an asymptomatic arthropathy.[12] The diagnosis is proven by joint aspiration demonstrating calcium pyrophosphate crystals. There is no associated biochemical abnormality.

Both the radiographic appearance and the location of the arthropathy are quite distinctive. Chondrocalcinosis is generally, although not invariably, found. Chondrocalcinosis may be in either hyaline or fibrocartilage, synovium, and capsule (Figs. 2-66, 2-67). The most common locations for chondrocalcinosis include the triangular fibrocartilage complex of the wrist, lunate-triquetral ligament of the wrist, menisci of the knee, symphysis pubis, and acetabular labrum. In patients with arthropathy, bone density is usually normal. There is uniform cartilage destruction. Although early disease shows erosive change, more advanced disease appears primarily productive with sclerosis, osteochondral fragments, and osteophytes. This appearance resembles OA, but the loca-

Key Concepts	**Pyrophosphate Arthropathy**

- It is a distinctive arthropathy, particularly by its distribution.
- Chondrocalcinosis is usually (although not invariably) present; look at the wrist, knee, and symphysis pubis.
- Exhibits mixed erosive/productive process, with productive features usually predominating.
- In the knee, patellofemoral disease predominates.
- In the wrist, radiocarpal disease predominates and can progress to a SLAC deformity.
- The hand shows specific involvement of the second and third MCPs.
- Large subchondral cysts may be a distinctive feature, occasionally even simulating neoplasm.

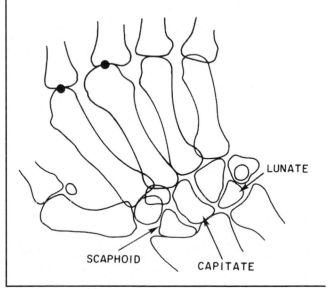

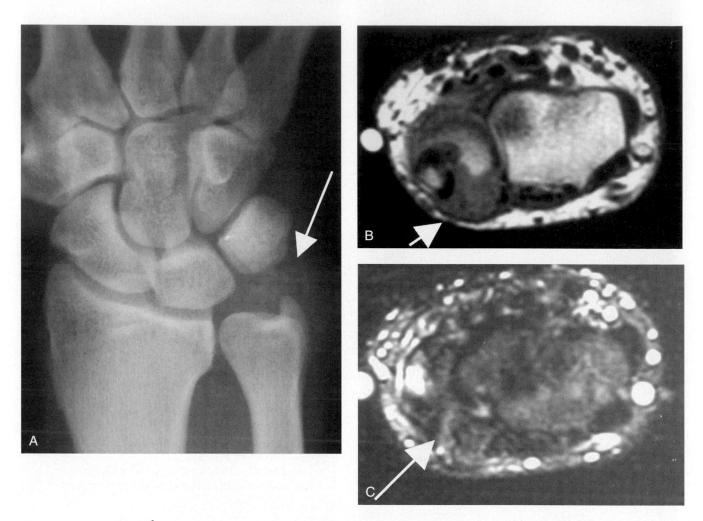

Fig. 2-65   Gout. **A,** The AP radiograph of a wrist in a 44-year-old male. It demonstrates a soft-tissue mass adjacent to the ulnar styloid and perhaps involving the TFCC (*arrow*). There is no associated osseous abnormality seen. Although a gouty tophus is in the differential diagnosis, it would be unusual for a male of this age. One would also consider synovial cell sarcoma or juxtacortical chondroma as possible diagnoses. **B,** The MRI is more suggestive of the diagnosis of gout, with the T1-weighted sequence (500/17) showing a low signal intensity soft tissue mass that has caused erosion of the distal ulna. **C,** T2-weighting shows the mass to remain low signal intensity, which is characteristic of gout (3000/99) (*arrow*). This case, as well as the previous two cases, illustrate the old adage that gout can look like anything. In the current case, the patient is Polynesian. This is an added risk factor for gout.

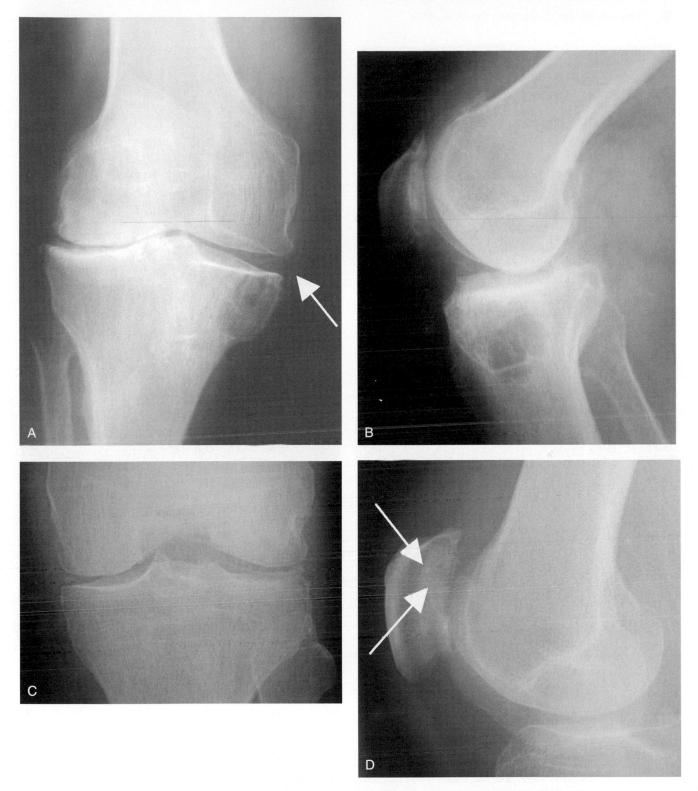

Fig. 2-66 Pyrophosphate arthropathy, knee. **A,** An AP radiograph of the knee in a 58-year-old male, demonstrating advanced pyrophosphate arthropathy. There is chondrocalcinosis in both the medial and lateral menisci, as well as in the deep fibers of the medial collateral ligament (*arrow*). There is a large subchondral cyst at the medial tibial plateau that was initially thought by the clinicians to represent a tumor. Even though degenerative changes are prominent at the medial and lateral compartments, they are even more prominently seen at the patellofemoral joint (**B,** lateral radiograph). Predominant patellofemoral joint involvement is also noted in another patient, with **C,** AP and **D,** lateral radiographs. In this case, the chondrocalcinosis is easily seen in both the hyaline and fibrocartilage of the knee on the AP film. The patellofemoral joint shows mixed erosive and productive change at the articular surface (*arrows* pointing at erosion). Again, patellofemoral disease predominates in pyrophosphate arthropathy of the knee.

153

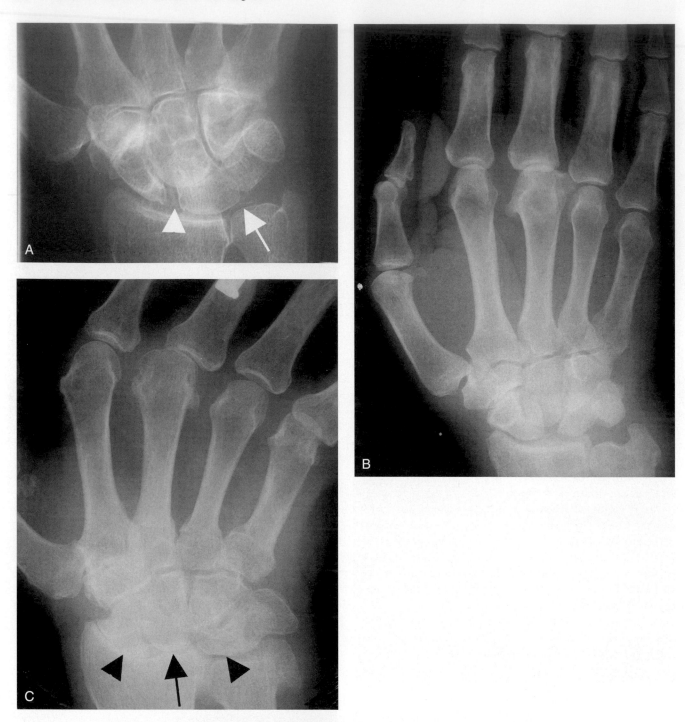

Fig. 2-67   Pyrophosphate arthropathy, hand and wrist. **A,** A PA radiograph of the wrist in an 81-year-old female with pyrophosphate arthropathy. Note the prominent chondrocalcinosis seen both in the TFCC (*arrow*) and scapholunate ligament (*arrowhead*). There is mild scapholunate disassociation (note the distance measures 3.5 mm at the scapholunate joint). There is mild radiocarpal cartilage loss and very prominent cyst formation in the scaphoid, capitate, and hamate. The findings are typical of pyrophosphate arthropathy. **B,** More advanced disease is seen in a PA radiograph in a 58-year-old male. In this case, the scapholunate disassociation is even greater, and the capitate is forcing its way between them in a configuration that is termed the SLAC wrist deformity. Although a SLAC wrist can be seen with other processes, the prominent productive change seen at the third MCP is so typical for pyrophosphate arthropathy, that the diagnosis can be made even without the presence of chondrocalcinosis. **C,** An even more advanced SLAC wrist deformity with complete separation of the scaphoid and lunate (*arrowheads*) and capitate articulation with the radius (*arrow*). In addition to the SLAC wrist deformity, we see prominent mixed erosive and productive change at the second and third MCPs. Again, this is typical for pyrophosphate arthropathy, even in the absence of chondrocalcinosis.

tion of abnormalities is distinctly different from OA. Subchondral cysts are a very distinctive feature, being both common and large, occasionally simulating a neoplasm.

The most frequently involved joints are the knee, wrist, and second and third MCP joints of the hand. The knee generally demonstrates chondrocalcinosis in the menisci, but deposition is also frequently seen in the hyaline cartilage, synovium, and capsule. The arthritic process may be present in all three compartments, but is usually seen earliest and most severely in the patellofemoral compartment, as opposed to the medial and lateral compartments (Fig. 2-66).

Pyrophosphate arthropathy involving the hand and wrist shows a unique distribution. First, the chondrocalcinosis is usually located in the triangular fibrocartilage complex (Fig. 2-67). However, close observation also may show chondrocalcinosis in the lunate-triquetral ligament and the hyaline cartilage of the wrist.[13] In addition, the arthropathy itself has a very specific distribution. Degenerative changes are specifically found in the radiocarpal joint, and late in the disease may be associated with scapholunate dissociation and scaphoid erosion into the distal radial articular surface. Proximal migration of the capitate between the dissociated scaphoid and lunate may result in a scapholunate advanced collapse (SLAC) wrist pattern (Fig. 2-67). A SLAC wrist deformity may certainly occur in the absence of CPPD and is not pathognomonic for that disease process. However, it should be noted that this radiocarpal distribution of joint involvement is significantly different from that seen in typical OA. Moreover, the second and third MCPs may specifically be involved (Fig. 2-67). The IPs are spared. This peculiar appearance and distribution is so typical that pyrophosphate arthropathy can often be diagnosed radiographically with a high degree of certainty.

Hip involvement is less frequent than knee and wrist, but if large subchondral cysts are seen with what otherwise appears to be OA, one should consider pyrophosphate arthropathy as the diagnosis and search for chondrocalcinosis (Fig. 2-68). Similarly, OA is uncommon in the shoulder and elbow in the absence of trauma or occupational injury and a degenerative joint pattern at these sites might suggest pyrophosphate arthropathy and chondrocalcinosis should be sought.

Hemochromatosis Arthropathy

Hemochromatosis arthropathy develops in up to 50% of patients who have hemochromatosis, presumably due to accumulation of iron and/or CPPD crystals in the joints. Hemochromatosis itself may be either primary owing to increased GI absorption of iron or secondary to blood transfusions, alcoholism, or excess iron ingestion. Onset

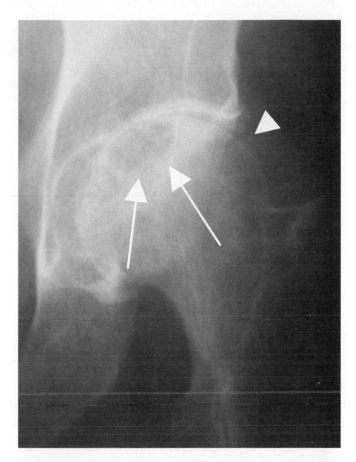

Fig. 2-68   Pyrophosphate arthropathy, hip. The AP radiograph shows a large subchondral cyst in the femoral head (*arrows*) and chondrocalcinosis at the labrum of the hip (*arrowhead*). This combination of findings makes the diagnosis of pyrophosphate arthropathy of the hip.

is usually in the middle age range and males are more frequently affected than females. The clinical triad of bronze skin, cirrhosis, and diabetes may be present.

The radiographic features of the arthropathy are essentially identical to that of pyrophosphate arthropathy. Thus, chondrocalcinosis is common. The disease is primarily productive, with large beaklike osteophytes typical at the MCP joints. However, some erosions may be seen (Fig. 2-69). Subchondral cysts are quite prominent, also similar to pyrophosphate arthropathy. The joints most commonly affected are identical to those with pyrophosphate arthropathy, including the radiocarpal joint, second and third MCPs, and the knee with the patellofemoral compartment predominating.

Wilson's Disease

Wilson's disease is an autosomal recessive process associated with abnormal accumulation of copper. It is seen more frequently in males than females and the rare arthropathy develops later in life. Radiographically, chondrocalcinosis may be present. The bones are osteopenic.

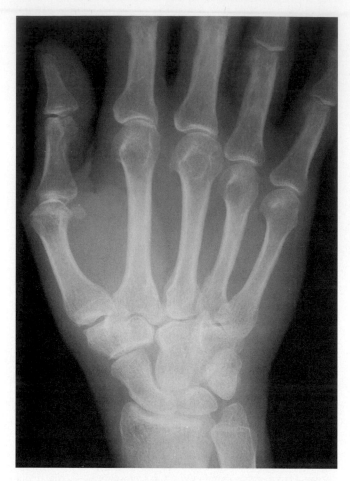

Fig. 2-69   Hemochromatosis. The PA radiograph of the hand and wrist demonstrate cartilage loss and large osteophytes at the second and third MCPs. This distribution is typical of either hemochromatosis or pyrophosphate arthropathy. In a younger male, as seen here, hemochromatosis is more probable.

Cartilage destruction occurs and the subchondral bone appears indistinct and irregular, with several small fragments or ossicles. This may give the appearance of osteochondritis. The joints most frequently affected are the wrist and hand, particularly the MCPs, followed by the foot, hip, shoulder, elbow, and knee.

Calcium Hydroxyapatite Deposition Disease (HADD)

Calcium hydroxyapatite deposition disease results in periarticular calcifications, is generally monoarticular, and results in an inflammatory reaction that is usually without structural joint abnormality. The etiology is unknown, but may relate to repeated minor trauma and calcium hydroxyapatite deposition in necrotic tissue. Hydroxyapatite deposition is seen in middle age and older individuals and affects men and women equally. The radiographic finding, which suggests the diagnosis, is a cloudlike and homogenous calcification occurring in per-

iarticular locations (tendon, ligament, capsule, or bursa). Occasionally the deposition is intra-articular, producing chondrocalcinosis. The calcification may change over time, showing enlargement or even disappearance.

The shoulder is the most frequently involved site, with calcification located at the sites of tendon insertion, particularly along the greater tuberosity, lesser tuberosity, as well as the origins of the biceps tendon and the subacromial-subdeltoid bursa. The hand may show periarticular deposits around the MCP and IP joints. The wrist may show hydroxyapatite deposition in any tendon insertion, but it is especially noted at the flexor carpi ulnaris insertion adjacent to the pisiform. Painful hydroxyapatite deposits may be treated by aspiration under fluoroscopic control or ultrasound guidance, and with injection of steroids.

Alcaptonuria (Ochronosis)

Ochronosis is a hereditary metabolic abnormality arising from the absence of homogentisic acid oxidase and consequent accumulation of homogentisic acid in various organs, including connective tissues. It affects males and females equally and the arthropathy generally occurs later in life. The radiographic findings are of dystrophic (hydroxyapatite crystal) calcification mostly involving the disks of the spine, but calcification is also occasionally seen in cartilage, tendons, and ligaments. The most specific radiographic appearance is in the spine, which appears osteoporotic with dense disk calcification. Other joints may be involved and show changes of mild DJD, but this is a much less specific appearance.

MISCELLANEOUS ARTHRITIC DISORDERS

Pigmented Villonodular Synovitis (PVNS)

Pigmented villonodular synovitis is a monoarticular process involving a proliferative disorder of the synovium, which results in hemorrhagic effusions and deposition of hemosiderin in the synovial tissues. PVNS is of

---

Key Concepts PVNS

- It is monoarticular.
- Exhibit hemorrhagic effusions, with hemosiderin deposition.
- The classic appearance of low signal intensity on both T1 and T2 imaging is seen in 80% of cases.
- Exhibits discrete erosion and prominent subchondral cyst formation.
- It is sparing of hyaline cartilage.
- The knee is the most frequent location.

unknown etiology and is seen as an intrasynovial process, as either intra-articular or tendon sheath disease. In the tendon it is called giant cell tumor of the tendon sheath. The two are histologically indistinguishable.

PVNS is a monoarticular process. It appears radiographically as an arthritis that causes erosions and particularly large subchondral cysts, whereas normal density and hyaline cartilage are preserved until very late in the disease process (Fig. 2-70). Only very rarely is a calcific metaplasia noted. The MRI appearance is often fairly specific, with the synovial masses demonstrating low signal intensity on both T1 and T2 sequences (Fig. 2-71). The diagnosis may be even more certain if gradient echo imaging demonstrates the "blooming" paramagnetic effect of hemosiderin deposition. The low signal intensity on T2 imaging, however, may not always be present owing to varying proportions of lipid, fibrous tissue, hemosiderin, pannus, fluid, cyst formation, and cellular elements. Intravenous gadolinium may more completely define the extent of the lesion but is not required for diagnosis. MRI is also valuable in demonstrating subtle erosions that may be present. It is important to accurately localize the entire lesion as that will affect the planning of therapy; lesions located posterior to the cruciate ligament, superior to the femoral condyles, or inferior to the

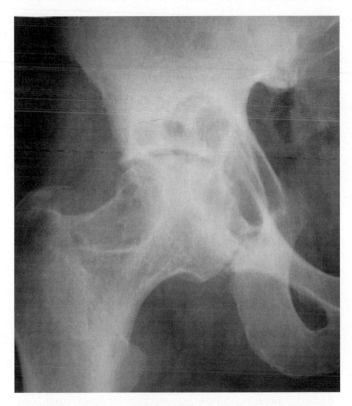

Fig. 2-70   Pigmented villonodular synovitis (PVNS). AP radiograph of the hip in this 45-year-old female demonstrates very prominent cyst formation involving both sides of the joint. These cysts are large, well defined, yet the cartilage remains intact. The findings are typical of PVNS.

tibial plateau are not accessible to arthroscopic synovectomy and must undergo an open procedure. In addition, if radiation synovectomy is planned, accurate localization of the abnormality is required.

PVNS presents in a wide age range, from adolescents to elderly patients. Eighty percent of cases of PVNS are found in the knee. Commonly affected joints include the hip and elbow. The differential diagnosis includes infection and other monoarticular arthritides such as gout. The signal intensity on MRI is not peculiar to PVNS and may be similar to that in gout, amyloid, or prominent synovitis.

Synovial Chondromatosis

Synovial chondromatosis is a synovial metaplasia of unknown etiology in which cartilaginous and osteocartilaginous nodules arise from metaplastic synovium. The nodules may grow and variably become loose or reattach to the synovium. Synovial chondromatosis is seen more frequently in males than females and generally in the third through fifth decades, although it can be seen in children or older adults as well. The process is most frequently seen radiographically as multiple round bodies of similar size and variable in mineralization, within an effusion. The round bodies occasionally appear lamellated and even trabeculated. The individual body size may range from 1 mm to 2 cms, but generally are fairly uniform within a single joint (Fig. 2-72).

Although there is usually not an arthritis associated with synovial chondromatosis, mechanical erosions can eventually be formed by the bodies and eventually secondary OA may occur. Synovial chondromatosis occurs most frequently in the knee, but is also seen in the hip, shoulder, and elbow. It is usually, although not invariably, monoarticular. Loose bodies seen with OA could be misdiagnosed as synovial chondromatosis, but loose bodies in OA are usually variably sized and few in number.

MRI is usually not required to make the diagnosis. However, on MRI one sees the effusion conforming to a distended joint capsule and multiple round bodies, which follow the signal of bone or cartilage on all sequences (Fig. 2-73). MRI is especially helpful in unusual presentation of synovial chondromatosis. Rarely, synovial chondromatosis is not detected radiographically owing to lack of mineralization of the bodies. An even more confusing picture might be that of erosive change due to synovial chondromatosis with unmineralized bodies. In either of these cases, MRI clarifies the diagnosis.

Osteochondroses

The osteochondroses represent an inelegant and artificial grouping of disease processes, all once believed

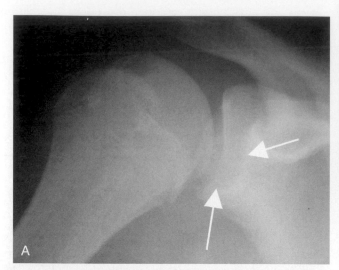

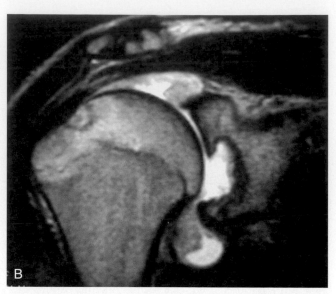

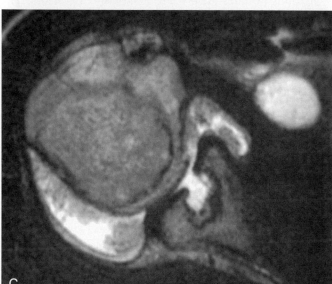

Fig. 2-71 PVNS. **A,** The AP radiograph of the shoulder in this 15-year-old male demonstrates an ill-defined erosion involving the glenoid (*arrow*). **B,** The T2-weighted MR in coronal and **C,** axial planes (2456/105), demonstrates the large erosion in the glenoid, as well as a second erosion in the humeral head. Note that the fluid in the glenohumeral joint contains soft-tissue masses that are low signal intensity. These remained low signal intensity on all sequences. Note that the low signal masses extend down the bicipital groove and surround the bicipital tendon. The findings are typical of PVNS.

to represent osteonecrosis. Only a few are true osteonecroses. Most are traumatically induced. Several are normal variants included as osteochondroses only by tradition and because they carry eponyms that suggest they are pathologic.

The osteochondroses arise in skeletally immature patients or young adults. With the exception of Freiberg's necrosis, males are affected more frequently than females. The traumatically induced osteochondroses often show bony fragments within a lucent bed, sometimes with flattening of a convex surface. The overlying cartilage is often intact.

Legg Calvé-Perthes Disease represents a true osteonecrosis of the hip, seen most frequently from age 4 to 8 when the vascular supply to the femoral head is most at risk. It is seen more frequently in males than females and may be bilateral in 10% of cases, although the presentation is usually asymmetric. The first radiographic sign may be effusion. Later, fragmentation and flattening of the ossification center may develop. Metaphyseal irregularity and "cysts" are manifestations of growth abnormality that results in a short, wide femoral neck (Fig. 2-74). Older patients at the time of diagnosis and females (who are generally more skeletally mature than males)

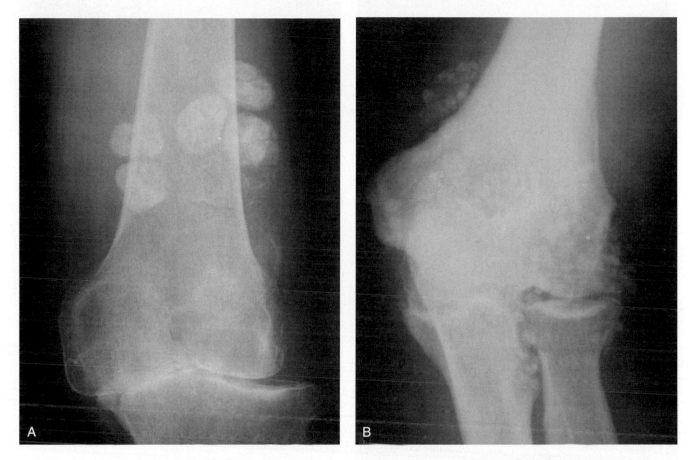

Fig. 2-72   Synovial chondromatosis. **A,** An AP radiograph of the knee in a 66-year-old male demonstrating multiple large round ossified bodies in the suprapatellar bursa. They are all of similar size and density. This is the usual appearance of synovial chondromatosis. However, the bodies can be of different size. **B,** An AP radiograph of the elbow in a 55-year-old male demonstrating many more bodies, all within the joint, and all much smaller.

Key Concepts	Synovial Chondromatosis

- Exhibits synovial metaplasia producing multiple round cartilaginous or osseous intra-articular bodies.
- Occurs most often in the knee, hip, elbow, shoulder.
- Bodies tend to be of uniform size within the joint.
- MRI is diagnostic if the bodies are not well enough mineralized to be seen radiographically.

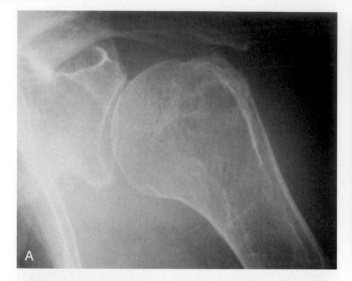

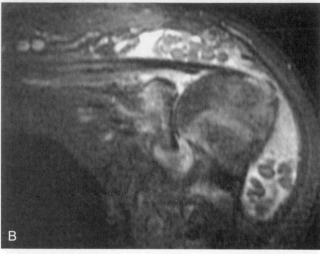

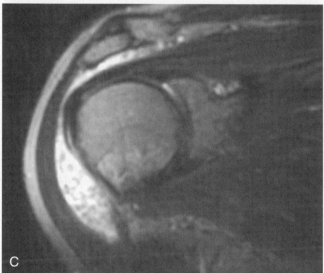

Fig. 2-73   Synovial chondromatosis. **A,** An AP radiograph of the shoulder in a 54-year-old female that demonstrates osteopenia and some mild erosive change, but no ossified bodies. The patient had a soft tissue mass. **B,** An MR, a T2-weighted (2500/80) image in the coronal plane shows multiple round bodies located in both the glenohumeral joint and the subacromial and subdeltoid bursa. This is a nice example of synovial chondromatosis that is not sufficiently ossified to be seen on the radiograph. **C,** A different patient who also had a normal radiograph. On this T2-weighted coronal MR (3600/75), we see multiple smaller round bodies in the subacromial and subdeltoid space, again a demonstration of synovial chondromatosis.

have a poorer prognosis. There have been several "head-at-risk" signs described, but all relate to lateral extrusion of the femoral head ossification center, seen radiographically as calcification lateral to the acetabular rim. This appearance indicates a lack of coverage of the femoral head and has a poor prognosis as the head and acetabulum are not congruent. MRI is used in assessing femoral head coverage in both the coronal and sagittal planes, as well as in diagnosing early bony bridging across the cartilaginous physeal plate, which could result in growth arrest or deformity.

Lunate malacia is also termed Keinbock's disease. This is also a true necrosis, believed to be related most frequently to trauma. It has been questionably associated with an ulnar minus variant (Fig. 2-75).

Freiberg's disease is a true necrosis, most commonly involving the second and third metatarsal heads (Fig. 2-76). It tends to be seen in teenage females and may be

related to the trauma of bearing weight in high-heeled shoes.

Osteochondritis dissecans is frequently found in the knee, most often affecting the lateral portion of the medial femoral condyle (Fig. 2-77). However, other articular locations are recognized, including sites on the femoral condyles anteriorly and on the patella (Fig. 2-78). Osteochondritis dissecans is believed to be related to repeated microtrauma. It appears as a concave subchondral fracture line, usually containing an osseous "body." If osteochondritis dissecans is symptomatic, it is important to demonstrate whether the "body" is loose or if the overlying cartilage is intact. This can be shown on MR imaging if an effusion tracks around the body and subchondral fracture line, or by MRI arthrography. Alternatively, after IV gadolinium injection and exercise, if there is high signal intensity surrounding the margin of the fragment, this is felt to represent granulation tissue around an unsta-

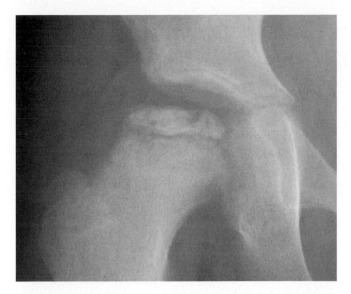

Fig. 2-74   AP radiograph of the hip in a 7-year-old female with Legg Perthes disease. The fragmented and flattened femoral capital epiphysis is seen.

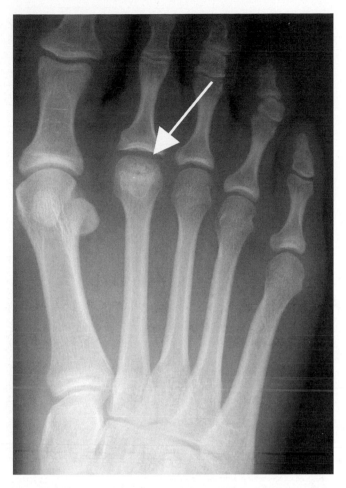

Fig. 2-76   Freiberg's necrosis. AP radiograph of the foot in a 26-year-old female demonstrates slight flattening and fragmentation of the head of the second metatarsal (*arrow*). This is a typical location, as well as gender prevalence, of this osteonecrosis.

ble fragment (Fig. 2-79). Osteochondritis dissicans should be differentiated from spontaneous osteonecrosis, which affects an older patient, who complains of acute onset of severe pain. Spontaneous osteonecrosis shows flattening on the weight-bearing surface of the femoral condyle, most frequently medial. It therefore is found in a different population and has a different radiographic appearance as well as subtly different location in the knee with respect to osteochondritis dissecans (Fig. 2-80).

Osgood-Schlatter's disease has been termed an osteochondrosis at the tibial apophysis. A true Osgood-Schlat-

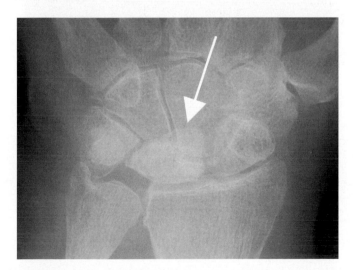

Fig. 2-75   Kienbock's disease. PA radiograph of the wrist demonstrates a dense, slightly flattened lunate (*arrow*), representing AVN, termed Kienbock's disease when it is in the lunate.

ter's disease is thought to be a traumatically induced avulsion. It is rarely complicated by either nonunion of the tibial tubercle or premature closure of the tibial tubercle with secondary development of genu recurvatum. However, the radiologist should be aware that several ossification centers may normally be seen at this apophysis, so that both soft tissue swelling and pain should be present in addition to bony fragmentation before the disease is suggested (Fig. 2-81). Sinding-Larsen-Johanssen disease is a similar process of the inferior pole of the patella in the same age group.

Blount's disease is considered by some to be an osteochondrosis of the medial aspect of the proximal tibial metaphysis. Fragmentation at this site results in a genu varum deformity (Fig. 2-82). The infantile type of Blount's disease is most common, especially among black children. It evolves when the normal physiologic bowing of the lower extremity worsens with weight bearing,

Text continued on p. 166

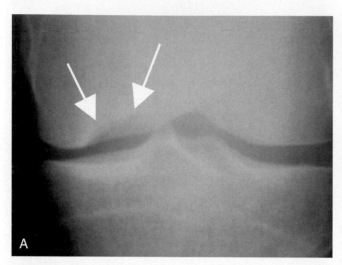

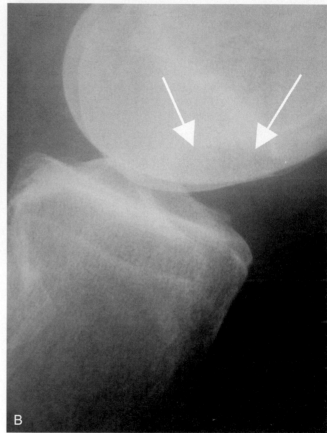

Fig. 2-77   Osteochondritis dissecans. **A,** The AP radiograph demonstrates a concavity in the lateral aspect of the medial femoral condyle with tiny, barely discernible fragments within it (*arrow*). **B,** The lateral view confirms the defect again, in a concave shape (*arrows*).

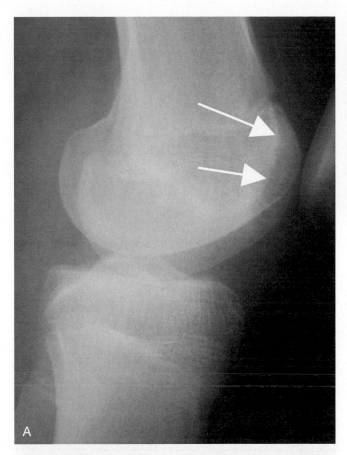

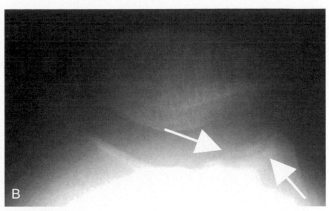

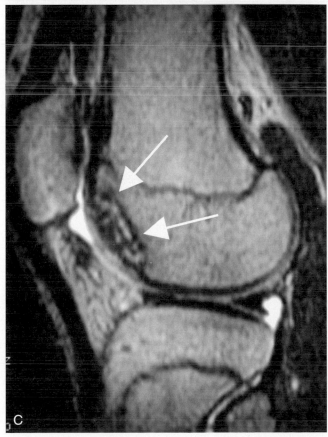

Fig. 2-78   Osteochondritis dissecans. The usual location of osteochondritis dissecans is demonstrated on the previous figure. However, occasionally osteochondritis is found in other locations, either on the femoral condyle or patella. **A,** In this case, the lateral radiograph shows irregularity and abnormal density on the anterior portion of the femoral condyle. **B,** This abnormality is confirmed on the sunrise view (*arrows*). **C,** A T2-weighted MRI (2500/80) of this knee in a sagittal plane. It is imaged following intra-articular injection of saline. The area of osteochondritis demonstrates that the fragments are granulating in, and there is no separation of the fragments from the underlying bone (*arrows*).

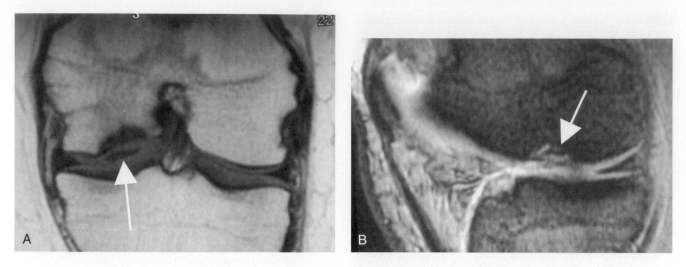

Fig. 2-79   Osteochondritis dissecans. **A,** A T1-weighted (600/15) coronal MRI demonstrating an osteochondral fragment in the typical location (*arrows*) for osteochondritis dissecans. This scan, along with the oblique gradient echo scan (**B**) demonstrates that the fragment is loose, with fluid surrounding it (*arrow*).

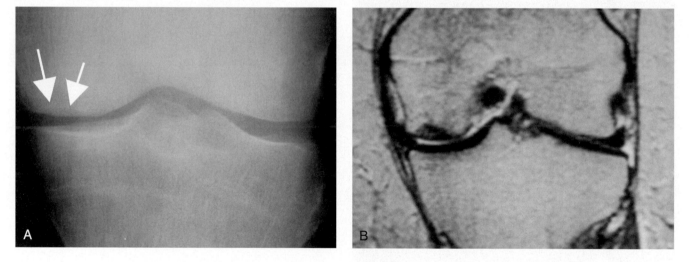

Fig. 2-80   Spontaneous osteonecrosis of the knee (SONK). **A,** An AP radiograph of the knee in a 72-year-old female, which demonstrates slight flattening of the medial femoral condyle (*arrow*). **B,** The MR shows low signal intensity on T2 imaging (2000/80).

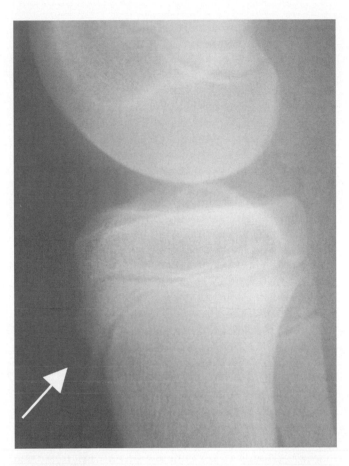

Fig. 2-81   Osgood-Schlatter's disease. Lateral radiograph of the knee in a skeletally immature patient demonstrates fragmentation of the anterior tibial apophysis (*arrow*). In the presence of pain as well as soft tissue swelling, this represents Osgood-Schlatter's disease. (Reprinted with permission from the ACR learning files.)

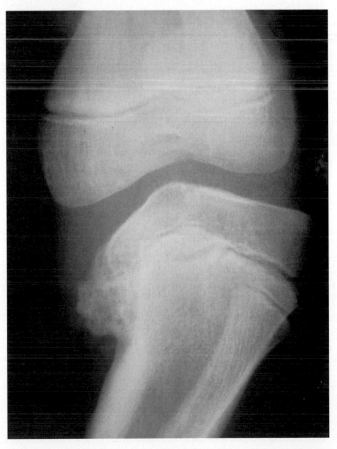

Fig. 2-82   Blount's disease. There is fragmentation and collapse of the medial tibial metaphysis in this 14-year-old male, demonstrating Blount's disease. (Reprinted with permission from the ACR learning file.)

especially in children who walk at an early age. This is not felt to be a true necrosis, but a result of persistent microtrauma of weight bearing and abnormal pressure resulting in fragmentation of the medial metaphysis. The findings are bilateral in greater than 50% of the cases. The adolescent type of Blount's disease is unilateral, and relates directly to either trauma or infection causing bony bridging of the medial growth plate.

Talar dome osteochondritis dissecans develops on the medial or lateral convex surface of the talus and is probably related to trauma and ankle laxity (Fig. 2-83).

Panner's disease is fragmentation of the capitellum. This is seen most commonly in adolescent fastball pitchers (Fig. 2-84). It generally is self-limited, with normal regeneration in most cases. However, hyperemia may lead to acceleration of maturation of the capitellum and radial head.

Scheuermann's disease may be classified as an osteochondrosis of the spine. The etiology is unknown but is felt not to be necrosis. There may be a congenital endplate weakness and/or repetitive microtrauma. With Scheuermann's disease, there is irregularity of the thoracic vertebral endplates, often associated with Shmorl's

nodes, resulting in a dorsal kyphosis. The normal thoracic kyphosis, measured between T4 and T12, should be between 20° and 40°. Scheuermann's disease is seen equally in males and females and preferentially affects the lower thoracic spine (Fig. 2-85).

There are several normal variants that show fragmented ossification centers in the skeletally immature patient and may simulate osteochondroses. The most frequently seen is that in the femoral condyle. This irregularity or fragmentation is located posteriorly on the femoral condyle in skeletally immature patients and may best be seen on the notch view (Fig. 2-86). This should not be confused with osteochondritis dissecans, which is more anterior in location. The normal variant condylar irregularity progresses to normal maturation of the femoral condyle and has normal overlying cartilage. Another location that may show a dense and fragmented apophysis is the calcaneus. This appearance has been termed Sever's disease, but this represents a normal variant. Similarly, the trochlea and lateral epicondyle, as well as the anterior tibial apophysis and tarsal navicular may ossify in a fragmented fashion quite normally. The tarsal navicular should be termed Kohler's disease only when fragmentation occurs in a previously seen normal tarsal navicular in a patient who complains of pain at that site. Similarly, irregularity can be found at the ischiopubic synchondrosis in the skeletally immature patient. This is a normal variant, despite being given the term Van Neck's disease.

Hypertrophic Osteoarthropathy (HOA)

Hypertrophic osteoarthropathy is a disease process of unknown etiology that presents clinically as arthritis with painful, swollen joints. Radiographically, the joints appear normal, with possible swelling and effusions but no erosive or productive changes. The major abnormality in fact is found on the "corner" of the film, where a symmetric periosteal reaction is seen. The reaction may show onion skinning, irregularity, or waviness, and its thickness and extent probably depend on the duration of the disease.

Hypertrophic osteoarthropathy (HOA) may be primary or secondary. The primary form is also termed pachydermoperiostitis, which is a spectrum of diseases ranging from mere periostitis to the complete process

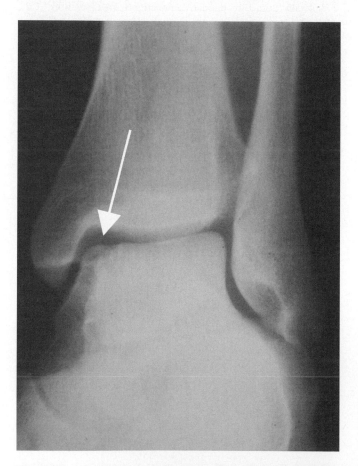

Fig. 2-83 Osteochondritis dissecans, talus. There is irregularity and concavity involving the medial aspect of the dome of the talus (*arrow*). Either the medial or lateral dome of the talus represent typical locations for trauma-induced osteochondritis.

Key Concepts	HOA

- Presents clinically as arthritis.
- Radiographically has normal joints.
- Thick periosteal reaction.
- Can be primary or secondary.
- Chest x-ray should be obtained to search for the primary cause.

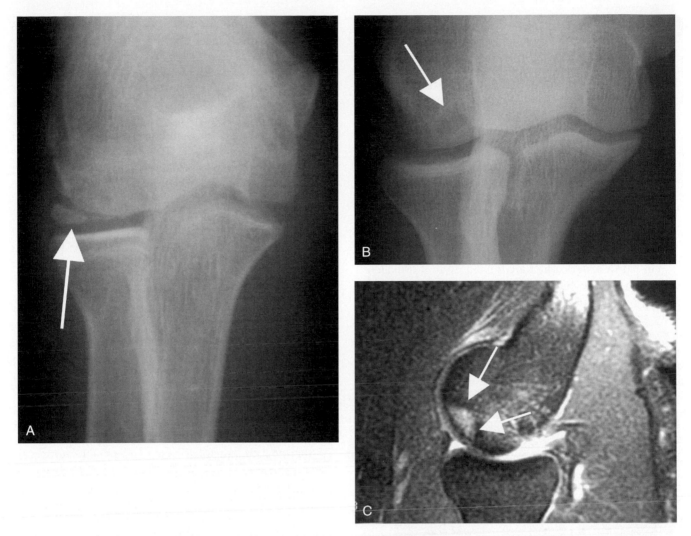

Fig. 2-84 Panner's disease. **A,** The AP radiograph of an elbow in a 13-year-old male demonstrates fragmentation and advanced maturation of the capitellum (*arrow*). **B,** A different patient, showing only an irregularity in the capitellum (*arrow*). A highly angled film (not shown) demonstrated that there is in fact fragmentation at this site. The patient was administered IV gadolinium, exercised the elbow, and a fat saturated T1-weighted sagittal MR image (753/16) demonstrates enhancement of the area of fragmentation (*arrow*). This indicates that it is a viable fragment.

of periostitis, clubbed digits, and thickening of the skin particularly at the forehead and dorsum of the hands (Fig. 2-87). Primary HOA is often familial and is much more common in males than females. The onset is in adolescence and there is usually spontaneous arrest of the process in young adulthood.

Secondary HOA is a painful periostitis in the extremities noted in patients with a number of disease processes, usually intrathoracic. These include bronchogenic carcinoma, as well as other malignant, benign, or chronic suppurative diseases of the lung. Secondary HOA can also be seen in patients with cyanotic heart disease, biliary cirrhosis, or IBD. The mechanism of the reaction is entirely unknown. Interestingly, a thoracotomy may lead to clinical remission almost immediately, with slower radiographic resolution. It is critical to recognize second-

ary HOA from periostitis and seek the underlying disease process, starting with the chest x-ray (Fig. 2-88).

The differential diagnosis of the periostitis seen in HOA includes thyroid acropachy, which can occur after surgical ablation of the gland for hyperthyroidism. The character of periostitis in thyroid acropachy is said to be more feathery and spiculated and predominately located on the hands and feet. Periosteal reaction in the lower limbs can also be seen in patients with vascular insufficiency.

Avascular Necrosis (AVN)

Avascular necrosis (AVN) of bone is a poorly understood phenomenon that may be related to trauma (interruption of vascular supply), marrow edema with impeded

Key Concepts	Avascular Necrosis

- Radiographic signs include sclerosis, followed by subchondral fracture and flattening.
- Cartilage remains normal until secondary degenerative disease.
- Most common etiologies include trauma, steroids, alcoholism, sickle cell disease.
- Most common sites are femoral head, lunate, proximal pole of the scaphoid, humeral head, vertebral body.
- Specific MRI sign: double line sign.

venous drainage, vascular compression, or intraluminal vascular obstruction. The most common etiologies of AVN in North America include trauma, steroid use, alcoholism, and sickle cell disease. It can be useful to try to detect the cause of AVN on the radiograph. An example of the traumatic etiology is found particularly in the hip, where delayed reduction of a dislocation or subcapital fracture can result in AVN. AVN related to steroids may be from either exogenous or endogenous (Cushing's disease) sources. It is thought that the mechanism of AVN with steroid use is an increase in the size of the fat cells and resultant increased marrow pressure, particularly in the femoral head. With steroid use, one sometimes sees a transplanted kidney in the iliac fossa on a film of the

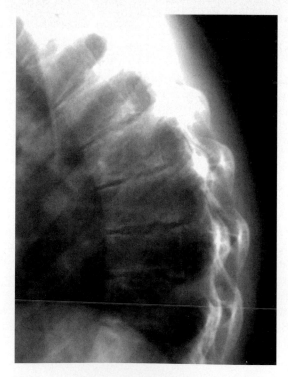

Fig. 2-85   Scheuermann's disease. The lateral radiograph in this 18-year-old female demonstrates mild anterior wedging of several thoracic vertebral bodies, along with irregularity of the end plates and resultant kyphosis.

pelvis taken to demonstrate AVN (Fig. 2-89). Patients who are alcoholics may develop avascular necrosis due to fat emboli and increased marrow pressure. Pancreatic calcification could suggest the diagnosis in this case. Patients with sickle cell disease develop AVN due to microvascular occlusion from the sickled cells. Pelvic films might also demonstrate diffuse abnormality in density or even calcified gallstones, which suggest the diagnosis of sickle cell disease (Fig. 2-90). The less common etiologies of AVN are interesting as well. With Gaucher's disease, the sinusoids are packed with Gaucher's cells, increasing marrow pressure; the related finding on the film may be hepatosplenomegaly (Fig. 2-91). With Caisson disease, nitrogen embolization following rapid decompression in a diver causes an increase in marrow pressure. Radiation has a direct toxic affect on vascular supply to the bone; abnormalities suggesting radiation necrosis, seen in a portlike configuration may lead to this diagnosis (Fig. 2-92). In patients with SLE, the vasculitis may be additive to the steroid therapy in causing AVN (see Fig. 2-39). AVN located in unusual sites such as the talus or humerus might suggest SLE as an etiology.

AVN of the hip is discussed here as the prototypical example of AVN as it is both common and debilitating. Initially, the articular cartilage is unaffected by AVN because it is nourished by synovial fluid. The first radiographic sign in hip AVN is sclerosis, generally in the center of the femoral head (Fig. 2-89). Initially, the sclerosis is relative in nature, as the necrotic bone initiates an inflammatory response in the surrounding vascularized bone, which results in osteoporosis surrounding the necrotic bone. Later in the process, a reactive interface develops, with bone formation and repair causing a zone of increased density. Following the sclerotic phase, the bone may develop a linear subchondral fracture, also termed a crescent sign. In the hip, this is best seen on a frog-leg lateral view, but is often discerned on an AP view as well (Fig. 2-93). With further subchondral fragmentation, flattening and bone deformity occur. Secondary degenerative change may occur much later. Radionuclide bone scan may initially show a photopenic region, but this is followed by increased activity with revascularization and repair.

MRI is the most sensitive imaging tool for detection of avascular necrosis. When the typical features are present, MR imaging may be highly specific as well. However, at some stages the MRI appearance may be nonspecific. Early edema changes of avascular necrosis are nonspecific and diffuse as seen on MRI. However, after initial edema, a specific, classic appearance may develop. The abnormality is located in the subchondral weight bearing area and shows a distinct marrow signal abnormality consisting of a peripheral low signal intensity rim on both T1 and T2 sequences, with an adjacent inner rim of increased signal intensity on T2, termed the "double rim"

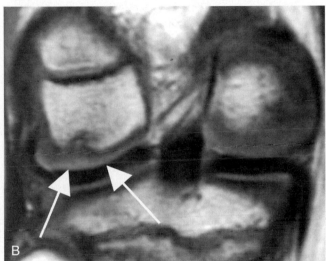

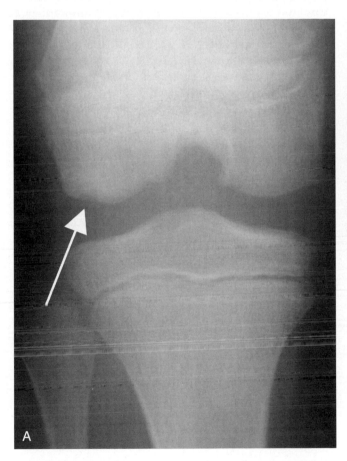

Fig. 2-86   Normal variant, irregularity of the femoral condyle. **A,** The AP notch radiograph demonstrates irregularity and apparent flattening of the posterior aspect of the lateral femoral condyle (*arrow*). **B,** The coronal proton density weighted (3200/18) MR image demonstrates normal cartilage (*arrow*) overlying this femoral condylar irregularity. This will ossify normally and should not be mistaken for osteochondritis dissecans.

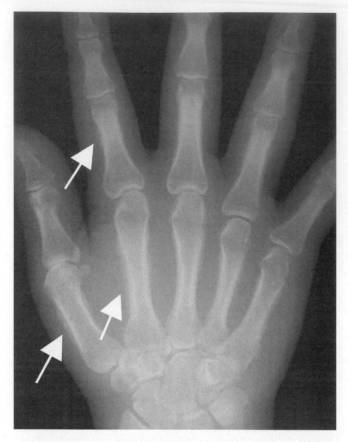

Fig. 2-87   Pachydermoperiostosis (primary hypertrophic osteoarthropathy). PA radiograph of the hand in this 26-year-old male demonstrates thick periosteal reaction along the proximal phalanges as well as metacarpals (*arrows*). The radiograph alone does not make the diagnosis of pachydermoperiostosis, but in combination with the thickening of the skin over the hands and forehead seen clinically, is in fact diagnostic.

sign (Fig. 2-94). The central signal within this rim is used to classify avascular necrosis. With Class A, the central signal is isointense to fat. In Class B, the central signal is isointense to hemorrhage. In Class C the central signal is isointense to fluid. Class D shows a central signal isointense to fibrous tissue or bone. These classes are roughly equivalent to the radiographic stages I–IV (I is normal, II shows trabecular changes without collapse, III shows collapse, and IV is AVN with secondary OA). It should be remembered that MRI has 98% specificity in differentiating normal from abnormal, but only 85% specificity in differentiating AVN from non-AVN disease.[14] It is also interesting to note that AVN may be clinically occult. One study of 100 asymptomatic renal transplant patients taking steroids showed 6% to have MRI evidence of AVN despite their asymptomatic state.[15] In another study, 14% had AVN by MRI but 33% of these resolved over 24 months.[16] Therefore the value of screening at-risk but asymptomatic patients has not been established, as the treatment is also not clear. Currently, treatment of symp-

tomatic hips with AVN consists of core decompression, seen radiographically as a cylindrical lucency extending from the femoral neck into the head. A vascularized fibular graft may be placed at this site to stimulate healing and revascularization (Fig. 2-95).

Very early in AVN, the MR imaging appearance may be entirely nonspecific, showing signal intensity of diffuse edema. There is another process that may have an identical appearance. Transient regional osteoporosis, seen radiographically as osteoporosis involving both sides of a joint with normal cartilage, also demonstrates abnormal uptake on bone scan and signal intensity of edema on MRI. Transient regional osteoporosis is a self-limited disease and may be migratory. Because treatment may be different for transient regional osteoporosis and AVN, diagnosis is important. With the MRI pattern of bone marrow edema in a painful hip, radiographs and timing may help make the distinction. If onset has been recent, waiting a few weeks and repeating radiographs may show the osteoporosis as typical of the transient regional type.

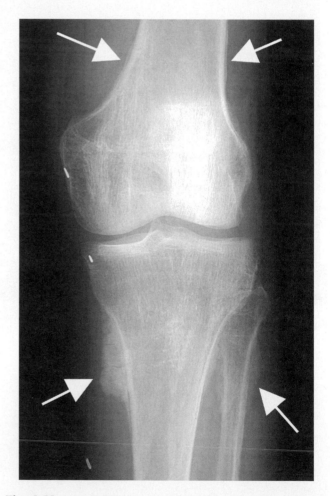

Fig. 2-88   Secondary hypertrophic osteoarthropathy. The AP radiograph of the knee in this 73-year-old male demonstrates prominent periosteal reaction, in both the femur as well as tibia and fibula (*arrows*). Chest film in this patient (not shown) demonstrated a lung tumor.

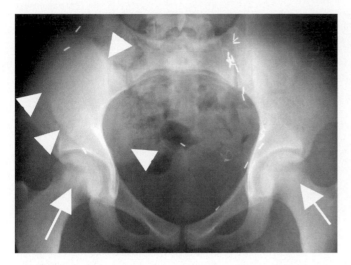

Fig. 2-89   Avascular necrosis. The AP radiograph of the pelvis in this 27-year-old female demonstrates central sclerotic areas within both femoral heads (*arrows*). The etiology of avascular necrosis is apparent, with the soft tissue mass of the renal transplant seen in the iliac fossa (*arrowheads*).

Survey radiographs of hip AVN include AP and frog-leg pelvis. MRI screening includes T1 coronal, T2 coronal, and either T1 or T2 sagittal. The evaluation should include not only the diagnosis, but also presence of flattening and OA. It is also important to indicate the extent and location of AVN in the coronal and sagittal planes, referring to locations with a clock-face description. This helps the surgeon determine whether the patient can be best treated by core decompression, osteotomy with realignment to a noncollapsed weight bearing portion, or prosthesis placement.

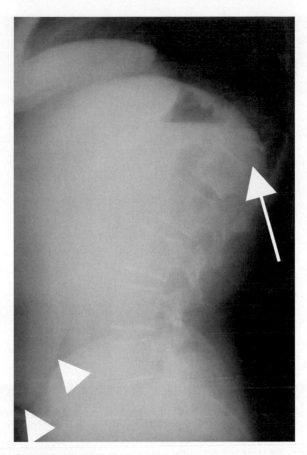

Fig. 2-91   Avascular necrosis: Gaucher's. This 31-year-old female has collapse of the T12 vertebral body (*arrow*). The patient has a nearly completely grey abdomen, with the edge of the tremendously enlarged liver and spleen outlined by arrowheads. This degree of organomegaly, in the presence of AVN, allows a diagnosis of Gaucher's disease.

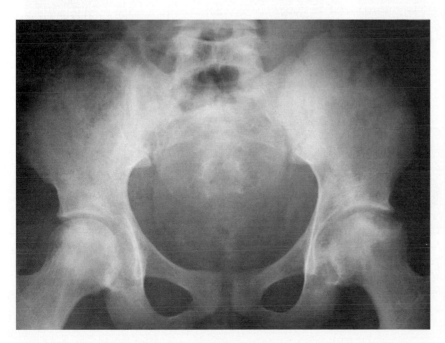

Fig. 2-90   Avascular necrosis, sickle cell disease. The AP radiograph of the pelvis in this 19-year-old male demonstrates abnormal density in the iliac wings due to bone infarct, as well as osteonecrosis of both femoral heads, with prominent collapse seen in the left femoral head. The combination of bone infarcts and avascular necrosis makes the diagnosis of sickle cell disease highly probable. (Reprinted with permission of the ACR learning file.)

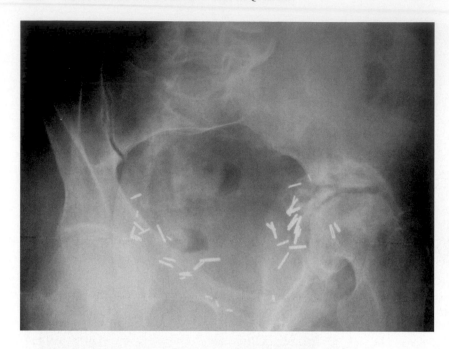

Fig. 2-92 Avascular necrosis: radiation injury. The left femoral head and acetabulum show the mixed sclerosis and lucency of radiation osteonecrosis, with collapse of the femoral head in this 64 year old male who was radiated for prostate cancer. The pelvic clips indicate a lymph node dissection.

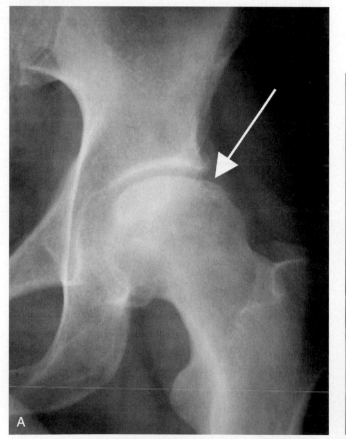

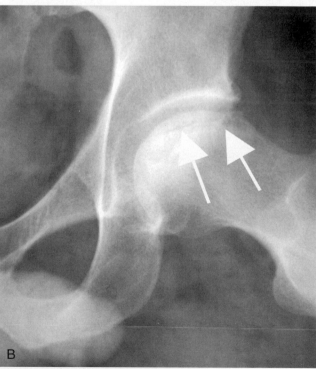

Fig. 2-93 Avascular necrosis: steroids. **A,** An AP radiograph of the left hip in this 37-year-old male demonstrates mild flattening (*arrow*) and subchondral fracture. **B,** The subchondral fracture is better demonstrated on the frogleg lateral (*arrows*). (Reprinted with permission of the ACR learning file.)

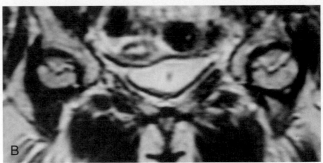

Fig. 2-94 Avascular necrosis, MRI. **A,** A coronal T1-weighted (700/20) image of the hips in a 19-year-old female with AVN. **B,** On the T2-weighted image (2000/70), the abnormal region is outlined by a low signal intensity outer rim and high signal intensity inner rim. This "double line" sign is considered pathognomonic for AVN. At this point, there is no flattening seen.

The most common sites of occurrence of AVN depend on the underlying etiology and include the femoral head, lunate, proximal pole of the scaphoid, and body of the talus in posttraumatic situations. The humeral head and talar sites may be seen particularly in sickle cell disease or

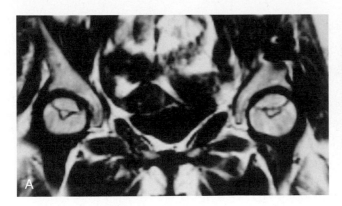

Fig. 2-95 Vascularized fibular graft. The AP radiograph of the hip demonstrates the packing of the femoral head with bone graft following decompression, as well as the placement of the vascularized fibular graft within the neck.

SLE. AVN of the spine may be nonspecific, with increased density of the vertebral body and collapse. However, if air is seen within the vertebral body, this is virtually pathognomonic for AVN. With MRI, this air vacuum may show high signal intensity on T2 imaging as, over the duration of the scan, a transudate crosses into this space (Fig. 2-96). Watch also for the "H-shaped" vertebra where the mid-portion of the superior and inferior endplates of osteonecrotic vertebrae are impacted, seen in AVN of the spine in sickle cell and Gaucher's disease.

DISH: Diffuse Idiopathic Skeletal Hyperostosis (Forestier's Disease)

DISH results in severe productive bony changes of the spine, including the annulus fibrosis, anterior longitudinal ligament, and paravertebral connective tissues, resulting in "flowing" ossification of the anterolateral aspect of the vertebral bodies. There is usually relative preservation of disk height of the involved segments. Degenerative disk disease as well as facet productive change is not prominent relative to the anterior ossifications (Fig. 2-97). The superior (nonarticular) portions of the SI joints are often bridged by ligamentous calcification, but the lower (articular) two-thirds of the SI joints are rarely affected. Therefore, DISH is usually easily differentiated from ankylosing spondylitis. The patient may also show prominent enthesophyte formation, especially in the pelvis, calcaneus, and the anterior surface of the patella. Additionally, pelvic ligaments (sacrotuberous and sacrospinus) may become calcified, as may the anterior and posterior longitudinal ligaments.

DISH occurs most frequently in middle aged and elderly persons, males more frequently than females. It is seen most commonly in the thoracic spine, although the cervical spine is frequently involved. Interestingly, while ossification of the posterior longitudinal ligament may be seen in association with DISH, there is a separately

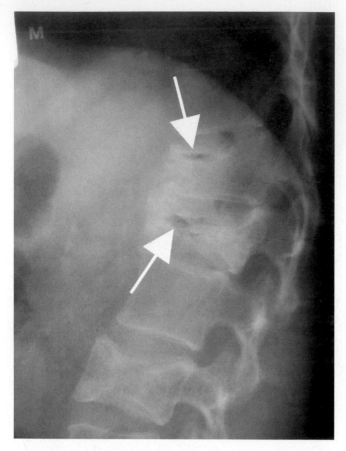

Fig. 2-96 Avascular necrosis: spine. This lateral radiograph of the spine in a male taking steroids for a heart transplant demonstrates a compression fracture at L3 but compression fractures at T12 and L1 which contain air within the bodies of the vertebra. This intra-body air (*arrows*) is considered pathognomonic for avascular necrosis of the spine.

named disease entity (OPLL, ossification of the posterior longitudinal ligament) that shows predominately posterior longitudinal ligament ossification, often with some bulky anterior osteophyte formation (Fig. 2-98). There is overlap between the two disease processes. OPLL predominately involves the cervical spine, whereas DISH more frequently is thoracic in location.

Retinoid arthropathy may be a consideration in patients using retinoic acid for skin diseases and who develop skeletal hyperostoses similar to those seen in DISH. In retinoid arthropathy, the cervical spine is the most common site of involvement, but thoracic and lumbar involvement is seen as well (Fig. 2-99). Eventually, along with the anterior osteophyte formation, anterior and posterior longitudinal ligament calcification may be seen.

Lead Arthropathy

Bullets lodged in bursal and joint spaces can result in lead poisoning due to dissolution of the lead by synovial fluid. With progressive degradation, the fragments are spread throughout the joint, lining the synovium and cartilage (Fig. 2-100). Synovial inflammation and foreign body mechanical damage to cartilage lead to productive change and secondary OA. Clinical lead poisoning requires sufficient breakdown of fragments for a large surface of lead to be reabsorbed. Lead bullets in extra-articular soft tissues dissolve much more slowly and are not associated with lead intoxication.

Acromegaly

Acromegaly results from an excess of growth hormone. In the skeletally immature patient, it produces a proportional increase in size of the bones, leading to giantism. In the skeletally mature patient, the bones cannot lengthen, but respond to growth hormone by tubular bone widening and acral growth.

In the adult, radiographic abnormalities include soft tissue thickening, especially over the phalanges and in the heel pad. The skull may show an enlarged sella due to the pituitary adenoma. The facial bones and mandible become quite prominent, as does the occipital protruberence. The paranasal sinuses may be enlarged and excessively pneumatized. The spine demonstrates an increased vertebral body and disk height and posterior vertebral body scalloping. There may be an exaggerated thoracic kyphosis.

In the appendicular skeleton, hand and foot changes predominate over those in the more proximal bones. The phalanges and metacarpals may be wide, with spadelike distal phalangeal tufts (Fig. 2-101). Excrescences at the tendon attachments along the phalanges may be prominent. The hyaline cartilage increases in width. Beaking osteophytes may eventually develop into secondary degenerative joint disease. In the remainder of the skeleton, there may be bony proliferation at the entheses.

Orthopedic Hardware: Joint Arthroplasty

Joint arthroplasties are common place today, especially in the hip and knee, but are also seen in several other joints. Imaging analysis of arthroplasties includes evaluation for anatomic placement, dislocation, loosening of the prosthesis, mechanical failure of the prosthesis, or infection. This section will concentrate on total hip arthroplasties for two reasons: first, this is the most frequent arthroplasty encountered and second, the principles of evaluation of the total hip arthroplasty are generalizable to other protheses.[17]

Failure of a total hip arthroplasty frequently relates to improper positioning of the components. In the total hip, the acetabular and femoral components should be placed in the expected anatomic site of each. The following parameters should specifically be assessed:

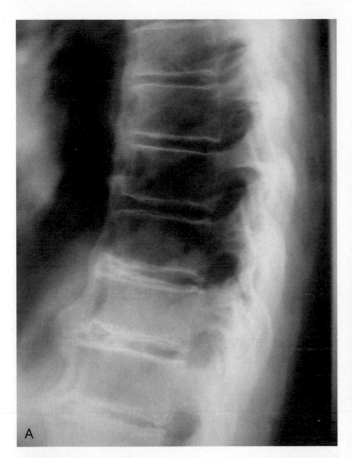

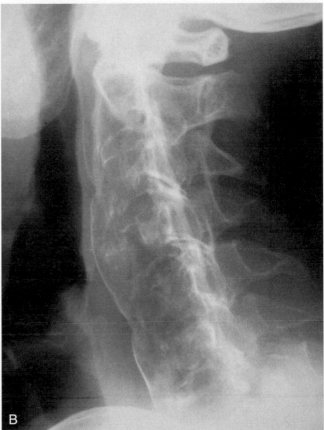

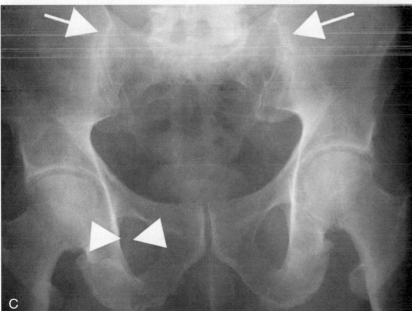

Fig. 2-97 DISH. **A,** The lateral thoracic spine shows the flowing anterior osteophytes that are so typical of DISH. **B,** The lateral cervical spine shows tremendously exaggerated flowing anterior osteophytes, also a manifestation of DISH. **C,** The AP radiograph of the SI joints shows normal inferior synovial SI joints, but fusion of the superior, nonsynovial portions of the SI joints (*arrows*). It also demonstrates ossification of the right sacrotuberous ligament. Both of these findings are typical of DISH.

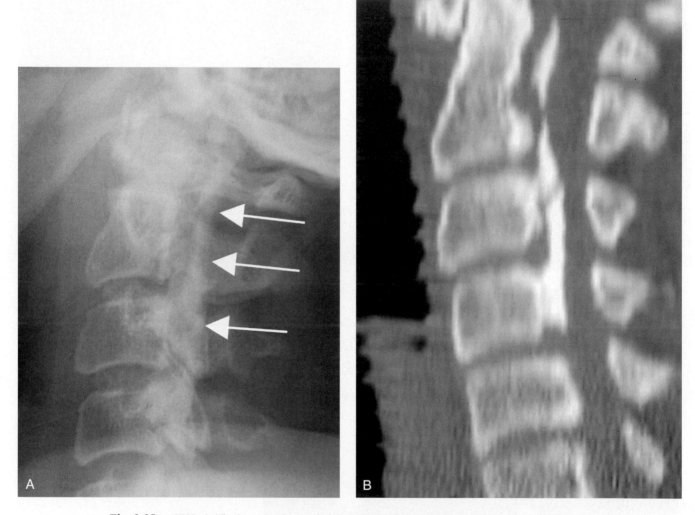

Fig. 2-98   OPLL. **A,** The lateral radiograph demonstrates the ossification of the posterior longitudinal ligament (*arrows*) in this patient's cervical spine. **B,** It is much more apparent on the sagittal CT reconstruction.

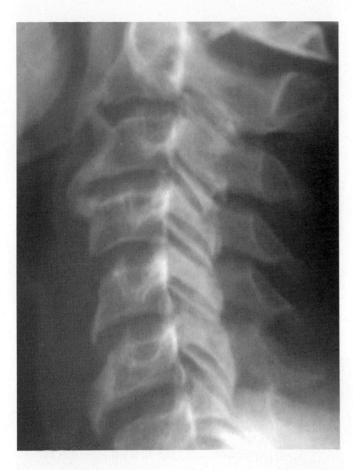

Fig. 2-99   Retinoid arthropathy. The lateral cervical spine in this 22-year-old male demonstrates prominent anterior osteophyte formation in the cervical spine, an incongruent finding in a patient of this age. He was using retinoids for a skin condition. (Reprinted with permission of the ACR learning file.)

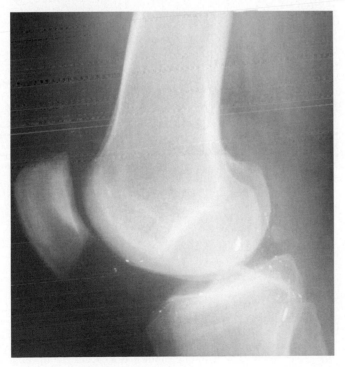

Fig. 2-100   Lead arthropathy. The lateral radiograph of the knee demonstrates fragmentation of a bullet that ended up within the knee joint. Note the tiny lead fragments lining the synovial surfaces of the joint. Fragmentation of bullets within a joint can result in lead poisoning.

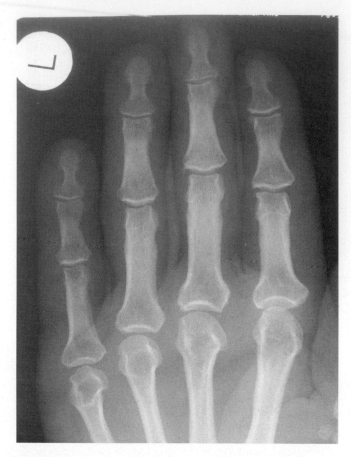

Fig. 2-101   Acromegaly. This PA radiograph demonstrates widening of the cartilage, overgrowth of the soft tissues, and overgrowth of the tuffs of the distal phalanges, all typical of acromegaly. (Reprinted with permission of the ACR learning file.)

1. The alignment of the acetabular component in the coronal plane is important. The lateral opening of the acetabulum (horizontal version) is measured as the angle of opening relative to the transischial line (a line drawn between the two ischial tuberosities, used throughout this section as a convenient landmark for measurement). The lateral opening angle of the acetabular component normally measures 40° +/− 10° (Fig. 2-102). An increased lateral opening angle puts the patient at risk for dislocation. A significantly decreased lateral opening limits abduction and may result in dislocation when the hip is placed in forced abduction.

2. The angle of the acetabulum in the lateral plane is also important. As seen on a groin lateral film, the acetabulum should be anteverted 10–15°. Zero degrees anteversion may be acceptable if there is anteversion at the femoral neck-shaft angle, but retroversion of the acetabular component is never acceptable and predisposes to dislocation. It is important to note that one can see on an AP radiograph that there is angulation of the acetabulum,

but one cannot determine whether the angulation is anteversion or retroversion without adding the information from the groin lateral film (Fig. 2-103).

3. Medial-lateral positioning of the acetabular component is also important. The acetabular component should be placed such that the horizontal center of rotation is similar to that of the normal femoral head (Fig. 2-102). If the acetabulum is too medialized, there may be excessive thinning of the medial wall and risk of failure. If the acetabular component is placed too far laterally, the iliopsoas tendon will cross medial to the femoral head center of rotation and muscle contraction will tend to force the head from the socket, increasing the probability of dislocation.

4. Equal limb length must be maintained. This can be evaluated by choosing a femoral landmark, such as the greater or lesser trochanter, and comparing it with the opposite side relative to the transischial line (Fig. 2-102, 2-104). Limb length can be affected by placement of the acetabulum, placement of the femoral component, length and size of the femoral neck and head, and thickness of the polyethylene liner. If the hip ends up too short, contracting muscles will be ineffective and the hip subject to dislocation. If the hip is placed such that there is over-lengthening of the limb, the neurovascular

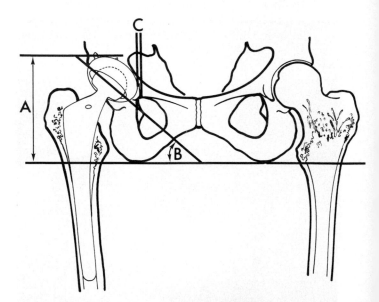

Fig. 2-102   Evaluation of total hip arthroplasty. The reference line for most of what should be evaluated in a THA is the transischial line. The distance labeled A is used to evaluate effective limb length; another way to evaluate this would be to compare the levels of the lesser trochanters with one another. B indicates the opening angle (lateral inclination) of the acetabular cup. The measurements between the lines indicated by C is used to evaluate for either excessive or lack of medialization of the cup.

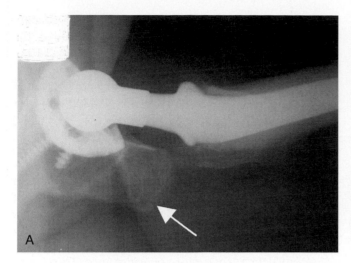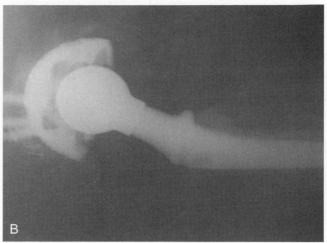

Fig. 2-103 Anteversion of the acetabular component. **A,** A groin lateral view demonstrating the ischium (*arrow*) that is a posterior structure and therefore showing anteversion (anterior angulation) of both the acetabular component and the femoral neck. **B,** A groin lateral film taken in a patient who chronically dislocates her hip. The reason for the dislocation is shown, with the acetabular component in a retroverted configuration.

bundle will be stretched and the muscles likely to spasm, again subjecting the hip to dislocation.

5. The femoral component should be placed in a neutral to slight valgus position (with the prosthesis resting against the lateral cortex proximally and against the medial cortex distally). A varus position predisposes a femoral component to loosening.
6. Inappropriate sizing of implant components may result in failure of the arthroplasty. The acetabular

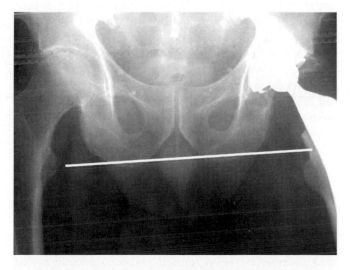

Fig. 2-104 Abnormal limb length. The transischial line is used for evaluation of effective limb length. Note that the patient's normal right hip shows the lesser trochanter to be at the level of the transischial line, whereas the total hip replacement results in the lesser trochanter extending beyond the line. The total hip results in an effective over-lengthening of the leg.

cups are sized for complete osseous coverage. Uncemented stems are chosen for optimal proximal fit rather than distal canal fit, with the goal of providing maximal surface contact to promote bone ingrowth and to prevent subsidence of the prosthesis (inferior movement of the implant into the femoral shaft).

In evaluating follow-up films of prostheses, it is crucial to have a comparison film taken at or around the time of placement of the prosthesis. Comparison with this index film may reveal subtle changes in position of a component, which may not be seen with the most recent comparison film (Fig. 2-105). Loosening can definitely be diagnosed when there is migration of a component (generally superiorly and medially with an acetabular component, inferiorly with a femoral component), or a change in alignment. Therefore, at follow-up, specific evaluation of limb length, lateral opening angle of the acetabulum, and positioning of the components relative to their position at the time of initial placement must be made. If there is no definite change in position or alignment, loosening may still be identified. In a cemented prosthesis, one may expect to see thin (1–2 mm) radiolucent zones at the cement interfaces. If these radiolucent zones are less than 2 mm wide at the bone-cement interface and are not continuous around the component nor progressive over time, they are considered normal. These lucencies are particularly common around the superolateral portion of the acetabular component and tip of the femoral stem. If however, that radiolucent zone measures greater than 2mm, or shows progressive widening, the prostheses is considered loose.

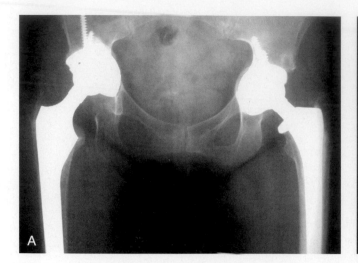
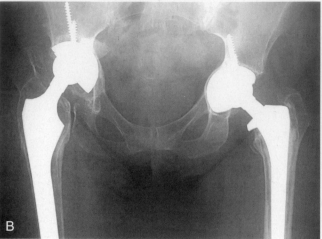

Fig. 2-105   Failed total hip arthroplasty. **A,** A cementless right total hip arthroplasty and hybrid left total hip arthroplasty, with the components appropriately aligned and showing no evidence of loosening. **B,** A film taken 4 years later shows a significant change, with loosening of all the components. The right acetabular component has tilted and is superiorly subsided. The right femoral component shows a lucency surrounding it at the bone component interface with subsidence of the component by approximately 2 cm. The left acetabular component shows a 2 mm lucency surrounding it, with slight tilt, indicating loosening. The left femoral component shows a 2–3 mm lucency surrounding the bone cement interface. This is loose as well. Finally, both acetabular components show offset of the femoral heads within them, indicating polyethylene wear.

Cement fractures also usually associated with loosening of the component (Fig. 2-106).

As with the cemented component, the most convincing sign of loosening in a cementless component is progressive change in position, either subsidence or tilt. However, there are other signs that may be of value and worth monitoring. First, it is important to note that prominent calcar resorption is common in cementless prostheses. Furthermore, a radiolucent zone between the bone and prosthesis is frequently seen, often with a sclerotic margin. Cortical thickening and endosteal sclerosis may be seen at the tip of the femoral prosthesis without implication of loosening of the stem.[18] However, such findings must be watched for progression. If the radiolucent zone at the bone prosthesis interface is greater than 2 mm in width, it is likely to represent loosening. Furthermore, excessive cortical hypertrophy and endosteal bone bridging at the stem tip or excessive endosteal scalloping also likely represent loosening, particularly if progression is shown (Figs. 2-107 and 2-108). Additionally, bead shedding (separation of microspheres from the component) suggest loosening. Progression and other signs should be watched for.

Besides loosening, failure of the construct itself may constitute a complication. Fracture of the prosthesis itself is uncommon, but when present tends to be of the distal stem. Separation of the polyethylene insert from its backing may be heralded by the presence of small wedge-shaped metallic fragments (Fig. 2-109). Fractures and displacement of the polyethylene can occasionally be seen, but rarely with enough clarity to illustrate in a textbook. Fracture of the host bone is uncommon and can occur in the pelvis as well as the femoral shaft. In the shaft, a fracture usually begins at the tip of the prosthetic stem and progresses longitudinally and anteriorly. This fracture pattern is seen most frequently in long stem femoral revisions, where the tip of the revision fractures the femoral cortex at its anterior bow. These fractures are usually nondisplaced and are easily overlooked.

Polyethylene wear is theoretically a trivial problem, but in practice occurs relatively frequently. Polyethylene wear can be subtle and asymmetric, and is revealed by offset of the femoral head within the acetabular cup, where the wear in the polyethylene occurs superolaterally in the weight bearing portion (Fig. 2-110). Polyethylene wear itself can cause mechanical symptoms. Additionally, the particles of polyethylene can cause a more serious problem, initiating a granulomatous reaction that can result in very impressive destruction of bone (Fig. 2-111). This osseous destruction related to granulomatous disease has been termed "massive osteolysis" or "particle disease." It is important to note that the source of the particles is immaterial; the particles may be polyethylene, cement, osseous debris, or even metallic microspheres. Rather than the material, the size of the particles seems to elicit the granulomatous reaction.

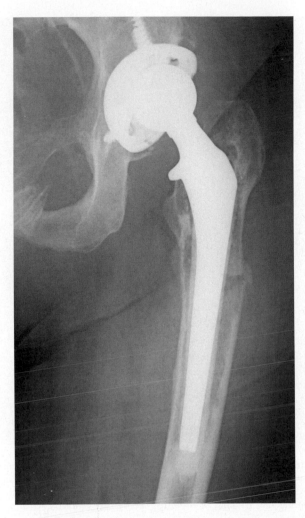

Fig. 2-106 Failed cemented femoral component. This AP radiograph demonstrates a wide lucency at the bone cement interface of the femoral component, with fracture in the proximal shaft of the femur. Additionally, there is polyethylene wear, with offset of the femoral head within the acetabular component.

Infection is a serious complication of total joint arthroplasty. Plain radiographic findings are usually not helpful nor specific in identifying prosthetic infections. The radiographs may either appear normal or may mimic loosening or particle disease. If infection is suspected, aspiration under strict aseptic condition, supplemented if necessary with nonbacteriostatic saline injection, enables detection of most prosthetic infections. Radionuclide imaging for detection of infection or loosening can be problematic as technetium uptake is a normal postoperative finding and expected for at least one year after surgery, with different uptake patterns observed for cemented and uncemented prostheses.

Many of the generalizations discussed above for total hip arthroplasty also apply to total knee arthroplasties.[19] The tibial component should be placed 90° +/− 5° to

the long axis of the tibial shaft on the AP radiograph and ranges from 90° to the long axis of the tibia to a slight posterior tilt on the lateral radiograph. The femoral component is placed in 5° +/− 5° to the long axis of the femoral shaft on the lateral, with 4–7° of valgus angulation of the knee as seen on the AP. Of all the components, the tibial is more likely to loosen. Early loosening is usually followed by tilting of the tibial component into a varus position with subsidence into the medial tibial plateau and collapse of the cancellous bone. Polyethylene wear, fragmentation, and dislocation may follow (Fig. 2-112). Patellar complications occur frequently, including subsidence, polyethylene wear, polyethylene dissociation from the metal backing, disintegration of the metal backing with metalosis (metal particles lining the polyethylene and capsule) (Fig. 2-113), and patellar AVN or fracture. An additional abnormality to watch for in followup of knee prostheses is a periprosthetic fracture. Patients who are osteoporotic with knee prostheses (for example, patients with RA) are particularly prone to developing fractures in the metaphyseal region of either the distal femur or proximal tibia. This may be seen as a minor change in contour or a sclerotic line of fracture

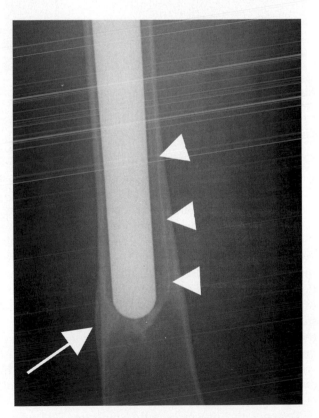

Fig. 2-107 Failed cementless femoral component. The AP radiograph demonstrates a wide lucency and sclerotic line surrounding the femoral component (*arrowheads*). Additionally, there is endosteal and periosteal hypertrophy (*arrow*).

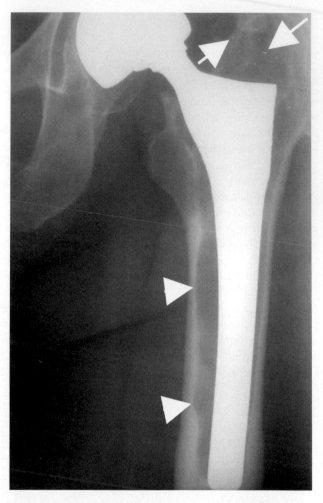

Fig. 2-108 Failed cementless femoral component. This AP radiograph demonstrates scalloping of the endosteum (*arrowheads*) as well as bead shedding (*arrows*), indicating failure of this cementless prosthesis. It has also subsided by approximately 1 cm.

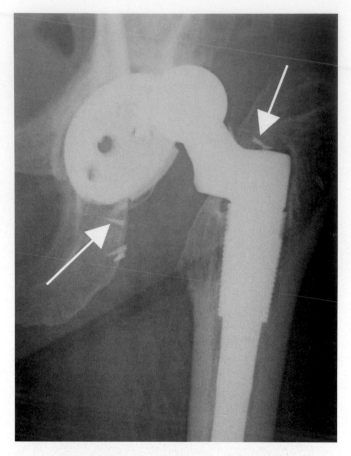

Fig. 2-109 Failed total hip arthroplasty. This patient has a dislocated total hip, with multiple wedge-shaped metallic densities (*arrows*). These spikes are used to hold the polyethylene within the metallic backing of the cup. Seeing them indicates failure of the cup.

healing (Fig. 2-114). If a patient has had a previous tibial tubercle transfer, proximal tibial fracture is even more likely following placement of a total knee arthroplasty.

Silastic arthroplasties are often placed, particularly at the MCP and MTP joints. If the arthroplasty is of the Swanson variety, it is most at risk for fracture at the thinnest part, that which acts as the "hinge" at the junction of the flange and the body. In addition dislocation of the flange may occur, especially in diseases such as RA that have soft tissue imbalance or contractures. Finally, as these prostheses are usually not cemented, repetitive motion results in particle breakdown and particle disease with prominent osteolysis can develop (Fig. 2-115). The same process can be seen with silastic carpal implants (Fig. 2-116).

Degenerative processes in the spine are often treated with anterior diskectomy and fusion. In the cervical spine, the ACDF (anterior cervical diskectomy and fusion) is performed with a bone plug placed between

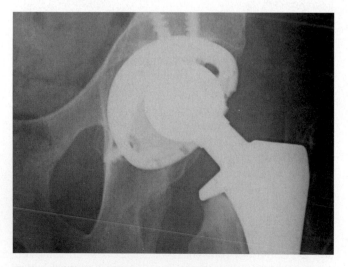

Fig. 2-110 Polyethylene wear. Polyethylene wear is indicated on this AP radiograph by the offset of the femoral head within the acetabular component.

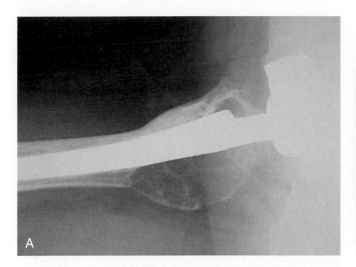

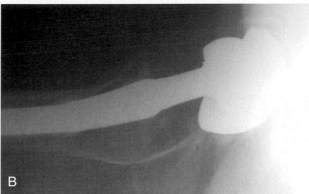

Fig. 2-111   Particle disease. **A,** The frogleg lateral demonstrates an expanded lytic lesion in the proximal femoral metaphysis. This osteolysis most frequently is related to particle disease. **B,** In this case, the source of the particles is seen only on the groin lateral, where offset of the femoral head within the cup is noted. Therefore, the osteolysis in this case is due to particle disease from polyethylene wear.

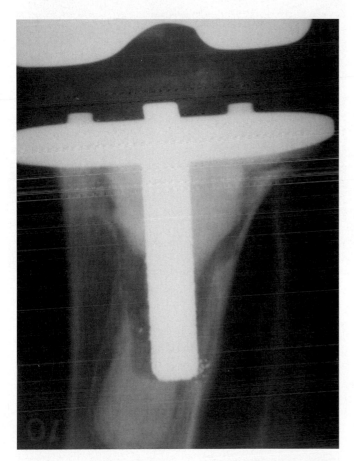

Fig. 2-112   Tibial component loosening. This AP radiograph demonstrates gross tibial component loosening, with medial tilt of the component, fracture of the cement, and bead shedding.

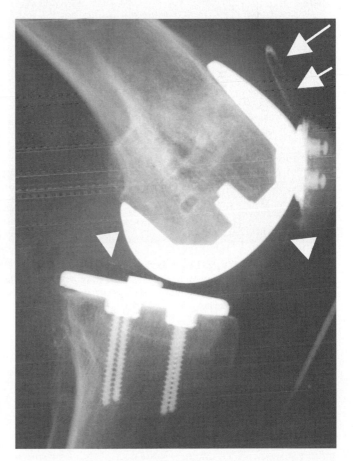

Fig. 2-113   Patellar component failure. This lateral radiograph demonstrates superior subsidence of the patellar component. It also shows dissociation of some of the metal backing, with displacement into the suprapatellar bursa (*arrows*). Finally, the patient is developing metallosis in the joint, with metallic fragments lining the polyethylene and joint capsule (*arrowheads*).

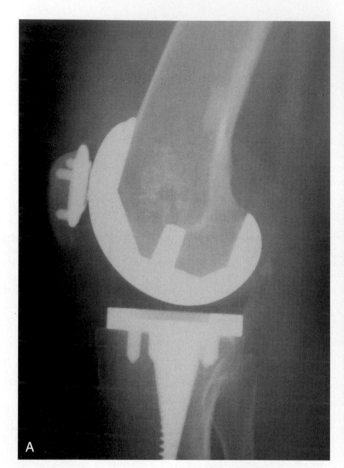
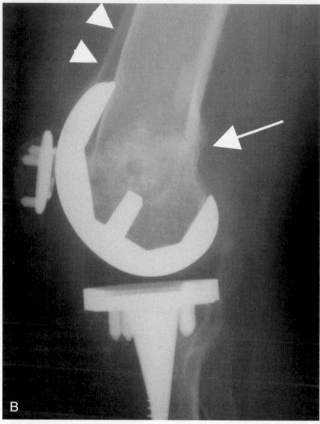

Fig. 2-114   Periprosthetic fracture. **A,** A lateral radiograph of the knee arthroplasty at the time of placement. **B,** The same knee several months later. The patient has developed a fracture in the distal femoral metaphysis (*arrow*), angulation at the fracture site, and healing reaction seen at the anterior femoral cortex (*arrowheads*).

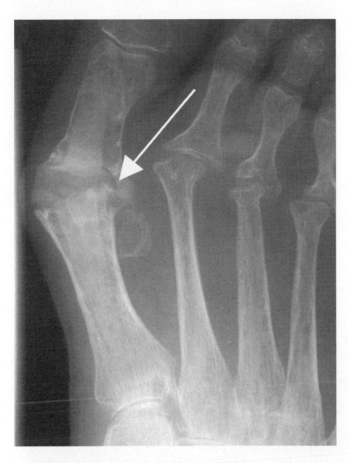

Fig. 2-115   Swanson prosthesis with particle disease. The AP radiograph of the great toe demonstrates a Swanson prosthesis placed at the first MTP. The prosthesis has failed, with fracture of the lateral body (*arrow*), and the resultant abnormal motion has allowed particle disease and osteolysis to occur in both the first metatarsal and proximal phalanx.

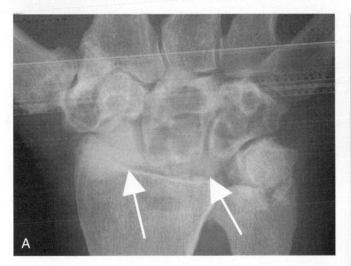

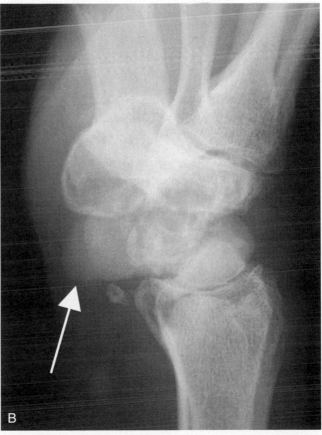

Fig. 2-116   Silastic carpal implant failure. **A,** A PA radiograph of the wrist demonstrating resection of the scaphoid and lunate and replacement by silastic prostheses (*arrows*). There is significant particle disease, with large cysts seen in the trapezium, capitate, and hamate. **B,** The lateral view shows dislocation of one of the carpal prostheses in a volar direction (*arrow*).

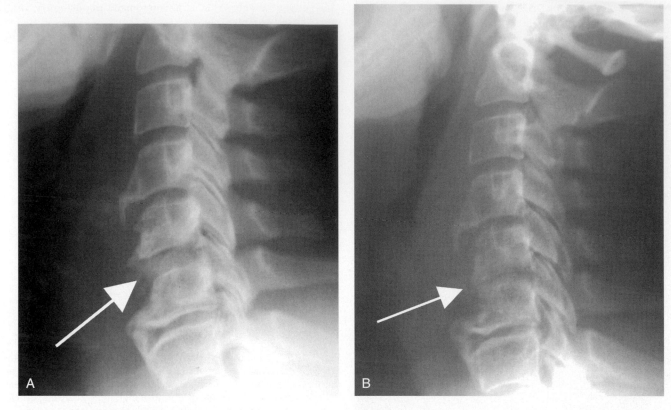

Fig. 2-117   ACDF complication. **A,** A lateral radiograph demonstrating an anterior discectomy and placement of bone graft at C5–6 (*arrow*). There is prevertebral soft tissue swelling, but this is expected on an immediate postoperative film. **B,** A film taken 3 weeks later shows continued prevertebral soft tissue swelling, and resorption of the bone graft, and new indistinctness of the endplates (*arrow*). This represents infection as a postoperative complication.

adjacent vertebral bodies. It may or may not be secured with an anterior plate and screw system. If there is an anterior plate, failure may be detected by backing out of the screws or shift in position of the plate. With or without the plate, the bone plug should be evaluated for shift in position (it can displace in any direction, but seems to displace most frequently in an anterior direction). An important additional complication to watch for is infection (Fig. 2-117).

REFERENCES

1. Murphey M, Wetzel L, Bramble J, Levine E, Simpson K, Lindsley H: Sacroiliitis: MR imaging findings, *Radiology* 180:239-244, 1991.
2. Bollow M, Braun J, Hamm B, et al: Early sacroiliitis in patients with spondyloarthropathy: Evaluation with dynamic gadolinium enhanced MR imaging, *Radiology* 194:529-536, 1995.
3. Weissman B, Rappaport A, Sosman J, et al: Radiographic findings in the hands in patients with systemic lupis erythematosis, *Radiology* 126:313-317, 1978.
4. Basset L, Blocka K, Furst D, et al: Skeletal findings in progressive systemic sclerosis (scleroderma), *AJR* 136:1121-1126, 1981.
5. Cobby M, Adler R, Swartz R, Martel W: Dialysis related amyloid arthropathy: MR findings in four patients, *AJR* 157:1023-1027, 1991.
6. Rafto S, Dalinka M, Scheibler M, Burk D, Kricun M: Spondyloarthropathy of the cervical spine and long term hemodialysis, *Radiology* 166:201-204, 1988.
7. Bock G, Garcia A, Weisman M, et al: Rapidly destructive hip disease: clinical and imaging abnormalities, *Radiology* 186:461-466, 1993.
8. Brower A, Allman R: Pathogenesis of the neurotrophic joint: neurotraumatic versus neurovascular, *Radiology* 139:349-354, 1981.
9. Bjorkengren A, Weisman M, Pathria M, Zlatkin M, Pate D, Resnick D: Neuroarthropathy associated with chronic alcoholism, *AJR* 151:743-745, 1981.
10. Wagner S, Schweitzer M, Morrison W, Przybylski G, Parker L: Can imaging findings help differentiate spinal neuropathic arthropathy from disk space infection? Initial experience. *Radiology* 214:693-699, 2000.
11. Yu J, Chung C, Recht M, Dailiana T, Jurdi R: MR imaging of tophacious gout, *AJR* 168: 523-527, 1997.

12. Steinbach L, Resnick D: Calcium pyrophosphate dihydrate crystal deposition disease revisited, *Radiology* 200:1-9, 1996.

13. Yang B, Sartoris D, Djukic S, Resnick D, Clopton P: Distribution of calcification in the triangular fibrocartilage region in 181 patients with calcium pyrophosphate dihydrate crystal deposition disease, *Radiology* 196:547-550, 1995.

14. Glickstein M, Burk D, Schiebler M, et al: Avascular necrosis versus other diseases of the hip: sensitivity of MR imaging, *Radiology* 169:213-215, 1988.

15. Tervonen O, Mueller D, Matteson E, Velosa J, Ginsberg W, Ehman R: Clinically occult avascular necrosis of the hip: prevalence in an asymptomatic population at risk, *Radiology* 182:845-847, 1992.

16. Kopecky K, Braunstein E, Brandt K, et al: Apparent avascular necrosis of the hip; appearance and spontaneous resolution of MR findings of renal allograft recipients, *Radiology* 179:523-527, 1991.

17. Manaster B: Total hip arthroplasty: radiographic evaluation, *Radiographics* 16:645-660, 1996.

18. Kaplan P, Montesi S, Jardon O, Gregory P: Bone in-growth hip prostheses in asymptomatic patients: Radiographic features, *Radiology* 169:221-227, 1988.

19. Manaster B: Total knee arthroplasty: Post-operative radiographic findings, *AJR* 165:899-904, 1995.

GENERALIZATIONS

DAVID A. MAY, M.D and DAVID G. DISLER, M.D.

BONE BIOMECHANICS

Mechanical forces that act upon bone can be distilled to three basic types. These are *compression, tension,* and *shear.* Compression is force that pushes two objects together. Tension is force that pulls two objects apart. Shear is force that slides two objects past one another. Within a single object, such as an appendicular bone, these forces act on a microscopic level. Any material, be

Key Concepts   Bone Biomechanics

- The three primary forces of trauma are compression, tension, and shear.
- Bones are most resistant to compression.
- The bones of children can bend or buckle without breaking into separate fragments.
- The bones of adults are stronger but stiffer, and break rather than permanently bending.

it metal, wood, or bone, has a unique threshold at which it will fail (fracture) with each of these forces. Bones and joints are *anisotropic.* This means that their mechanical properties are different when loaded in different directions. Specifically, bones and joints are weaker in tension than in compression.

Another important biomechanical property of bone is that it can deform (bend) while under load and then return to its original shape after the load is removed. However, a sufficiently powerful force can permanently deform the bone or cause it to fracture. In normal adult bones, the fracture threshold is lower than the permanent deformation threshold, so bending deformity is generally not seen. In younger children's bones, the opposite is true, so fractures in the form of bending injuries can occur as well as complete fractures.

A fracture can be caused by just one of the three basic mechanical forces, or by a combination. An example of a fracture due to isolated *tension* is the transverse fracture of the patella, in which violent contracture of the extensor mechanism of the thigh places the patella under extreme tension. If the patella fails, the resulting fracture will be transverse (Fig. 3-1). This example illustrates the general rule that fracture lines resulting from tension occur perpendicular to the direction of the applied force. The common avulsion fracture is another example of a tension fracture. Isolated *compression* force in a long bone usually produces an oblique fracture (Fig. 3-2), and in the spine produces a vertebral body compression (Fig. 3-3). *Shear* forces tend to create fracture lines oblique to the line of force. Shear forces are present on a microscopic level in most fractures because the multi-

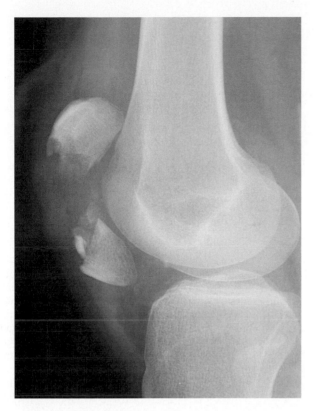

Fig. 3-1   Transverse fracture of the patella caused by tension failure during extreme quadriceps contraction.

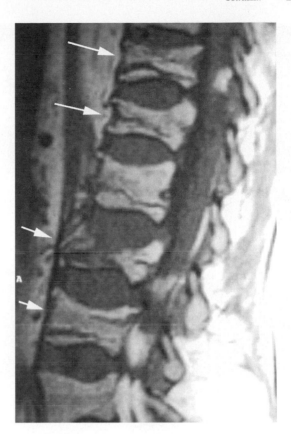

Fig. 3-3   Multiple compressions of the lumbar vertebral bodies (*arrows*) in a patient with osteoporosis (sagittal T1-weighted image). The irregular low signal lines within the vertebral bodies represent fracture lines.

directional bone trabeculae are placed under shear stress regardless of whether the primary force is compression or tension.

Many fractures are caused by a combination of the three basic mechanical forces. One such example is bending. If a bone is bent, tension forces develop along the convex portion of the curve while compressive forces develop along the concave portion of the curve. Bone is better able to withstand compression forces than tension forces, so the convex margin will fail first. Examples of bending-type fractures are a childhood plastic deformation (Fig. 3-4A), childhood greenstick fracture (Fig. 3-4B), and a butterfly-shaped comminuted fracture in adults (Fig. 3-5). Another combination force is a twisting or rotational injury in which rotational force is applied around the circumference of a bone. This mechanism combines compression, tension, and shear, resulting in a spiral fracture (Fig. 3-6).

An additional important biomechanical property of bone is that the fracture threshold is inversely related to the rate at which a load is applied. In other words, bone is more resistant to a slowly increasing force than to rapidly increasing force. A rapidly delivered, sharp impact such as from a bullet or a direct blow to a bone is more

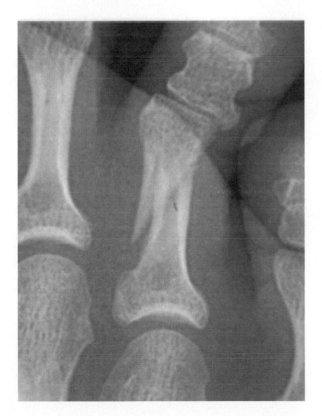

Fig. 3-2   Oblique fracture of the fourth toe proximal phalanx.

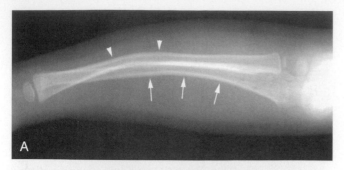

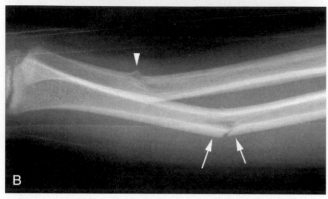

Fig. 3-4   Bowing fractures in children. **A,** Pure plastic bowing fracture of the forearm in a 5 year old. The ulna is laterally bowed (*arrows*) and the radius is dorsally bowed (*arrowheads*). These bones are normally mildly bowed in these directions, but the degree of bowing, combined with a history of fall and forearm pain establishes the diagnosis. **B,** Greenstick fracture. Note the distraction on the convex side of the radius fracture (*arrows*). Also note the buckle fracture on the concave (compression) side of the ulna (*arrowhead*).

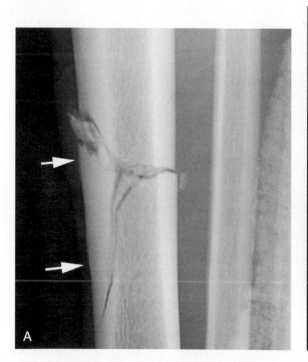

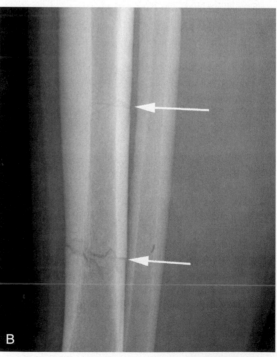

Fig. 3-5   Comminuted fractures. **A,** Adult equivalent of bowing fracture: butterfly comminution fracture. The *arrows* point to the butterfly fragment in a tibial fracture. **B,** Segmental fracture. Lateral view of the tibia shows two fracture sites (*arrowheads*) separated by a segment of normal bone.

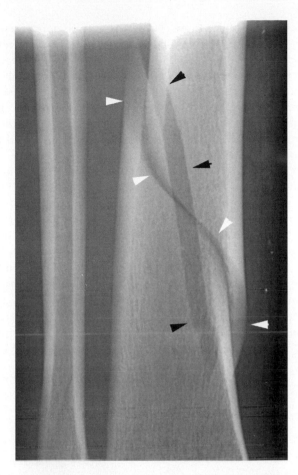

Fig. 3-6   Spiral fracture. Note the typical combination of a spiral component (*white arrowheads*) and a straight, longitudinal component (*black arrowheads*).

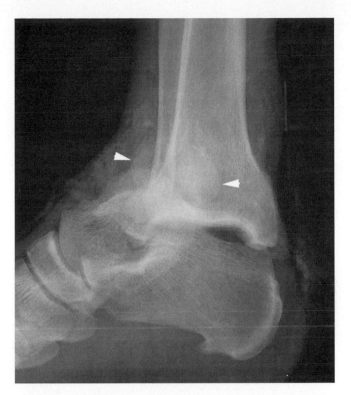

Fig. 3-7   Fracture-dislocation of the ankle. Note that the tibia is seen in the AP projection, but the foot is seen in the lateral projection. Also note two fracture fragments (*arrowheads*) that other views (not shown) revealed to be portions of the malleoli.

likely to cause a fracture than a greater force that builds slowly. However, even a slowly increasing force can eventually exceed a bone's fracture threshold, often with severe damage to the bone as a great deal of force is present. In the soft tissues, a rapidly applied force also is more likely to cause tissue failure. This is why a high velocity injury such as a gunshot wound can cause so much damage to the soft tissues. Small defects within a bone such as a screw tract will concentrate forces at a single point called a *stress riser* that lowers the threshold for fracture.

The ligaments provide joint stability by resisting tension. Forces applied across a joint may cause ligament failure (tear) or fracture of the ligamentous attachment, with transient or chronic subluxation or dislocation. *Subluxation* is partial loss of contact between the articular surfaces. *Dislocation* is complete loss of contact between the articular surfaces. *Diastasis* is separation or widening of a slightly mobile joint such as the acromioclavicular joint or the symphysis pubis. (This term is also used less precisely to describe gaps between articular surface fragments of an intraarticular fracture.) Traumatic dislo-

cation and diastasis generally imply the presence of significant ligamentous injury and the potential for chronic joint instability. Traumatic dislocation often disrupts both ligaments and bones (Fig. 3-7). The causes of subluxation include an acute or chronic ligamentous injury, laxity due to a generalized process such as Ehlers-Danlos syndrome (discussed in Chapter 5), or articular cartilage thinning in the setting of arthritis. Ligamentous injury that does not cause complete disruption is termed a *sprain*. Ligament sprains may be graded based on the MR imaging features, but the gold standard is clinical examination.

FRACTURE DESCRIPTION TERMINOLOGY

Open versus Closed Fracture

In a *closed fracture,* osseous fragments do not breach the skin surface. In contrast, an *open fracture* is a fracture

Key Concept	Fracture Description Terminology

- Consistent use of the precise language of fractures allows clear communication of the findings in a fracture.

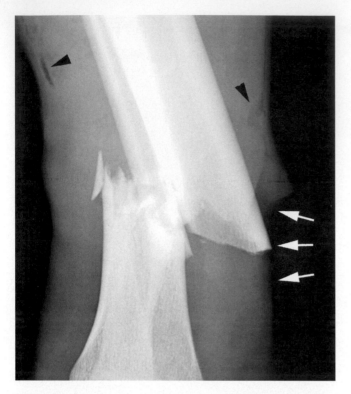

Fig. 3-8   Open fracture of the tibia. Note bone fragment projecting through skin wound (*white arrows*). Also note the subcutaneous gas (*black arrowheads*) that can be an important tell-tale sign of skin disruption in subtler cases of open fracture.

that is associated with skin disruption and exposure of a bone fragment (Fig. 3-8). This substantially increases the risk for infection and is considered an emergent situation for surgical reduction and lavage of the fracture site. As a rule of thumb, the risk of osteomyelitis is increased if the skin wound is more than 1 cm in size, and significantly increased if the wound is more than 10 cm in size. Wound contamination also increases the risk of infection.

Incomplete versus Complete Fractures

Incomplete fractures are those in which the fracture line does not circumferentially disrupt the cortex. Such fractures occur most often in children because of the different mechanical properties of bone in children compared with that of adults, in which bone can bend before fracture. Most incomplete fractures involve some deformity of the bone, although an incomplete fracture can be nondisplaced, such as a toddler's fracture (Fig. 3-9). Three major types of displaced incomplete fractures are buckle, greenstick, and plastic bowing deformity. A *buckle fracture* is focal compression of cortex due to an axial load (Figs. 3-10, 3-4B). A *torus fracture* is a complete (circumferential) type of buckle fracture, but these terms are often used interchangeably. A *greenstick fracture* results from bending force with tension failure of the

convex side of the bone (Fig. 3-4B). A pure *plastic bowing deformity* is a bending of bone without a discrete fracture line (Fig. 3-4A). This injury represents innumerable microfractures of a long segment of bone. Incomplete fractures in adults are unusual, and often have unusual mechanisms (Fig. 3-11). *Complete fractures,* unlike incomplete fractures, result in fracture lines extending across all cortical margins of bone and are described as *transverse, oblique,* or *spiral.*

Comminution indicates that the bone is fractured into more than two fragments. A *segmental* comminuted fracture is one in which the same bone is fractured in two remote sites, with an intact segment of bone separating the fracture sites (Fig. 3-5B). A butterfly-comminuted fracture is one in which a wedge-shaped fragment of intervening bone is present (Fig. 3-5A). The butterfly fragment occurs on the side in which a greater degree of compression has occurred. Butterfly compression fractures are more prone to displacement and telescoping of fracture fragments and thus a greater propensity for instability.

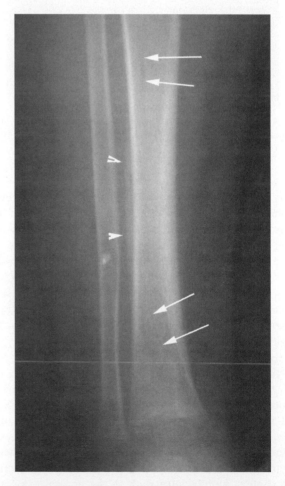

Fig. 3-9   Toddler's fracture. Note the subtle nondisplaced fracture of the tibial shaft (*arrows*) and the lateral periosteal reaction (*arrowheads*) indicating that the fracture is healing. (Courtesy of L. Das Narla, M.D., Richmond, VA.)

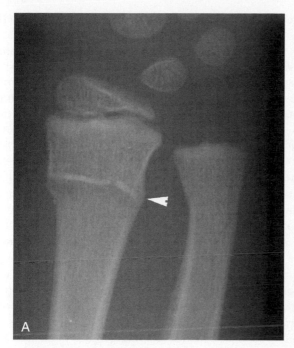

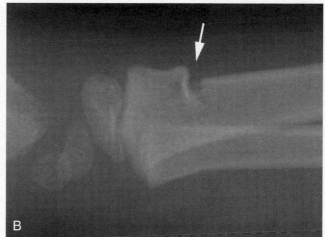

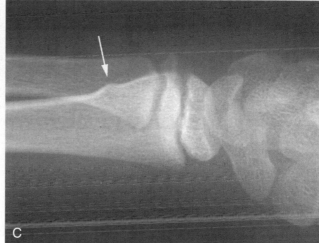

Fig. 3-10   Childhood buckle fracture **A, B,** PA (**A**) and lateral (**B**) views show a dorsal distal radial metaphyseal buckle fracture (*arrows*). **C,** Subtle dorsal buckle in an older child (*arrow*).

Hence, internal or external fixation is often used to treat these fractures.

Position

In addition to a description of the degree of comminution, an accurate description of relative position of bone fragments is extremely important and requires conventional language to facilitate communication of the findings. First, it is useful to localize a long bone fracture by dividing the length of the bone into thirds. Thus, a fracture can be located in the proximal third, the junction of the proximal and middle thirds, the middle third, the junction of the middle and distal thirds, or the distal third. A long bone fracture can also be described as being epiphyseal, metaphyseal, metadiaphyseal, or diaphyseal. It is important to describe whether fractures extend to articular margins because such fractures greatly increase the need for surgical intervention and lessen the likelihood of a normal outcome. One of the most important complications of intraarticular fractures is posttraumatic

osteoarthritis. In skeletally immature patients, it is important to describe whether a fracture extends to or through a physis, as such fractures increase the likelihood for growth plate arrest, limb length discrepancy, and angular deformities. Physeal fractures and the Salter-Harris classification system are discussed below.

Once the exact position of the fracture fragments has been identified, it is important to describe deformities of *position and alignment*. It is unusual for a fracture to be anatomic (normal) in position. More commonly, fractures are displaced. By convention, *displacement* is described by the relative position of the more distal fragment compared to the more proximal fragment. Displacement can occur in any direction and the amount of displacement should be described. Again by convention, the amount of transverse displacement is described as a percentage of the cross-sectional diameter of the dominant osseous fragment. If displacement is greater than 100% of the shaft diameter, the fracture fragments can slide past one another. Muscle pull usually results in overlap of the fragments, a finding termed *bayonet appo-*

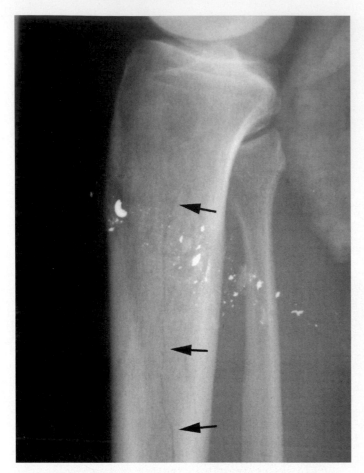

Fig. 3-11   Incomplete tibial fracture in an adult (*black arrows*) due to a gunshot wound. Note the metal fragments that mark the bullet tract.

quate, but CT can be helpful in difficult cases (see Fig. 5-75).

Avulsion fractures are caused by tension (traction) by a tendon or ligament. The term *chip fracture* may be used to describe any small cortical fragment, but is more precisely limited to fractures caused by focal impaction or shearing rather than avulsion.

An *intraarticular fracture* extends through an articular surface. Intraarticular extension can be surprisingly subtle, for example in the proximal tibia, requiring oblique views and sometimes CT or MRI for diagnosis. Such fractures usually produce the nonspecific finding of a hemarthrosis, which may produce a fluid-fluid level on a horizontal beam radiograph due to settling of the cellular components of blood. A *fat-fluid* level, caused by escape of marrow fat into a joint space, is much more specific for an intraarticular fracture, but is less commonly seen. Sometimes three levels are seen, with the fat on top and the cellular layer on the bottom (Fig. 3-12). Attention to alignment along the articular surface is important, as step-offs or separation of fracture fragments by more than 2 mm is associated with posttraumatic OA. The presence of such malalignment may prompt the surgeon to choose surgical reduction and fixation.

Stress Fractures

In precise usage, a *stress fracture* occurs as either a fatigue fracture or an insufficiency fracture, but the terms stress fracture and fatigue fracture are often used interchangeably. A *fatigue fracture* occurs when abnormal stresses, usually in the form of multiple and frequent

sition. The length of any such overlap should be included in the report. In contrast, *distraction* is longitudinal separation of the fracture fragments along the long axis of the bone.

Angular deformity refers to a directional change in the long axis of the fracture fragments. This can be described by the direction of the apex of the angle formed by the fracture fragments or by the orientation of the distal fracture fragment. Orthopedic surgeons more commonly describe angular deformities by the angular displacement of the distal fracture fragment. For example, *medial,* or *varus angulation* means that the distal fracture fragment is pointing toward the midline of the body. *Lateral,* or *valgus angulation* refers to the distal fracture fragment that is pointing away from the midline of the body.

Rotation, or torsion, refers to twisting of one fracture fragment relative to another around the long axis of a bone. Rotational deformity is important, but can be difficult to determine with radiographs. It is necessary to image the entire length of a fractured bone as well as the joint at either end. Clinical evaluation is usually ade-

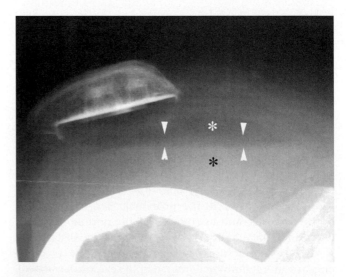

Fig. 3-12   Fat-fluid-fluid level. Cross table lateral view in a patient with an intraarticular distal femur fracture and a knee arthroplasty. Note the low attenuation fat layer on top (*white asterisk*), with a water density serum layer in the middle (between the *white arrowheads*), and a slightly denser layer containing serum and blood cells at the bottom (*black asterisk*).

repetition of otherwise normal stress, are placed on normal bone. Several factors contribute to the development of a fatigue-type stress fracture. First, the muscles, tendons, and ligaments normally help to redistribute forces applied to the bones and joints. However, muscle fatigue during prolonged exercise results in less protection of the bones and joints. Second, increased bone loading stimulates a normal adaptive process that leads to new bone formation. This observation is known as *Wolff's law*. The mechanism of this phenomenon is not completely understood, but on a microscopic level appears to be stimulated by microfractures. New bone formation requires the activity of both osteoblasts and osteoclasts, as the weaker or injured old bone is replaced with stronger new bone. Unfortunately, the osteoclasts begin first, so, paradoxically, an increase in physical activity at first results in the bones becoming weaker for a few weeks before ultimately becoming stronger. This creates a window of vulnerability during which time the microfractures can coalesce into a discrete fracture.

Thus, stress fractures evolve over time. Early stress injuries tend to be distributed along a long segment of the cortex. Radiographs at this stage are usually normal, but faint cortical resorption or periosteal reaction may be seen. This stage is sometimes termed a *stress reaction* or, in the tibia, a *shin splint,* but the terminology is not standardized. With ongoing microfractures, a focal segment within the stress reaction may weaken more rapidly. This weaker segment becomes a focal point for bone deformation during repeated loading because it is less able to resist deformation than the remainder of the bone. This concentration of microscopic bone deformation at the focally weakened segment has two important consequences. First, the stresses applied to the remainder of the bone are partially relieved, allowing it to heal. Second, the microfractures in the weakened segment are subject to greater deformation, so they are more likely to progress. In any terminology, this is a true stress fracture (Fig. 3-13). A bone scan at this stage will show intense tracer uptake confined to one portion of the cortex. Radionuclide bone scan has high negative predictive value in that a negative bone scan virtually excludes the possibility of a stress fracture. (However, regarding diagnosis of an *acute* fracture in the elderly, a bone scan may be falsely negative in the first 72 hours after injury in up to 20% of cases.) Radiographs may reveal focal periosteal reaction or fuzzy sclerosis at or near the weakened segment, but remain much less sensitive than a bone scan. Linear sclerosis, often perpendicular to major trabecular lines, may be seen in a healing phase. MRI is highly sensitive because of the associated marrow edema, and can be specific if a low signal fracture line is seen. If untreated, a stress fracture can progress to a complete fracture. Stress fractures can occur in almost any weight-bearing bone. Classic locations are the

femoral neck and tibial shaft in runners, the metatarsals of new military recruits (*march fracture,* Fig. 3-13C), and the bones of the feet in a variety of athletes. Lumbar spondylolysis, discussed in Chapter 5, probably also is a form of stress fracture.

Treatment of a stress fracture requires rest and, in more advanced cases, immobilization. Successful treatment also requires the cooperation of the patient. Many stress fractures are self-inflicted overuse injuries, in which patients ignore the warning signs because of their passion for the injurious activity. Knowledge that earlier intervention results in more rapid healing may help to persuade the injured patient to allow their injury to heal.

An *insufficiency fracture* occurs when normal stresses are placed on bone that is demineralized, typically by osteoporosis or metabolic bone disease. The multiple osteoporotic compressions in Figure 3-3 are examples of insufficiency fracture. Like a fatigue-type stress fracture, an insufficiency fracture can often be diagnosed by clinical history, but imaging is helpful for confirmation. Detection of a nondisplaced insufficiency fracture on radiographs can be quite difficult due to osteopenia. Initial films are negative about 80% of the time. Bone scan is sensitive but nonspecific unless a specific pattern of tracer uptake can be identified, such as the H-shaped pattern of activity in a sacral insufficiency fracture (discussed in Part III). MR imaging is highly sensitive to the presence of a fracture and is more specific than radionuclide imaging because a fracture line usually can be shown (Fig. 3-3). Though less sensitive than MRI, CT imaging can also be helpful, especially if MR images are dominated by extensive edema that obscures a fracture line. In this setting, CT often shows a lucent fracture line and evidence of early bone healing, which are specific for the presence of fracture.

The more general term *pathologic fracture* includes any fracture that occurs with normal stresses in an abnormal bone. Technically speaking, an insufficiency fracture is a type of pathologic fracture. However, the term pathologic fracture is usually reserved to describe a fracture through bone weakened by a tumor (Fig. 3-14).

FRACTURE REDUCTION, HEALING, AND COMPLICATIONS

Fracture reduction is restoration of anatomic (normal) alignment. *Closed reduction* is achieved by manipulation of the fractured extremity and casting. *Open reduction* involves operative access to the injured bone, often for the purpose of applying fixating hardware (*internal fixation,* Fig. 3-15) or assessment of the alignment of intraarticular fragments. *Internal fixation* is usually achieved by placement of a cortical plate fixed with transverse screws on the surface of the bone, pin or screw placement across

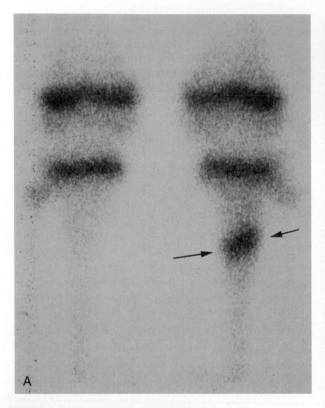

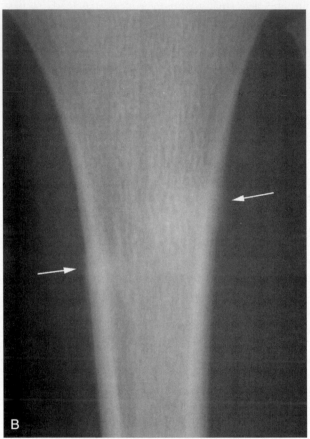

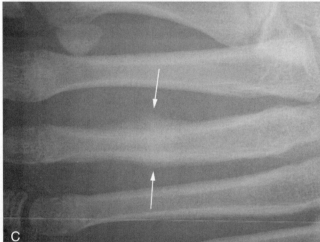

Fig. 3-13 Stress fractures. **A, B,** Tibial stress fracture. Bone scan (**A**) shows oblique transverse stress fracture in the proximal tibia (*arrows*). AP radiograph (**B**) shows very subtle perisoteal new bone formation in the same site (*arrows*). This example illustrates the superb sensitivity of bone scan in detection of long bone diaphyseal stress fractures. **C,** March fracture in a different patient. Note the periosteal new bone formation (*arrows*) and the subtle sclerosis caused by healing response to the fracture. (Courtesy of William Howard, M.D., San Antonio, TX.)

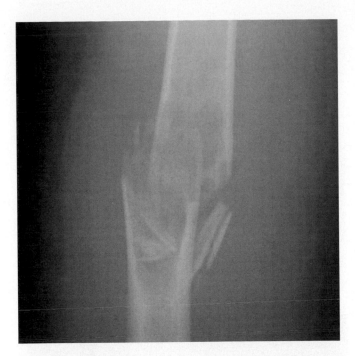

Fig. 3-14   Pathologic fracture through a unicameral bone cyst in the humerus of a child.

the fracture, or rod or nail within the medullary space along the long axis of the bone. *External fixation* is achieved by pins placed through the skin into the bone remote from the fracture site. The pins are fixed to one another externally (Fig. 3-16). External fixation is often used when the fracture site may be infected, or for fractures near the end of a bone. Regardless of reduction and immobilization, the main bone fragments must be in contact to allow healing. Compression across the fracture improves contact between the fragments and reduces the risk of nonunion. A variety of techniques may be used to achieve such compression (Fig. 3-15). On the other hand, compression must sometimes be limited, for example in comminuted long bone fractures that would telescope and shorten if compressed. The length of the bone can be controlled by fixation with a cortical plate or an intramedullary nail (rod) with proximal and distal interlocking screws.

Dynamic fixation means that fragment motion is allowed in one direction, but constrained in all others. Examples are a dynamic hip screw (discussed further in

---

Key Concepts | **Fracture follow-up radiographs**

The key issues are:
- Has the fracture changed in position or alignment?
- Is the fracture healing?
- Has a complication occurred? If hardware is present, is there evidence for a hardware-related complication?

Part III of this chapter) and "dynamizing" an intramedullary nail. In the latter, after a fracture has partially healed and gained a degree of stability, bone apposition may be improved by removal of the interlocking screws at one end of the nail. This allows the fragments to slide along the nail and impact against one another (Fig. 3-17), thereby improving bone apposition and healing.

When reducing a fracture, the orthopedic surgeon *reverses* the forces that caused the fracture. For example, a Colles fracture is caused by compression of the dorsal aspect of the distal radius. When reducing a Colles fracture, the surgeon must distract the dorsal radius, which is accomplished by distraction and palmarflexion of the wrist. Although the goal of fracture reduction is restoration of anatomic alignment, compromises must often be made to achieve the best possible outcome. A host of factors determine the desired fragment positions after reduction, including maximizing the likelihood of healing or minimizing the risk of complications. Postreduction radiographs of a Colles fracture may show exaggerated palmar tilt of the distal radius. However, the dorsal radius will tend to collapse before healing is complete, so the initial over-correction of the fracture will resolve before the fracture heals.

After the initial reduction, the purpose of subsequent imaging is to assess for the presence of healing and the occurrence of complication. Normal fracture healing is a predictable process, although it is affected by several factors including the age of the patient, the degree of local bone and soft tissue devitalization, the location of the fracture, the degree of immobilization and apposition of bone fragments after reduction, and the presence of complicating factors including infection, tumor at the site of fracture, bone necrosis, and systemic factors such as nutritional status, cigarette smoking, and corticosteroid treatment.

In the earliest phases of healing, a hematoma forms at the fracture site and induces a healing response associated with the release of growth factors and neovascularization. This initially results in localized bone demineralization around the fracture site. In addition, the bone at the margins of the fracture is necrotic, and is removed by osteoclasts. These changes cause blurring of the fracture margins as one of the first findings in fracture healing. Subsequently, immature bone called callus is formed within the hematoma, and between the apposing margins of the fracture fragments. Over time, the callus is remodeled into mature lamellar bone and biomechanical stability is restored (Fig. 3-18).

The rate of fracture healing depends on several variables. Healing is generally slower in the elderly, the malnourished, and cigarette smokers. Corticosteroid treatment retards fracture healing. Microscopic motion at the fracture site stimulates healing. Extremely rigid fixation with orthopaedic hardware can slow the rate of healing

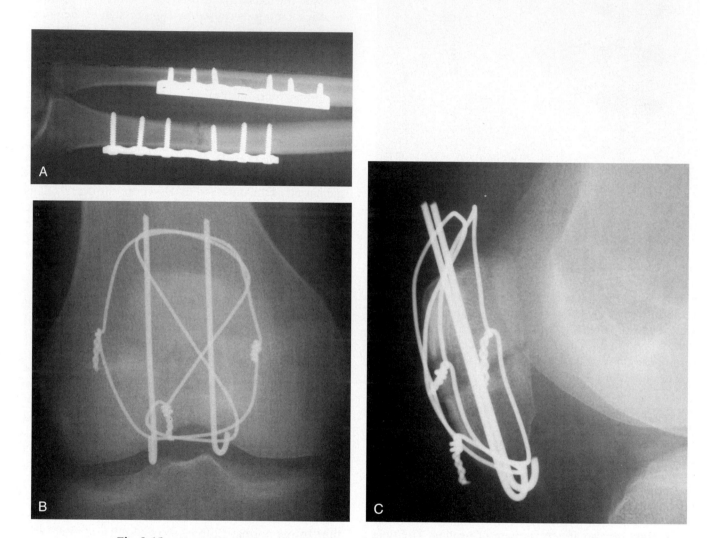

Fig. 3-15   Internal fixation. **A,** Adult both bones forearm fractures fixed with cortical compression plates. The slots for the screw heads are designed to force the fragments towards the center of the plate. Such compression increases apposition of bone fragments and thus speeds healing. **B,** (AP) and **C,** (lateral) views of compression wiring fixation of patellar fracture. Same patient as Fig. 3-1.

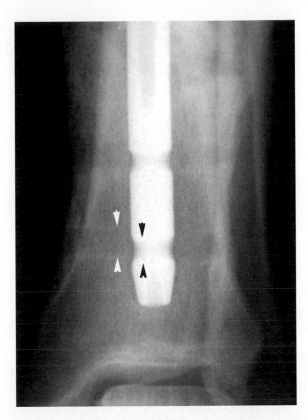

Fig. 3-17 Dynamized intramedullary nail. This distal tibial fracture is in the late stages of healing. The fracture was initially fixed with an intramedullary nail with proximal and distal interlocking screws. After the healing process had begun and partial fracture stability achieved, the distal interlocking screws were removed. This allowed the distal fragment to slide proximally along the nail until fully impacted against the proximal fragment, causing the old screw tracts (*white arrowheads*) shift proximally relative to the screw holes in the nail (*black arrowheads*).

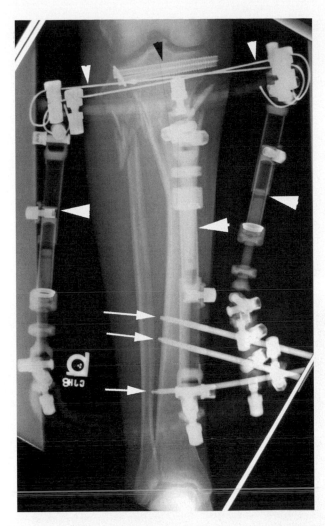

Fig. 3-16 External fixation. Note the fixation of the main proximal tibial fragment with crossing wires (*small white arrowheads*), the main distal fragment with pins (*white arrows*), and the adjustable external frame (*large white arrowheads*). This patient also has a tibial plateau fracture that is fixed with two transverse screws (*black arrowhead*).

by removing this stimulus. On the other hand, inadequate fixation causes abundant callus formation, but the callus cannot mature into biomechanically stable bone. The site of the fracture also affects the rate of healing. The tibia normally takes months to heal, in contrast with 6 to 8 weeks in most other bones. The term *delayed union* should be used with caution by a radiologist, because it may be incorrectly applied to a fracture that is healing slowly but satisfactorily. *Nonunion,* however, is a radiographic diagnosis in which one fails to see any evidence of bridging bone, and in which the fracture fragments at the apposing end become rounded and sclerotic (Fig. 3-19). Nonunion may be *hypertrophic,* that is, sclerotic and associated with excessive bone deposition, or *atrophic,* that is, associated with demineralization.

Malunion is fracture healing with angular or positional deformity. Malunion can result in a limb length

discrepancy or limb deformity that may limit function or cause pain. Not all malunion is equally disabling. The patient is more likely to tolerate some angular deformity if it is in the plane of motion of adjacent joints. For example, anterior angulation of a tibial fracture can be compensated at the knee and ankle. Anterior or posterior angular deformities in children may be corrected over time by the normal remodeling of ongoing bone growth. However, varus or valgus angular deformity in children tends to remodel less well, and rotational deformity very little.

Avascular necrosis (AVN) occasionally occurs after a fracture and is more common in bones or portions of bones in which there is tenuous blood supply. Examples include the proximal pole of the scaphoid, the talar dome, and the head of the femur. These bones have in common an extensive covering of articular cartilage, which limits the available sites for a blood vessel to enter the bone. If a bone's vascular supply is disrupted by a fracture, the affected bone does not develop the expected finding of demineralization related to hyperemia

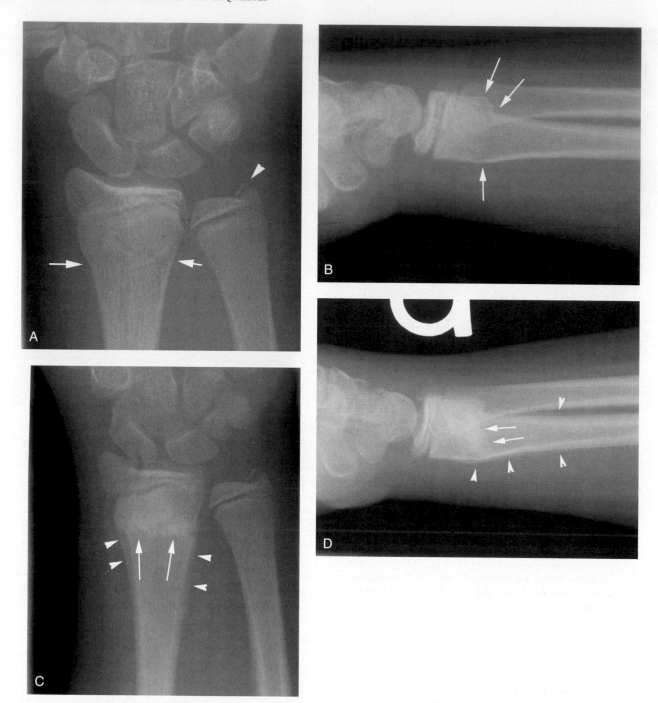

Fig. 3-18   Fracture healing in a child. PA (**A**) and lateral (**B**) views show an acute distal radius buckle fracture (*arrows*). Also note the ulnar styloid avulsion (*arrowhead* in **A**). **C, D,** Follow-up views 3 weeks later show trabecular healing seen as increased density along the fracture line (*arrows*). Also note the periosteal new bone formation (*arrowheads*). The periosteum is loosely adherent to the underlying bone in children, except at the physis, where it is tightly attached. Childhood fractures often result in periosteal elevation due to hematoma associated with the fracture. The elevated periosteum begins to form new bone soon after the fracture.

Continued

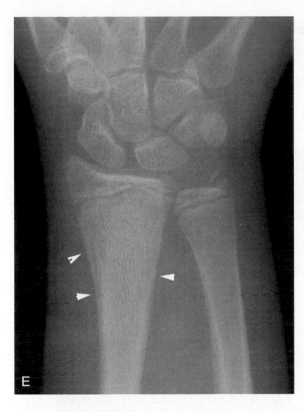

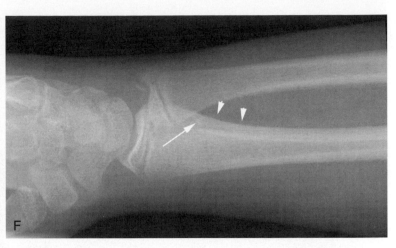

Fig. 3-18, cont'd   **E, F,** Follow-up views 5 weeks later show further maturation and remodeling of the periosteal new bone and remodeling of the old fractured cortex (*arrow* in **F**). On subsequent radiographs (not shown), the bone remodeled to anatomic alignment with no evidence that the fracture had ever occurred.

around the fracture site. The necrotic fragment remains dense while the vascularized surrounding bone becomes osteopenic. Although increased density is generally a sign of AVN, mild sclerosis of the proximal pole of the scaphoid can be a normal finding in a healing scaphoid fracture.

Osteomyelitis is a potential fracture complication after an open fracture or orthopedic hardware placement. Open fractures are at high risk for osteomyelitis and should be followed carefully for the development of soft tissue gas or for radiographic signs of osteomyelitis. Osteomyelitis can be caused by percutaneous pin placement. This is usually manifest as an area of osteolysis surrounding the pin or tract enlargement on follow-up imaging after removal of a pin.

Orthopedic hardware failure is another potential complication. Hardware failure can occur in three settings. The first setting occurs with inadequate fracture reduction, which results in undue strain on applied hardware. The second setting is inadequate hardware. The third setting occurs in noncompliant patients who place excessive loads on their reduced fractures and hardware before the bone can heal (Fig. 3-20). Unless the bone heals, even the strongest hardware may eventually fail.

Reflex sympathetic dystrophy is another posttraumatic complication in which there is a poorly understood alteration in the sympathetic nervous system affecting a limb in which severe regional hyperemia is accompanied by osteoporosis, soft tissue trophic changes, and alteration in temperature control.

Myositis ossificans and *heterotopic ossification* are poorly understood potential complications of fractures and fracture treatment (Fig. 3-21). These conditions are not identical, but both involve a rapid onset of soft-tissue ossification after soft-tissue injury. Myositis ossificans initially presents as a masslike lesion that must not be biopsied at this stage because the histology resembles an aggressive sarcoma. During the ensuing weeks, maturing peripheral ossification will reveal the true, benign nature of this process. Over the course of weeks to months the new bone migrates toward and ultimately merges with the adjacent bone. Heterotopic ossification is a radiologically similar process but is not confined to skeletal muscle. Heterotopic ossification often occurs after a hip arthroplasty or placement of an intramedullary nail in the femur. It also occurs more frequently in patients with a severe neurologic injury such as paraplegia. The heterotopic bone can limit the range of motion of an adjacent joint, or can bridge across the joint, resulting in joint fusion.

CHILDHOOD FRACTURES

Children's bones are different than those of adults. First, as indicated earlier in this chapter, they have greater

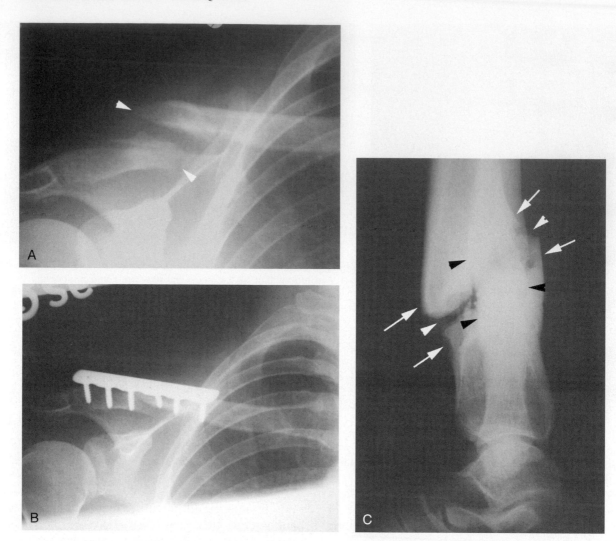

Fig. 3-19   Fracture nonunion. **A, B,** Atrophic nonunion of a clavicle fracture. Note the smooth, tapering margins of the fragments (*arrowheads* in **A**). Surgical fixation was required (**B**). **C,** Hypertrophic nonunion of a tibial fracture. Note the dense new bone on both sides of the fracture (*white arrows*) that is separated by radiolucent fibrous tissue. The healed fibula fracture (*black arrowheads*) projects over the tibial fracture, but no bridging bone across the tibial fracture is present. Surgery to remove the fibrous tissue and produce apposition of the osseous fragments was required.

potential for remodeling after fracture healing. The exact cause for this is unclear although is dependent on the age of the child, as it is more likely to occur with younger age and with a metaphyseal fracture. Angular deformity in the plane of movement of the adjacent joint is more likely to remodel than deformity perpendicular to the plane of movement.

Second, the biomechanical properties of children's bones are different than those of the adult. The propensity for incomplete fracture with bowing or buckling was discussed earlier. This plasticity decreases with age. "Bones are like bagels" (Robert Wilkinson, M.D., personal communication). The bones of a newborn are like a fresh bagel, soft and easily bent with only minimal

disruption of the outer surface. As a child grows, the bones become progressively stronger and stiffer, like a bagel that has been left out on the kitchen counter for a few days. The bagel is stiffer but can still be bent, but only with considerable disruption of its outer surface. By adulthood, the bones are like a bagel that has been on the counter for weeks. It is strong enough to support a stack of cookbooks, but it cannot bend (at least not perceptibly). If enough bending force is applied, the bagel will break, but it will not bend.

Another important biomechanical feature of the bones of children is the presence of a cartilaginous *physis* (epiphyseal plate, growth plate) near the ends of the long bones. The anatomy of the physis is discussed in Chapter

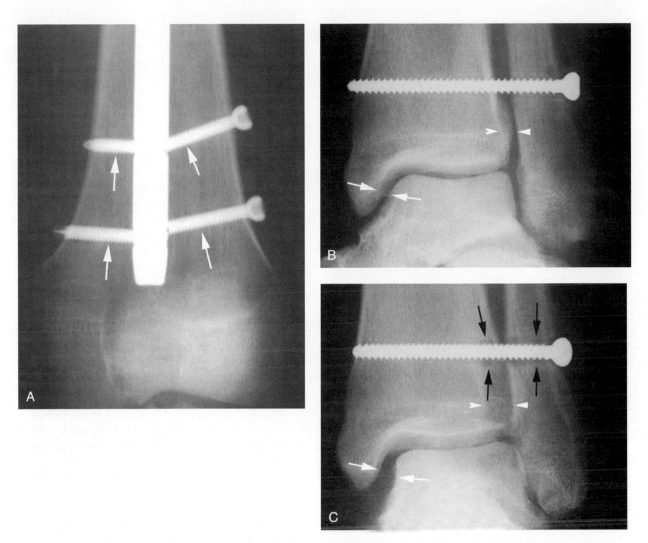

Fig. 3-20   Hardware complications. **A,** Hardware failure (fracture). This patient had a femoral shaft fracture that was fixed with an interlocking intramedullary nail. He resumed weight bearing earlier than advised, which placed shearing force on the interlocking screws. The distal screws failed (*arrows*). **B, C,** Hardware loosening. Initial radiograph (**B**) shows an intact syndesmotic screw fixing a distal tibiofibular diastasis injury. Note the the normal alignment of the distal tibiofibular joint (*arrowheads*) and the medial ankle mortise (*arrows*). Repeat radiograph (**C**) several weeks later now shows lucency around the lateral aspect of the screw, especially in the fibula, indicating bone resorption (*black arrows*). Note the widening of the distal tibiofibular joint (*arrowheads*) and the medial mortise (*white arrows*). Infection or mechanical loosening could cause this appearance. No infection was found in this case.

5. The physis is the weakest part of a bone in terms of resistance to shearing and torsional forces, but it is not exceptionally weak in terms of resistance to compression. Physeal fractures account for 15% of pediatric fractures. The percentage is not higher because most pediatric fractures are caused by compression resulting from a fall. Fractures that extend across or through a physis are classified by the Salter-Harris system. A Salter-Harris I fracture involves only the physis. If the fracture also extends through a portion of the metaphysis, it is classified as Salter-Harris II. This is the most frequent pattern, accounting for about 85% of physeal fractures. Salter-

Harris III fractures involve the physis and epiphysis. A Salter IV fracture is a fracture through the epiphysis, physis, and metaphysis. The rare Salter-Harris V fracture results from a compression injury of the physis, which may be missed or confused with a Salter-Harris I fracture.

Initial detection of physeal fractures is usually made with physical examination and radiographs. Ultrasound can be useful in infants, as it provides excellent visualization of unossified cartilage. MRI can be used in problem cases in which the diagnosis is not established with radiographs. Bone scan is hampered by the normal, intense tracer uptake at the physis. Pinhole imaging and careful

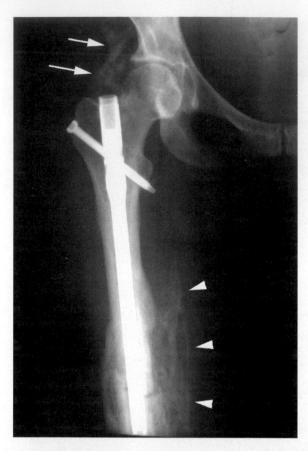

Fig. 3-21   Posttraumatic heterotopic ossification (*arrows*) and myositis ossificans (*arrowheads*). The myositis ossificans is merging with the medial femur, indicating that it is in an advanced stage.

comparison with the contralateral side improve the accuracy of bone scintigraphy.

The major complication of physeal fractures is growth arrest. Only a tiny fraction of physeal injuries result in this complication. Growth arrest can be caused by malunion with direct apposition of a metaphyseal and an epiphyseal fragment or by development of a bony bridge across the physis (Fig. 3-22). A bony bridge can either completely or focally arrest growth at a physis. The former can result in limb length discrepancy. The latter can result in angular deformity or a ball in cup deformity as the remainder of the physis continues to grow (Fig. 3-22A). The growth recovery line associated with the fracture may merge with the bony bridge (Fig. 3-22A). The risk of significant physeal injury is greatest at the distal tibia, followed by the distal femur. For any given physeal fracture, a higher Salter-Harris classification number indicates a greater risk for physeal injury.

The goal of treatment of focal growth arrest is to prevent the development of deformity. If the damaged physis was already close to completion of growth, then it can be surgically fused (epiphyseodesis) to prevent development of angulation. On the other hand, if the

child is young and several years of additional growth is anticipated, then the physis is salvaged by obliteration of the bony bridge with a drill using an oblique approach. Preoperative MR imaging can be helpful in planning this procedure, as it allows precise localization of the bridge (Fig. 3-22B). Salvage procedures for angular deformity and leg length discrepancy include osteotomies and leg lengthening procedures, discussed in Chapter 5.

The growth plate is also a site prone to stress injury. This can be considered as a chronic Salter I injury and can be recognized on radiographs by widening and irregularity of the growth plate. These injuries occur as overuse injuries in high-performance child and adolescent athletes. Specific situations in which these injuries arise are in the distal radius and ulna of gymnasts (Fig. 3-23), the proximal humerus of baseball pitchers and the lower extremities of runners. Patients usually improve with conservative therapy.

CHILD ABUSE

Knowledge of the potential radiologic findings in child abuse (nonaccidental trauma, battered child syndrome, shaken baby syndrome, trauma X) is essential for any radiologist who interprets pediatric images. This discussion will briefly review the skeletal findings that are most specific for child abuse. Other organ systems, notably the central nervous system, may also suffer injuries that are fairly specific for child abuse.

Proper radiographic assessment of a possibly abused infant or young child includes a complete set of high quality radiographs of the entire body (Table 3-1). As recommended by Paul Kleinmann, M.D., we prefer to obtain the views of each extremity separately, which results in a total of 19 images. Obtaining these radiographs is time consuming and requires a highly skilled and diplomatic technologist. A repeat examination after 2 weeks is helpful in children less than 2 years of age to detect healing fractures that were originally occult. Bone scintigraphy becomes useful by age 2 years, either as a primary screen or as an adjunct to the radiographic series. The examination can be tailored in many older children who can communicate "where it hurts," but some sort of whole body screening may still be appropriate. MRI and ultrasound (US) can be helpful in detecting marrow edema, subperiosteal hematoma, or fractures of epiphyseal cartilage.

Skeletal findings associated with child abuse have been thoroughly described by Paul Kleinmann, M.D. in his textbook *Diagnostic Imaging of Child Abuse,* and are summarized in Table 3-2. The *classic metaphyseal lesion* is the metaphyseal corner fracture and the bucket handle fracture. These actually are the same injury, seen from different perspectives (Fig. 3-24A, B). The classic metaph-

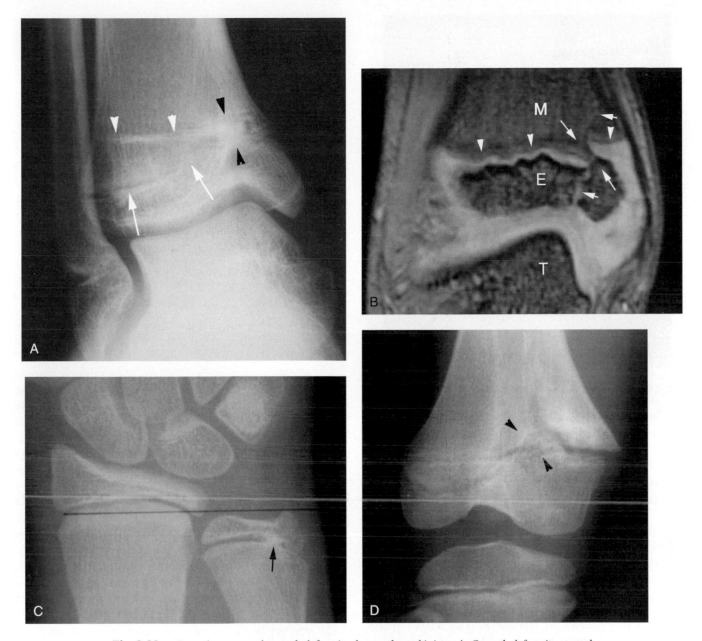

Fig. 3-22   Growth arrest and growth deformity due to physeal injury. **A,** Growth deformity caused by a post-traumatic bony bridge. This AP view was obtained several months after a distal tibia fracture that healed with casting. Note the osseous healing across the medial physis, forming a continuous bony bridge between the metaphysis and epiphysis (*black arrowheads*). Also note the growth recovery line in the distal tibial metaphysis that was formed as a result of the fracture (*white arrowheads*). Since the fracture, there has been normal growth laterally, but absent growth medially due to physeal tethering by the bony bridge. As a result, the growth recovery line is seen to merge with the physis (*white arrows*) at the bony bridge. **B,** Coronal MR image of a bony bridge in the distal tibia in a different patient. Gradient echo MR image (3-D SPGR with fat suppression) displays cartilage with high signal intensity. Note the bony bridge (*long arrows*), old Salter IV fracture line (*short arrows*) and the physis (*arrowheads*). M, metaphysis; E, epiphysis; T, talus. (Courtesy of Rodney Bell, RTR and Patrick Sorek, M.D., Kalamazoo, Michigan.) **C,** Ulnar shortening without other deformity due to a bony bridge (*arrow*). **D,** Bony bridge in the distal femur after a Salter IV fracture (*arrowheads*).

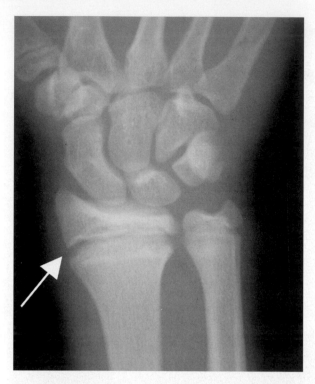

Fig. 3-23   Chronic Salter 1 injury of the distal radius in a young female gymnast. Note the sclerosis and irregularity around the physis (*arrows*).

yseal lesion is radiographically similar to a Salter-Harris II fracture, but the transverse component extends through the immature bone of the distal metaphysis rather than through the cartilaginous physis as in a true Salter-Harris II fracture. The mechanism is a combination of twisting and tension, as can occur when a child is violently shaken or when an extremity is violently, simultaneously pulled and twisted. Fractures around the infant thorax, especially the posterior ribs, result from forceful squeezing of the thorax by adult hands (Fig. 3-24C). Cardiopulmonary resuscitation of infants generally does not cause these fractures because their bones are so flexible. Other types of fractures are frequently seen in child abuse, but are less specific (Table 3-2, Fig. 3-24D).

Table 3-1 Radiographic series for suspected child abuse	
AP skull	AP humeri
Lateral skull	AP forearms
Lateral cervical spine	Oblique hands
AP thorax	AP femora
Lateral thorax	AP tibias
AP pelvis	AP feet
Lateral lumbar spine	

Table 3-2   Specificity of radiology findings for child abuse
High Specificity
Classic metaphyseal lesions
Rib fractures, especially posterior
Scapular fractures
Spinous process fractures
Sternal fractures
Moderate Specificity
Multiple fractures, especially bilateral
Fractures of different ages
Epiphyseal separations
Vertebral body fractures and subluxations
Digital fractures
Complex skull fractures
Common But Low Specificity
Subperiosteal new bone formation
Clavicular fractures
Long bone shaft fractures
Linear skull fractures

Source: Kleinman P. *Diagnostic Imaging of Child Abuse*, St. Louis, 1998, Mosby.

Radiologists are often asked to date healing fractures. This is an inexact science, but some generalizations can be made. Subperiosteal new bone formation generally does not appear until 4–10 days after a fracture and resolves by 2–3 weeks. Immature endosteal callus develops along the fracture, resulting in increased density, within 10–14 days and is maximal at 2–3 weeks. The endosteal callus matures and is subsequently removed by remodeling by 7–13 weeks after the fracture. Remodeling of a deformity begins by 3 months and can take up to 2 years. Repeated injury can prolong all of these time periods.

The main differential diagnosis of radiographic evidence of child abuse is osteogenesis imperfecta, discussed in Chapter 5. Other, exceedingly rare syndromes also may produce findings suggestive of child abuse in the absence of true abuse. Examples of such conditions include Caffey disease (discussed in Chapter 5), Menke's syndrome (abnormal copper metabolism leading to weak bones), and congenital indifference to pain. Congenital infection (e.g., due to syphilis), scurvy, and rickets also may produce features suggestive of child abuse. The clinical and laboratory work-up is usually adequate to diagnose or exclude all of these conditions.

MUSCLE INJURY

MR imaging is the most sensitive modality for evaluating most types of muscle injuries. Inversion recovery or T2-weighted images with fat suppression reveal edema, masses and fluid collections. T1-weighted images may reveal the presence of fatty infiltration, a finding that

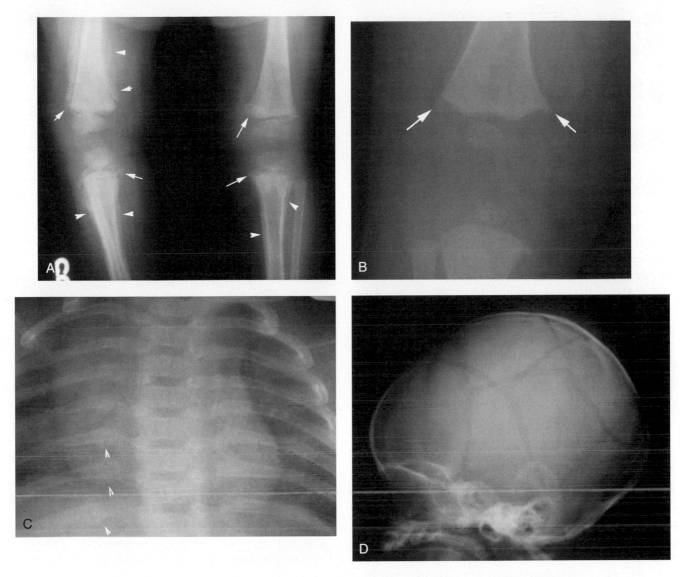

Fig. 3-24   Child abuse. **A, B,** Classic metaphyseal lesions (*arrows*). Also note the extensive periosteal new bone formation of varying maturity in **A** (*arrowheads*), reflecting fractures of different ages. **C,** Posterior rib fractures. The fracture lines are not visible, but the callus formation indicates their presence (*arrowheads*). These can be undetectable at the time of injury, illustrating the usefulness of followup radiographs. Even on delayed radiographs, subtle fractures of child abuse may remain very subtle and must be carefully sought. **D,** Multiple skull fractures. This finding is less specific for child abuse than the classic metaphyseal lesion and posterior rib fractures.

indicates chronic and generally irreversible muscle injury. Radiographs and CT display intramuscular calcification that can be a subacute or late finding after many types of muscle injury. These modalities also allow assessment of the pattern of calcification, for example, the peripheral calcification of myositis ossificans.

Traumatic muscle injury may be produced by an extrinsic force such as a direct blow, or by intrinsic force generated by the muscle itself. Extrinsic injuries include contusion and intramuscular hematoma, and, in extreme cases, myonecrosis. Any of these lesions may lead to myositis ossificans, discussed in Chapter 1. A muscle

contusion produces intramuscular edema and small fluid collections, usually centered at the site of injury. An intramuscular hematoma may contain a fluid-fluid level and have high signal on T1-weighted images due to the presence of methemoglobin. An older hematoma may have a low signal intensity rim due to the presence of hemosiderin. The classic intrinsic muscle injury is the *muscle strain*. A strain represents microscopic muscle fiber tearing at the musculotendinous junction, and is caused by forceful contraction while under load. Strains are most common in muscles that elongate while they contract, such as the hamstrings and the biceps. MR images of a mild muscle strain show edema centered along the musculotendinous junction (Fig. 3-25). Moderate strains have more extensive edema and minute fluid collections. Severe strains involve disruption of the musculotendinous junction. MR images reveal this disruption along with fluid collections and extensive regional edema.

Chronic complete tendon tears cause muscle retraction and, over time, atrophy. Atrophy is seen as a decrease in muscle bulk with increased signal on T1-weighted images due to fatty infiltration.

A common overuse muscle injury, termed delayed onset muscle soreness (DOMS), is often an affliction of recreational athletes ("weekend warriors"). DOMS is a type of microscopic muscle injury that becomes clinically evident a few days after the overuse event, and slowly resolves with rest. MR images reveal fairly uniform muscle edema, without fluid collections. However, severe cases can lead to rhabdomyolysis and myonecrosis, with bizarre MR findings due to multifocal intramuscular hemorrhage and edema.

Neuromuscular conditions such as muscular dystrophy and autoimmune muscle injury in dermatomyositis and polymyositis cause muscle degeneration that is initially seen as diffuse muscle edema, but over time progresses to fatty atrophy. Denervation produces a similar temporal progression, with the initial muscle edema first appearing about 2–4 weeks after denervation. If normal innervation is restored, muscle returns to normal both clinically and on MR images. However, after several weeks to months, fatty atrophy develops, indicating irreversible injury.

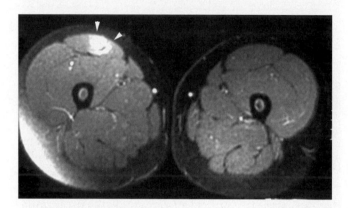

Fig. 3-25 Rectus femoris muscle strain. T2-weighted image with fat suppression shows high signal intensity along the musculotendinous junction of the right rectus femoris muscle (*arrowheads*).

SOURCES AND SUGGESTED READINGS

Bergquist T, ed: *Imaging of orthopedic trauma*, ed. 2, New York, 1992, Raven.

Chew FS: *Skeletal radiology: The bare bones*, ed. 2, Baltimore, 1997, Williams & Wilkins.

Chem RK, Cardinal E eds: *Guidelines and gamuts in musculoskeletal ultrasound*, New York, 1999, Wiley-Liss.

Kleinmann P: *Diagnostic imaging of child abuse*, St. Louis, 1998, Mosby.

Manaster BJ: *Handbook of skeletal radiology*, ed 2, St Louis, 1997, Mosby-Yearbook.

May DA, Disler DG, Jones EA, Balkissoon A, Manaster BJ: Abnormal signal within skeletal muscle in magnetic resonance imaging: patterns, pearls, and pitfalls, *Radiographics* 20:S295–315, 2000.

Rockwood CH, Green DP, Bucholz RW, Heckman JD, eds: *Fractures in adults*. ed. 4, Philadelphia, 1996, Lippincott-Raven.

Rockwood CH, Wilkins KE, Beaty JH, eds: *Fractures in children*. ed. 4, Philadelphia, 1996, Lippincott-Raven.

Rogers LF: *Radiology of skeletal trauma*, New York, 1992, Churchill Livingstone.

CHAPTER 3 · Trauma

UPPER EXTREMITY TRAUMA

PART II

DAVID A. MAY, M.D.

INTRODUCTION

This section reviews traumatic conditions of the upper extremity. The joints, especially the shoulder, are emphasized, owing to their complexity and to the frequent use of cross sectional imaging of the joints in routine clinical practice. Radiography and MRI are emphasized, but applications of CT and US to upper extremity trauma also are discussed. Each sub-section includes a review of normal anatomy and anatomic variants. Reference to an anatomy atlas may be helpful as you read each anatomy review.

SHOULDER

The shoulder girdle is composed of the scapula, the proximal humerus, the lateral clavicle, and related muscles and connective tissues. Joints of the shoulder girdle include the glenohumeral, acromioclavicular, and scapulothoracic joints. The sternoclavicular joint is also included in this discussion.

The glenohumeral joint is the most mobile, least stable major joint in the body, and consequently is a frequent site of pain and dysfunction. Despite having a fairly simple appearance on radiographs, the articulation of the humerus and the scapula is remarkably complex due to numerous supporting soft tissue structures. Modern imaging, most notably MRI and MR arthrography and to a lesser degree CT and US, now allow noninvasive or minimally invasive assessment of these structures, and orthopedic surgeons have come to expect their colleagues in radiology to have a good understanding of this complex joint. Most referrals for shoulder cross sectional imaging are made for suspected rotator cuff pathology or for shoulder instability and often-related injuries such as labral tears; therefore these conditions are emphasized. Due to the complex 3-dimensional and functional anatomy of the shoulder, this section begins with a review of normal shoulder anatomy and anatomic variants, followed by a discussion of specific shoulder maladies. This approach results in repetition of some key points.

Imaging Techniques

Dozens of radiographic projections of the shoulder have been described. Routine radiographic positions often include AP in internal and external rotation, axillary, trans-scapular Y, and Grashey (true AP) views, discussed below. Radiographs identify dislocations, most fractures, many of the osseous findings associated with rotator cuff impingement, and tell-tale signs of a prior dislocation such as Hill-Sachs and Bankart fractures. Conventional arthrography allows demonstration of a complete rotator cuff tear, and partial thickness inferior surface tears.

Plain CT is useful in characterizing fractures, complex dislocations, and soft tissue calcifications such as calcific tendinitis. CT arthrography allows evaluation of the anterior and posterior labrum, joint capsule, and rotator cuff tears. US can reliably diagnose joint effusions, many rotator cuff tears, and biceps long head tendon tears and dislocations. US of the shoulder requires a high degree of operator experience and requires more physician time than MRI. Nonetheless, shoulder US is gradually increasing in popularity, although it has not yet gained wide acceptance.

MRI of the shoulder is accomplished in planes parallel to the rotator cuff and parallel to the articular surface of the glenoid, that is, oblique coronal and oblique sagittal planes, respectively, as well as in the axial plane. Sequence selection is to a large degree a matter of personal preference and the capabilities of the available MRI scanner, but always includes a T1-weighted sequence to assess marrow signal and a long TE sequence in the oblique coronal plane to assess for abnormal signal within the rotator cuff tendons. We prefer a fat suppressed T2-weighted fast spin echo sequence performed in all three planes for assessment of rotator cuff signal. The use of fat suppression enhances detection of subtle marrow and rotator cuff edema. Use of a moderate TE with this sequence (approximately 60 msec) also enhances assessment of articular cartilage defects. The technique of shoulder arthrography is discussed in Appendix 1. MR imaging performed after arthrography ("MR arthrography") is the gold standard radiologic examination of the labrum. Depending on whether gadolinium or saline was injected, T1-weighted or T2-weighted imaging is emphasized, respectively. "Indirect arthrography" can be accomplished by intravenous injection of gadolinium, followed by exercise a delay of 15–20 minutes before imaging to allow the gadolinium to diffuse across the synovium into the joint. Indirect arthrography is less invasive than direct arthrography, but is less reliable in delivering contrast into the joint, and does not distend the joint. This limits its usefulness in assessing the joint capsule and glenohumeral ligaments.

Normal Anatomy, Normal Anatomic Variants, and Fractures

Clavicle The clavicle is S-shaped, with an anterior convex margin along its medial half. The clavicle articulates medially with the manubrium and laterally with the acromion process of the scapula. The *rhomboid fossa* is a variable, frequently irregular concavity in the undersurface of the medial clavicle above the costal cartilage of the first rib (Fig. 3-26). This normal variant should not be mistaken for a lytic or erosive process. In both children and adults, most clavicle fractures are caused by a fall on an outstretched hand, and most fractures occur through the middle third. The fracture fragments are frequently displaced because traction by the sternocleidomastoid muscle displaces the medial fragment superiorly and the weight of the arm, transmitted through the acromioclavicular and coracoclavicular ligaments, pulls the distal fragment inferiorly (Fig. 3-19A). The muscles that attach the shoulder to the chest wall such as the pectoralis major and latissimus dorsi often medially dis-

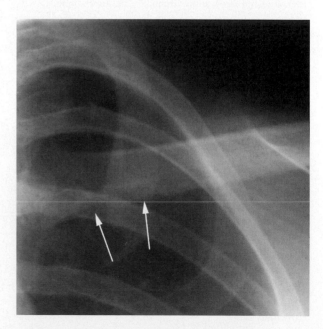

Fig. 3-26   Rhomboid fossa. Note the irregular defect in the inferior medial clavicle adjacent to the first rib (*arrows*).

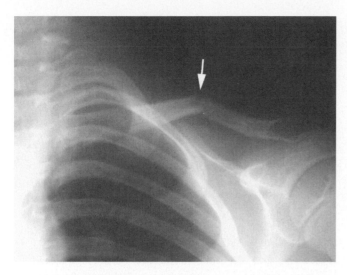

Fig. 3-27 Clavicle fracture in a child (*arrow*). As in an adult, the sternocleidomastoid muscle pulls the proximal fragment superiorly.

place the distal fragment, causing the fragments to override. Despite such displacement, the large majority of clavicle fractures heal rapidly and without complication with minimal immobilization. Childhood clavicle fractures may be incomplete (Fig. 3-27). Surgical fixation of clavicle fractures is usually reserved for open fractures, fractures in high-level athletes, cases of delayed union or nonunion, and distal fractures associated with acromi-

oclavicular or coracoclavicular ligament disruption (Fig. 3-19B).

Proximal humerus The proximal humerus is comprised of the articular surface or head that is bordered by the anatomic neck, the lesser and greater tuberosities, and the vertically oriented intertubercular or bicipital groove between the tuberosities. The surgical neck is the ill-defined, transverse junction of the humeral shaft and the tuberosities. Radiographic anatomy of the shoulder depends on the projection. AP radiographs in external rotation profile the greater tuberosity laterally and the articular surface medially. The lesser tuberosity projects over the center of the humeral head. Internal rotation projects the greater tuberosity over the head, resulting in a rounded contour (Fig. 3-28). A true AP or Grashey view is obtained at a 40° medolateral angle. This view profiles the glenohumeral joint (Fig. 3-29A). An axillary view is obtained with the x-ray beam passing caudocraniad with the arm abducted (Fig. 3-29B). If normally located, the humeral head aligns with the glenoid on this view. A trans-scapular Y view is obtained by angling the x-ray beam parallel to the scapula (Fig. 3-29C). This view superimposes a normally located humeral head and the glenoid. The "Y" is formed by the scapular spine superiorly and posteriorly, the coracoid superiorly and anteriorly, and the scapular body inferiorly. Unlike the axillary view, the Y view does not require manipulation of the shoulder. Many other specialized views have been described.

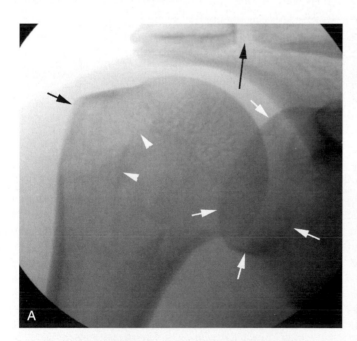
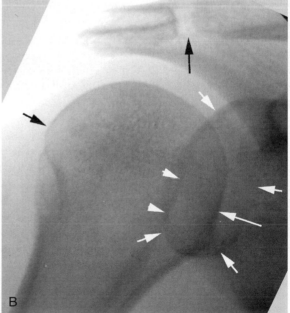

Fig. 3-28 Shoulder normal radiographic anatomy: AP views in external (**A**) and internal (**B**) rotation. Greater tuberosity (*short black arrow*); lesser tuberosity (*long white arrow in* **B**); glenoid rim (*short white arrows*); bicipital groove (*white arrowheads*); acromioclavicular joint (*long black arrow*).

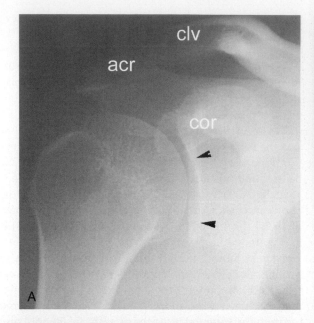

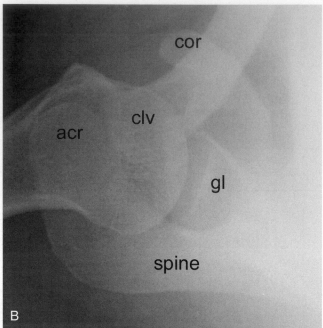

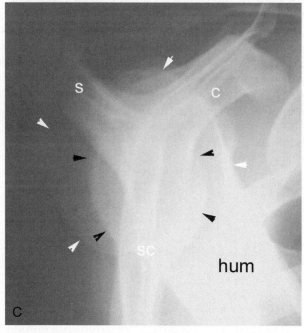

Fig. 3-29 Shoulder radiographic anatomy: Grashey (true AP) (A), axillary (B), and Y (C) views. **A,** Grashey (true AP) view is obtained 40° oblique in the horizontal plane. This aligns the x-ray beam with the glenohumeral joint. Note the acromion (acr), clavicle (clv), coracoid process (cor) and the glenoid (*black arrowheads*). **B,** Axillary view is obtained with the arm abducted and the beam passing vertically through the shoulder. Note the acromion (acr), clavicle (clv), coracoid process (cor) and the glenoid (gl). **C,** Trans-scapular Y view is obtained with the patient turned approximately 45° oblique to the x-ray beam with his hand resting on the opposite shoulder. The humeral head (*white arrowheads*) should be centered over the glenoid (*black arrowheads*). The "Y" is formed by the spine of the scapula posteriorly (s), the coracoid process anteriorly (c), and the body or blade of the scapula (sc). Also note the humeral shaft (*hum*).

Proximal humeral fractures are much less common in children than adults. Buckle or torus fractures of the surgical neck and proximal shaft region may be seen (Fig. 3-30). The head and greater tuberosity are formed from separate ossification centers that unite during childhood, resulting in an inverted "V" shape of the combined physis that may simulate a fracture (Fig. 3-30). True Salter-Harris-type fractures are most frequently type I fractures in preschoolers up to about 5 years of age (Fig. 3-31) or type II fractures in pre-teens.

Proximal humeral fractures are common in adults, especially in osteoporotic bones. Fractures of the surgical neck are the most common (Fig. 3-32A). A widely used

classification of proximal humeral fractures in adults was described by the orthopedic surgeon Neer. The Neer system provides prognostic information and aids in treatment planning. This system is based on recognition of four potential fracture sites: the anatomic neck, the lesser tuberosity, the greater tuberosity, and the surgical neck. Each of the four fracture sites results in a potential fragment, or "part." A fracture fragment is not considered to be a separate part in the Neer system unless it is displaced by more than 1 cm or rotated by more than 45°. Thus, a single fracture line could result in a 1-part fracture or a 2-part fracture, depending on the degree of fragment displacement (Fig. 3-32A, B). A comminuted

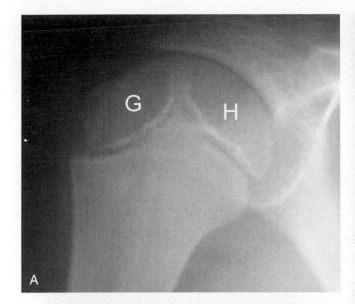

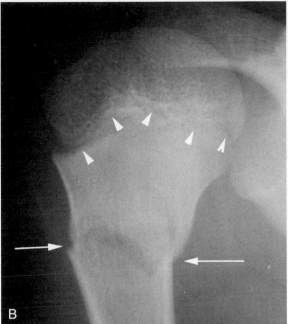

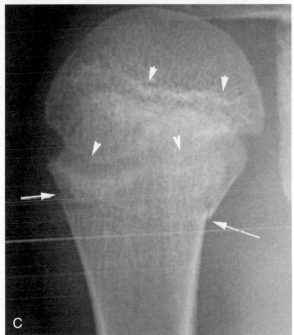

Fig. 3-30 Normal proximal humeral physis and metaphyseal fractures. **A,** External rotation, normal appearance. Separate ossification centers for the humeral head (H) and the greater tuberosity (G) result in an inverted V shape of the physis. **B,** External rotation view in a child with a metaphyseal fracture. Note the physis (*arrowheads*) and the more distal fracture (*arrows*). **C,** Internal rotation view in a different child with a metaphyseal fracture. The physis has a complex appearance (*arrowheads*) that should not be confused with a fracture. Note the subtle metaphyseal fracture (*arrows*).

proximal humerus fracture could range from a 1-part fracture to a 4-part fracture, depending on fragment displacement or angulation. Anatomical neck fractures are rare and have a poor prognosis, because the blood supply to the head is completely disrupted. In contrast, the more common surgical neck fracture has a good prognosis because the blood supply to the head is preserved.

Pseudosubluxation of the shoulder is inferior and lateral subluxation of the humeral head. "Pseudo" is a misnomer, as the subluxation is quite real. In the setting of trauma, this finding usually reflects transient deltoid atony, although a hemarthrosis or joint effusion also may cause this finding (Fig. 3-33).

Scapula The scapula consists of the body, the spine, the acromion process, the scapular neck, the glenoid, and the coracoid process. Two important landmarks adjacent to the scapular neck are the spinoglenoid notch posteriorly and the suprascapular notch superiorly. The neurovascular supply to the supraspinatus and infraspinatus muscles passes through these notches. A mass lesion such as a ganglion cyst or a displaced fracture fragment in this region can compress this neurovascular bundle and simulate rotator cuff pathology. This is discussed further below.

Fractures of the scapula are rare in children. In both children and adults, scapular fractures are usually the

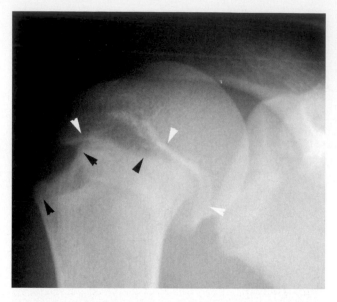

Fig. 3-31 Salter-Harris I proximal humerus fracture. The arrowheads mark the epiphyseal (*white arrowheads*) and metaphyseal (*black arrowheads*) margins of the physis.

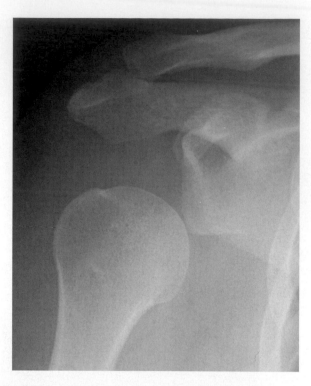

Fig. 3-33 "Pseudosubluxation" of the shoulder of a stroke victim. The subluxation is real and is due to muscle atony.

result of direct blunt trauma. Scapula fractures can be a challenge to identify on radiographs obtained in the acute trauma setting owing to overlapping anatomy and support equipment as well as the frequent presence of other fractures. Knowledge of the mechanism of injury and careful scrutiny of the scapula is needed (Fig. 3-34). Scapular body fractures are usually treated with immobilization. Fractures of the glenoid, scapular neck, and coracoid process are often treated with surgical reduction and fixation. One should not hesitate to obtain a CT scan if these fractures are present or suspected.

The normal development of the scapula from numerous separate ossification centers can simulate a fracture in children, adolescents, and young adults. Separate ossifications centers form the tip of the coracoid process, the acromion process, the glenoid rim, the inferior angle of the scapular body, and the vertebral border of the scapular body. Failure of fusion of the acromial ossifica-

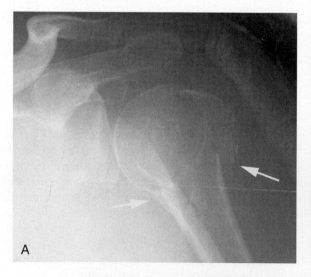

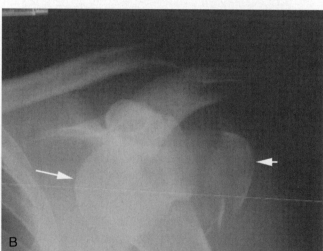

Fig. 3-32 Proximal humerus fractures in adults. **A,** Surgical neck fracture (*arrows*). **B,** Fracture dislocation. The humeral head (*long arrow*) is anteriorly dislocated. The greater tuberosity (*short arrow*) was sheared off and is laterally displaced from the remainder of the proximal humerus by greater than 1 cm, making this a Neer 2 fracture.

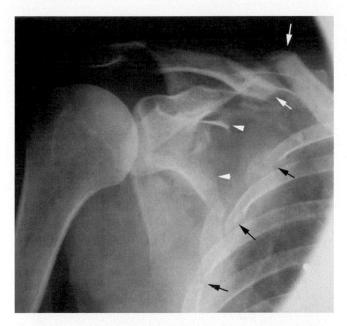

Fig. 3-34 Scapula fracture (*white arrowheads*). Also note the rib fractures (*black arrows*) and the clavicle fracture (*white arrows*).

tion center results in the normal variant *os acromiale.* Although os acromiale is a normal variant, it is associated with rotator cuff impingement and therefore should be noted when observed on imaging studies. Os acromiale is most readily identified on axillary shoulder radiographs and axial CT or MR images, where it is seen as a coronally

oriented linear defect traversing the acromion. Os acromiale may be distinguished from an acromial fracture by its smooth, straight, and frequently uniformly sclerotic margins (Fig. 3-35). Os acromiale is present in 2%–3% of the population and is bilateral in 60% of cases.

Another normal variant of the scapula that may simulate a lytic process is a *scapular foramen.* A scapular foramen is a well circumscribed "hole" in the center of the scapular body. A similar finding occasionally occurs in the iliac wings. This normal variant occurs in flat bones that have strong opposing muscles on each side of the bone.

Glenoid dysplasia, also termed *glenoid hypoplasia,* or *scapular neck dysplasia,* is a developmental deformity of the scapular neck caused by failure of formation of the glenoid neck ossification center (Fig. 3-36A). The glenoid is wide and medially positioned. This appearance suggests a healed impaction fracture of the glenoid neck. Glenoid dysplasia may have associated acromial or humeral head deformity. It usually is asymptomatic, but may be associated with shoulder instability. *Erb's Palsy* may resemble glenoid dysplasia radiographically (Fig. 3-36B), but would be readily distinguished by the history of shoulder and arm weakness since birth.

Sternoclavicular joint The *sternoclavicular* (SC) *joint* is the articulation of the medial-inferior clavicle with the superior-lateral manubrium. The SC joint is lined with fibrocartilage and contains a small fibrocartilage disc. The SC joint is difficult to evaluate with radiographs owing

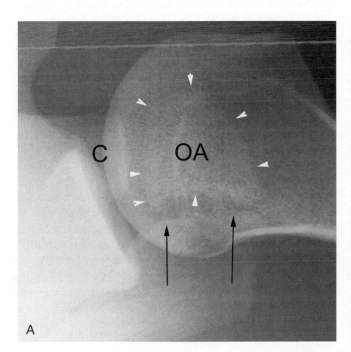
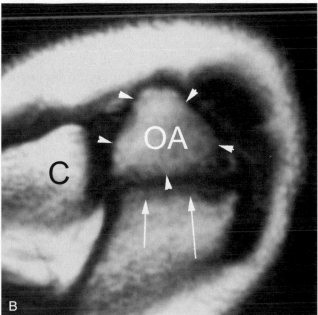

Fig. 3-35 Os acromiale. Axillary radiograph (**A**) and axial T2-weighted MR image (**B**) in different patients show an os acromiale (OA, *white arrowheads*). Note the slightly irregular but straight margins between the os acromiale and the remainder of the scapula (*arrows*). **C,** marks the distal clavicle.

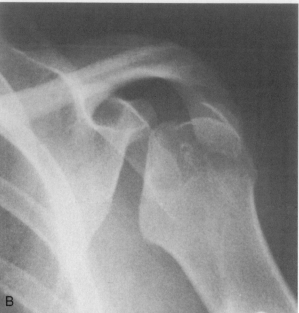

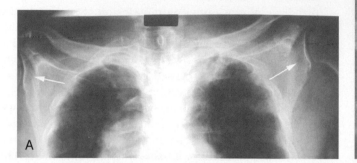

Fig. 3-36   Glenoid dysplasia. **A,** Bilateral glenoid dysplasia (*arrows*). **B,** Erb's Palsy. The dysplastic glenoid and flat humeral head resemble glenoid dysplasia, but the clinical history allows distinction of these conditions.

to overlapping spine, ribs, and mediastinum. AP and lordotic views can be helpful, but thin section CT is usually superior.

Important pathologic processes that involve the SC joint are dislocation and infection. A high-speed motor vehicle crash or similarly violent injury can cause dislocation of the SC joint (Fig. 3-37). The medial clavicle can dislocate in any direction. Superior dislocation may be detected with radiographs, but posterior dislocation, which can result in compression of the great vessels or trachea, usually requires CT for diagnosis. An important

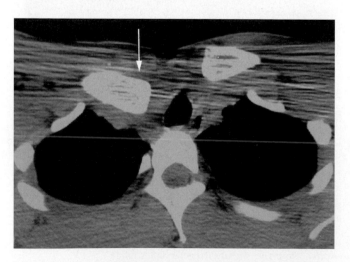

Fig. 3-37   Sternoclavicular joint posterior dislocation (*arrow*). The left side is in normal position.

potential pitfall is that the medial clavicle epiphysis does not begin to ossify until 18–20 years of age and does not fuse with the remainder of the clavicle until about 25 years of age. Because SC dislocations occur most frequently in this age range, Salter-Harris 1 or 2 fractures may be misinterpreted as SC dislocations or vice versa. Careful attention to the CT images for a smoothly marginated, calcified epiphysis or an irregularly marginated fracture fragment can avoid this pitfall.

SC joint infection occurs most frequently in intravenous drug abusers and elderly patients. SC infection may clinically simulate a traumatic injury, as both result in joint pain, tenderness and soft tissue swelling. CT of an infected sternoclavicular joint may reveal cortical destruction. If infection is suspected, aspiration of the joint is the best diagnostic test.

Acromioclavicular joint   The *acromioclavicular (AC) joint* is tightly invested with connective tissue, resulting in a strong joint with limited mobility. The nearby, strong coracoclavicular ligaments add to the stability of the AC joint. The AC joint is a synovial joint, and like any other synovial joint is vulnerable to OA. Osteophytes projecting inferiorly from the AC joint can narrow the subacromial space and cause rotator cuff pathology, discussed further below. Traumatic injury to the AC joint is graded by clinical and radiographic findings.

Radiographs of a normal AC joint show the inferior margins of the acromion and clavicle to form a continuous line or arc across the joint, with symmetric appearance of the right and left AC joints. Traumatic injury disrupts the rela-

Key Concepts	AC Joint Injuries

- Compare both sides.
- Grade 1: AC ligament sprain.
    Radiographs: normal or near-normal.
- Grade 2: AC ligament rupture. Coracoclavicular ligaments intact.
    Radiographs (may need traction on arm): wide (>5 mm) or malaligned AC joint, normal coracoclavicular distance (<11–13 mm).
- Grade 3: AC and coracoclavicular ligaments rupture.
    Radiographs: wide or malaligned AC joint, wide coracoclavicular distance.
- Grade 4: Clavicle dislocated posteriorly. Can compress supraspinatus muscle.
    Radiographs: AP view may be normal. Axillary view or CT needed.

tively weaker AC ligaments before the relatively stronger coracoclavicular ligaments, resulting in a predictable pattern of injury that is described by a grading system (Fig. 3-38). A grade 1 AC injury is an AC joint sprain without gross disruption of the AC joint. The AC joint is painful and tender. Radiographs may be normal or may show mild AC mild joint laxity with minimal subluxation or widening. A grade 2 AC injury or separation is complete disruption of the AC ligaments with intact coracoclavicular ligaments. Radiographs reveal discontinuity or widening of the AC joint, but a normal coracoclavicular distance. A grade 3 AC injury or separation is complete disruption of both the AC and coracoclavicular ligaments. Passive inferior traction on the arm, usually accomplished by attaching a weight of about 7.5 kg to the wrist, may reveal or upgrade an AC injury that is not apparent without traction. Useful rules of thumb are that the AC joint space is usually no more than 5 mm wide, with right and left differing by no more that 2–3 mm. The coracoclavicular distance is usually no wider than 11–13 mm, with right and left differing by no more that 5 mm. Although these numbers are worth remembering as useful guidelines, clinical findings and comparison with the uninjured side may reveal a ligament injury despite "normal" measurements, or conversely may reveal intact ligaments despite measurements that exceed the "normal" range. A 50% difference between the two sides is considered to be significant. Thus, radiography of both the injured and uninjured sides is recommended, as normal variation may simulate or mask an injury.

The distal clavicle also may dislocate posteriorly relative to the acromion into or through the trapezius muscle, sometimes described as a grade 4 AC injury (Fig. 3-38C). The posteriorly displaced clavicle can compress the supraspinatus muscle against the scapula, causing pain and dysfunction. Surgical correction is required. Radiographic diagnosis of posterior dislocation requires an axil-

lary radiograph, and CT may be needed for precise determination of the clavicle position and identification of possible associated fractures. An unusual form of AC separation is inferior dislocation of the distal clavicle below the coracoid process and posterior to the biceps short head tendon. This injury also requires surgical correction.

Old AC injuries may heal with persistently abnormal alignment. The injured ligaments often calcify or ossify.

Finally, recall that a widened AC joint may also result from erosion of the distal clavicle due to rheumatoid arthritis, hyperparathyroidism, and infection. It may also appear widened from traumatic osteolysis, and cleidocranial dysplasia. Clinical correlation and careful inspection of radiographs of the distal clavicle for erosion, irregularity, or absence of the subchondral cortex usually leads to the correct diagnosis.

Glenohumeral joint anatomy Figures 3-39, 3-40, and 3-41 review the normal anatomy of the glenohumeral joint.

The glenohumeral joint is a ball and socket joint. The osseous glenoid is oval in shape, with its long axis oriented in a roughly superior–inferior direction. The subchondral bone of the glenoid is nearly flat, with a shallow central depression. The overlying glenoid articular cartilage is thinnest at its central portion, slightly increasing the concavity of the glenoid fossa. The fibrocartilaginous glenoid labrum forms a rim around the glenoid that contributes about 3 mm of additional depth to the glenoid fossa and increases the joint contact area. This anatomy results in a shallow socket that allows for extraordinary mobility, but with poor intrinsic stability. Glenohumeral joint stability depends on a combination of several static and dynamic mechanisms that are discussed in the following paragraphs: compressive force applied by the rotator cuff and biceps long head tendons, the labrum, the joint capsule, the glenohumeral ligaments, and negative pressure at the area of contact of the articular surfaces. The latter is due to complex osmotic effects within the joint that may be likened to a suction cup applied to a pane of glass.

The glenoid fossa, when viewed *en face,* may be compared to the face of a clock, with the superior glenoid at 12 o'clock, the inferior glenoid at 6 o'clock, the anterior glenoid at 3 o'clock, and the posterior glenoid at 9 o'clock (Fig. 3-39). The reader should note that the clock-face convention used here places anterior to the viewer's right, opposite of the usual convention on oblique sagittal MR images of placing anterior to the viewer's left. The orientation used here is that used in the orthopedic literature, and is recommended when reporting imaging findings to orthopedic surgeons.

The muscles of the *rotator cuff* originate from the medial scapula and insert on the proximal humerus. The rotator cuff tendons are broad and sheetlike at their humeral insertions. The *supraspinatus* muscle is located above the

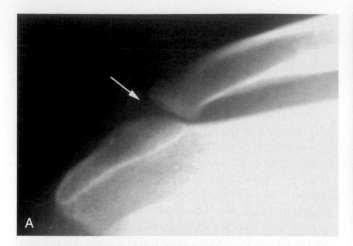

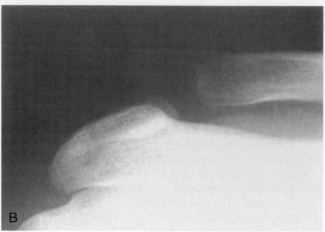

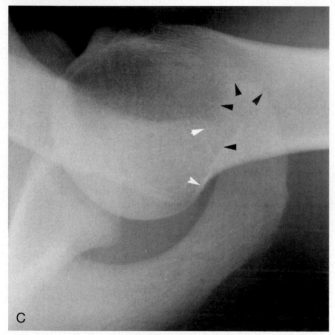

Fig. 3-38 Acromioclavicular joint injury **A, B,** Grade 2 AC sprain. AP radiograph without (**A**) and with (**B**) distraction of the AC joint (*arrow* in **A**) shows widening in **B. C,** Grade 4 AC separation. AP view (not shown) showed no definite abnormalities. Axillary view (**C**) shows the distal clavicle (*white arrowheads*) is displaced posteriorly relative to the acromion (*black arrowheads*).

scapular spine and superior to the humeral head. The *infraspinatus* muscle is located below the scapular spine and superior–posterior to the humeral head. The *teres minor* muscle is located inferoposteriorly, below the infraspinatus. The supraspinatus, infraspinatus, and teres minor muscles insert onto the greater tuberosity. The *subscapularis* muscle is the only rotator cuff muscle located anterior to the scapula and it alone inserts onto the lesser tuberosity. Some subscapularis fibers extend beyond the lesser tuberosity to contribute to the *transverse humeral ligament* that traverses the intertubercular groove to the greater tuberosity. The transverse humeral ligament assists in containing the biceps long head tendon within the intertubercular groove. The subscapularis is the largest rotator cuff muscle, about as large as the infraspinatus and teres minor muscles combined. The *rotator interval* is a thin membrane between the supraspinatus and subscapularis tendons. It is a part of the rotator cuff and

superior joint capsule. The coracohumeral ligament and the superior glenohumeral ligament (discussed below) also contribute to the rotator interval.

The biceps muscle has two heads. The biceps short head originates from the coracoid process. The biceps long head tendon originates from the supraglenoid tubercle and the glenoid labrum at the one o'clock position within the joint capsule, arches over the humeral head within the joint capsule, then courses inferiorly in the intertubercular groove. This anatomy allows the biceps long head tendon to resist anterior and superior humeral head subluxation and thus contributes to glenohumeral joint stability. The synovial sheath of the biceps long head tendon in the intertubercular groove communicates with the glenohumeral joint.

The rotator cuff muscles and the biceps individually contribute to shoulder motion. The subscapularis internally rotates the shoulder, the teres minor and infraspi-

Key Concepts | **Glenohumeral Joint Anatomy**

- Coracoacromial arch
- Subacromial space contains subacromial subdeltoid bursa and rotator cuff.
- Rotator cuff:
    Supraspinatus superiorly
    Infraspinatus posteriorly
    Teres minor inferior to infraspinatus
    Subscapularis anteriorly
    Rotator interval between supraspinatus and subscapularis tendons
- Biceps long head tendon originates from superior labrum at biceps labral complex.
- Labrum:
    Fibrocartilage
    Deepens glenoid fossa and serves as attachment for biceps tendon and glenohumeral ligaments.
    Highly variable superior anterior portion.
- Joint capsule and the glenohumeral ligaments:
    Contribute to glenohumeral stability.
    Superior GHL: glenoid (variable origin) to capsule.
    Contributes to rotator interval.
    Occasionally absent.
    Middle GHL: anterior labrum to subscapularis tendon. Highly variable, may be absent.
    Inferior GHL: labrum to humerus with anterior and posterior bands.
    Anterior band originates from anterior labrum from 2–4 o'clock position.
    Posterior band originates for posterior labrum at 7–9 o'clock position.
    Most important of the glenohumeral ligaments because of contribution to joint stability, but hardest to image (MR-arthrography best).
    Coracohumeral ligament. Contributes to rotator interval.
- Synovial outpouchings:
    Axillary recess or pouch
    Subscapularis (subcoracoid) recess

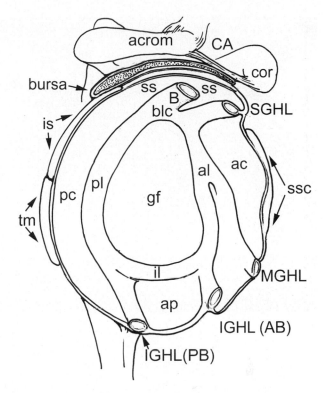

Fig. 3-39   Glenohumeral joint anatomy. This diagram views the glenoid fossa *en face* with the humeral head removed. Anterior is to the viewer's *right*, by a convention used by orthopedic surgeons. The MR images in this chapter display anterior to the viewer's *left*, by a convention often used by radiologists.
Key to Figures 3-39, 3-40, 3-41.
Bones: acrom, acromial arch; cor, coracoid process; lt, lesser tuberosity; gt, greater tuberosity; sgn, spinoglenoid notch (posterior scapular neck); ssn, suprascapular notch (superior scapular neck); sp, spine of scapula; cl, clv, clavicle.
Muscles and tendons: B, biceps long head; ss, supraspinatus; is, infraspinatus; tm, teres minor; ssc, subscapularis; ri, rotator interval.
Ligaments: CA, coracoacromial ligament; SGHL, superior glenohumeral ligament; MGHL, middle glenohumeral ligament; IGHL, inferior glenohumeral ligament; IGHL (AB), inferior glenohumeral ligament anterior band; IGHL (PB), inferior glenohumeral ligament posterior band.
Capsule: ac, anterior capsule; ap, axillary pouch; pc, posterior capsule; ap, axillary pouch; scr, subscapular recess or bursa (subcoracoid recess).
Labrum: blc, biceps labral complex; al, anterior labrum; il, inferior labrum; pl, posterior labrum. *Subacromial subdeltoid bursa,* bursa. *Glenoid fossa,* gf.

natus externally rotate the shoulder, and the supraspinatus abducts the shoulder. The biceps long head contributes to shoulder flexion. However, the primary function of the rotator cuff is to resist glenohumeral subluxation. To understand the importance of the rotator cuff in maintaining glenohumeral stability, consider the effect of contraction of the powerful deltoid muscle during shoulder abduction. Deltoid contraction applies a superior subluxing force to the humeral head, which, if not counterbalanced, would result in impingement of the supraspinatus and infraspinatus tendons between the humeral head and the coracoacromial arch. The muscles of the rotator cuff, operating as a unit and assisted by the biceps long head tendon, apply compressive force across the glenohu-

meral joint to maintain normal glenohumeral joint alignment.

The normal labrum is quite variable in terms of shape and fixation to the glenoid. The labrum is most frequently triangular in cross section, but the posterior labrum often has a rounded lateral contour. Small articular surface irregularities such as small clefts may occur as a normal variant. The peripheral margin of the labrum is fixed to the glenoid periosteum, and usually to the joint capsule and underlying glenoid articular cartilage as well. However, labral fixation to the glenoid may be loose or entirely

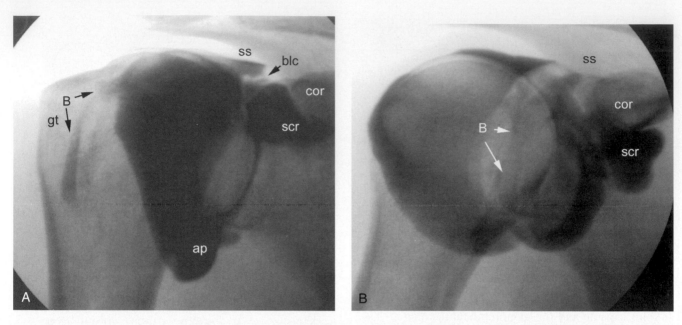

Fig. 3-40   Glenohumeral joint: normal arthographic anatomy. Arthrogram of the same patient as Figure 3-28. **A,** AP external rotation. **B,** AP internal rotation. (See Key with Fig. 3-39.)

absent in the superior–anterior labrum between 12 and 3 o'clock. Several specific patterns of this normal variation occur fairly commonly. A *sublabral foramen* is absent fixation of the labrum between 1 and 3 o'clock (Fig. 3-42). A *sublabral recess* or sulcus is a cleft between the superior labrum and the glenoid (Fig. 3-43) as a result of normal variation in the biceps labral complex. The biceps labral complex is the attachment of the biceps long head tendon to the superior labrum. The biceps tendon can originate entirely from the superior labrum, or partially from the labrum and partially from the osseous glenoid. The latter arrangement is associated with a meniscus-like superior labrum that is fixed to the biceps tendon and the glenoid periosteum, but not to the underlying glenoid articular cartilage. The less common *Buford complex* is an absent anterior superior labrum and a thickened, cordlike middle glenohumeral ligament that may simulate a labral detachment (Fig. 3-44). In contrast, absent labral fixation below 3 o'clock or posterior to about 12 o'clock generally indicates labral pathology, especially in young adults. However, minimal partial detachments may be seen as an age-related finding in older individuals.

The glenohumeral joint capsule is difficult to assess on imaging studies unless the capsule is distended by a joint effusion or during arthrography. The capsular anatomy is fairly simple and constant posteriorly, but is quite complicated and variable anteriorly. The posterior joint capsule is attached to the glenoid labrum and adjacent glenoid periosteum, and is bounded by the rotator cuff. The anterior capsule may also attach to the glenoid rim, or may insert onto the scapula medial to the labrum. A classification system may be used to describe the position of the

anterior capsular attachment to the scapula (Fig. 3-45). A type 1 anterior capsular insertion is attachment of the anterior joint capsule to the lateral glenoid. A type 2 insertion is attachment of the capsule to the scapular neck up to 1 cm medial to the labrum. A type 3 insertion is attachment of the capsule more than 1 cm medial to the labrum. Type 2 and especially type 3 anterior capsular insertions may occur as a normal variant or a consequence of a previous anterior shoulder dislocation that stripped the capsule and periosteum off of the glenoid. The latter condition may be associated with other evidence of a prior shoulder dislocation and is further discussed below. Regardless of the etiology, capsular attachment medial to the labrum is associated with shoulder instability and therefore should be noted when observed on imaging studies. The glenohumeral joint capsule also is variable in terms of the redundancy of its tissues. Excessive redundancy predisposes the shoulder to instability, dislocation, rotator cuff degeneration and tears, and labral tears. However, some capsular redundancy is required to allow for a normal range of motion. Conversely, an overly tight joint capsule, as can occur after inflammatory processes ("adhesive capsulitis," Fig. 3-46) or surgical "tightening" procedures performed to correct shoulder instability, can cause pain and reduced shoulder mobility. Estimation of capsular laxity on imaging studies is subjective and arguably should be avoided unless the findings are extreme. Normal synovial recesses, or pouches, extending from the glenohumeral synovial compartment include the subscapularis (subcoracoid) recess (for bursa) anteromedially and the axillary pouch or recess inferiorly (Fig. 3-40). These recesses are nearly always distended during shoulder arthrography, and should not be confused with capsular laxity or redundancy.

Text continued on p. 225

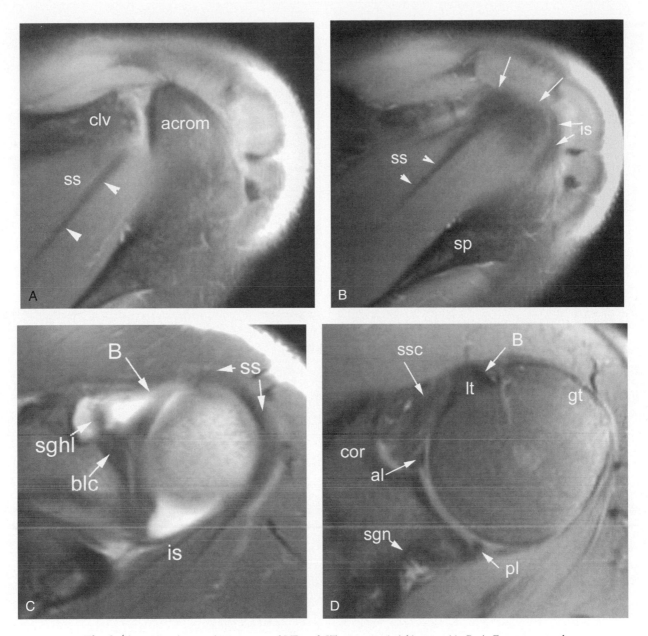

Fig. 3-41   Glenohumeral joint: normal MR and CT anatomy. Axial images (*A-I*). **A,** Fat suppressed proton density image through the acromioclavicular joint. The most superior image should include this joint to assess for os acromiale and anterior spurs. Note the central slip of the supraspinatus tendon (*arrowheads*). The oblique coronal scans should be aligned with this portion of the tendon. **B,** (Just below *A,* same study). Note how the supraspinatus tendon becomes broad distally, like a cuff (*long arrows*). **C,** MR arthrogram image through the top of the humeral head is perpendicular to the supraspinatus tendon as it curves over the head towards its insertion onto the greater tuberosity. For this reason, distal supraspinatus tears may be best seen on axial images. **D,** Fat suppressed proton density image at the level of the base of the coracoid.

Continued

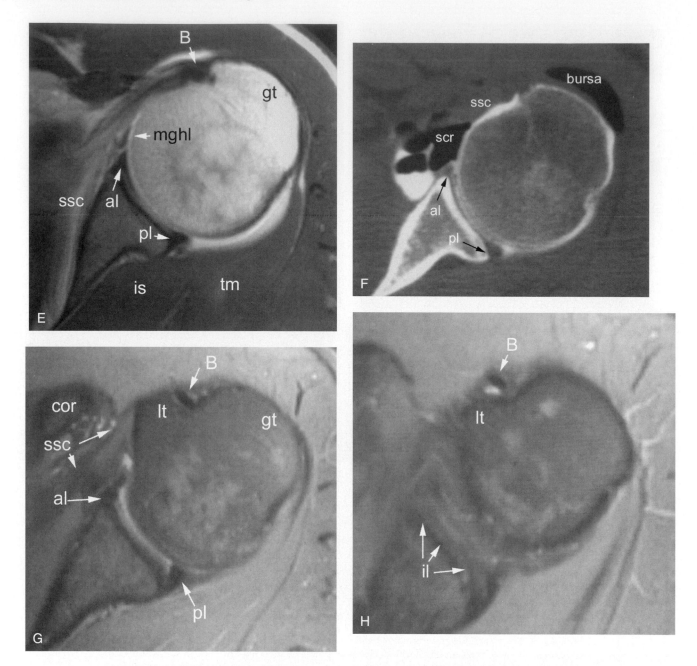

Fig. 3-41, cont'd   **E,** T1-weighted MR arthrogram image at approximately the 9 and 3 o'clock level. The increased signal intensity in the subscapularis tendon and muscle was due to a combination of harmless contrast extravasation from the joint and direct injection during needle placement. **F,** CT air contrast arthrogram in a different patient at approximately the same level as **E.** The gas in the subdeltoid bursa was due to a rotator cuff tear (not shown). **G,** Fat suppressed proton density image at approximately the 4 o-clock–8 o-clock level. **H,** Fat suppressed proton density image through the inferior glenoid.

Continued

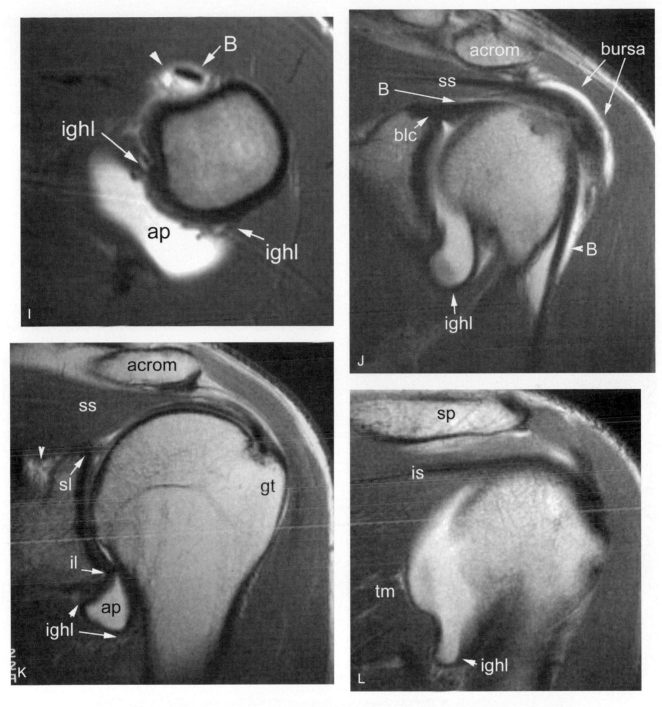

Fig. 3-41, cont'd   I, T1-weighted MR arthrogram image through the axillary pouch. Note that contrast fills the biceps tendon sheath (*arrowhead*), a normal finding. Oblique coronal images (*J-L*). **J, K, L,** All images are T2-weighted arthrogram images from the same study. **J,** Anterior image; **K,** Central image. Note the suprascapular notch (*arrowhead*) that contains the suprascapular nerve that innervates the supraspinatus and infraspinatus muscle. **L,** Posterior image. Oblique sagittal images (*M-P*).

Continued

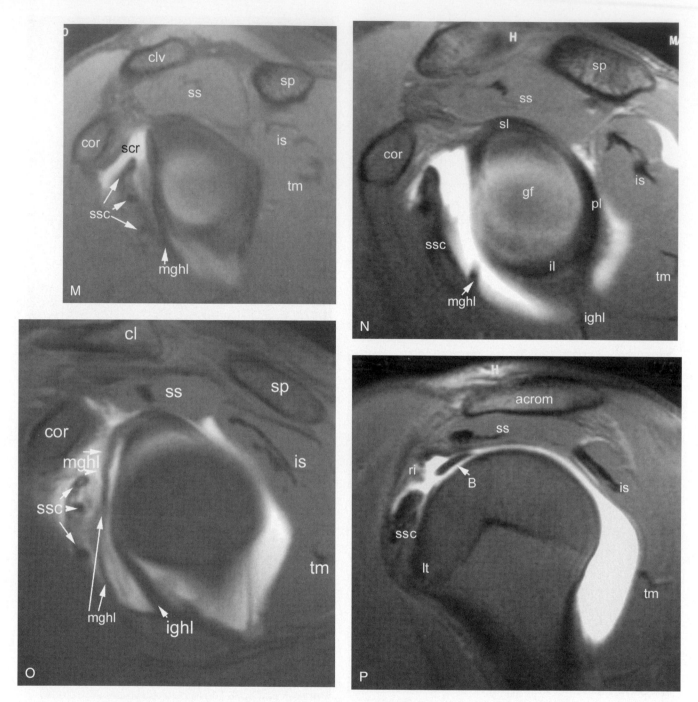

Fig. 3-41, cont'd M, N, O, P, All images are T1-weighted MR arthrogram images, but not from the same study. **M,** Slightly medial to the glenoid fossa. **N,** At the glenoid fossa. **O,** Lateral to the glenoid fossa. **P,** Through the center of the humeral head. (See Key with Fig. 3-39.)

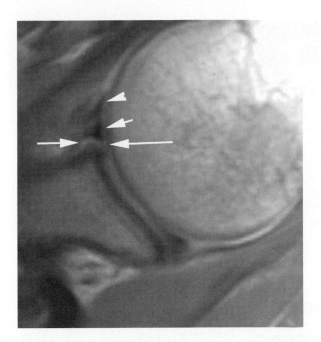

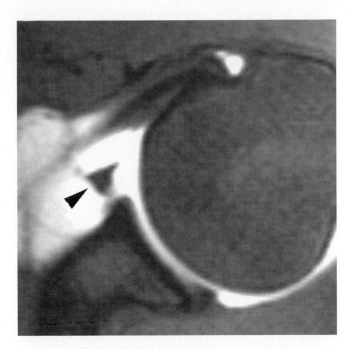

Fig. 3-42 Normal variant sublabral foramen. Axial T2-weighted MR arthrogram image shows contrast (*long arrows*) passing between the anterior labrum (*short arrow*) and the glenoid. This finding is a normal variant only between 1 and 3 o'clock. Also note the middle glenohumeral ligament (*arrowhead*). Contrast between this ligament and the labrum should not be mistaken for a labral tear.

Fig. 3-44 Buford complex. Note absent anterosuperior labrum and thick middle glenohumeral ligament (*arrowhead*).

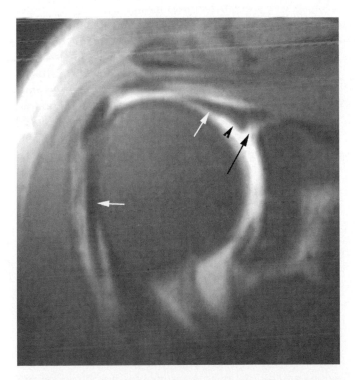

Fig. 3-43 Sublabral sulcus (*black arrow*). Note the biceps long head tendon (*white arrows*) and the meniscus-like superior labrum (*black arrowhead*).

The three glenohumeral ligaments (GHL) are thick fibrous bands within the anterior portion of the joint. The GHLs are important contributors to anterior shoulder stability. The thickest and most important is the inferior glenohumeral ligament (IGHL), which extends from the glenoid labrum to the proximal humeral shaft in a slinglike arrangement of thick anterior and posterior bands connected by a thin membrane. The IGHL is lax and redundant when the arm is adducted, contributing to the normal axillary pouch (Figs. 3-40, 3-41). However, when the arm is abducted 90°, the IGHL tightens and becomes the primary stabilizer of the glenohumeral joint. The highly variable middle glenohumeral ligament (MGHL) originates at the superior portion of the anterior labrum or adjacent glenoid neck, and attaches to the base of the lesser tuberosity of the humerus with the subscapularis muscle. The MGHL is absent in about one-fourth of patients. When present, the MGHL may be of variable thickness and is occasionally duplicated. The normal variant Buford complex of an absent anterior–superior labrum and thick MGHL was noted in the previous discussion of labral anatomy (Fig. 3-44). The superior glenohumeral ligament (SGHL) originates from the superior–anterior labrum, MGHL, or the biceps long head tendon, and attaches distally to the superior aspect of the lesser tuberosity. The middle and superior glenohumeral ligaments contribute to anterior glenohumeral stability, but are not as critical to shoulder stability as the IGHL. The GHLs are best demonstrated on imaging studies with distension of the joint capsule using CT or MR arthrography.

The acromion process and the coracoacromial ligament form the *coracoacromial arch* (Fig. 3-47). The

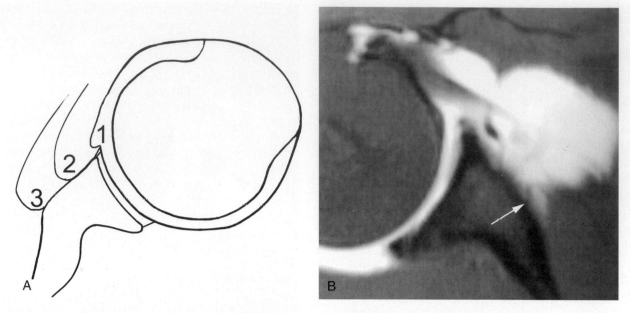

Fig. 3-45   Anterior capsule insertion variation. **A,** Classification:
Type 1: Capsule attached to anterior labrum
Type 2: Capsule attached to scapula up to 1 cm medial to anterior labrum
Type 3: Capsule attached to scapula more than 1 cm medial to anterior labrum.
(From Massengill AD, Seeger LL, Yao L, et al. Labrocapuslar ligamentous complex of the shoulder: normal anatomy, anatomic variation, and pitfalls of MR imaging and MR arthrography. *Radiographics* 1994; 14:1211–1223). **B,** Axial T1-weighted fat suppressed MR arthrogram image shows a type 3 anterior capsular insertion (*arrow*).

coracoacromial ligament is variable in thickness, ranging from about 2 to 5 mm. It is seen on MR images as a low signal intensity structure that can be traced between the anterior acromion process and the coracoid on sequential images. The coracoacromial arch contributes

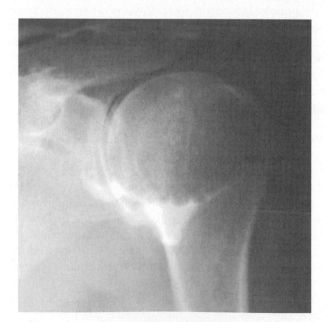

Fig. 3-46   Adhesive capsulitis. Arthrogram shows a very low capacity joint capsule.

to shoulder stability by limiting superior subluxation of the humeral head. This anatomy also makes the coracoacromial arch a major factor in rotator cuff impingement. The *subacromial space* is the space between the humeral head and the coracoacromial arch. Important contents of the subacromial space, from superior to inferior, are the subacromial bursa, the supraspinatus and infraspinatus tendons, and the joint capsule. The subacromial bursa communicates with the more lateral subdeltoid bursa, and for practical purposes, they may be considered as a single bursa (subacromial subdeltoid bursa). This bursa allows the rotator cuff to glide beneath the coracoacromial arch and the deltoid muscle. Any process that narrows the subacromial space has the potential to compress the soft tissues in the subacromial space. This is discussed further below in the discussion of rotator cuff impingement.

Rotator Cuff Impingement

Rotator cuff impingement syndrome is shoulder pain related to impingement (compression) of the rotator cuff, the biceps long head tendon and the subacromial bursa between the humeral head and the coracoacromial arch. Rotator cuff impingement syndrome occurs in both young and old patients. A cardinal feature of rotator cuff impingement is reproducible pain with overhead maneu-

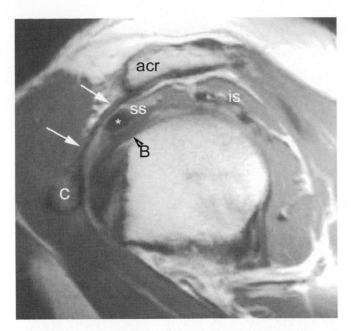

Fig. 3-47   Coracoacromial arch. Oblique sagittal MR image happens to include the entire coracoacromial ligament on one image (*arrows*, c, coracoid process; acr, acromion). Note that the supraspinatus tendon (ss) is deep to the coracoacromial ligament, which is often a factor in supraspinatus impingement. In this case, the supraspinatus tendon is focally thickened (*asterisk*) due to chronic impingement. Also note the infraspinatus (is), and biceps long head tendon.

vers. Not surprisingly, impingement occurs more frequently in individuals who perform repetitive overhead activities, such as throwing athletes or certain workers. Although rotator cuff impingement syndrome is a clinical diagnosis, many of the anatomic factors that contribute to rotator cuff impingement may be seen on imaging studies, which can assist in the diagnosis.

The large majority rotator cuff tendon tears are the result of chronic tendon impingement. Therefore, most rotator cuff tears occur in older individuals. Chronic impingement causes tendon degeneration and weakening, leading to tendon disruption after seemingly trivial trauma. The supraspinatus tendon is the most vulnerable of the rotator cuff tendons to impingement, degeneration, and tear simply because of its anatomic location at the most frequent site of impingement between the anterior acromion and the humeral head.

Several anatomic and dynamic factors contribute to rotator cuff impingement. At least one, and often several are present in a patient who develops a rotator cuff tear. The shape of the acromion process is often the single most important anatomic factor. Acromial features associated with impingement include spurs, a hooked anterior undersurface of the acromion, and AC joint degenerative changes.

An anterior acromial spur is a traction spur (enthesophyte) at or adjacent to the acromial attachment of the coracoacromial ligament. This spur may be seen on an AP radiograph or an AP radiograph angled 30° caudally, or occasionally an axillary radiograph. It extends anteriorly, medially, and inferiorly from the anterior acromion process (Fig. 3-48A). Acromial spurs at the attachment of the coracoacromial ligament can be distinguished from the ligament on sagittal oblique MR images because they contain marrow fat (Fig. 3-48B).

The morphology of the inferior surface of the acromion can be determined by an outlet radiograph or by sagittal oblique MR images (Fig. 3-49). The Bigliani classification describes the acromial undersurface as flat (type

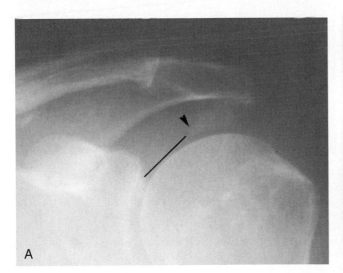

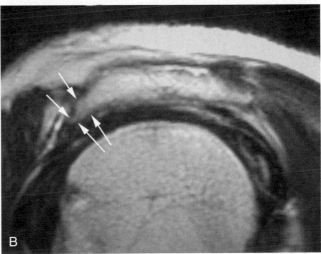

Fig. 3-48   Anterior acromial spur. **A,** AP radiograph shows an unusually long an enthesophyte (acromial spur, *black arrowheads*). The black line marks the location of the coracoacromial ligament. **B,** Oblique sagittal T2-weighted MR image shows a spur (*arrows*) at the attachment of the coracoacromial ligament. Note that the spur contains marrow, which allows it to be distinguished on MR images from the coracoacromial ligament, which has low signal intensity on all sequences.

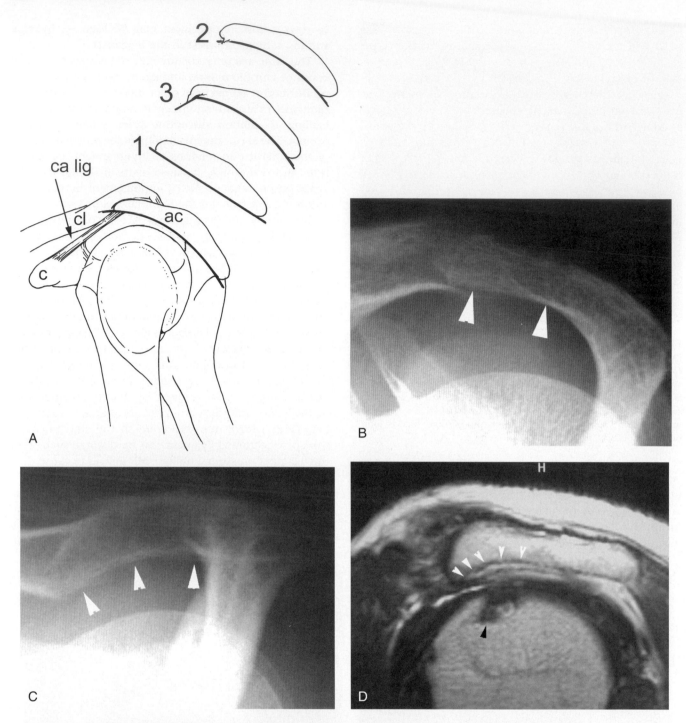

Fig. 3-49 The Bigliani classification of the shape of the undersurface of the acromion. **A,** Diagram with anterior to the viewer's left shows the contour of type 1 (flat), type 2 (concave), and type 3 (anterior hook). c, coracoid process; ac, acromion; cl, clavicle; ca lig, coracoacromial ligament. **B,** Type 1. Outlet view shows a flat acromial undersurface (*arrowheads*). **C,** Type 2. Outlet view shows a concave acromial undersurface (*arrowheads*). **D,** Type 3. Oblique sagittal T2-weighted MR image shows anterior hook (*white arrowheads*). Also note the humeral head marrow signal changes (*black arrowhead*) caused by chronic impingement. The subacromial space is narrow because there is a complete rotator cuff tear with retraction (not shown).

1), concave, that is, matching the contour of the humeral head without focal subacromial space narrowing (type 2), or hooked anteriorly with associated narrowing of the subacromial space (type 3). Type 3 morphology is strongly associated with rotator cuff impingement. The reader is cautioned that the apparent contour on sagittal oblique MRI images is somewhat dependent on the orientation of the images, as well as which image is selected. Relatively medial images (adjacent to the AC joint) may suggest an anterior hook when none is present.

The slope or orientation of the acromion process, specifically lateral or anterior downsloping, also can narrow the subacromial space and cause rotator cuff impingement.

AC joint OA, with associated inferiorly oriented osteophytes, callus, or soft tissue hypertrophy, can markedly narrow the subacromial space (Fig. 3-50). The developmental variant os acromiale (Fig. 3-35), discussed earlier, is associated with rotator cuff impingement, but only as a minor factor.

A prior humeral head fracture that heals with deformity may cause rotator cuff impingement.

Chronic impingement can cause secondary changes in the acromion and humeral head. The cortex of the anterior acromion and the superior aspect of the greater tuberosity may become irregular, vaguely suggestive of erosive disease. Small "cysts," best appreciated on MR images, may develop within the greater tuberosity near the rotator cuff insertion and the acromion (Figs. 3-49D, 3-51). The greater tuberosity may become rounded and sclerotic. The acromial undersurface may become sclerotic and acquire a concave contour that matches the

contour of the humeral head. This finding suggests that a chronic large rotator cuff tear is present.

Subacromial bursitis is associated with rotator cuff impingement, both as a cause and an effect. An example of the former is bursal enlargement due to rheumatoid arthritis that effectively narrows the subacromial space available for the rotator cuff tendons. Bursitis also may occur as a direct consequence of impingement. MR images and US reveal increased fluid in the bursa, a nonspecific finding that may also be seen in the presence of a full thickness rotator cuff tear (Fig. 3-52).

Special mention must be made of calcific bursitis and calcific tendinitis. Although the two conditions are not necessarily related, bursitis often follows tendinitis as part of an interesting progression (Fig. 3-53). Initially, small asymptomatic calcium deposits, usually calcium hydroxyapatite, form in the rotator cuff tendons ("silent phase"). Such clinically silent calcium deposition is surprisingly common. However, if the calcium deposits enlarge, associated mass effect effectively narrows the subacromial space, and impingement symptoms of variable degree develop ("mechanical phase"). The calcium deposits may subsequently erupt from the tendon into the joint space, the subacromial bursa, the greater tuberosity, or into periarticular tissues. Intrabursal rupture causes a clinical syndrome of acute bursitis. Eruptions of calcific deposits from the tendon may occur repeatedly until the tendon is cleared of such deposits. Bursal fibrosis can occur as a late stage complication. Diagnosis of calcific tendinitis and bursitis is readily made with radiographs (Fig. 3-53A). MR images may reveal low signal intensity on all imaging sequences (Fig. 3-53B).

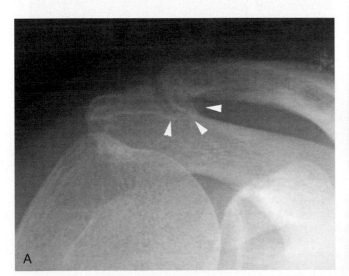

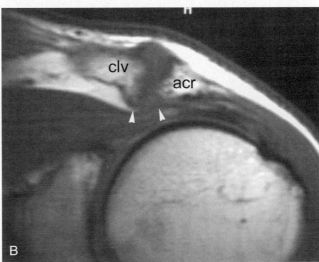

Fig. 3-50   Acromioclavicular osteophytes. AP radiograph (**A**) and oblique coronal T1-weighted MR image in a different patient (**B**) show spurs projecting inferiorly from the AC joint (*arrowheads*). (clv, clavicle; acr, acromion in **B**).

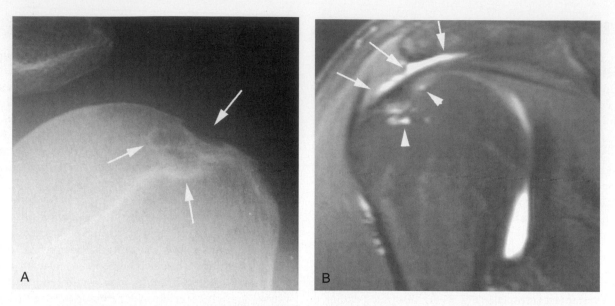

Fig. 3-51   Chronic rotator cuff impingement. **A,** AP radiograph in internal rotation shows cystlike lucencies in the posterior-superior humeral head and adjacent greater tuberosity. **B,** Oblique coronal fat suppressed T2-weighted MR arthrogram image shows tiny cystlike lesion in the posterior-superior lateral humeral head (*arrowheads*). The patient also has a rotator cuff tear (not shown) that has resulted in contrast entering the subacromial bursa (*arrows*).

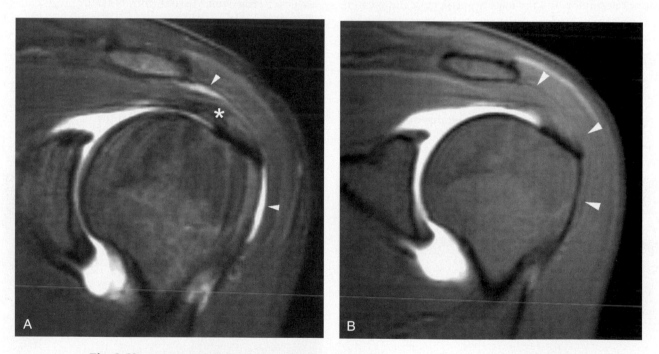

Fig. 3-52   Subacromial bursitis. MR arthrogram. Sagittal T2-weighted MR coronal image with fat suppression (**A**) shows fluid in the subacromial subdeltoid bursa (*arrowheads*) as well as thickening and increased signal intensity within the supraspinatus tendon (*asterisk*). These findings suggest that a complete rotator cuff tear is likely to be present. However, note that the bursal fluid does not have increased signal intensity (*arrowheads*) on the corresponding fat suppressed coronal T1-weighted MR arthrogram image (**B**) from the same study. Thus, there is no communication between the joint and the bursa, so the cause of the bursal fluid is bursitis rather than rotator cuff tear.

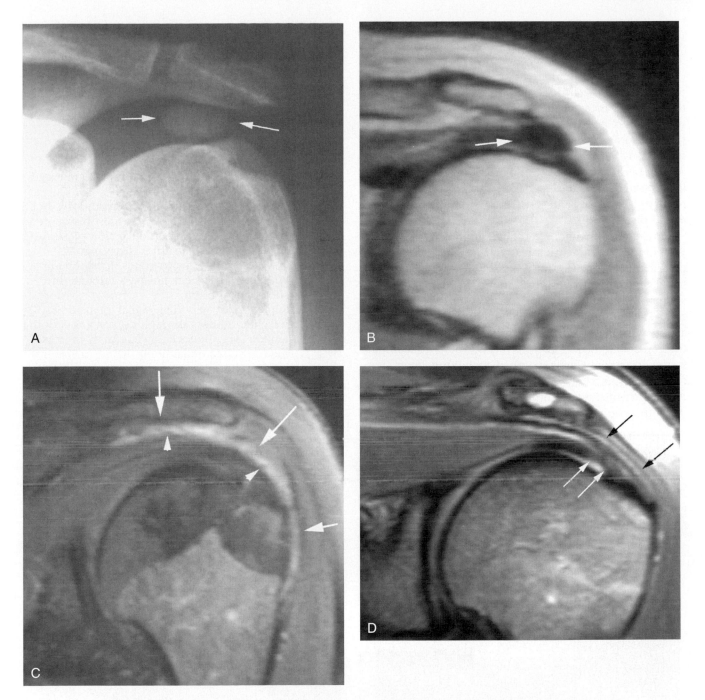

Fig. 3-53   Calcific tendinitis. **A, B,** Mechanical phase. AP radiograph (**A**) shows typical amorphous calcification of calcific tendinitis (*between arrows*). Oblique coronal proton density-weighted MR image obtained in a low field magnet (**B**) shows supraspinatus tendon thickening and very low signal intensity in the region of mineralization (*between arrows*). These findings were also present on T1-weighted, T2-weighted, and inversion recovery MR images (not shown). The patient subsequently underwent surgical debridement of the calcific tendinitis with significant symptomatic improvement. **C,** Followup oblique coronal fat suppressed T2-weighted MR image obtained about 4 months later shows a more normal appearance of the rotator cuff tendons (*arrowheads*). Radiographs (not shown) also showed resolution of the calcium deposit. However, now note the bursal fluid (*arrows*) with tiny low signal intensity filling defects thought to represent residual hydroxyapatite crystals and other debris. The patient was only mildly symptomatic. **D,** Oblique coronal fat suppressed T2-weighted MR image obtained 2 months later shows only a trace amount of fluid in the subacromial bursa (*black arrows*) and mild findings of supraspinatus tendonopathy (*white arrows*). Bursal fibrosis can develop as a late stage complication of calcific tendinitis, but this patient clinically did not have such fibrosis.

A distinct and much less common form of rotator cuff impingement is posterior–superior glenoid impingement that is seen in throwing athletes, especially baseball pitchers. The extreme abduction and external rotation that occurs during the "cocking" phase of throwing, when the elbow is most posterior, just before beginning forward motion of the arm, causes compression of the posterior and superior soft tissues. The superior labrum, rotator cuff, IGHL, greater tuberosity and glenoid may be injured by such impingement. Posterior-superior glenoid impingement in skeletally immature baseball pitchers can result in irregularity and sclerosis of the posterior aspect of the physis.

Surgical treatment of rotator cuff impingement usually is accomplished by acromioplasty, that is, surgical decompression of the subacromial space (Fig. 3-54). Acromioplasty is frequently performed during rotator cuff repair surgery in order to correct the cause of the rotator cuff tear. The inferior surface of the acromion is resected, along with any associated acromial and AC spurs, and the coracoacromial ligament is released at its attachment to the acromion. Current surgical technique favors performing this procedure through an arthroscope placed in the subacromial bursa, termed arthroscopic subacromial decompression (ASD).

Rotator Cuff Degeneration and Tear

Recurrent impingement causes tendon edema and hemorrhage, and can lead to tendinitis, fibrosis, and degeneration. "Tendinitis" is a bit of a misnomer, as inflammatory cellular infiltrates within the symptomatic

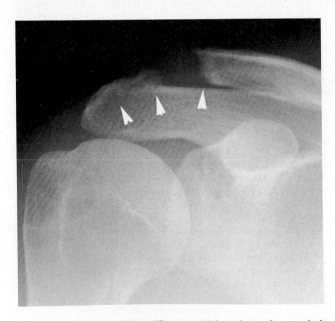

Fig. 3-54 Acromioplasty. The acromial undersurface and the AC joint (*arrowheads*) were resected as treatment for rotator cuff impingement.

Key Concepts	Rotator Cuff Tear

- Most tears are due to chronic impingement.
- Other causes: Rheumatoid arthritis (pannus), acute injury.
- Supraspinatus distal insertion most frequent site.
- Infraspinatus, less frequently subscapularis, also tear.
- MRI findings:
    Normal: Low signal intensity.
    Tendinosis (degeneration/tendinitis): increased signal on T2-weighted images.
    Partial tear: may be identical to tendinosis, but often higher signal intensity, possibly centered on bursal (upper) or articular (lower) surface. Articular (inferior) surface tears may be detected on MR arthrograms if gadolinium enters tear but does not pass through into subacromial bursa.
    Complete tear: Very high signal intensity on T2-weighted images through the thickness of the tendon. May be focal or extensive. Increased fluid in subacromial bursa. Range in size from tiny focal tendon perforations to massive tears. Large tears may have tendon retraction
    Chronic tears: muscle atrophy and fatty infiltration
- Imaging pitfalls:
    Magic angle on short TE sequences causes increased tendon signal intensity 55° to magnet bore. Solution: evaluate rotator cuff tendons with T2-weighted (long TE) images
    MR findings of tendinosis may be seen in asymptomatic individuals
    Bursitis: Increased bursal fluid can suggest full thickness cuff tear
    Prior rotator cuff surgery: small rotator interval defect not repaired at surgery
- Clinical pitfalls:
    Suprascapular nerve injury or neuritis (MRI shows muscle signal changes of denervation, may show cause)
    Nondisplaced greater tuberosity avulsion fracture (MRI shows the fracture)
    Bursitis (MRI shows bursal fluid, intact rotator cuff)

---

tendon are usually not a prominent feature. The alternative umbrella terms "tendinopathy" or "tendinosis" are preferable, as they do not attempt to distinguish tendonitis, fibrosis, and degeneration. However, the term "tendinitis" remains popular because the acuity of clinical features in some patients is suggestive of an acute inflammatory process. Regardless, all of these changes result in an increase in free water within the tendon that is seen on MR images as increased signal intensity on both T1 and T2-weighted sequences (Fig. 3-55). Healing is possible, but is limited by poor tendon blood supply that consists primarily of tiny vessels that extend from the muscle belly and the humerus. Ongoing tendon impingement in the presence of one or more of the anatomic factors discussed earlier can result in a partial thickness tendon tear. A partial thickness tear may occur in the bursal or articular surface, or within the substance of the tendon (intrasubstance tear), or as a combination. A partial thickness tear may have a similar appearance to tendinosis on MR images, or may be seen as a discrete defect on the bursal or articular surface, usually with higher signal intensity than tendon degeneration (Fig. 3-56). A partial tear can progress to a full thickness (complete) tear. A full thickness tear is fairly reliably detected on MR imaging as a defect in the tendon. The tear fills with joint fluid or granulation tissue, both of which have very high signal intensity on T2-weighted images (Fig. 3-51, 3-57). Increased fluid in the subacromial bursa is frequently seen as an associated finding. Careful attention to window and level settings and correlation of the oblique coronal images with the oblique sagittal and axial images is often helpful in confirming a subtle partial or full thickness tear. If a full thickness tear extends across the tendon, the proximal margin of the torn tendon and muscle belly can retract medially. A chronically retracted muscle belly becomes atrophic and infiltrated with fat, a situation that is best appreciated on T1-weighted MR

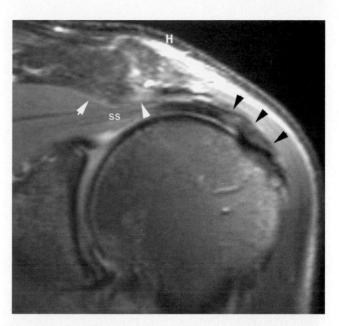

Fig. 3-56 Rotator cuff partial thickness tear. Oblique coronal fat suppressed T2-weighted MR image shows supraspinatus tendon thickening with increased signal intensity that is greatest along the bursal (superior) surface (*black arrowheads*). Note the acromioclavicular osteophytes (*white arrowheads*) that deflect the supraspinatus musculotendinous junction (ss). When the arm is abducted, these spurs compress the distal supraspinatus tendon. (This is the same study as Figure 3-50B.) Arthroscopy revealed partial thickness tearing, felt to be due to impingement by the acromioclavicular spurs.

images. Muscle retraction, atrophy and fatty infiltration indicate a chronic tear that will not benefit from surgical repair.

Ultrasound also can detect such tears (Fig. 3-58). Conventional arthrography is extremely accurate in detecting full thickness tears. Contrast injected into the glenohumeral joint flows through the tear into the subacromial bursa (Fig. 3-59).

Most rotator cuff tears occur in the supraspinatus tendon, often at its anterior insertion onto the greater tuberosity. Rotator cuff tears can and do occur in other locations. The so-called *"critical zone,"* approximately 1-cm proximal to the distal insertion, is the watershed between the humeral and muscular blood supplies and is vulnerable to degeneration and tearing due to its poor blood supply. Massive tears involving more than one tendon most frequently begin in the anterior supraspinatus tendon and extend posteriorly into the infraspinatus tendon and inferiorly through the rotator interval into the subscapularis tendon. A chronic massive rotator cuff tear with retracted tendons results in a chronically high riding humeral head. Radiographs may reveal the subacromial space to be obviously narrowed (6 mm or less), and may reveal remodeling of the acromial undersurface into a concave contour that matches the contour of the humeral head due to chronic impaction.

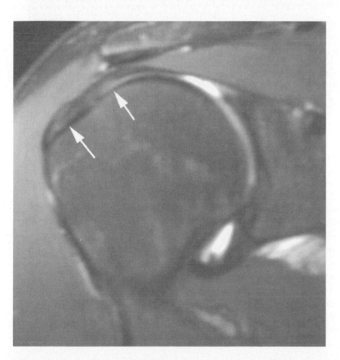

Fig. 3-55 Rotator cuff tendinosis (tendonopathy). Oblique coronal T2-weighted MR arthrogram image with fat suppression shows increased signal in the supraspinatus tendon (*arrows*). Arthroscopy showed no tear. The signal changes likely are due to tendon degeneration.

Text continued on p. 237

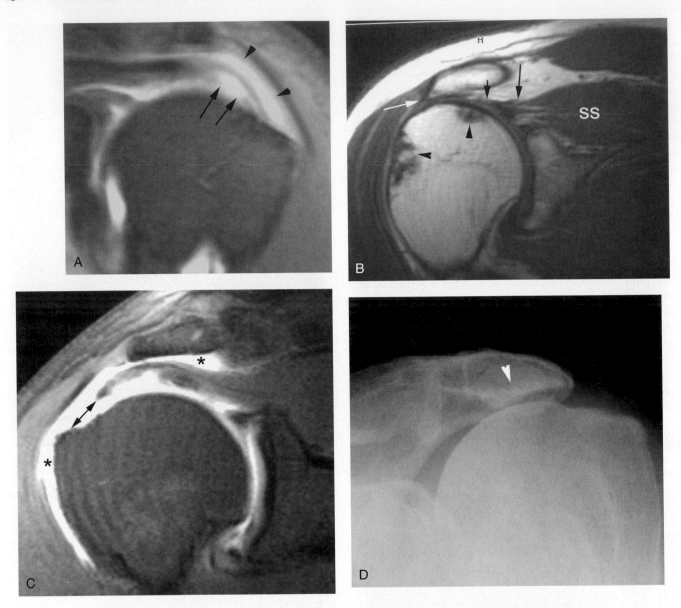

Fig. 3-57   Rotator cuff complete (full thickness) tear. **A,** Oblique coronal T1-weighted MR arthrogram image shows a large undersurface partial tear in the supraspinatus tendon (*arrows*). The contrast in the subacromial subdeltoid bursa (*arrowheads*) indicates that a full thickness tear in the rotator cuff must be present. Arthroscopy revealed a small perforation associated with the undersurface defect shown here. **B,** Oblique coronal T1-weighted MR image shows a complete tear of the supraspinatus tendon. Note the retracted edge of the tendon (*short black arrow*) and musculotendinous junction (*long black arrow*). Also note the narrow subacromial space. There is no atrophy or fatty infiltration of the supraspinatus muscle belly (*SS*), suggesting that the retraction is not chronic. Also note the findings associated with rotator cuff impingement: the acromial spur (*white arrow*), and the humeral head marrow findings related to chronic impingement (*black arrowheads*). **C,** Oblique coronal fat suppressed T1-weighted MR arthrogram image shows a massive rotator cuff tear with retraction of the supraspinatus tendon (*double arrow marks the defect*). Note the contrast in the subacromial subdeltoid bursa (*asterisks*). **D,** Radiograph in a patient with a chronic, retracted rotator cuff tear shows narrow subacromial space and sclerosis of the acromial undersurface (*arrowhead*) related to chronic impaction by the humeral head.

Continued

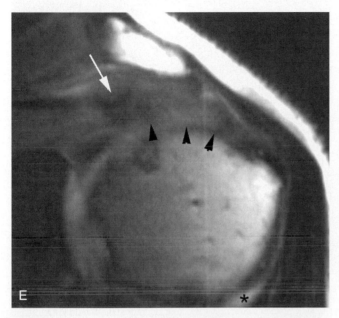

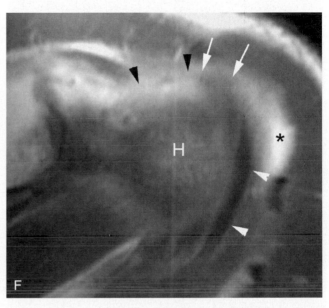

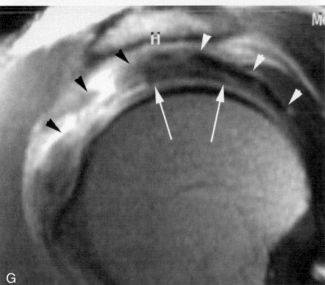

Fig. 3-57, cont'd   E, F, G, Value of correlation of images different planes. **E,** Oblique coronal T1-weighted MR arthrogram image with partial fat suppression shows amorphous high signal in the anterior supraspinatus tendon (*black arrowheads*). Note the more normal low signal intensity of the proximal supraspinatus tendon (*white arrow*). Note the contrast in the subacromial bursa (*asterisk*), indicating that a rotator cuff tear is present. **F, G,** Axial (**F**) and oblique sagittal (**G**) T1-weighted images confirm the tear (*black arrowheads*) and help to determine the size of the tear. (*White arrows,* intact posterior portion of supraspinatus tendon; *white arrowheads,* infraspinatus tendon; H, humeral head; *, contrast in the subdeltoid bursa).

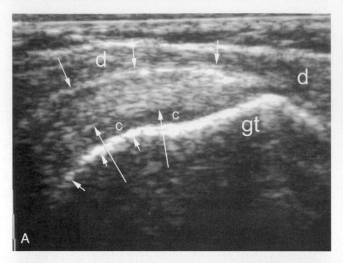

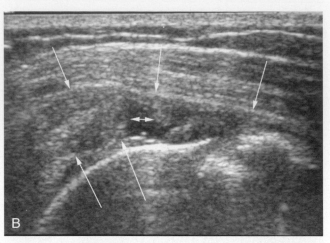

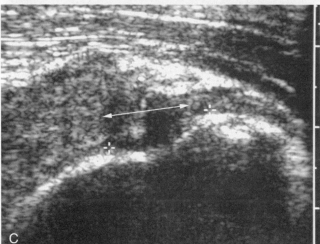

Fig. 3-58   Rotator cuff tears: ultrasound findings. The scans are obtained with the arm adducted and internally rotated. This position moves the distal supraspinatus tendon out from under from the acromion, allowing it to be imaged with ultrasound. **A,** Normal supraspinatus tendon (*long arrows*). Also note the greater tuberosity (gt), deltoid muscle (d), subchondral cortex of the humeral head (*short arrows*) and the articular cartilage (c). **B,** Partial thickness undersurface tear (*double arrow marks the defect*) seen as hypoechoic defect within the supraspinatus tendon (*arrows*). **C,** Complete tear (*double arrow marks the defect*) (Courtesy of Doohi Lee, M.D., Richmond, VA.)

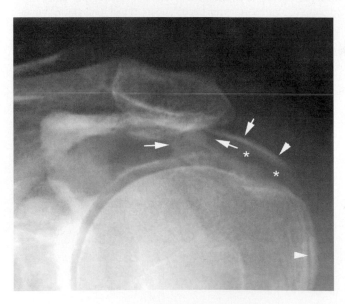

Fig. 3-59   Rotator cuff tear: arthrographic findings AP spot view shows contrast passing through a supraspinatus tear (*between arrows*) into the subacromial subdeltoid bursa (*arrowheads*). Note the "filling defect" of the distal supraspinatus tendon (*asterisks*). Also note that the acromion downslopes laterally, a finding associated with rotator cuff impingement.

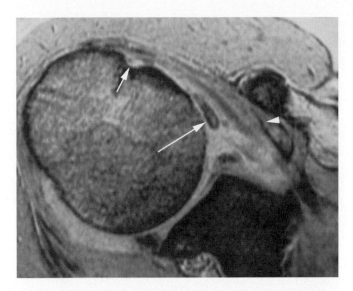

Fig. 3-60 Biceps long head tendon dislocation. Axial gradient echo MR image shows the biceps long head tendon (*long arrow*) to be medially dislocated out of the bicipital groove (*short arrow*). Note the partial tear of the subscapularis tendon (*arrowhead*).

Biceps Tendon Pathology

The biceps long head tendon originates at the biceps labral complex at the 12 to 1 (usually 1) o'clock position of the superior-anterior glenoid. Superior labral tears (discussed below) can involve the biceps tendon. The intraarticular portion of the biceps tendon is vulnerable to impingement, degeneration, and tearing by the same mechanism as the rotator cuff. Impingement may cause tendon degeneration, fraying, partial or complete tearing,

or occasionally thickening. Biceps tendon dislocation or subluxation from the intertubercular groove indicates interruption of the transverse ligament. Because the transverse ligament receives fibers from the subscapularis tendon and coracohumeral ligament, biceps subluxation is associated with injury to these structures. An empty intertubercular groove, containing only joint fluid, may indicate biceps long head dislocation or complete tendon tearing with retraction (Fig. 3-60). Tenosynovitis also causes the tendon sheath to fill with fluid. However, this finding is nonspecific as the tendon sheath usually communicates with the glenohumeral joint and a finding of tendon sheath fluid thus may be secondary to a joint effusion.

Clinical Mimickers of Rotator Cuff Pathology

There are numerous conditions that share clinical features with rotator cuff impingement and tear. Imaging studies in these patients can exclude rotator cuff disease, and frequently can identify the true cause of the patient's symptoms. A fall in a patient with healthy rotator cuff tendons can result in a nondisplaced avulsion fracture of the greater tuberosity. Such a fracture can be virtually imperceptible on radiographs. MRI is diagnostic (Fig. 3-61). Suprascapular nerve dysfunction can cause a syndrome of supraspinatus and infraspinatus denervation that clinically mimics a rotator cuff tear. Denervation results in diffuse muscle edema beginning about 2–4 weeks after the initial insult (Fig. 3-62). Chronic denervation causes irreversible fatty infiltration and atrophy. The suprascapular nerve may be injured by traction, neuritis, and compression. In our experience, suprascapular nerve

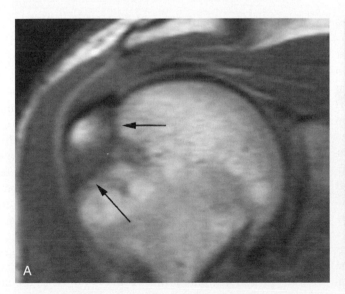
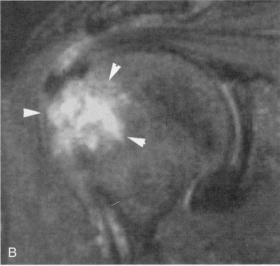

Fig. 3-61 Greater tuberosity fracture. Radiographs (not shown) did not reveal a fracture. Oblique coronal T1-weighted (**A**) and fat suppressed T2-weighted (**B**) MR images show a nondisplaced fracture, seen as a low signal line in **A** (*arrows*) with extensive surrounding edema in **B** (*arrowheads*).

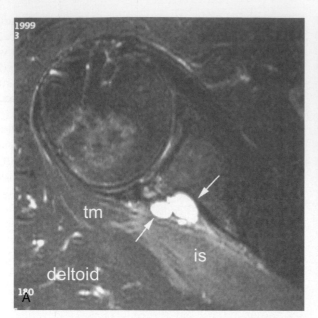
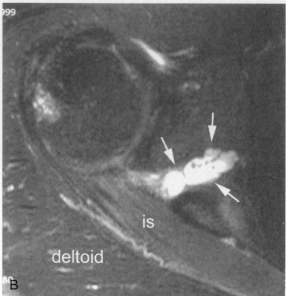

Fig. 3-62   Infraspinatus denervation caused by a paralabral cyst. The patient had clinical findings suggestive of a rotator cuff tear. Axial fat suppressed T2-weighted MR images at the level of the spinoglenoid notch (**A**) and one cut higher at the level of the suprascapular notch (**B**) show a multilobulate high signal mass (*arrows*) consistent with a ganglion cyst that fills these notches. The cyst is compressing the suprascapular nerve that innervates the supraspinatus and infraspinatus muscles. The infraspinatus and supraspinatus (not shown) muscle denervation results in diffusely increased signal intensity (muscle edema). Contrast the infraspinatus (is) with the normal deltoid and teres minor (tm) muscles. A ganglion cyst in this location is usually associated with a labral tear (paralabral cyst). (Reproduced with permission from May DA, et al: Abnormal signal within skeletal muscle in magnetic resonance imaging: patterns, pearls, and pitfalls. *Radiographics* 2000; 20:S295–315).

trauma due to traction injury is the most frequent cause of suprascapular nerve dysfunction. Brachial neuritis, also known as Parsonage Turner syndrome can cause selective suprascapular nerve dysfunction. Parsonage Turner syndrome is an idiopathic, possibly viral-related condition that occurs most frequently in young adult men. Most cases spontaneously resolve. The suprascapular nerve is vulnerable to entrapment in the spinoglenoid notch on the posterior scapular neck and the adjacent suprascapular notch on the superior scapular neck. A mass or displaced fracture fragment may cause such compression. Special mention must be made of a paralabral cyst, that is, a ganglion or synovial cyst adjacent to the glenoid labrum, as a potential cause of suprascapular nerve entrapment. Such cysts are frequently a consequence of a labral tear. In this situation, the labral tear functions as a one-way valve, allowing joint fluid to pass through the tear out of the joint but not back in, allowing the formation of a fluid-filled cystic mass. A paralabral cyst can progressively enlarge into the spinoglenoid notch and/ or the suprascapular notch (Fig. 3-62).

Glenohumeral (Shoulder) Dislocation, Instability, and Labral Tears

Dislocation   The shoulder is the most frequently dislocated major joint. Glenohumeral dislocation may occur in almost any direction, but the large majority of dislocations are anterior (95%). The most frequent mechanism of anterior shoulder dislocation is forced extension, abduction, and external rotation of the arm. A direct blow to the posterior shoulder or anterior distraction also can result in anterior dislocation. Radiographs are diagnostic (Fig. 3-63). A trans-scapular Y, axillary, or transthoracic view is necessary in any traumatized patient as these views reliably demonstrate or exclude a dislocation. Radiographs of anterior shoulder dislocation reveal the humeral head to be positioned anterior, medial, and slightly inferior to the glenoid fossa. Once dislocated, the superior–posterior humeral head is in contact with the anterior inferior glenoid rim. This may result in a wedge-shaped humeral head impaction fracture, termed a *Hill-Sachs lesion* (Fig. 3-64). A Hill-Sachs lesion may only be

| **Key Concepts** | **Glenohumeral Joint Instability** |

- Glenohumeral joint is highly mobile but intrinsically unstable.
- Stability depends on static and dynamic factors:
    Static: labrum, capsule, glenohumeral ligaments, suctionlike effects.
    Coracohumeral arch also limits superior subluxation
    Dynamic: rotator cuff, biceps long head tendon
- Anterior instability.
    Prior history of anterior dislocation frequent.
        Potential associated findings:
        Bankart lesion (soft tissue)
            Anterior labral tear or detachment
            Torn glenohumeral ligaments
            Anterior capsular stripping, medial attachment to scapular neck or body
        Bankart fracture
        Hill-Sachs fracture
- Multidirectional instability.
    Capsular laxity
    Dyscoordination of rotator cuff muscles
- Pitfalls:
    Findings not visible without joint capsule distension
    Contrast extravasation during CT or MR arthrography may simulate anterior capsular stripping
    Normal variant form of medial anterior capsular insertion may simulate anterior capsular stripping
    Normal variation in SGHL and MGHL may simulate a tear
    Normal flattening or cleft in posterior humerus just above surgical neck simulates a Hill-Sachs lesion on CT or MRI axial images. Always look for Hill-Sachs at or above coracoid process.
    Labral tear mimickers:
        Normal variations in anterior superior labrum (Sublabral foramen, Buford complex)
        Normal variant mild irregularities on articular surface of labrum
        Pseudotears of labrum:
            Close apposition of a GHL and labrum (space between simulates a tear)
            Normal finding of articular cartilage between labrum and osseous glenoid
            Magic angle causes increased labral signal (short TE only)

apparent on radiographs obtained after the dislocation is reduced, and even then may be quite subtle. Radiographs in internal rotation are more sensitive than external rotation because the lesion is located posterolaterally. CT and MR images are highly sensitive in detection of Hill-Sachs lesions. These modalities reveal a wedge shaped defect in the posterolateral superior humeral head at or just above the level of the coracoid process (Fig. 3-64). MR images of fractures less than 6–8 weeks old also typically reveal adjacent humeral marrow edema. The size of a Hill-Sachs lesion should be noted, as larger lesions are more strongly associated with subsequent anterior glenohumeral instability.

Anterior dislocation also injures the anterior soft tissue structures of the shoulder. The *Bankart lesion* is a tear or separation of the anterior inferior glenoid labrum classically, but not necessarily, with a chip fracture from the glenoid rim. Associated soft tissue injuries include GHL tears, coracohumeral ligament tear or avulsion, subscapularis tears with possible subluxation of the biceps long head tendon or avulsion fracture of the lesser tuberosity, and stripping of the anterior joint capsule from its glenoid attachment. The presence of glenoid marrow edema indicates that a Bankart lesion is likely to be acute. A Bankart fracture may be a subtle finding on radiographs but is easily identified with CT (Fig. 3-65).

Bankart lesions and related soft tissue injuries are the most important sequellae of an anterior shoulder dislocation, because they damage the anterior glenohumeral stabilizers, with resulting anterior glenohumeral instability and the potential for recurrent anterior dislocations. Anterior dislocation in a teenager or young adult is particularly likely to result in extensive anterior soft tissue injury and chronic anterior instability. These soft tissue injuries are difficult to detect on routine MR images unless the joint capsule is distended by an effusion or after an arthrogram. Careful scrutiny of the anterior joint structures is required. Findings to look for include tears or fraying of the glenohumeral ligaments and anterior inferior labrum, subscapularis tendon tear or muscle atrophy, subluxation of the biceps long head tendon, anterior capsular stripping, subluxation of the humeral head, and Hill-Sachs and Bankart fractures (Fig. 3-65).

There are several potential pitfalls that may falsely suggest anterior capsular injury on MR arthrograms. Differentiation of traumatic capsular stripping from atraumatic, normal variant medial capsular attachment can be difficult. The appearance of the joint capsule on imaging studies is dependent upon the amount of fluid in the joint and the position of the humerus. If the joint is distended with fluid, a previously stripped joint capsule may be seen to join the scapula at a shallow angle, whereas an atraumatic, normal variant medial capsular attachment often forms an obtuse angle (Fig. 3-65C). Alternatively, injected contrast may "extravasate" along the anterior-medial scapula, simulating capsular stripping. Such extravasated contrast often dissects into the subscapularis muscle, resulting in a distinctive pattern that may be distinguished from the more homogeneous signal intensity of intracapsular contrast (Figs. 3-41E, 3-65E). Normal subcoracoid and axillary capsular recesses should not be mistaken for a redundant capsule. Small

Text continued on p. 244

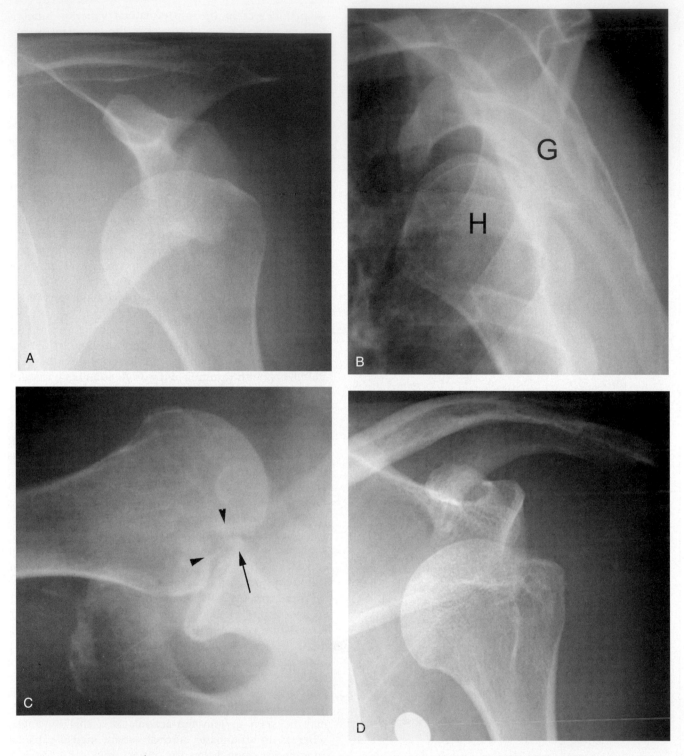

Fig. 3-63   Anterior shoulder dislocation. **A,** AP view shows the humeral head inferior to the coracoid. **B,** Y view shows the humeral head (H) anterior to the glenoid (G). **C,** Axillary view in a different patient shows a Hill-Sachs fracture (*arrowheads*) caused by impaction against the anterior labrum (*arrow*). **D,** Grashey (true AP) view in a different patient also shows the subcoracoid and medial position of the humeral head.

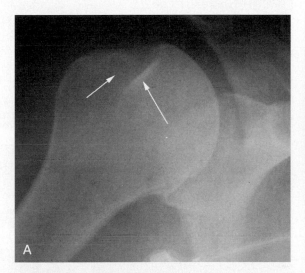

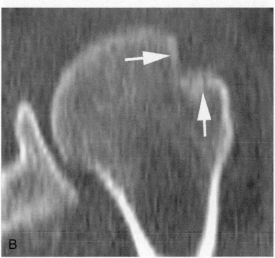

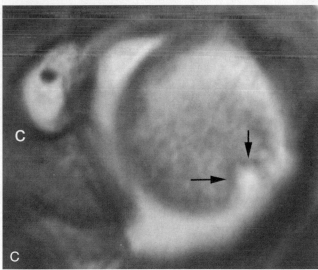

Fig. 3-64   Hill-Sachs fractures in three patients. **A,** AP view in internal rotation shows a notchlike defect in the superoposterior humeral head (*arrows*). **B,** CT coronal reconstruction shows similar finding (*arrows*). **C,** Axial T1-weighted MR arthrogram image also shows notchlike defect. Note that the Hill-Sachs fracture is seen at the level of the base of the coracoid process (c). A Hill-Sachs fracture generally does not occur below this level, although it often occurs above.

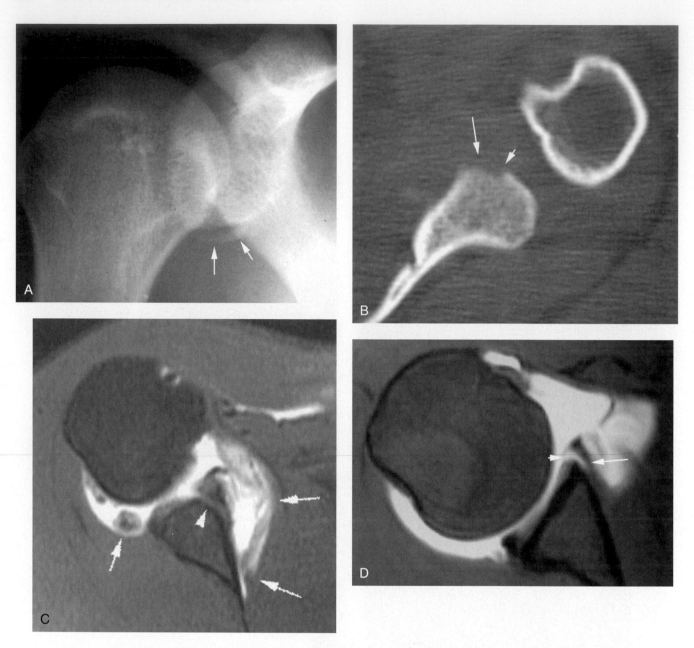

Fig. 3-65 Bankart lesion and variants. **A, B,** Radiograph (**A**) shows a subtle chip fragment inferior to the glenoid (*arrows*). CT image (**B**) shows the donor site at the anterior inferior glenoid (*arrows*). **C,** Axial fat suppressed T1-weighted MR arthrogram image in a different patient shows Bankart fracture (*arrowhead*). Also note anterior capsular stripping (*arrows*) and intraarticular body (*short arrow*). **D,** Soft tissue Bankart lesion (Perthes variant). The anteroinferior labrum is torn (*arrowhead*). In this variant, the labrum remains attached to the perisoteum, which is partially stripped off of the anterior glenoid, but not completely torn away (*arrow*).

Continued

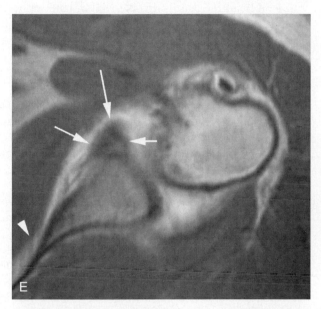

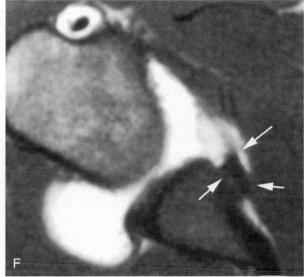

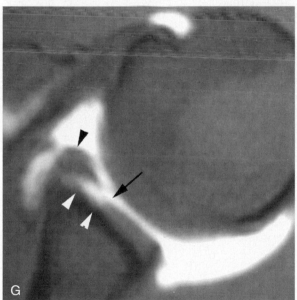

Fig. 3-65, cont'd   E, "GLOM" sign (GLenolabral Ovoid Mass, *arrows*) on a T1-weighted axial MR arthrogram image. This appearance indicates avulsion of a portion of the anterior labrum. Also note the incidental extravasation of contrast into the subscapularis anterior to the scapula (*arrowhead*). **F,** AL-PSA lesion (Anterior Labral Periosteal Sleeve Avulsion, *arrows*). This lesion may be thought of as a medially displaced Perthes lesion. The labrum and associated stripped periosteum have displaced medially and healed in this abnormal location (*arrows*). This Bankart variant has a high association with recurrent shoulder dislocation. **G,** GLAD lesion (GLenolabral Articular Disruption). The anteroinferior labrum and the underlying cartilage have stripped away from the glenoid as a unit (*black arrowhead*). Note the bare subchondral bone of the glenoid (*white arrowheads*), the sharp margin between the normal glenoid articular cartilage posteriorly, and the defect anteriorly (*black arrow*). (**C.** Courtesy of William Morrison, M.D., Philadelphia, PA.)

clefts in the anterior labrum are a frequent normal variant that may simulate a labral tear. Similarly, the anterior superior labrum may not be attached to the glenoid (sublabral foramen), or may be entirely absent (Buford complex), as discussed earlier. The SGHL and especially the MGHL are variable in their size and course, and may be absent in normal individuals. The IGHL is more constant, with the anterior band usually thicker than the posterior band. However, this situation may be reversed, with the posterior band being thicker. The posterior-lateral humeral head has a normal indentation above the surgical neck, potentially simulating a Hill-Sachs fracture. This indentation occurs below the level of the coracoid process, whereas Hill-Sachs fractures are seen at or above the level of the coracoid process. Normal synovial folds or inadvertently injected air bubbles may simulate an intraarticular loose body. Shoulder surgery can leave extensive metal artifact in and around the shoulder, especially if metallic suture anchors were placed (Fig. 3-66).

Posterior glenohumeral dislocation is much less common than anterior dislocation. Posterior dislocation is caused by forceful muscle contraction (seizure or electrocution, potentially resulting in bilateral dislocations), or a fall on a flexed and adducted arm. The humeral head usually dislocates directly posteriorly and is locked in internal rotation. AP radiographs may be misleading, as the posteriorly dislocated humeral head can project over its normal position in this projection. A transscapular Y or axillary view is diagnostic (Fig. 3-67). Associated osseous and soft tissue injuries mirror those of anterior dislocation. The posterior joint capsule is stripped off of the glenoid and the posterior labrum is often torn or separated from the glenoid, resulting in posterior glenohumeral instability and leaving the patient vulnerable to recurrent posterior dislocations. The anterior humeral head impacts against the posterior glenoid rim and a humeral head fracture ("reverse Hill-Sachs fracture") or a posterior glenoid rim chip fracture ("reverse Bankart fracture," Fig. 3-67C, D) may result. A reverse Hill-Sachs fracture may be appreciated on an AP radiograph as a vertically oriented linear impression (*"trough sign,"* Fig. 3-67C).

Shoulder dislocation in other directions is unusual. A distinctive form of inferior dislocation termed *luxatio erecti* results in fixed abduction of the arm.

Shoulder instability Shoulder instability, or more precisely glenohumeral instability, is a tendency of the humeral head to sublux or dislocate. Glenohumeral instability can occur in any direction, but the most common pattern is anterior instability. Anterior instability is usually the consequence of prior anterior shoulder dislocation, with disruption of the anterior shoulder stabilizers, as discussed above. Recurrent anterior dislocations are a classic feature of anterior instability. However, a history of dislocation is not present in all individuals with anterior instability.

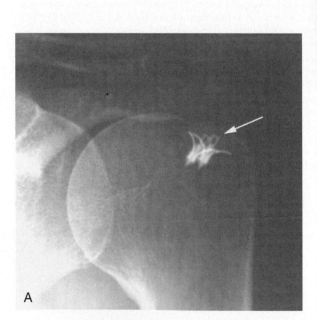
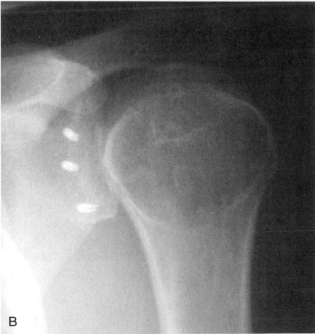

Fig. 3-66 Postoperative shoulder. **A,** Rotator cuff repair with metallic suture anchors in the greater tuberosity (*arrow*). The suture anchors provide a site to reattach the torn supraspinatus tendon. **B,** Anterior capsular repair. The suture anchors were placed in the anterior glenoid, to allow reattachment of a stripped anterior capsule.

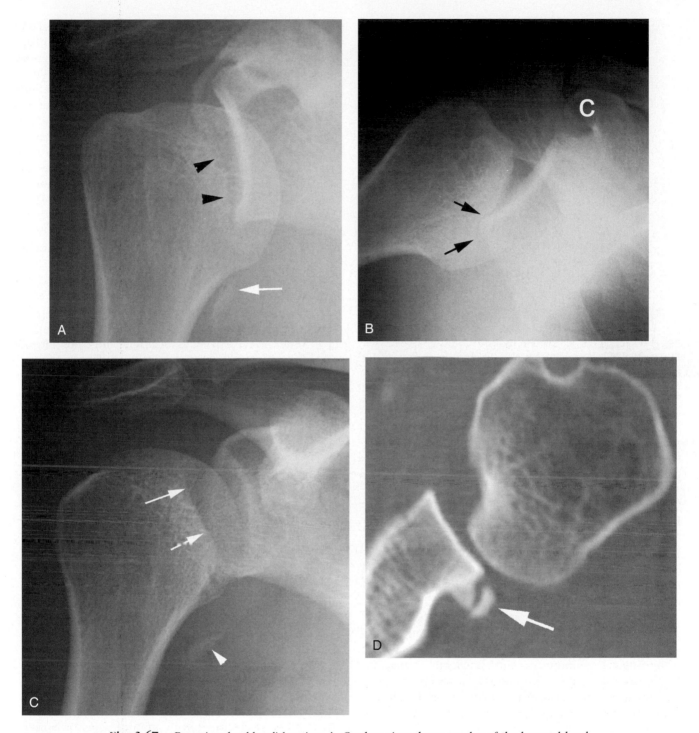

Fig. 3-67   Posterior shoulder dislocation. **A,** Grashey view shows overlap of the humeral head and glenoid, indicating that a dislocation is present. Note the subtle humeral head impaction fracture (*black arrowheads*) and the small reverse bony Bankart chip fracture (*white arrow*). **B,** Oblique axillary view shows reverse Hill-Sachs impaction fracture (*arrows*). Note that the dislocation is remote from the coracoid process (c), unlike an anterior dislocation. **C,** Post-reduction AP view shows the classic "trough sign" of a reverse Hill-Sachs fracture (*arrows*). Also note the reverse bony Bankart chip fracture fragment (*arrowhead*). **D,** Axial CT image in a different patient shows a slightly displaced reverse bony Bankart fracture (*arrow*) and posterior subluxation of the humeral head.

Continued

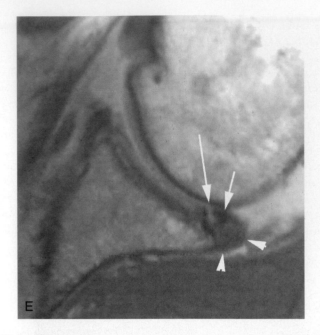

Fig. 3-67, cont'd   E, Reverse Bankart soft tissue lesion. Axial T1-weighted MR arthrogram image. In this case, the posterior band of the inferior glenohumeral ligament (*short arrow*) is torn from its labral origin (*long arrow*). Note the intermediate signal mass of granulation tissue and fibrosis (*arrowheads*).

Posterior instability, like posterior dislocation that may precede it, is relatively rare. MR findings include disruption of the posterior labrum, lax posterior joint capsule, and interruption of the posterior band of the IGHL (reverse Bankart lesion). Treatment is also surgical. The Bennett lesion is a rim of calcification immediately posterior to the posterior osseous glenoid rim, best demonstrated by CT, that is associated with posterior labral injuries and posterior rotator cuff injuries. The calcification is thought to represent an enthesophyte in the posterior band of the IGL.

Treatment of anterior or posterior instability is usually surgical. The goal is to restore normal anatomy by repairing the damaged structures. If this is not possible, or if the original anatomy was not sufficiently stable, the orthopedic surgeon may choose from a variety of procedures that enhance shoulder stability by tightening the joint capsule or shortening the subscapularis muscle (Fig. 3-66B).

Multidirectional instability (MDI) is glenohumeral joint laxity due to a lax joint capsule, often exacerbated by poorly coordinated action of the rotator cuff muscles. MDI is frequently bilateral, and most patients are young. Generalized joint laxity may be present. A patient with multidirectional instability may be able to sense laxity in their glenohumeral joint during routine activities such as holding a briefcase. Humeral head subluxation can result in pain, labral injuries, and rotator cuff impingement. Imaging findings are often absent, although the labrum

may be small and the capsule lax and redundant. Treatment consists of rotator cuff strengthening exercises. Surgical tightening of the joint capsule is sometimes needed.

Labral tears   Discussion of labral tears is included with the discussion of shoulder dislocation and instability because most labral tears occur in association with these conditions. The Bankart lesion, discussed above, is the classic example of a labral tear caused by shoulder dislocation. However, labral tears can occur in the absence of shoulder instability. In particular, only about 20% of superior labral (SLAP tears) are associated with shoulder instability.

Imaging diagnosis of labral tears is complicated by the normal variation of labral shape and fixation to the glenoid,

---

Key Concepts   Labral Tear

- Detection increased on MRI with joint effusion or arthrograms.
- Anterior tear: strong association with prior anterior dislocation and anterior instability, especially in a young patient (Bankart lesion, with numerous variants).
  - Pitfalls:
    - Sublabral foramen between 1 and 3 o'clock
    - Normal finding of articular cartilage between labrum and osseous glenoid
    - Magic angle
    - Perthes lesion resembles normal labrum
    - Mild partial labral detachments may be incidental in older individuals
- SLAP tear (Superior labral anterior and posterior)
  - Occurs at biceps labral complex. Tears may extend into biceps tendon, glenohumeral ligaments, anterior labrum, posterior labrum.
  - Only 20% are associated with instability.
  - Oblique coronal images: tend to be oriented from superior-lateral to inferior-medial.
  - Pitfalls:
    - Sublabral recess: follows contour of articular cartilage, oriented from superior-medial to inferior lateral.
    - Chronically high riding shoulder may develop a SLAP-like cleft that is not an acute SLAP tear and does not benefit from surgery.
    - Normal variations in anterior superior labrum (foramen, Buford complex).
    - Normal variant mild irregularities on articular surface of labrum.
    - Pseudotears of labrum:
      - Close apposition of a GHL and labrum (gap between simulates a tear).
      - Normal finding of articular cartilage between labrum and osseous glenoid.
      - Magic angle causes increased labral signal (short TE only).

particularly the anterior–superior labrum discussed above. The normal labrum has low signal intensity on all MRI sequences. Magic angle phenomenon results in increased signal intensity on short TE sequences in portions of the labrum oriented 55° from the bore of the magnet. Linear or amorphous high signal intensity suggests a labral tear. CT and MR arthrography are superior to conventional MRI in revealing a labral tear, because contrast flows into the tear, increasing its conspicuity. CT and MR arthrography also are the best imaging studies to demonstrate a labral detachment. Detection of an anterior labral tear is slightly improved by placing the arm in the "ABER" position (ABduction and External Rotation) by placing the patient's forearm behind his or her head. This position

pushes the humeral head against the anterior labrum, which can "pry open" an anterior labral tear.

SLAP tears (Superior Labral Anterior and Posterior) are tears of the biceps labral complex (Fig. 3-68). The superior labrum, proximal biceps tendon, and biceps attachment to the labrum are variably involved. SLAP tears occur during rapid arm abduction during a fall or during the deceleration phase of throwing, and are an occupational hazard of throwing athletes such as baseball pitchers. The anatomy of SLAP tears is complex (Table 3-3) and is evolving. Classification of the subtype of SLAP tear requires high-quality imaging, preferably with MR arthrography. Detection of a SLAP tear is increased if MR imaging is performed with downward traction on the

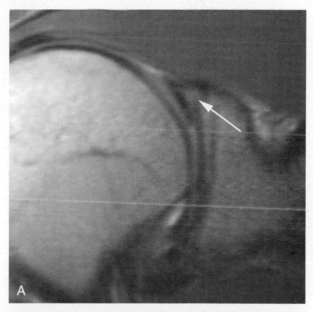
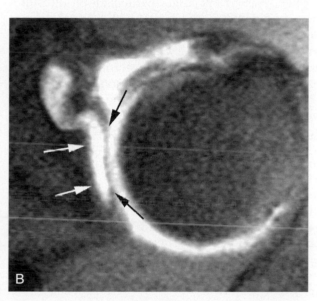
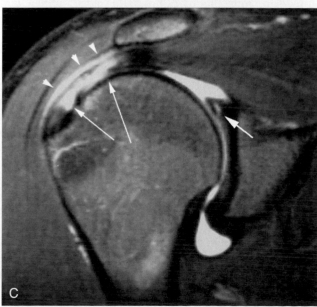

Fig. 3-68   SLAP tears. **A,** Oblique coronal T2-weighted MRI image shows high signal intensity within the superior labrum oriented towards the acromion (*arrow*). Other images (not shown) showed this pattern to extend into the posterior superior labrum, consistent with a SLAP tear. **B,** Axial T2-weighted saline arthrogram image at the level of the inferior margin of the superior labrum in a different patient shows fluid tracking between the labrum (*black arrows*) and the glenoid (*white arrows*). The separation of the labrum and the glenoid extends farther posteriorly than the 12 or even 11 o'clock positions and therefore is likely to represent a SLAP tear rather than a sublabral sulcus. **C,** Oblique coronal T2-weighted MR arthrogram image shows a SLAP tear (*short arrow*). This patient also has an extensive partial thickness rotator cuff tear (*long arrows*). The bursal fluid (*arrowheads*) indicates that a complete rotator cuff tear also is present.

Table 3-3   Arthroscopic classification of superior labral (SLAP) tears

Type 1 Degenerative superior labral fraying. Normal biceps tendon.
Type 2 Superior labral and biceps tendon avulsion
Type 3 Superior labral bucket handle tear. Biceps tendon normal, remains attached to torn labrum
Type 4 Labral bucket handle tear extending into biceps tendon

arm. This can be accomplished with a strap around the wrist attached to a weight suspended from the end of the couch by a rope and pulley arrangement.[1]

The diagnosis of SLAP tears by MRI can be difficult for several reasons. MR images, particularly on MR arthrograms, frequently reveal a "defect" in the superior labrum oriented in an anterior–posterior direction, which in many cases is the normal variant sublabral sulcus discussed previously (Fig. 3-43). This normal variant is typically oriented in a superomedial to inferior lateral direction (points towards the patient's head). In contrast, many (but not all) SLAP tears are oriented in a superior-lateral to inferior-medial direction (points towards the acromion). Alternatively, a SLAP tear, like any other labral tear, may escape detection. Detection of SLAP tears at MRI is improved by scanning with the arm in external rotation or under traction. Another pitfall in diagnosis of SLAP tears is that a chronically high riding shoulder, such as can occur with chronic rotator cuff tear, can cause a SLAP-like lesion that is not treated surgically.

Miscellaneous Shoulder Conditions

Osteochondral injuries of the shoulder include bony Bankart, reverse Bankart, and GLAD (glenolabral articular disruption, Fig. 3-65G) injuries already discussed. Although the shoulder is not a weight bearing joint, considerable loads are placed across the shoulder joint during abduction, and osteochondritis dissecans or articular cartilage injuries may result. Most articular cartilage defects of the glenohumeral joint occur in the setting of OA. The subscapularis muscle occasionally avulses the lesser tuberosity.

Shoulder arthoplasty is performed for painful arthritis or severe humeral head fractures. A humeral hemi-arthroplasty is often used, although a glenoid component may also be placed (Fig. 3-69).

ARM

The anatomy and injuries of the proximal humerus, including the Neer classification of proximal humerus fractures, are discussed previously in this chapter.

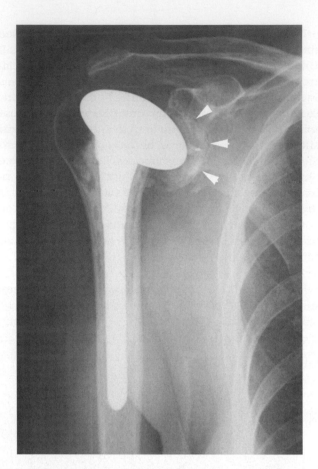

Fig. 3-69   Total shoulder arthroplasty. Note the cemented glenoid component (*arrowheads*).

The humeral shaft includes the broad deltoid tuberosity on its proximal lateral surface (Fig. 3-70). The ulnar, median, musculocutaneous, and radial nerves course through the arm. When performing a percutaneous biopsy of the humerus, these nerves may be avoided by choosing an anterolateral approach. A *supracondylar process,* or avian spur, is a rare (about 1 in 200) developmental variant, seen as a bony excrescence on the anterior-medial distal humeral shaft (Fig. 3-71). An associated ligament of Struthers can connect the supracondylar process to the medial epicondyle, where it may entrap the median nerve.

Fractures of the humeral shaft are predictably displaced by traction by the muscles that insert at different locations on the humerus (Fig. 3-72). The surgical neck is the most frequent site of a humerus fracture in adults. Surgical neck fractures can result in abduction of the proximal fragment by the rotator cuff. Fractures between the pectoralis major and deltoid insertions result in adduction of the proximal fragment by the pectoralis. Fractures distal to the deltoid insertion result in abduction of the proximal fragment by the deltoid (Figs. 3-72,

3-73). Humeral fractures, or attempts at closed reduction of a humeral fracture, may injure the radial nerve as it courses posterior to the shaft. Treatment of humeral shaft fractures is usually accomplished by placement of a hanging cast, that is a cast that immobilizes the elbow and extends part way up the arm. Most patients tolerate less-than-anatomic alignment quite well, as the highly mobile shoulder joint can compensate for some rotational and angular deformity. Internal fixation is usually reserved for severe or complex fractures such as segmental or intraarticular fractures, or if there is associated neurovascular injury.

The quadrilateral space is formed by the teres minor muscle superiorly, the teres major muscle inferiorly, the humerus laterally, and the triceps muscle medially. The axillary nerve courses through the quadrilateral space, where it is vulnerable to entrapment due to mass lesions, fracture, or abduction of the arm. Such entrapment results in denervation of the deltoid and teres minor muscles that may become evident as atrophy and weakness of these muscles.

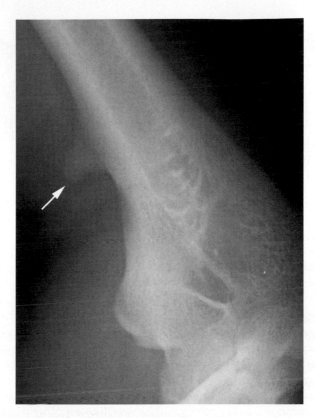

Fig. 3-71   Supracondylar process (avian spur). This normal variant bony excrescence (*arrow*) projects anteriorly and slightly medially from the distal humeral shaft.

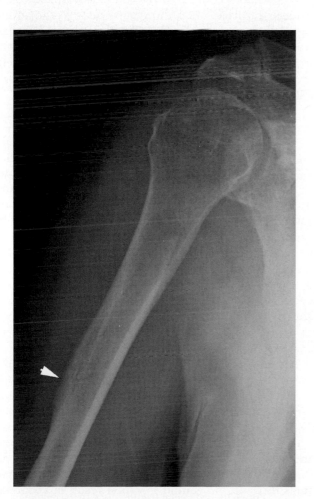

Fig. 3-70   Normal deltoid tuberosity (*arrow*).

ELBOW

The elbow is formed by the articulations of the radial head with the humeral capitellum and the proximal ulna with the humeral trochlea, the proximal radioulnar joint, and related muscles and connective tissues.

Imaging Techniques

Radiographic evaluation of the traumatized elbow should include at least AP and lateral views, the latter obtained with the elbow flexed 90° in order to assess for a joint effusion. AP oblique views can increase detection of subtle fractures. An oblique radial head view is useful if a radial head fracture is suspected. US and arthrography are used less commonly, but can be useful in some situations. US is useful in assessing for a joint effusion and identifying fractures of unossified cartilage in children. Arthrography can identify full thickness collateral ligament tears and some articular surface partial thickness collateral ligament tears, as well as some chondral defects. Arthrography also can characterize chondral fractures in children and assist in characterizing osteochondritis dissecans lesions for fragment fixation.

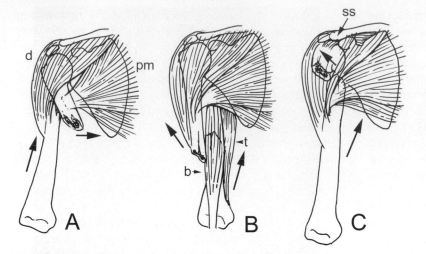

Fig. 3-72   Displacement of humeral fractures. **A,** Fractures between the pectoralis major (pm) and deltoid (d) insertions result in adduction of the proximal fragment by the pectoralis. **B,** Fractures distal to the deltoid insertion result in abduction of the proximal fragment by the deltoid (see also Figure 3-73). The fragments may override, as shown in the diagram. The distal fragment is pulled proximally by the biceps (b) and triceps (t) muscles and medially by the pectoralis major muscle. **C,** Displaced surgical neck fractures can result in abduction of the proximal fragment by the supraspinatus muscle (ss) as well as proximal displacement of the distal fragment, similar to **B.**

CT is useful for characterizing complex articular fractures and posttraumatic complications in adults such as intraarticular bodies, osteophytes and fracture fragment malalignment. CT arthrography combines the advantages of conventional arthrography and CT, and offers superior assessment of intra-articular bodies.

MRI of the elbow is performed in the coronal, sagittal, and axial planes with the elbow extended. Use of a surface coil that allows the elbow to be scanned at the patient's side enhances patient comfort, but places the elbow away from the "sweet spot" of the magnet isocenter. Placing the elbow in a knee, temperomandibular joint or head coil with the arm fully abducted (elbow above the patient's head) is an alternative if off axis imaging is unsuccessful. Imaging sequences include T1 and T2-weighted sequences, the latter often with fat suppression to more readily detect marrow or soft tissue edema.

A volume-acquisition T2-weighted gradient echo sequence is often used to provide high resolution images with thin sections of 1–3 mm, to allow optimal assessment of the collateral ligaments. A volume-acquisition T1-weighted gradient echo sequence with fat suppression provides thin section, high resolution assessment of the articular cartilage. MR arthrography adds to the advantages of conventional CT and CT arthrography. MR arthrography technique is reviewed in Appendix 1. MR arthrography is the preferred technique for assessment of collateral ligament injury in athletes and osteochondral lesions such as osteochondritis dissecans.

Elbow Anatomy

The normal radiographic anatomy of the elbow is illustrated in Figure 3-74. The distal humeral shaft widens

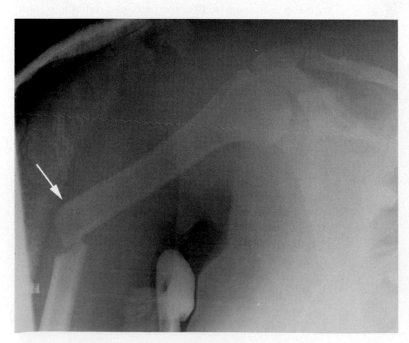

Fig. 3-73   Humeral fracture distal to the deltoid tuberosity (*arrow*) results in abduction of the proximal fragment.

Key Concepts	Normal Elbow Radiographic Anatomy

- AP view checklist:
    Radial head aligned with capitellum.
    Ulna aligned with trochlea.
    Radial head articulates with ulna.
    Normal valgus ("carrying angle"), ~ 165°.
    Children: ossification centers normally positioned.
- Lateral view checklist:
    Radial head aligned with capitellum
    Anterior humeral line intersects middle third of capitellum
    Ulna congruent with trochlea
    Any fat density anterior to humerus has straight anterior margin
    No fat density posterior to humerus

medially and laterally to form the epicondyles. The lateral epicondyle is the common origin of the wrist extensor (dorsiflexor) muscles, and the medial epicondyle is the common origin of the wrist flexor muscles. The humeral condyles are the rounded capitellum laterally and the V-shaped trochlea medially. The condyles are anteriorly positioned relative to the epicondyles. A line drawn along the anterior humeral shaft cortex, the *anterior humeral line,* normally passes through the middle third of the capitellum (Fig. 3-75). Variation from this arrangement is evidence for a fracture. The distal humerus has concavities on both its anterior and posterior surfaces. The shallow coronoid fossa anteriorly accommodates the ulnar coronoid process during elbow flexion. The deeper olecranon fossa posteriorly accommodates the ulnar olecranon process during elbow extension. A normal variant foramen may connect the coronoid and olecranon fossae. The normal variant supracondylar process was discussed earlier (Fig. 3-71).

The cylindrical radial head articulates with the rounded capitellum and the concave lateral margin of the proximal ulna. A line drawn through the center of the radial shaft should bisect the capitellum on any view (Fig. 3-75). This line is called the *radiocapitellar line.* If this line does not bisect the capitellum, then a radial dislocation is present. The radial tuberosity on the proximal medial radial shaft is the insertion site of the biceps tendon. This medial insertion allows the biceps to function as a wrist supinator (turns palm forward) as well as an elbow flexor. When viewed *en face,* the radial tuberosity may simulate an aggressive lytic lesion (Fig. 3-76). The

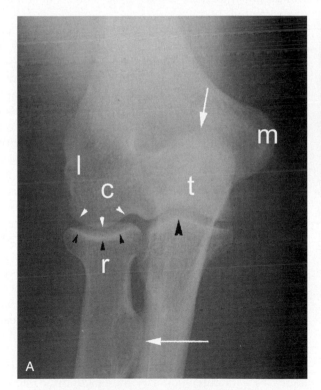

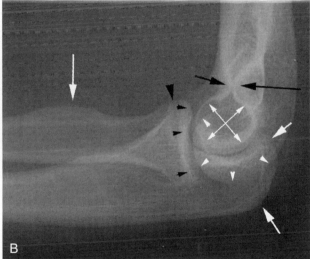

Fig. 3-74 Elbow: normal radiographic anatomy **A,** AP view. **B,** Lateral view. Small black arrowheads, radial head proximal articular surface; small white arrowheads, capitellum articular surface; large black arrowhead, coronoid process of the ulna; short white arrow, olecranon process of the ulna; long white arrow, radial tuberosity (insertion site of biceps). AP view (**A**): r, radial neck; c, capitellum; t, trochlea (superiposed over the olecranon); m, medial epicondyle: l, lateral epicondyle. Short black arrow (**B** only), coronoid fossa; long black arrow (**B** only), olecranon fossa; white double arrows (**B** only) trochlea.

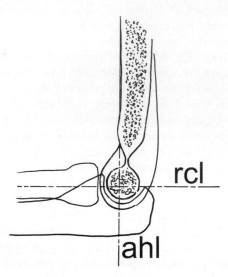

Fig. 3-75 Radiocapitellar and anterior humeral lines. The *anterior humeral line* (ahl) is drawn along the anterior cortex of the humeral shaft cortex. If this line does not pass through the middle of the capitellum, then a fracture is likely. The *radiocapitellar line* (rcl) is drawn along the center radial shaft. If this line does not bisect the capitellum, then a radial head dislocation or subluxation is present. This diagram also illustrates the normal relationship of the trochlea (seen in cross section) and the ulna. Note that the capitellum articular surface projects slightly anterior to the trochlea.

characteristic location of this finding and the exophytic contour on an orthogonal view reveal the benign nature of this finding.

The proximal ulna includes the olecranon process posteriorly and the coronoid process anteriorly, and broad articular contact with the humeral trochlea. A small notchlike defect or groove may be seen on the ulnar articular surface, usually appreciated only on MR images,

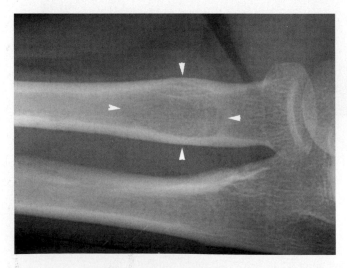

Fig. 3-76 Pseudolesion of the proximal radius (*arrowheads*) caused by the normal appearance of the radial tuberosity when seen *en face.*

at the base of the coronoid process (Fig. 3-77). A similar pseudodefect may be noted on the dorsal capitellum (Fig. 3-78). The triceps tendon inserts on the posterior olecranon (Fig. 3-77B). Distal triceps injury and avulsion of the triceps tendon insertion are often clinically apparent, but MRI can assist in determining the extent of injury.

The "carrying angle" is the angle formed by the humerus and the ulna in the coronal plane when the elbow is extended. The normal fully extended elbow joint is in about 165° of valgus alignment, slightly greater in women and less in men. (Think of this as allowing the upper extremity to match the contour of the waist and hips with the arms at one's side.) A related angle in children is *Baumann's angle* formed by the humeral shaft and the capitellar physis (Fig. 3-79). *Cubitus varus* is abnormally increased carrying angle (i.e., loss of valgus), and *cubitus valgus* is abnormally decreased carrying angle (i.e., too much valgus).

The subcutaneous olecranon bursa overlies the olecranon process and is the most common site of bursitis in the body. Olecranon bursitis whether due to direct trauma, hemorrhage, or inflammatory process such as rheumatoid arthritis causes pain and swelling over the olecranon process (Fig. 3-80). The extensor surface of the elbow and proximal forearm is one of the more common sites of rheumatoid nodules.

A fat pad normally resides within the olecranon fossa when the elbow is flexed. This fat pad is normally not visible on lateral radiographs obtained with 90° elbow flexion because it is superimposed on the dense bone of the distal ulna. However, a hemarthrosis or any other process that distends the joint capsule (joint effusion, pus, synovitis as in rheumatoid arthritis, Pigmented Villonodular Synovitis) can displace this fat pad superiorly and posteriorly out of the olecranon fossa, producing the *posterior fat pad sign* on a lateral radiograph (Figs. 3-81, 3-82). A separate fat pad *anterior* to the distal humerus is a normal finding on lateral radiographs. The anterior fat pad normally has a straight anterior contour. Distension of the elbow joint can alter this contour into a "spinnaker sail sign" or "anterior fat pad sign" due to anterior and superior displacements of the fat pad. The anterior fat pad sign is more sensitive, but less specific for the presence of elbow joint distension. In the setting of acute trauma, a posterior fat pad sign in an adult nearly always indicates that a fracture is present. This finding is less specific in children as soft tissue injuries may cause an effusion. The absence of a fat pad sign does not exclude a significant injury, as a fracture such as some epicondylar fractures may be extraarticular, and a severe injury can lacerate the joint capsule and allow a hemarthrosis to decompress into the extraarticular soft tissues.

The *os supratrochleare dorsale* is a small ossicle that resides in the olecranon fossa. Although generally consid-

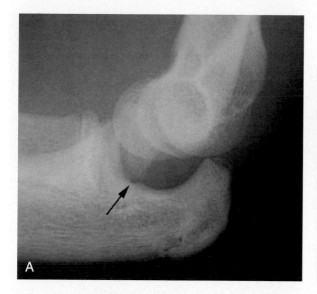

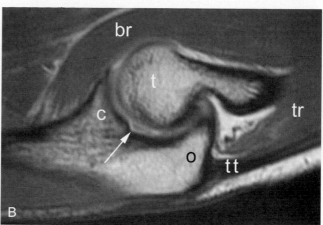

Fig. 3-77 Normal variant "pseudodefect" of the ulna at the base of the olecranon process. **A,** Lateral radiograph in a patient with an elbow dislocation shows a small notchlike defect in the subchondral bone at the base of the coronoid process (*arrow*). **B,** Sagittal T1-weighted MR arthrogram image also demonstrates the normal variant pseudodefect (*arrow*). This image also illustrates normal anatomy (br, brachialis muscle; t, trochlea; c, coronoid process; o, olecranon; tt, triceps tendon; tr, triceps muscle).

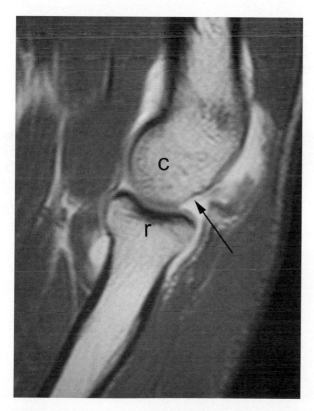

Fig. 3-78 Normal "pseudodefect" of the capitellum. Sagittal T1-weighted MR arthrogram image from the same study as Figure 3-77A shows a shallow concave "defect" in the dorsal capitellum (*arrow*). This normal variant should not be confused with an osteochondral defect. C, capitellum; r, radial head.

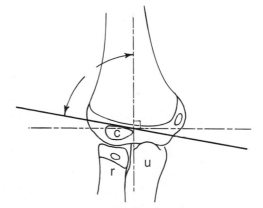

Fig. 3-79 Measurement of Baumann's angle in children. Two lines are drawn, one along the shaft of the ulna, and one parallel to the distal humeral physis along the proximal capitellum (c). The angle formed is measured as shown in the diagram. Both sides are compared. A difference of ≥5° is significant and may alter therapy. An increase in Baumann's angle indicates varus alignment, and a decrease, valgus alignment. r, radius; u, ulna.

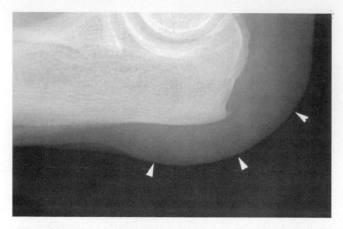

Fig. 3-80   Olecranon bursitis. Lateral radiograph shows soft tissue swelling centered over the dorsal proximal ulna (*arrowheads*). This case was due to hemorrhage into the bursa caused by direct trauma.

ered to be a normal variant, the os supratrochleare dorale can cause impingement and pain during elbow extension. An intraarticular osseous body can have an identical appearance and also may cause impingement (Fig. 3-83). The distinction is not important, because a symptomatic ossicle will be removed, and an asymptomatic ossicle generally will not.

Elbow Fractures in Children

Most elbow fractures in children are the result of a fall on an outstretched hand. Compression injuries are unusual, but the axial load can result in forced hyperextension or valgus. Hyperextension can cause the ulna to lever against the distal humerus like a bottle opener removing a bottle cap (Fig. 3-84). This mechanism causes the most

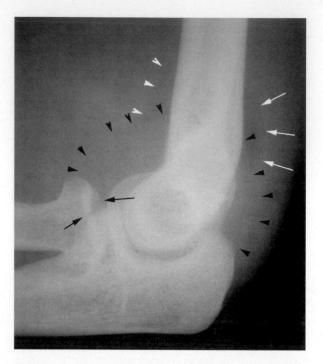

Fig. 3-82   Fat pad sign in an adult with a radial head fracture (*black arrows*). Lateral radiograph shows posterior (*white arrows*) and anterior (*white arrowheads*) fat pad signs due to hemarthrosis. Black arrowheads mark the distended joint capsule.

common elbow fracture of children, the *supracondylar fracture,* that is a fracture of the distal humerus proximal to the humeral condyles (Fig. 3-85). Supracondylar fractures can range from obvious to subtle on radiographs, but two cardinal signs are often present: a posterior fat

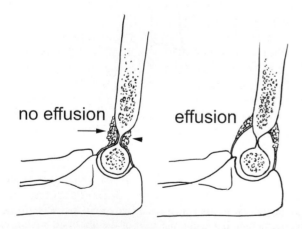

Fig. 3-81   The fat pad sign. Diagram shows how distention of the elbow joint capsule displaces the posterior fat pad (*arrowhead*) out of the olecranon fossa, making it visible on a lateral view, and distorts the anterior fat pad (*arrow*), potentially causing it to have a convex margin anteriorly.

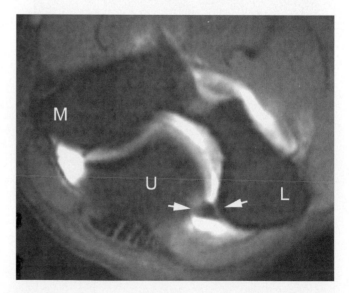

Fig. 3-83   Intraarticular body. Axial fat suppressed T1-weighted MR arthrogram image shows a small filling defect (*between arrows*) between the ulna (u) and humerus in the lateral aspect of the olecranon fossa. This body caused pain with elbow extension and therefore was removed. L, lateral epicondyle; M, medial epicondyle.

Key Concepts	Elbow Fractures in Children

- Fat pad sign usually present, but is less sensitive and specific for fracture than in adults.
- Supracondylar (65%):
    Fall on an outstretched hand causes elbow hyperextension.
    Abnormal anterior humeral line.
- Medial epicondylar avulsion (10%):
    Fall on an outstretched hand causes valgus stress.
    Possible entrapment—don't miss it!!!
    Little leaguer's elbow = chronic avulsive injury to medial epicondyle physis.
- Lateral condylar (15%):
    Lateral fall with arm at side causes varus stress across elbow.
    May be incomplete, involving only part of the physis.
    Most involve lateral metaphysis (at least Salter-Harris II).
    Important variants
        Salter-Harris IV through capitellum ossification center (rare).
        Fracture through condylar cartilage (resembles Salter-Harris II) Unstable if complete
- Separation of the condyles from the metaphsis (complete Salter-Harris I, may be Salter-Harris II):
    Infants: birth injury, child abuse
    Toddlers: child abuse, twisting injuries
- Radial head dislocation:
    Congenital
    Jerked (nursemaid's) elbow

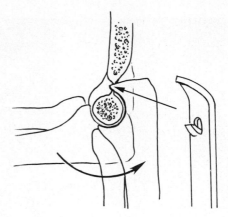

Fig. 3-84 Mechanism of the pediatric supracondylar fracture. A fall on an outstretched hand can result in elbow hyperextension, especially in children as they have lax ligaments and more flexible joints. Hyperextension concentrates tension and shearing force across the relatively weak supracondylar distal humerus, analogous to the leverage applied to a bottle cap by a bottle opener, resulting in fracture with apex anterior angulation.

pad sign, and posterior displacement of the capitellum relative to the anterior humeral line (Fig. 3-75). Alignment on the AP radiograph should also be assessed for evidence of abnormal cubitus valgus or varus as either of these findings may alter therapy. Comparison with the contralateral elbow may be required. A quantitative approach is to measure Baumann's angle formed by the humeral shaft and the capitellar physis (see Fig. 3-79). The injured and uninjured sides are measured. A difference of 5° or more is considered to be significant.

Fractures of the lateral humeral condyle are the second most common type of elbow fracture in children. Lateral condyle fractures are caused by varus stress. Varus stress across the elbow may be produced by a lateral blow to the forearm, or if a child falls laterally with his arm at his side. Varus stress causes distraction force across the lateral side of the elbow that can result in an avulsion-like fracture that may be complete or incomplete. Typically, these fractures extend along or across the lateral distal humeral physis, usually with a small metaphyseal fragment (Fig. 3-86). The distal extent of the fracture is more variable. If incomplete, the fracture may not extend be-

yond the physis, or the fracture may extend distally into the lateral condyle, either through the ossified portion of the capitellum (true Salter-Harris IV) or, far more frequently, medial to the capitellum through unossified cartilage (Fig. 3-87). Incomplete lateral condyle fractures generally are stable and are treated with casting. However, if the fracture line continues distally to the articular surface, the fracture is complete. Complete lateral condyle fractures generally are unstable and require operative fixation. Distinguishing a complete fracture from an incomplete fracture can be difficult because most of the fracture extends through cartilage and is therefore not visible on radiographs. Additional imaging with US, MRI, or arthrography can be helpful.

Valgus stress, whether repetitive or a single event, can result in *avulsion of the medial epicondyle ossification center* (Figs. 3-88 to 3-90). Valgus stress causes traction on the medial epicondyle by the strong medial collateral ligament and the wrist flexor-pronator muscle group. The medial epicondyle physis is the weakest link of the elbow medial stabilizers, and it yields before the other structures are injured. The avulsed medial epicondyle is displaced distally by the pull of the medial collateral ligament and the flexor-pronator muscles. Radiographs reveal displacement of the medial epicondyle ossification center, which may be subtle and require comparison with the uninjured side for confident diagnosis, or may be obvious and require no further imaging. A hemarthrosis may not be present because the injury can be entirely extraarticular. US or MRI can be helpful in diagnosing avulsion of an unossified medial epicondyle in a younger child. Prompt

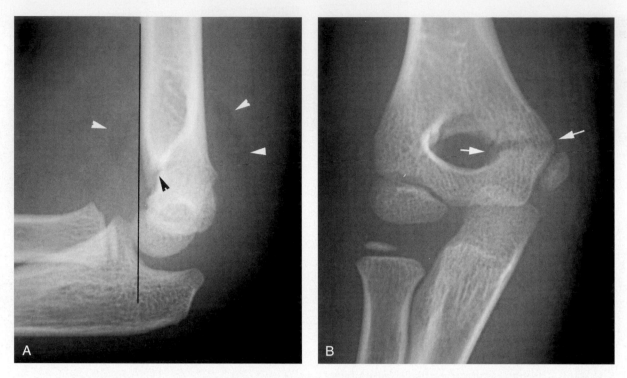

Fig. 3-85   Displaced supracondylar fracture. **A,** Lateral view shows displaced anterior and posterior fat pads (*white arrowheads*) and posterior displacement of the capitellar growth center relative to the anterior humeral line. A portion of the fracture line is faintly seen (*black arrowhead*). **B,** AP view shows the lateral aspect of the fracture line. The AP view of a supracondylar fracture often does not show the fracture. Careful attention to the appearance of the fat pads and alignment on the *lateral* view is necessary to make the diagnosis.

healing with normal function is achieved simply by placing the arm in a sling, although radiographs often reveal persistent widening and irregularity of the injured physis. Surgical repair is generally reserved for high-level athletes or elbow instability. Displacement of the medial epicondyle by greater than 5 mm is more likely to require fixation.

An important exception to this generally happy situation is *medial epicondyle entrapment.* The elbow often transiently dislocates posterolaterally during a medial epicondylar avulsion. The medial aspect of the elbow joint may open transiently, allowing the avulsed medial epicondyle fragment to slip between the trochlea and ulna, where it becomes entrapped after the humerus and ulna attempt to return to their normal positions (Figs. 3-88, 3-90). Rapid identification of this condition is essential, because an entrapped medial epicondyle will fuse to the ulna within a few weeks, resulting in permanent disability. Radiographs of medial epicondylar entrapment may be deceptive. A fat pad sign may not be present. The entrapped medial epicondylar ossification center may simulate a normal trochlear ossification center if the

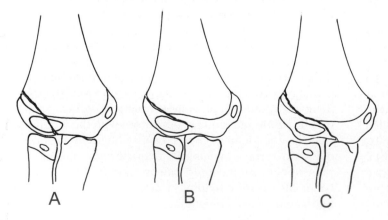

Fig. 3-86   Diagram of childhood lateral humeral condylar fractures. **A,** True Salter-Harris IV with osseous fracture of the capitellar growth center. **B,** Incomplete fracture with extension into the condylar cartilage. The fracture line might also terminate within the physis without extension into the condylar cartilage. **C,** Complete fracture through the condylar cartilage. This fracture can be difficult to diagnose with radiographs. This pattern is more common than **A,** and is also potentially unstable.

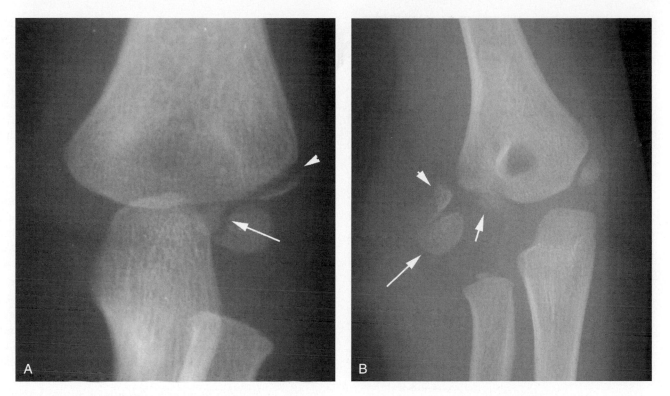

Fig. 3-87   Lateral condylar fracture. **A,** Salter Harris IV fracture. AP radiograph shows the fracture extending through the distal lateral metaphysis (*arrowhead*) and the capitellar growth center (*arrow*), similar to Figure 3-86A. **B,** Complete fracture. The fragment is displaced laterally and rotated. Note the small metaphyseal fragment (*arrowhead*) and the capitellar growth center (*long arrow*). Although the capitellar growth center appears to be intact on this view, there is a small nondisplaced capitellar fragment (*short arrow*). Also note the extensive lateral soft tissue swelling. (**B,** Courtesy of L. Das Narla, M.D., Richmond, VA.)

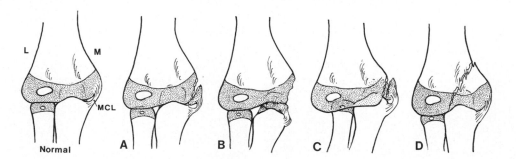

Fig. 3-88   Diagram shows types of fractures involving medial epicondyle in children. Right elbow is illustrated. (MCL, medial collateral ligament; M, medial; L, lateral.) **A,** simple avulsion of medial epicondyle. **B,** avulsion with entrapment of medial epicondyle between ulna and trochlea. **C,** avulsion in association with elbow dislocation. **D,** Salter-Harris IV fracture of medial humeral condyle. (Reprinted with permission from May DA, Disler DG, Jones EA, Pearce DA. Using sonography to diagnose an unossified medial epicondyle avulsion in a child. *AJR* 2000; 174:1115-1117. Modified with permission from Rogers LF. *Radiology of Skeletal Trauma.* New York: Churchill Livingstone, 1992:772-779).

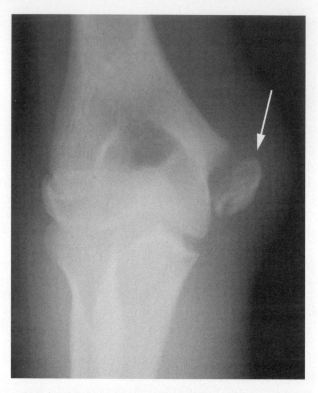

Fig. 3-89   Medial epicondyle avulsion AP radiograph shows medial and slight distal displacement of the medial epicondyle ossification center (*arrow*). Note the surrounding soft tissue swelling.

trochlea is unossified. Knowledge of the normal maturation of the elbow ossification centers is necessary to avoid this pitfall. The order of appearance on radiographs of the six ossification centers of the elbow may be recalled with the mnemonic CRITOE (Fig. 3-91). The *c*apitellum begins to ossify at about age one year, followed by the *r*adial head after age 3 years, followed by the medial ("*i*nternal") epicondyle at about age 4-5 years, followed, sometimes closely, by the *t*rochlea at about age 7-8 years, followed by the *o*lecranon at age 8-10 years, followed by the lateral ("*e*xternal") epicondyle at age 9-13 years. Ossification of each center tends to begin a year or two earlier in girls than boys. The exact ages actually are fairly variable and aren't terribly important. Rather, it is the *order of appearance* of the ossification centers that is important to know. If what appears to be a normal trochlear ossification center is seen without a normally positioned, partially ossified medial epicondylar center, the diagnosis of medial epicondylar entrapment is likely. If this diagnosis is suspected in a younger child, in whom neither the medial epicondyle nor the trochlea have begun to ossify, then US, MRI, or arthrography can be used.

The term *little leaguer's elbow* is often generically to describe any traumatic abnormality of the medial epicondyle in a child. A more specific use of this term refers to a chronic repetitive traction injury seen in young

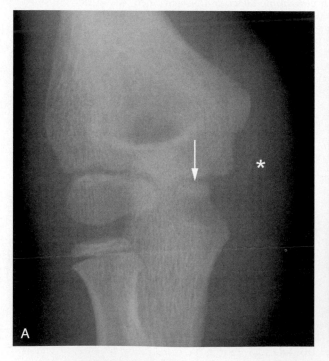

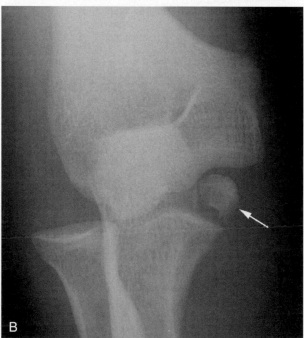

Fig. 3-90   Medial epicondyle entrapment. **A,** The entrapped medial epicondyle simulates a normal trochlear ossification center (*arrow*). The medial soft tissue swelling is a clue to the diagnosis, but the important finding is that a normal medial epicondyle growth center is not seen (*asterisk*). **B,** Entrapped medial epicondyle in an older child after spontaneous partial reduction of an elbow dislocation. Diagnosis in this case is easier than **A.** Note that all of the other ossification centers have fused. The medial epicondyle is the last elbow center to fuse.

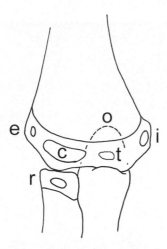

Fig. 3-91 Diagram of the order of appearance of ossification centers around the elbow ("CRITOE"). c, capitellum; r, radial head; i, medial ("internal") epicondyle; t, trochlea; o, olecranon; e, lateral ("external") epicondyle.

baseball pitchers, other throwing athletes, and hockey players. Radiographs reveal displacement, fragmentation, and/or sclerosis of the medial epicondyle. Because the medial epicondyle is the last elbow secondary ossification center to fuse, little leaguer's elbow can occur late into adolescence.

Fracture-separation of the entire distal humeral physis, also termed *separation of the humeral condyles* is a displaced Salter-Harris I (or rarely Salter-Harris II) fracture of the distal humerus. Displacement is usually medial or posteromedial, in contrast with the posterolateral displacement usually seen in adult elbow dislocation. Significant force is required, often with a twisting component. This injury can occur during a difficult delivery, and is associated with child abuse in infants and toddlers. Clinical and radiographic diagnosis can be difficult, especially in infants, because the displaced tissues are unossified, and the condition is difficult to distinguish from elbow dislocation. Ultrasound can reveal the diagnosis in infants and toddlers. Radiographic diagnosis is easier after the capitellum ossifies, as the displacement of the capitellum relative to the humerus and the normal radiocapitellar alignment can be appreciated.

Childhood elbow dislocation can also occur on a congenital basis, either as a sporadic finding (Figs. 3-92, 3-93), or in association with onycho-osteodysplasia (discussed in Chapter 5). In chronic congenital radial head dislocation, the radial head becomes overgrown and dysplastic, allowing easy distinction from a post-natal traumatic dislocation. The elbow is the most frequently traumatically dislocated joint in children younger than age 10 years. Complete dislocation of both the ulna and radius occurs after a fall with the elbow slightly flexed. The radius and ulna usually dislocate posteriorly, although

displacement in virtually any direction may occur. If only the radial head is dislocated, then a proximal ulnar fracture (Monteggia fracture) must be excluded (Fig. 3-94).

Subluxation of the head of the radius, also termed *jerked elbow, pulled elbow,* or *nursemaid's elbow,* is subluxation or dislocation of the radial head in a young child with no or only partial disruption of the annular ligament. A distracting force applied to the forearm or hand with the arm extended can allow the radial head to slip out of the collar formed by the annular ligament. The force required is not excessive. The typical child with this condition is between 2 and 3 years of age, although it may occur in older children up to 6 or 7 years of age. Careful scrutiny of radiographs may reveal subtle subluxation of the radial head, but radiographs are frequently normal. A fat pad sign or other radiographic abnormality is usually absent. Subluxation of the head of the radius is painful. The child holds the injured elbow in flexion and pronation, and refuses to allow extension. Fortunately, the condition is usually self limited, with eventual spontaneous reduction of the radial head to its normal position within the annular ligament. Closed reduction by elbow extension and supination is usually elected for patient comfort. Such reduction may be unintentionally achieved by the radiographer who coaxes the child to extend her elbow for the AP radiograph.

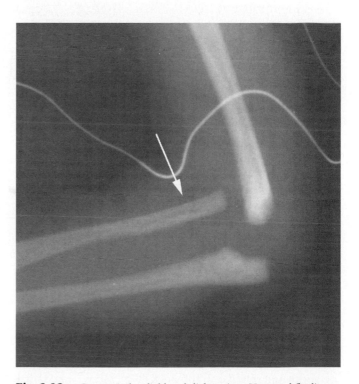

Fig. 3-92 Congenital radial head dislocation: Neonatal findings. Lateral radiograph in a newborn shows volar displacement of the proximal radius (*arrow*). The humerus and ulna are normally aligned.

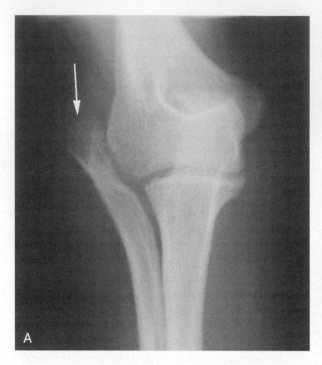 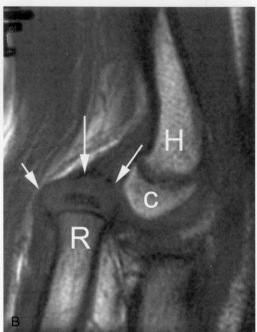

Fig. 3-93 Chronic congenital radial head dislocation. **A,** Radiograph in an older child with congenital radial head dislocation shows lateral dislocation and overgrowth in the form of elongation of the proximal radius. **B,** Sagittal T1-weighted MR image in a different child shows anterior dislocation with mild overgrowth of length and anteroposterior size (*arrows*). Note the dysplastic capitellum (c), with angular contours rather than the normal semicircular cross section. (H, humerus; R, radial shaft).

Elbow Fractures in Adults

A fall on an outstretched hand is the most common cause of *radial head and neck fractures* in adults. The axial load associated with a fall causes impaction of the capitellum against the radial head. Two patterns are most frequently seen. A single longitudinal fracture line may occur through the articular surface of the radial head, often with distal impaction of a portion of the head (Fig. 3-82). These fractures can be subtle, but a fat pad sign is almost always present and the patient is tender over the radial head. Additional views at different oblique angles may be needed to reveal the fracture. Treatment is by immobilization with a sling. However, fracture displacement resulting in an articular surface stepoff of 2 mm or greater is associated with development of secondary OA, especially if a large portion of the radial head is displaced, so open reduction with internal fixation is sometimes used. The second common fracture pattern is impaction of an intact radial head into the radial neck. The radial head articular surface is preserved, but may be angulated relative to the neck (Fig. 3-95). Some radial head fractures are quite subtle radiographically, and may be detected on an MRI study performed for elbow pain (Fig. 3-96).

Key Concepts | **Elbow Fractures in Adults**

- Fat pad sign: sensitive and specific in the setting of trauma.
- Radial head and neck (50%):
    May be subtle — get additional views
    Tender over radial head
    More than 2-mm articular surface displacement is significant
    Associations:
        Capitellar fractures
        Posterior elbow dislocation
        Essex-Lopresti fracture: comminuted radial neck and/or head, tear of the interosseous ligament of the forearm, dislocated distal radioulnar joint
        Monteggia fracture: proximal ulna fracture, radial head dislocation
        Coronoid process fracture
- Olecranon fracture: may be distracted by triceps pull.
- Intercondylar T or Y fracture
    Comminuted with extension into joint through trochlear ridge.
- Transcondylar fracture: older patients with osteoporosis.

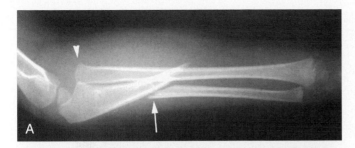

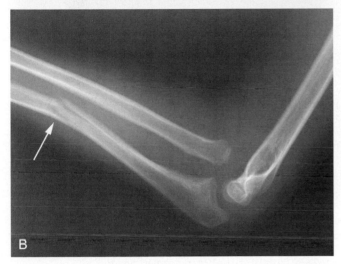

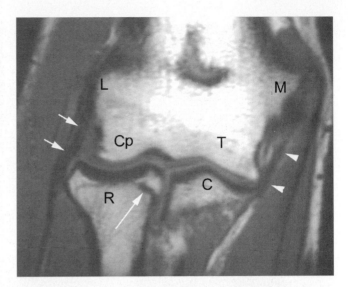

Fig. 3-96   Radiographically occult radial head fracture: diagnosis with MRI. Coronal T1-weighted MR image shows an incomplete radial head fracture seen as a low signal line (*long arrow*). It is not terribly important to diagnose such fractures, so MR is rarely used. This image also demonstrates normal elbow anatomy. Short arrows, radial collateral ligament; arrowheads, ulnar collateral ligament; L, lateral epicondyle; M, medial epicondyle; R, radial head; Cp, capitellum. Note its normal rounded contour; T, trochlea. Note its normal V-shaped contour; C, coronoid process of the ulna.

Fig. 3-94   Monteggia fracture dislocation. **A,** Lateral view of the forearm shows anterior dislocation of the radial head (*arrowhead*) and a fracture of the proximal ulna (*arrow*). **B,** In this case the ulna fracture is a greenstick fracture (*arrow*). (**B,** Courstesy of L. Das Narla, M.D., Richmond, VA.)

A comminuted radial head and neck fracture is caused by high-force trauma such as a high-speed motor vehicle crash. This fracture is associated with additional elbow and forearm injuries such as capitellar and coronoid process fractures, elbow dislocation (usually posterior), and

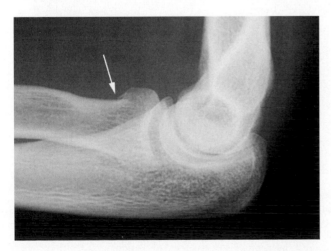

Fig. 3-95   Radial head fracture in adults (see also Figure 3-82). The fracture is often nondisplaced and therefore subtle (*arrow*).

the *Essex-Lopresti fracture.* The Essex-Lopresti fracture is an acute tear of the interosseous ligament of the forearm, comminuted fracture of the radial head and neck, and dislocation of the distal radioulnar joint (Fig. 3-97). It is important to identify this unstable fracture because resection of the radial head and neck fragments, a frequent treatment for comminuted fractures, will allow the radius to migrate proximally, resulting in abnormal alignment at the wrist.

Elbow dislocation is less frequent in adults than in children. As in children, the radius and ulna usually dislocate posteriorly, although displacement in virtually any direction may occur. Associated fractures are frequent, and there often is significant associated ligamentous, neurovascular, and other soft tissue injury. Myositis ossificans in the muscles that surround the elbow, notably in the brachialis muscle, is a frequent sequellum of elbow dislocation (Fig. 3-98). Prompt reduction of the elbow dislocation reduces the risk of posttraumatic ossification and associated reduced range of motion.

Intraarticular fracture of the olecranon can occur as a result of avulsion of the olecranon process by the triceps tendon (Fig. 3-99). Traction by the triceps displaces the proximal fragment proximally, potentially resulting in wide diastasis. This fracture is treated with internal fixation with an olecranon screw, or wires and a figure-of-eight tension band (Fig. 3-99B).

Distal humerus fractures in older, osteoporotic patients are often simple transverse fractures. Fractures in

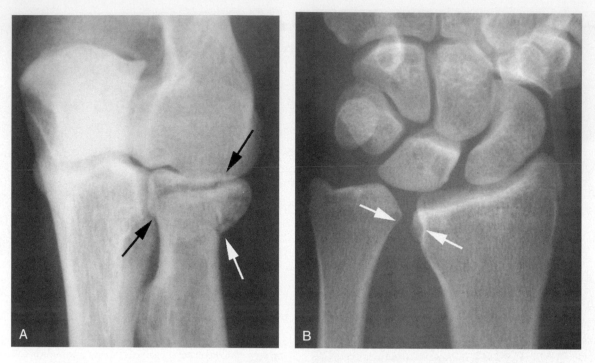

Fig. 3-97 Essex-Lopresti fracture dislocation. The elbow (**A**) shows a comminuted radial head fracture (*arrows*). The wrist (**B**) shows distal radioulnar joint dislocation seen as joint widening and distal displacement of the ulna (*arrows*). The primary injury is an acute tear of the interosseous ligament of the forearm. This is an unstable fracture that requires specialized orthopedic management.

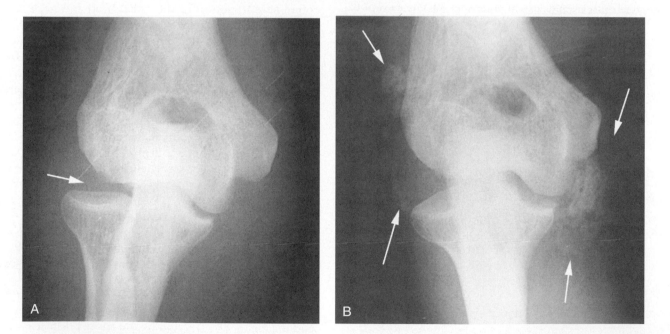

Fig. 3-98 Soft tissue calcification after elbow dislocation. **A,** Initial AP view after reduction of an elbow fracture. Note that the radiocapitellar articulation is wide (*arrow*), indicating that reduction was not complete. Because this patient suffered a severe neurologic injury, it was elected not to complete the reduction. **B,** 3 weeks later, calcification can be seen around the elbow (*arrows*). The calcification is due to myositis ossificans and calcification in other soft tissues. The patient's neurologic injury with associated absence of motion of this joint likely contributed to the rapidity and severity of the soft tissue calcification.

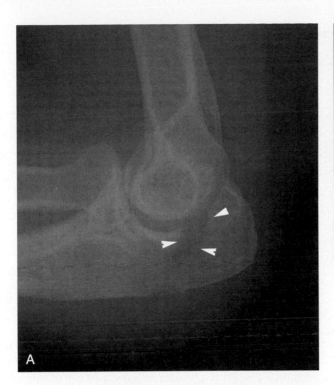

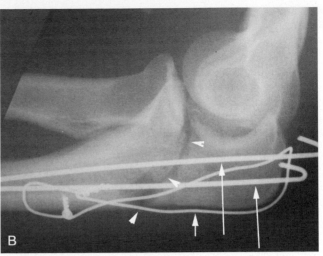

Fig. 3-99   Olecranon avulsion. **A,** Transverse fracture due to avulsion by the triceps muscle. **B,** Postoperative appearance in a different patient. Fixation can be accomplished with a longitudinal screw or, as in this case, wires (*long arrows*) with a figure of eight tensioning band (*short arrows*). Note the fracture (*arrowheads*).

younger adults usually also include a longitudinal component in a "Y" or "T" configuration. The intraarticular fracture line usually extends through the trochlea. Surgical fixation is required, usually accomplished with transcondylar screws and medial and lateral plates. An intraarticular approach through an olecranon osteotomy is often used during this repair. The repaired osteotomy is similar in appearance to an internally fixed olecranon fracture, except that an osteotomy has straight, smooth margins (Fig. 3-100).

Elbow Ligaments and Tendons

The major ligaments of the elbow are the *medial or ulnar collateral ligament (MCL) complex,* and the *radial or lateral collateral ligament (LCL) complex* that blends into the *annular ligament* that surrounds the radial head (Figs. 3-96, 3-101 to 3-104).

The most important, and fortunately easiest to image component of the MCL complex is the cordlike *anterior bundle or band* that attaches the medial epicondyle to the anterior medial ulna on the coronoid process (Fig. 3-96, 3-101). The anterior bundle is sometimes referred to simply as the MCL. The anterior bundle is vulnerable to injury with acute or chronic valgus stress. The anterior bundle is best seen on coronal MR images obtained with the elbow extended. A normal anterior bundle has sharp

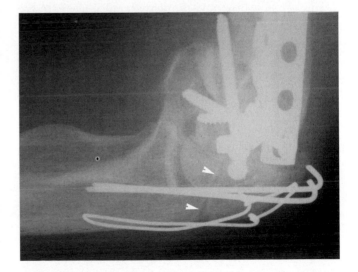

Fig. 3-100   Olecranon osteotomy. This patient suffered a comminuted intra-articular distal humerus fracture that required open reduction with internal fixation. An olecranon osteotomy was performed to provide access to the articular surface of the humerus during reduction. The method of fixation of the osteotomy is similar to the olecranon fracture in Figure 3-99B, but note the straight margins of the osteotomy (*arrowheads*). The presence of extensive fixation hardware in the distal humerus provides another clue that the ulna was not fractured.

Key Concepts   Elbow Ligaments and Tendons

- Ligaments:
    - Medial (ulnar) collateral ligament complex
        - Complex anatomy; anterior bundle is most important component
        - Extends from medial epicondyle to medial coranoid process
        - Well seen on MRI and MR arthrography
        - Injured with valgus stress, such as baseball pitchers
    - Annular ligament
        - Wraps around radial head, attached to ulna
        - Injured with radial head dislocation in adults, but intact or only partially torn in childhood subluxation of the radial head (jerked elbow).
    - Lateral (radial) collateral ligament.
        - Inserts into annular ligament.
        - Injured with varus stress
- Tendons:
    - Common flexor-pronator tendon origin on medial epicondyle
        - Tendinitis, tears (e.g., carpenters, baseball pitchers)
    - Common extensor supinator tendon origin on lateral epicondyle
        - Tendinitis, tears (e.g., carpenters, tennis elbow)
    - Biceps tendon
        - Inserts on radial tuberosity of proximal radius.
        - Injured with overuse. Weakened by steroids, rheumatoid arthritis.
        - MR diagnosis: serial axial images through tendon from muscle belly to radial insertion are essential to diagnose or exclude a tear.

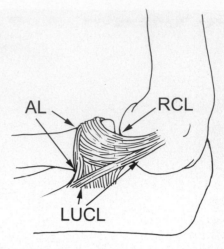

Fig. 3-102   Diagram of lateral ligaments of the elbow. AL, annular ligament; RCL, radial (lateral) collateral ligament. Note that the RCL blends into the annular ligament. LUCL, lateral ulnar collateral ligament.

margins and low signal intensity on all sequences (Fig. 3-96). Partial tears or sprains of the anterior bundle are seen on T2-weighted images as increased signal intensity within the ligament. A recent therapeutic injection may have a similar appearance. Intraarticular contrast may enter but not pass completely through a partial thickness tear. Complete tears reveal interruption and possibly laxity of ligament fibers, with escape of joint fluid or injected contrast into the surrounding extraarticular soft tissues (Fig. 3-105).

The other components of the MCL complex are the *posterior bundle* and the *oblique band or transverse ligament* (Figs. 3-101, 3-104A). The oblique band connects the medial proximal olecranon to the coronoid process just posterior to the anterior bundle insertion. The posterior bundle originates at the medial epicondyle and spreads fanlike to the proximal ulna. The posterior bundle and the oblique band form the floor of the cubital tunnel and are adjacent to the ulnar nerve (Fig. 3-104A). These ligaments are thin and closely apposed to the trochlea and ulna, making them difficult to distinguish as distinct structures even with high resolution MR images. However, tears of these ligaments can be inferred if joint fluid or intraarticular contrast escapes from the medial aspect of the elbow with a normal appearing anterior band.

The *lateral collateral ligament* (LCL) extends from the lateral epicondyle in a fanlike configuration to the annular ligament (Figs. 3-96, 3-102, 3-105). The *lateral ulnar collateral ligament* extends from the posterior aspect of the LCL origin on the lateral epicondyle around the posterior aspect of the radial head and neck to the posterolateral ulna. This ligament is an important posterolateral elbow stabilizer. Lateral ligament injuries have a similar appearance on MR images as medial ligament injuries but are less common.

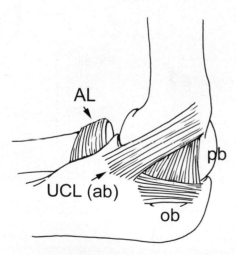

Fig. 3-101   Diagram of medial ligaments of the elbow. AL, annular ligament; UCL (ab), ulnar (medial) collateral ligament anterior bundle or band. This is the strongest and most important component of the UCL. pb, posterior bundle of the UCL; ob, oblique (transverse) band of the UCL.

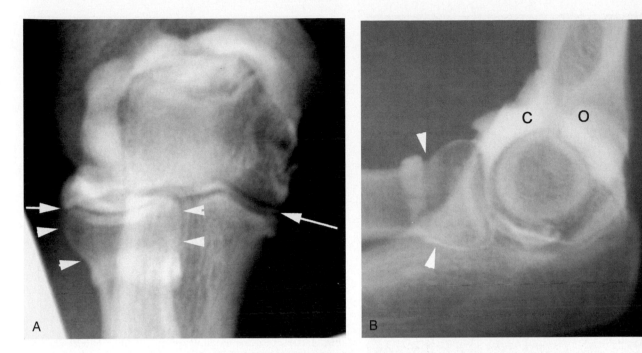

Fig. 3-103   Normal arthrographic anatomy of the elbow. A, AP view. B, Lateral view. Arrowheads, impression from annular ligament around radial head. Short arrow in A, position of radial collateral ligament. An RCL tear would allow contrast to flow laterally. Long arrow in A, position of ulnar collateral ligament. A UCL tear would allow contrast to flow medially. C, coronoid fossa in B. O, olecranon fossa in B.

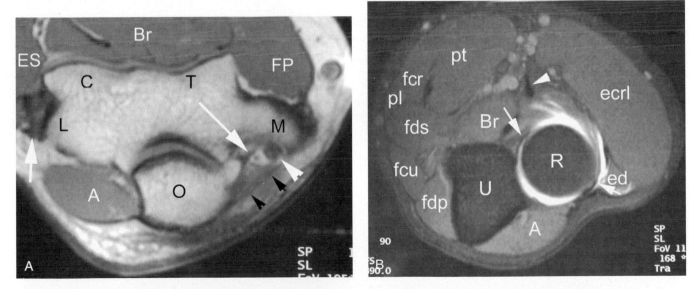

Fig. 3-104   Normal MR anatomy of the elbow: axial images. **A,** Axial T1-weighted MR image through the distal aspect of the humeral epicodyles. White arrowhead, ulnar nerve; black arrowheads, cubital tunnel retinaculum; short white arrow, common extensor tendon; long arrow, floor of the cubital tunnel formed by the transverse and posterior bands of the UCL. **B,** Fat suppressed T1-weighted MR arthrogram image more distal than A, through the radial head. Arrowhead, biceps tendon; Short arrows, annular ligament. *Muscles:* A, anconceous; Br, brachialis; ES, extensor-supinator group; FP, flexor pronator group; ecrl, extensor carpi radialis longus; ed, extensor digitorum; fcr, flexor carpi radialis; fcu, flexor carpi ulnaris; fdp, flexor digitorum profundus; fds, flexor digitorum superficialis; pl, palmaris longus; pt, pronator teres.
Bones: L, lateral epicondyle; M, medial epicondyle; R, radial head; C, capitellum; T, trochlea; o, olecranon; u, ulna.

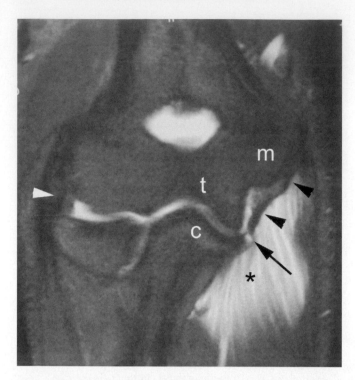

Fig. 3-105   Ulnar collateral ligament tear. Coronal fat suppressed T2-weighted MR arthrogram image in a professional baseball pitcher who developed medial elbow pain while pitching. Note the focal tear (*black arrow*) in the distal UCL with extension of contrast into the medial musculature (*). Also note the normal low signal intensity of the remainder of the UCL (*black arrowheads*) and the normal radial collateral ligament (*white arrowhead*). C, coronoid process; t, trochlea; m, medial epicondyle.

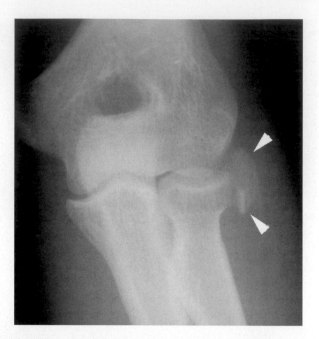

Fig. 3-106   Calcific tendinitis of the common extensor tendon (*arrowheads*). Clinically, this patient had "tennis elbow," with lateral epicondyle pain exacerbated by wrist dorsiflexion.

The *annular (orbicular) ligament* of the radius is attached to the ulna and wraps around the radial head in the transverse plane, forming a collar that prevents radial head dislocation (Figs. 3-101, 3-104). The annular ligament is disrupted by radial head dislocation in adults.

Lateral epicondylitis ("*tennis elbow*") is tendinitis of the common origin of the wrist dorsiflexors and supinators at the lateral epicondyle. Lateral epicondylitis is caused by repetitive motion, and is an affliction of carpenters, golfers, and many other active individuals in addition to tennis players. The large majority of cases recover with conservative therapy. MR imaging can be helpful in refractory cases in assessing the extent of injury, as surgical debridement can be helpful in some cases. Tendinitis is seen as increased signal intensity on T2-weighted images and/or tendon thickening. A therapeutic injection performed within the previous few weeks can produce identical findings. Radiographs may reveal calcification (Fig. 3-106). A tear is seen as a focus of very high signal intensity on T2-weighted images filling a defect within the tendon (Fig. 3-107). The high signal intensity may represent fluid or blood within a tendon defect, granulation tissue, or a combination. Ultrasound also may be used to diagnose tears of this tendon (Fig. 3-108).

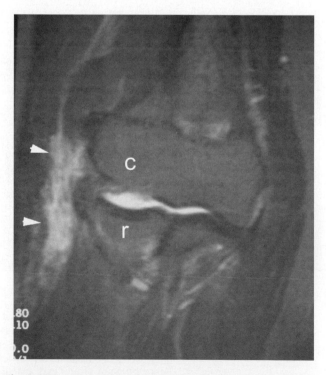

Fig. 3-107   Tear of the common extensor tendon. Coronal inversion recovery MR image shows high signal intensity in and adjacent to the tendon (*arrowheads*). C, capitellum; r, radial head.

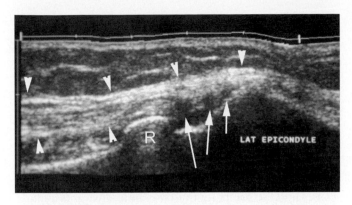

Fig. 3-108 Partial thickness tear of the common extensor tendon: Ultrasound diagnosis. Coronal image reveals hypoechoic defects in the deep portion of the proximal tendon (*arrows*). Note the normal sonographic appearance of the remainder of the tendon (*arrowheads*). R, radial head. (Courtesy of Doohi Lee, M.D., Richmond, VA.)

Medial epicondylitis is tendonitis of the common origin of the wrist flexors and pronators at the medial epicondyle. The MR imaging features are identical to lateral epicondylitis. Medial epicondylitis occurs in professional baseball pitchers and tennis players. An associated traction spur at the coronoid insertion of the anterior bundle of the MCL may be seen. Chronic avulsive irregularity of the medial epicondyle physis (little leaguer's elbow) in skeletally immature throwing athletes may also occur in association with medial epicondylitis.

The *distal biceps tendon* can undergo degeneration and tear. Most biceps tendon tears occur in men and are due to repetitive stress. Rheumatoid arthritis, previous local steroid injection, and use of anabolic steroids increase the risk of biceps tendon tear. A chronically degenerated tendon may completely tear spontaneously or after a seemingly trivial injury. Complete rupture of the distal biceps tendon is usually clinically evident owing to retraction of the muscle belly, but some cases are difficult to

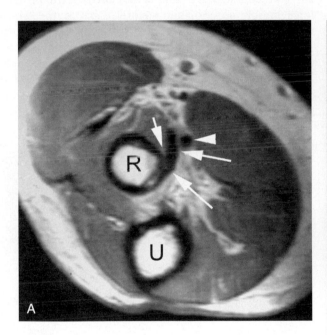

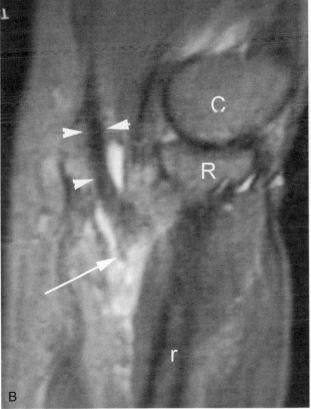

Fig. 3-109 Biceps tendon insertion. **A,** Normal distal biceps tendon. Axial T2-weighted MR image shows the distal tendon (*long arrows*) inserting onto the radius (R). Most biceps tendon tears occur at the insertion. The short arrow marks the location of the cubital bursa, which is normal in this case and therefore is not seen. Inflammation of this bursa causes local fluid accumulation and can clinically simulate a distal biceps tear or tendinitis. The arrowhead marks the ulnar artery. U, ulna. **B,** Biceps tendon tear. Sagittal inversion recovery image shows retracted and frayed torn margin of the biceps tendon (*arrow*). Note the normal appearing biceps tendon more proximally, with low signal intensity (*arrowheads*). R, radial head; r, radial shaft; C, capitellum.

diagnose clinically. Most disruptions occur at the tendon insertion onto the radial tuberosity, but more proximal tears may occur. MR images of a degenerated or partially torn tendon reveal increased signal intensity on all sequences, tendon thickening, and surrounding edema. A partially or completely torn distal biceps is often surrounded by fluid. A tendon rupture is seen on MR images as interruption of tendon fibers. Sagittal images may allow demonstration of the torn and retracted tendon on a single image (Fig. 3-109), but serial axial images extending from the musculotendinous junction to the radial tuberosity are more reliable in detection or exclusion of a biceps tendon tear. Therefore, it is essential that an axial sequence extends distally to the radial tuberosity. The normal biceps courses anterior to the brachialis muscle before curving posteriorly to the radial tuberosity (Figs. 3-104, 3-109).

Several clinical and imaging pitfalls are associated with biceps tendon tears. An associated hematoma may lead to clinical suspicion of an underlying sarcoma. MR images will reveal a mass with bizarre signal characteristics related to the hemorrhage, potentially misleading the radiologist as well. Some of the proximal medial biceps tendon fibers form the flat, broad *biceps aponeurosis* (*lacertus fibrosis*) that inserts into the medial fascia of the forearm. A distal tendon rupture can be clinically masked if the biceps aponeurosis remains is intact, because the intact aponeurosis limits tendon retraction and allows for limited biceps function. Chronic inflammation of the small *cubital bursa* may be both a cause and an effect of biceps tendon rupture. This bursa is located between the distal tendon and the medial radius (Fig. 3-109A). MR images reveal fluid distension of the bursa. Radiographs may reveal reactive changes in the adjacent radius, suggesting an aggressive process such as a neoplasm. All of these potential pitfalls may be avoided with careful scrutiny of the biceps tendon.

Triceps tendon injuries are unusual. Complete tears are usually diagnosed by physical examination and radiographs. More frequently, the olecranon fractures and is displaced proximally, as discussed above (see Fig. 3-99). MRI or US can be used to characterize a partial tendon tear or degeneration.

Miscellaneous Elbow Injuries

Compression and entrapment neuropathies of the elbow *Cubital tunnel syndrome* is ulnar neuropathy caused by trauma in the cubital tunnel located posterior to the medial epicondyle. The cubital tunnel is formed by the medial epicondyle, proximal ulna, and the overlying retinaculum. Causes of cubital tunnel syndrome include ulnar nerve subluxation, nerve traction, ulnar bone spurs, a ganglion or other mass lesion, fibrosis, fracture, inflammatory process, or anatomic derangements. Clinical

features include weakness of the flexor carpi ulnaris muscle and the intrinsic muscles of the hand. MRI may reveal a causative lesion, or simply signal alteration in the fat that normally surrounds the ulnar nerve within the tunnel. T2-weighted and inversion recovery MR images may reveal nerve or perineural edema (Fig. 3-110). Treatment depends on the cause. Offending masses are resected. The retinaculum may be released and the nerve transferred out of the cubital tunnel.

The radial nerve is vulnerable to a compressive neuropathy just distal to the elbow where the deep branch passes into the supinator muscle. Clinical features include weakness of finger extensor muscles and pain and tenderness adjacent to the lateral epicondyle. The latter symptoms may simulate lateral epicondylitis. Potential causes include previous elbow dislocation or fracture, a mass lesion, or fibrosis. MR images may reveal a masslike lesion such as a hematoma or neoplasm, but usually are unrevealing.

The median nerve is vulnerable to entrapment neuropathy as it courses between the two heads of the pronator teres muscle anterior and slightly distal to the elbow. Clinical features include weakness of the first three fingers and pain with writing, weightlifting, and other activities that use the pronator teres muscle. As with radial nerve entrapment, MR images are usually unrevealing unless a mass lesion is present. The median nerve may be entrapped proximal to the elbow by a ligament of

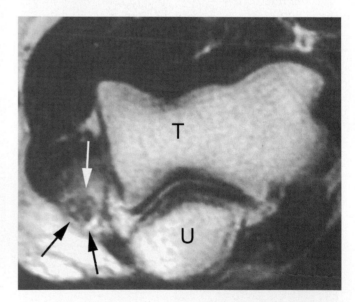

Fig. 3-110 Ulnar nerve injury. Axial T2-weighted MR image distal to the medial epicondyle shows thickening and heterogeneously increased signal intensity in the ulnar nerve (*black and white arrows*). T, trochlea; U, proximal ulna. The cause of the injury in this case was trauma due to repetitive overstretching of the nerve. The ulnar nerve must normally stretch to accommodate elbow flexion. In this case, a portion of the nerve was fixed by fibrosis in the cubital tunnel, which focused the stretching forces on a short segment of the nerve.

Struthers, as discussed earlier in the section on the arm. The median nerve is also vulnerable to a compressive neuropathy just distal to the elbow as it passes through the flexor carpi ulnaris muscle. Imaging findings are usually absent, although a mass may be seen.

Osteochondritis dissecans (OCD, Fig. 3-111) of the capitellum can be considered to be a variant type of traumatic elbow injury. The distal and posterior portions of the capitellum are vulnerable to direct impaction when the elbow is flexed. This mechanism is a likely cause of capitellar OCD.

FOREARM

Traumatic conditions of the proximal and distal ends of the ulna and radius are discussed separately in the sections on the elbow and wrist.

Isolated fracture of the ulnar shaft ("*nightstick fracture*") is caused by a direct blow. A classic nightstick fracture occurs when the forearm is raised to protect the head from a blow from a blunt object such as a policeman's nightstick.

Most forearm shaft fractures usually include both bones, either with fracture of both (Fig. 3-112) or fracture of one and dislocation of the other. *Both bones* fractures are of the ulna and radius and are treated with casting in children. These factures heal rapidly and can remodel after the fracture has healed. Adult both bones fractures are usually treated by internal fixation of each bone (Fig. 3-15A). *Post-traumatic radioulnar synostosis,* that is, osseous union of the ulna to the radius is an unusual complication of a both bones fracture. Treatment is resection of the synostosis.

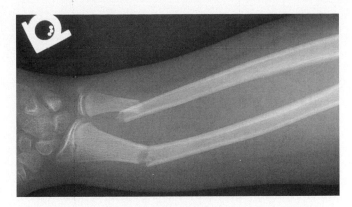

Fig. 3-112   Both bones forearm fracture in a child.

The *Galeazzi* fracture is a fracture of the radial shaft and dislocation of the distal ulna (Fig. 3-113). The distal radioulnar joint is injured and may develop chronic instability. The *Monteggia* fracture is dislocation of the radial head and fracture of the proximal ulnar shaft (Fig. 3-94).

The important Essex-Lopresti fracture (Fig. 3-97) was discussed earlier.

The volar forearm muscles are invested in indistensible fascia and hence are vulnerable to *compartment syndrome* similar to the compartments of the leg. Forearm fracture, supracondylar fracture, soft-tissue crush injury, knife wound to the forearm, and osteotomy of the radius or ulna can cause muscle swelling or hemorrhage that leads to a viscious cycle of increasing intracompartmental pressure, ischemia, nerve injury, and ultimately tissue necrosis. *Volkmann's contracture* is a devastating result of volar forearm compartment syndrome. The fingers and wrist develop progressive fixed flexion deformity due to fibrosis of the necrosed forearm muscles. Early detection is imperative to avoid this devastating outcome. When acute compartment syndrome is suspected, direct measurement of intracompartmental pressure is the appropriate test. This should not be delayed in order to obtain an MRI or other imaging study. Treatment of acute compartment syndrome is by decompression of the affected compartment by fasciotomy.

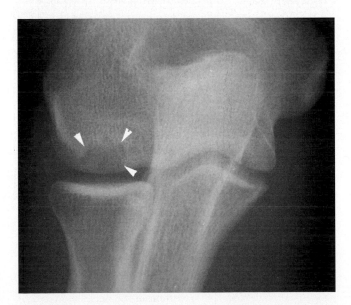

Fig. 3-111   Osteochondritis dissecans of the capitellum. Note the irregular lucent defect in the subchondral bone (*arrowheads*).

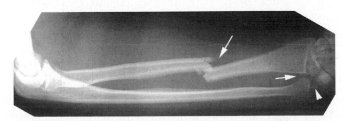

Fig. 3-113   Galeazzi fracture. Note the radial shaft fracture (*long arrow*) and distal ulnar dislocation (*short arrow*). This patient also has an ulnar styloid fracture (*arrowhead*).

WRIST

The wrist connects the hand to the forearm and elbow. The wrist includes the tissues between the proximal aspect of the distal radioulnar joint and the base of the metacarpals, a region that includes the distal ulna and radius, the eight carpal bones, the proximal metacarpals, the triangular fibrocartilage, and numerous related ligaments, tendons and synovial compartments. The wrist is a marvelously, maddeningly complex joint, made all the more challenging for the radiologist by the comparatively small size of many important soft tissue structures that test the limits of our scanners and our diagnostic skills. This section begins with a brief discussion of imaging techniques, followed by a review of anatomy and pathol-ogy of the wrist beginning proximally in the distal forearm and continuing distally to the carpometacarpal joints.

Imaging Techniques

Radiographic evaluation of the traumatized or painful wrist should include, at a minimum, PA and lateral radiographs, the latter obtained with wrist in neutral position to properly assess carpal alignment. Dedicated views of the scaphoid are required if the patient has snuff box tenderness or any other evidence of a scaphoid fracture. Scaphoid imaging is reviewed further in the discussion of the carpal bones. A variety of other specialized radiographic projections of the wrist have been described. US is useful when assessing for a joint or tendon sheath effusion, tendon pathology, or for a mass lesion in the

---

Key Concepts | **Wrist Anatomy Overview**

- Distal Radioulnar Joint (DRUJ)
    Allows supination/pronation.
    Separate synovial compartment, bounded distally by the triangular fibrocartilage.
    Arthrogram capacity: 1 cc.
- Distal Ulna and Radius
    Ulna slightly shorter than radius.
    Radius has approximately 20°–25° ulnar inclination and 11° palmar tilt (normal range 2°–20°).
    Scaphoid and lunate fossae: shallow impressions on distal radial articular surface.
- Triangular Fibrocartilage Complex (TFCC)
    Fibrocartilage "disk" fixed to radius and ulnar styloid.
    Functionally extends articular surface of radius medially.
- Radiocarpal Joint
    Bounded proximally by the radius and TFCC, distally by proximal carpal row and scapholunate and lunotriquetral interosseous ligaments.
    Arthrogram capacity: approx. 3–5 cc.
- Carpal bones
    Two rows form smooth arcs.
    Dual rows allow great range of motion.
    Proximal row functions as a linkage ("intercalated segment") between radius and distal carpal row.
    Lateral view: scaphoid tilted palmar 45°. Lunate aligned with capitate.
    Lunate and capitate form *central carpal column*.
    Forces transmitted and carpal motion occurs across the central column.
- Intercarpal (midcarpal) joint
    Bounded proximally by the scapholunate and lunotriquetral interosseous ligaments.
    Can communicate distally with the carpometacarpal joints.
    Arthrogram capacity: approximately 3–5+ cc.

- Carpometacarpal joints
    Form a zig-zag pattern on AP radiograph.
- Pisotriquitral joint
    Palmar
    Arthrogram capacity: approximately 1 cc. (Not routinely evaluated during arthrography.)
    May communicate with radiocarpal joint as a normal variant.
- Capsular ligaments
    Volar and Dorsal sets. Volar generally are stronger.
    Complex and incompletely understood.
    Essential components of wrist stability.
    Difficult to image.
  Tendons
    Dorsal: extensors
    Multiple separate compartments.
    Extensor carpi ulnaris tendon sheath contributes to carpal stability and is a component of the TFCC.
    Palmar: flexors
- Carpal tunnel
    Contains wrist flexor tendons and median nerve.
    Bounded:
        Medially by pisiform and hook of hamate
        Laterally by scaphoid
        Dorsally by the wrist capsule
        Palmarly by the flexor retinaculum
- Guyons' canal
    Contains ulnar nerve.
    Palmar and medial to carpal tunnel.

carpal tunnel. Fluoroscopy can provide a great deal of evidence about the functional status of ligaments and tendons, based on the alignment and motion of the carpal bones. Arthrography can reveal tears of the lunotriquetral and scapholunate interosseous ligaments and the triangular fibrocartilage. CT is useful for characterizing complex fractures, and posttraumatic complications such as malunion or nonunion of the scaphoid.

MRI of the wrist is extremely sensitive in the detection of fractures, AVN, tenosynovitis, and mass lesions. These abnormalities may be detected in a cooperative patient with almost any scanner. However, assessment of carpal ligaments and the triangular fibrocartilage complex requires extremely high quality imaging with a dedicated coil and a high field magnet. Imaging sequences are a matter of personal preference, but generally include coronal high resolution T2-weighted or gradient echo images to assess the interosseous ligaments and the triangular fibrocartilage complex, and T1-weighted and fat suppressed T2-weighted images to assess the bone marrow for edema or fracture. Axial images are needed to assess the nerves and tendons, notably those in the carpal tunnel. MR arthrography enhances detection of ligament and triangular fibrocartilage complex tears.

Normal wrist anatomy is reviewed in Figures 3-114 and 3-115.

The Distal Forearm

The articular surface of the distal radius is normally tilted towards the ulna by approximately 20° to 25° and towards the palm by approximately 11° (Fig. 3-114). Deviation from this pattern most frequently is due to an old fracture that healed with deformity, although developmental conditions such as Madelung deformity (see Fig. 5-45) also should be considered. The articular surface of the radius frequently contains two shallow depressions that correspond to the scaphoid and lunate bones, respectively termed the *scaphoid fossa* (or facet) and the *lunate fossa* (or facet). These are useful landmarks when describing an intraarticular fracture of the distal radius.

The distal ulna is normally no longer than the adjacent radius, and may be a few mm shorter. The term *ulnar positive* (or *ulnar plus*) *variance* indicates that the distal ulna is longer or extends more distally than the radius. A long ulna can impact against the triangular fibrocartilage and the medial lunate. *Ulnar negative* (or *ulnar minus*) *variance* indicates that the distal ulna is more than a few millimeters shorter than the distal radius. Ulna minus is associated with an increased risk of *Kienböck's disease*, also termed lunatomalacia or avascular necrosis of the lunate (Fig. 2-75). Accurate identification of ulnar variance requires a properly positioned PA radiograph with the wrist and forearm in neutral alignment (Fig. 3-116). Wrist dorsiflexion with the hand pressed against the film cassette will cause the more dorsal ulna to project distally, simulating ulna positive variance. Wrist supination "shortens" the ulna and wrist pronation "lengthens" the ulna relative to the distal radius.

The Distal Radioulnar Joint (DRUJ)

The distal radioulnar joint (DRUJ) is anatomically and functionally distinct from the more distal synovial compartments around the carpal bones. The DRUJ, paired with the proximal radioulnar joint at the elbow, allows wrist pronation and supination. The distal ulna has a cylindrical contour that articulates with a concave depression in the distal radius, the *sigmoid notch*, exactly the reverse of the arrangement at the elbow between the smaller, cylindrical radial head and the proximal ulna.

The DRUJ has a relatively small volume and is well distended at arthrography by injection of just 1 cc of contrast (Fig. 3-115). The DRUJ is bounded distally and separated from the radiocarpal joint by the triangular fibrocartilage. Communication between the DRUJ and the radiocarpal compartment at arthrography indicates a perforation in the triangular fibrocartilage complex. Communication between the DRUJ and the extensor carpi ulnaris tendon sheath can occur following wrist trauma with capsular injury or in RA.

DRUJ subluxation and instability can occur as an isolated injury or as a component of a more complex injury such as a Colles' fracture or a Galeazzi or Essex-Lopresti fracture-dislocation. The distal ulna is normally slightly posterior relative to the radius. In most instances of DRUJ subluxation, the distal ulna subluxes further dorsally. Diagnosis is suggested by physical examination, and CT or MRI can be used for confirmation. A suggested protocol is to obtain limited axial images through the DRUJ with the wrist in neutral, extreme pronation and extreme supination. The convex articular surface of the lateral distal ulna should be congruent with the sigmoid notch of the medial distal radius, regardless of wrist position. Wrist pronation tends to accentuate any subluxation. Imaging the uninjured side for comparison purposes is suggested, as there may be some normal variation.

Distal Forearm Fractures

Distal forearm fractures are among the most common musculoskeletal injuries. Most are the result of a fall on an outstretched hand. The age of the patient is an excellent predictor of the fracture pattern. Children usually suffer a transverse fracture of the metaphysis of the distal radius, often a fracture of the distal ulna as well. These fractures are frequently buckle or torus fractures, and are proximal to the physis (Figs. 3-10, 3-18). Adolescents have stronger bones, so the fracture almost always extends partially through the comparatively weak physis, usually in a Salter-Harris II pattern. Also seen in pre-teens and adolescent gymnasts is a Salter-Harris I variant stress injury of

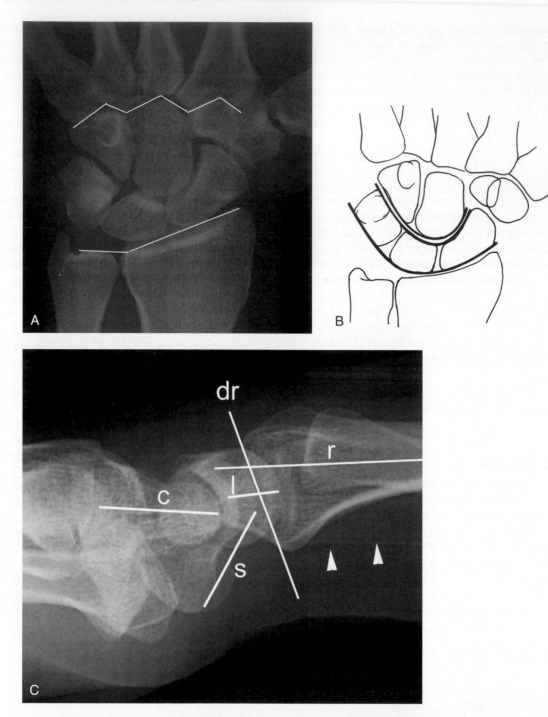

Fig. 3-114   Normal radiographic anatomy of the wrist. **A,** PA view. Note the normal ulnar inclination of the distal radius (*long white line*). Also note the approximately equal length of the distal ulna and radius (*short transverse line*), and the "zig-zag" contour formed by the carpometacarpal joints. **B,** Diagram of the normal smooth carpal arcs. Interruption of one of these arcs is evidence of an ligamentous injury or carpal dislocation. **C,** Lateral view. The long axes of the radius, capitate, scaphoid and lunate are marked with lines (r, c, s, and l, respectively). Note how the long axis of the scaphoid is estimated by connecting the two most volar projections. The radius, capitate and lunate are approximately colinear. The scaphoid is angled approximately 45° palmar compared to the lunate. The long axis of the scaphoid is easiet to determine as drawn here, by drawing a line along the palmar aspect of this bone. Note the palmar tilt of the distal radial articular surface (dr). Also note the normal fat pad volar to the pronator quadratus muscle (*arrowheads*).

Key Concepts	Common Wrist and Distal Forearm Fractures

- Age 4–10 years: Distal radius and ulna
  Transverse metaphyseal.
  Often incomplete (buckle or torus).
  Outcome is uniformly good. Remodel back to anatomic alignment.
- Age 11–16 years: Distal radius
  Usually Salter II.
  Dorsal displacement—best seen on lateral view.
- Age 17–40: Scaphoid, occasionally triquetrum or both
  May be occult on radiographs—requires high index of suspicion.
  Special views: oblique, ulnar deviation.
  MRI, CT, or bone scan for problem cases.
  Associated ligamentous injuries can lead to pain, disability, early osteoarthritis.
- Age 40+: Colles' fracture of distal radius
  Dorsal displacement and angulation.
  May have: associated ulnar styloid component.
    Comminution frequent
    Intraarticular extension into DRUJ, radiocarpal joint
    Intraarticular stepoff of 2 mm or greater increases risk for secondary osteoarthritis.
  More frequent in women.
  Associated with osteoporosis.
  Other common distal radial fractures in adults:
    Smith's: reverse Colles
    Barton's: dorsal rim with dorsal displacement of the fragment and the carpus (carpal bones as a unit). Unstable
    Reverse Bartons: volar rim fracture with displacement of the fragment and the carpus (carpal bones as a unit). Unstable.
    Hutchinson (Chauffeur's): intraarticular radial styloid

the distal radial physis. Radiographs in these children reveal widening of the physis with irregular, sclerotic margins (Fig. 3-23). After closure of the physes in young adults, most wrist fractures involve the scaphoid. As middle age approaches, the distal radius again becomes the most common site of fracture. The fractures seen in children and adolescents may be subtle, but are usually straight-forward to describe and treat. Fractures in adults are more variable in terms of comminution, alignment, intraarticular extension, and treatment.

Several "named" distal radius fracture patterns are so deeply ingrained in the orthopaedic and radiology lexicon that radiologists should be familiar with these injuries. *Colles* fracture, with apex volar angulation and dorsal impaction, is by far the most frequent wrist fracture in middle aged and older adults (Fig. 3-117A, B). The clinical deformity that accompanies a Colles fracture is sometimes likened to an upside-down fork, with the forearm representing the handle and the wrist and hand representing the tines. Colles fracture is more common in women owing to relatively weaker bones, and is associated with hip and proximal humerus fractures in elderly patients. The dorsal impaction often worsens after casting, owing to compressive forces across the wrist from the dorsal and palmar tendons. Even with external fixation, anatomic alignment may be difficult to maintain. Thus, Colles fractures often heal with loss of normal palmar tilt and ulnar inclination, and frequently heal with dorsal tilt, as well as loss of radial length. This alteration in radial articular surface alignment, combined with frequently coexisting ligamentous injuries, results in alteration of wrist mechanics with potential for development of chronic pain and early osteoarthritis. Reflex sympathetic dystrophy and acquired ulna positive variance with ulnar impaction syndrome also may occur after a Colles or any other distal radius fracture. Intraarticular extension increases the risk for these complications. *Smith's* fracture is a reverse Colles fracture, with apex dorsal angular deformity resulting in volar tilt of the distal radius articular surface. *Barton's* fracture is an unstable intraarticular fracture of the dorsal lip of the radius, with dorsal subluxation of the carpus along with the dorsal radius fragment. Surgical reduction and fixation are required. A *reverse Barton's* fracture is a similar injury with volar displacement (Fig. 3-117C). A *Hutchinson's* fracture (*chauffeur's fracture*) is an intraarticular fracture of the radial styloid (Fig. 3-117D). Hutchinson's fractures are caused by avulsion by the radial collateral ligament, or a direct blow. The latter often is association with a fracture dislocation. Hutchinson's fractures are associated with scapholunate ligament tears. This fracture is also known as a chauffeur's fracture because it was an affliction of chauffeurs before the introduction of electric starters. The chauffeur was required to start the car with a crank inserted through the front grill into the engine. If the engine suddenly misfired or started during cranking, the crank would violently accelerate in the hands of the chauffeur, placing an enormous load across the radial styloid. A fall on an outstretched hand is the most frequent cause of this fracture today.

Numerous classification systems of distal radius fractures have been described, each having advantages and disadvantages. It may be worth learning a system used by your local orthopaedic surgeons (if there is one), in order to enhance communication of abnormal findings. Otherwise, it is suggested that you limit your report to a clear description of the findings, with specific reference to the presence or absence of articular extension into the DRUJ or into the radiocarpal joint. The presence of an ulnar styloid fracture also should be noted. If intraarticular extension is present, articular step-off or diasta-

Text continued on p. 276

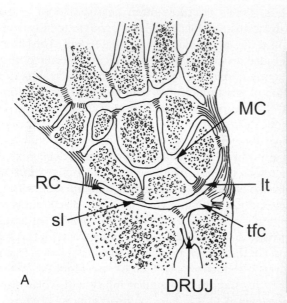

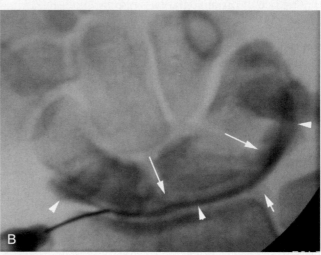

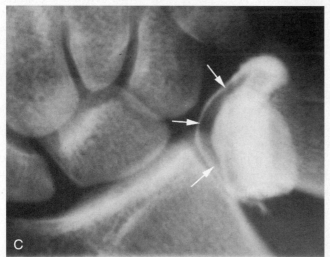

Fig. 3-115   Wrist compartmental anatomy. **A,** Diagram shows the synovial compartments of the wrist. MC, midcarpal joint; RC, radiocarpal joint; DRUJ, distal radioulnar joint; Note the structures that separate the compartments: the scapholunate (sl) and lunotriquetral (lt) interosseous ligaments separate the radiocarpal and midcarpal compartments. The triangular fibrocartilage complex (tfc) separates the radiocarpal joint from the distal radioulnar joint. Note the ligamentous fixation of the triangular fibrocartilage to the radius, ulna, and medial joint capsule. **B,** Normal radiocarpal arthrogram. Fluoroscopic spot view shows contrast filling a normal radiocarpal joint (*arrowheads*). Note that contrast does *not* flow through the interosseous ligaments of the proximal carpal row (*long arrows*) or the triangular fibrocartilage (*short arrow*). **C,** Normal distal radioulnar joint arthrogram. Note the radiolucent articular cartilage of the distal ulna (*arrows*).

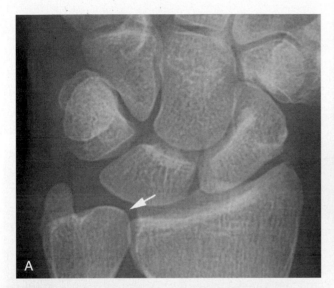

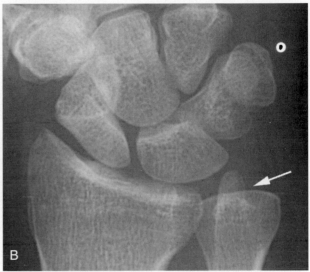

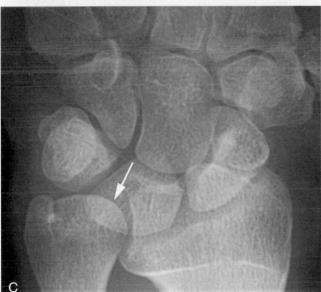

Fig. 3-116   Effect of wrist position on apparent ulnar variance. All images are of the same patient. A properly positioned PA radiograph is obtained with the wrist in neutral position. Pronation (**A**) causes apparent lengthening of the ulna (*arrow*). Supination (**B**) causes apparent shortening of the ulna (*arrow*). Wrist dorsiflexion (**C**), as can occur with the hand flat on the x-ray cassette but with the elbow elevated, causes apparent lengthening of the ulna (*arrow*).

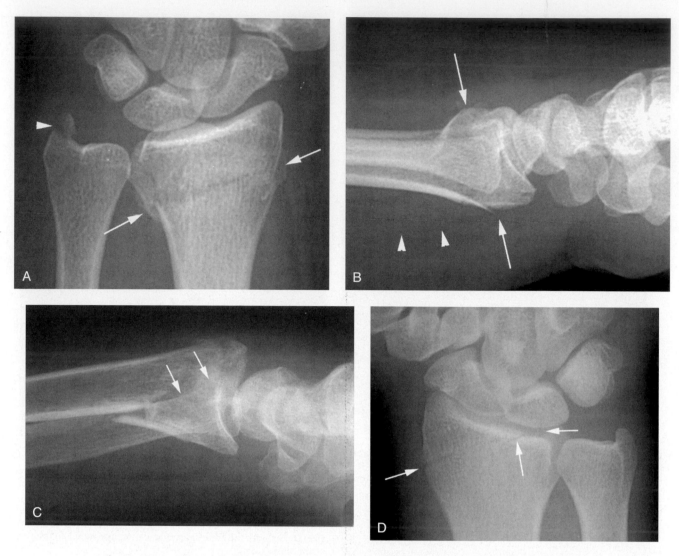

Fig. 3-117   Distal radius fractures. **A, B,** Colles fracture PA (**A**) and lateral (**B**) views show a dorsal impaction fracture of the distal radius (*arrows*) that results in dorsal, rather than the normal palmar tilt of the articular surface of the distal radius. Also note the ulnar styloid fracture (*arrowhead in* **A**). On the lateral view (**B**), the normal pronator fat pad is absent (*arrowheads* mark normal position of this fat pad). **C,** Reverse Barton's fracture of the volar lip of the radius (*arrows*), with volar subluxation of the carpus along with the radius fragment. This is an unstable fracture. **D,** Hutchinson's (chauffeur's) fracture of the radial styloid (*arrows*).

sis of 2 mm or greater should be noted, as such deformity is associated with development of posttraumatic osteoarthritis and thus is an indication for operative reduction.

The Triangular Fibrocartilage Complex

The *triangular fibrocartilage complex* (TFCC) is located between the distal ulna and the proximal carpal row. The TFCC is the primary stabilizer of the DRUJ and also allows wider distribution of forces across the radiocarpal joint. The TFCC consists of several components that are not discrete structures, but rather blend continuously from one structure to the next. The TFCC includes a central disk-shaped fibrocartilagenous portion, termed the *triangular fibrocartilage* (TFC). The TFC blends into the thick, strong dorsal and volar *radioulnar ligaments* that fix the TFC to the radius laterally and to the ulnar head and styloid process medially. The extensor carpi ulnaris tendon sheath and the medial portions of the wrist capsular ligaments also are components of the TFCC. Many TFCC injuries occur during a wrist fracture and are not immediately apparent. Tears of the TFCC cause ulnar sided wrist pain and weakness. A click or pop with wrist motion may be present. Arthrography or MRI may reveal a defect in the TFC or communication between the radiocarpal joint and the DRUJ (Fig. 3-118).

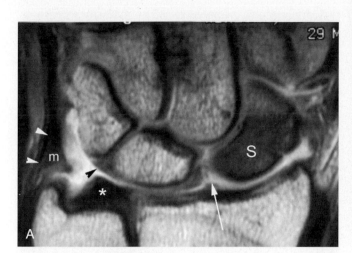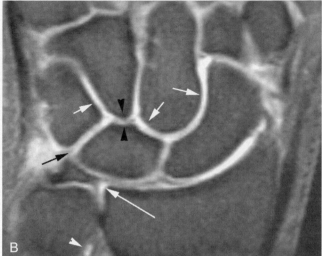

Fig. 3-118   The triangular fibrocartilage complex. **A,** Coronal T1-weighted MR arthrogram image shows normal appearance of the triangular fibrocartilage (*), with low signal intensity and smooth margins. This patient has a normal variant "meniscal homologue" (m) attached to the ulnar collateral ligament (*white arrowheads*). The meniscal homologue is composed of fibrocartilage and is triangular in cross section, hence its name. Also note the scapholunate ligament tear (*white arrow*) but intact lunotriquetral ligament (*black arrowhead*) and the low signal intensity of the scaphoid marrow (S), due to edema related to a healing scaphoid fracture. (Courtesy of Charles Pappas, M.D., Burlington, VT.) **B,** Triangular fibrocartilage complex tear. Coronal fat suppressed T1-weighted MR arthrogram image obtained after radiocarpal injection shows the triangular fibrocartilage to be avulsed from its radial attachment (*white arrow*). Contrast has entered the distal radioulnar joint through this defect (*white arrowhead*). Also note the high signal intensity within the midcarpal joint (*short white arrows*) due to contrast passing through a lunotriquetral ligament tear (*black arrow*). This patient has a common normal variant in which the hamate articulates with the lunate (*black arrowheads*), termed a type 2 hamate. This normal variant is associated with accelerated articular cartilage degeneration at this articulation. (A type 1 hamate does not articulate with the lunate.)

Patterns of TFCC tears are complex, but generally occur as a perforation of the TFC, or a tear of the TFC fixation to the radius, ulna, or dorsal or volar joint capsule. Occasionally, similar, asymptomatic defects may be observed in older individuals, thought to represent a consequence of "normal" age-related degeneration. This potential pitfall of false positive diagnosis is similar to age-related partial separations of the glenoid labrum of the shoulder, small perforations in the lunotriquetral and scapholunate interosseous ligaments of the wrist, and signal alterations in the menisci of the knee.

Ulnar impaction syndrome is impingement of the distal lateral ulna against the TFCC and the proximal carpal row, in particular the proximal medial lunate (Fig. 3-119). Chronic/repetitive impingement causes degeneration of the TFC and lunate cartilage. Clinical features are similar to a TFCC tear. Radiographs may reveal ulna positive variance and subchondral cysts, sclerosis or osteophytes in the proximal medial lunate, proximal radial triquetrum, and/or distal ulna. An old radial fracture as the cause of the ulnar positive variance may be evident. TFCC tears or degeneration may be documented by arthrography or MRI. Treatment is by surgical shortening of the ulna.

Ulnar impingement syndrome is impaction, often with pseudarthrosis, of a markedly shortened ulna against the distal metaphysis of the radius. Clinical features may mimic ulnar impaction, but are often more severe. Ulnar impingement is a potential complication of ulnar growth arrest, surgical ulnar shortening, or any traumatic or growth abnormality that reduces the length of the ulna.

The Radiocarpal Joint

The radiocarpal joint is a synovial compartment that is bounded by the proximal carpal row distally and the radius and the triangular fibrocartilage proximally (Fig. 3-115). Motion across the radiocarpal joint is complex and is described in the following discussion of the carpal bones and ligaments. The capacity of the radiocarpal joint at arthrography is approximately 3–5 cc. Communication between the radiocarpal and midcarpal joints indicates that there is a tear of the scapholunate and/or the lunotriquetral interosseous ligament. Such tears usually are sig-

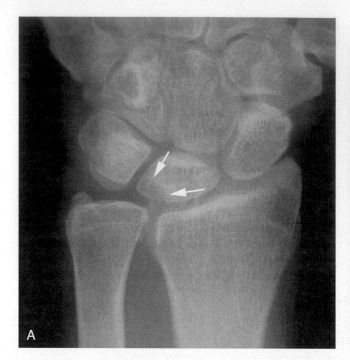

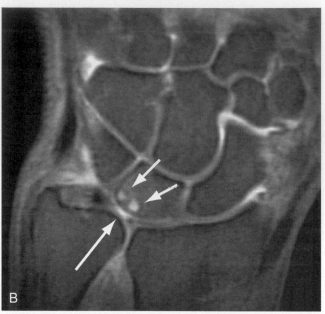

Fig. 3-119   Ulnar impaction syndrome with triangular fibrocartilage tear. **A,** PA radiograph shows mild ulna positive variance. Note the small cystlike lucencies in the proximal medial lunate (*arrows*). The lunate lesions are due to impaction by the ulna. **B,** Coronal fat suppressed T2-weighted MR arthrogram image in the same patient confirms the cystlike lesions in the lunate (*short arrows*) and shows a related triangular fibrocartilage tear (*long arrow*). (Courtesy of William Morrison, M.D., Philadelphia, PA.)

nificant in younger individuals, but also can occur in the form of asymptomatic perforations in older individuals. Communication between the radiocarpal joint and the DRUJ indicates a perforation of the TFCC, which is less frequently seen as an incidental, age-related finding. As with the DRUJ, wrist trauma or rheumatoid arthritis can cause communication between the radiocarpal joint and the extensor carpi ulnaris tendon sheath.

The Carpal Bones

A useful approach to understanding the anatomy of the carpus (the carpal bones as a unit) begins with the concept of carpal rows. The carpal bones are arranged in two rows. The proximal carpal row consists of the triquetrum, lunate, and scaphoid. The distal carpal row consists of the hamate, capitate, trapezoid, and trapezium. (The pisiform is positioned palmar to the triquetrum.) A PA radiograph of a normal wrist reveals the margins of the carpal rows to form smooth arcs, termed *carpal arcs* or *Gilula's arcs* in honor of the radiologist Louis Gilula, M.D., who described them (Fig. 3-114). The lateral view of the wrist superimposes most of the carpal bones. However, a well-positioned lateral wrist radiograph will allow identification of the radius, lunate, capitate, and third metacarpal. These bones should be

roughly colinear when the wrist is in neutral alignment (*not* dorsiflexed, Fig. 3-114C). The scaphoid is seen on the lateral view, normally in approximately 45° palmar flexion.

Carpal motion is complex, but may be simplified by again considering the concept of carpal rows. A useful simplification is that each carpal row functions as a unit, with carpal motion occurring at the radiocarpal joint and the *midcarpal joint* between the carpal rows. Approximately 50% of wrist flexion and extension occurs at the radiocarpal joint and 50% at the midcarpal joint. Motion in the coronal plane, that is, ulnar and radial deviation, is more complex (Fig. 3-120), because the carpus pivots around a center of rotation in the proximal capitate. When the wrist is in neutral position, the lunate straddles the junction of the radius and the TFC. Ulnar deviation slides the proximal carpal row *radially* (laterally) as the hand angles medially. In addition, the scaphoid and lunate tilt dorsally during ulnar deviation. The lunate articulates completely with the radius when the wrist is in ulnar deviation. Radial deviation slides the proximal carpal row *medially* as the hand angles laterally. In addition, the scaphoid and lunate tilt volarly during radial deviation. Only about 30%–50% of the lunate articulates with the radius when the wrist is in radial deviation. Variation from these normal carpal alignment and motion patterns

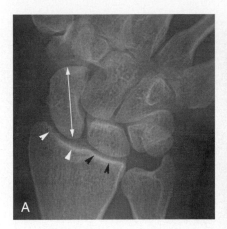
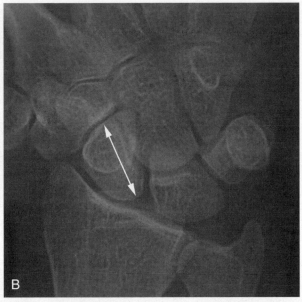

Fig. 3-120   Normal carpal motion in ulnar (**A**) and radial (**B**) deviation. Note that the proximal carpal row slides along the radius. Also note that the scaphoid "shortens" with radial deviation (**B**) as it tilts more volarly, and "elongates" with ulnar deviation, as it tilts less volarly. The spaces between the scaphoid, lunate and triquetrum change only slightly between the two images. Also note that the concavities in the articular surface of the distal radius. These are the normal scaphoid and lunate fossae, marked with white and black arrowheads, respectively in **A**. These fossae may be well developed, as in this patient, or nearly absent. Slight angulation of the x-ray beam also can make these fossae more or less apparent.

may be the only telltale sign of a significant ligamentous injury and/or carpal instability, further discussed below.

Carpal Bone Fractures and Dislocations

The most frequently fractured carpal bone is the scaphoid (Fig. 3-121). Most scaphoid fractures occur through the waist (midportion) and are nondisplaced. Like other bones that are largely covered with articular cartilage such as the femoral head and the talar dome, the proximal pole of the scaphoid has a tenuous blood supply and is vulnerable to avascular necrosis, delayed union, or nonunion if the blood supply is interrupted by trauma.

Key Concepts	Carpal Trauma

- Scaphoid is the most commonly fractured carpal bone.
    Waist and proximal pole fracture potential complications: AVN, delayed union, nonunion, humpback deformity
- Triquetral fracture: chip fracture from dorsal aspect. May only be seen on lateral or oblique view.
- Lesser arc = dislocation zone. Surrounds lunate.
- Greater arc = fracture dislocation zone. Transscaphoid perilunate dislocation most common.

The distal pole has an excellent blood supply and heals promptly. In an unfortunate anatomic arrangement, the blood supply to the proximal pole enters the scaphoid at the waist and courses proximally within the bone. Therefore, a scaphoid waist or proximal pole fracture has a high likelihood of injuring the only available blood supply to the proximal pole. A delay in immobilization increases the risk that this blood supply will be interrupted. Thus, prompt diagnosis and treatment are essential. Some scaphoid fractures are simply not visible on initial radiographs, even with dedicated views. Negative radiographs in the presence of snuff box tenderness and a history of wrist trauma require immobilization or further imaging with limited CT or MRI (Fig. 3-121C). If immobilization is selected (it usually is), repeat radiographs after 7–10 days usually reveal bone resorption or faint sclerosis around a fracture. Some fractures remain radiographically occult. Scaphoid waist and proximal pole fractures may take up to two years to heal. Cystic changes and fragmentation along the fracture margins can occur in slowly healing fractures and in cases of nonunion (Fig. 3-121A). Screw fixation and bone grafting are occasionally required (Fig. 3-121E). In addition to the complications of delayed union, nonunion, and AVN, a scaphoid fracture may heal with apex dorsal angulation, termed the *humpback* deformity (Fig. 3-121D). Thin section CT sections obtained parallel to the long axis of the scaphoid exqui-

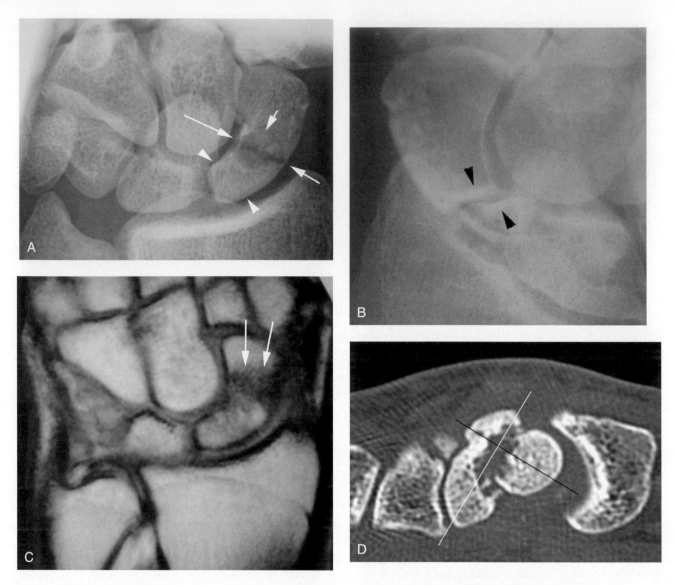

Fig. 3-121 Scaphoid fracture. **A,** Subacute scaphoid fracture. Note the fracture line (*long arrows*), cystic changes around the fracture line (*short arrow*), and the diffusely increased density of the proximal pole (*arrowheads*). The proximal pole sclerosis does not necessarily imply avascular necrosis and a poor prognosis. This case healed well with casting. **B,** Nonunion. Note the sclerosis and smooth margins of the old fracture (*arrowheads*), indicating that this is a chronic finding. **C,** MR diagnosis. This patient had snuff box tenderness after a fall, but radiographs were negative, even in retrospect. Coronal T1-weighted MR image shows a low signal intensity band traversing the scaphoid waist (*arrows*), representing a nondisplaced fracture and adjacent edema. **D,** Humpback deformity. Oblique coronal CT image aligned with the scaphoid shows dorsal tilt of the proximal fragment (*black line*) and palmar tilt of the distal fragment (*white line*), resulting in the "humpback" deformity. Other images (not shown) showed that the fracture had healed in this position.

Continued

sitely demonstrate complications such as the humpback deformity, and allow detailed assessment of presence or absence of fracture healing.

The second most frequent carpal bone fracture is an avulsion fracture of the joint capsule from the dorsal triquetrum. This fracture is usually visible only on a lateral or slightly off-lateral radiograph, where it is seen as a small cortical chip displaced a few millimeters from the triquetrum (Fig. 3-122). Point tenderness over the fracture is an important clue to this diagnosis. Transverse fractures across the capitate and proximal hamate can be seen as part of complex fracture-dislocations. The hook of the hamate (hamulus) can fracture with a direct blow to the palm or as a stress fracture in carpenters or golfers. The hook is seen on end on PA radiographs as a dense "C" projecting over the mid-distal hamate. If the

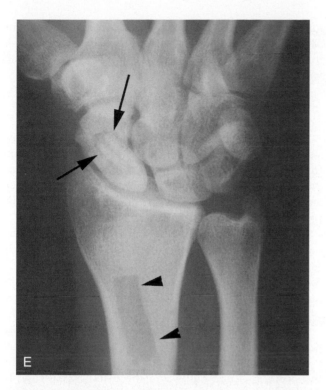

Fig. 3-121, cont'd **E,** Delayed union of this scaphoid fracture was successfully treated with bone grafting. Note the graft fragments (*arrows*) and the graft donor site in the distal radius (*arrowheads*).

hook is displaced, this "C" may not be seen. A carpal tunnel view or other dedicated views may reveal this fracture (Fig. 3-123). CT is definitive. Lunate fractures are rare. However, the lunate is vulnerable to avascular necrosis (Kienbock's disease, Fig. 2-75), especially in the presence of negative ulna variance, which can lead to lunate fragmentation and collapse.

Carpal trauma concentrates disruptive forces along arcs that run perpendicular to Gilula's arcs (Fig. 3-124). *Greater arc* injuries extend through the radial styloid and scaphoid, and across the proximal capitate, hamate, triquetrum, and ulnar styloid, or through the ligaments adjacent to these bones. This accounts for the relative frequency of scaphoid and radial and ulnar styloid fractures, as well as the ligamentous injuries that can accompany these fractures. *Lesser arc* injuries are confined to the ligaments surrounding the lunate. A relatively common greater arc injury is the *transscaphoid perilunate fracture-dislocation,* in which the arc of injury passes through the scaphoid waist, across the ligaments fixing the distal carpal row and the triquetrum to the lunate, and the ulnar styloid. Other greater arc injuries include the transscaphoid, transcapitate, perilunate fracture-dislocation (Fig. 3-125), and the rare and severe transscaphoid, transcapitate, transhamate, transtriquetral fracture-dislocation. Restoration of normal function is difficult in any of these injuries. The bones can be restored to their proper positions, and the fractures can heal, but the extensive associated ligamentous damage often results in abnormal carpal motion with pain and loss of function (Fig. 3-125C).

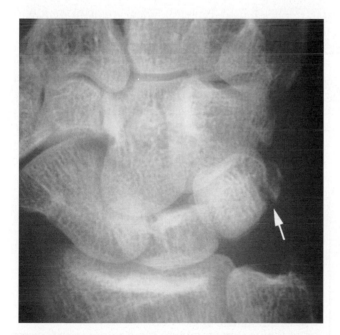

Fig. 3-122 Triquetral dorsal avulsion fracture (*arrow*). Small triquitral fractures can sometimes be difficult to identify on PA and lateral views. An oblique view as illustrated here often helps to demonstrate the fracture.

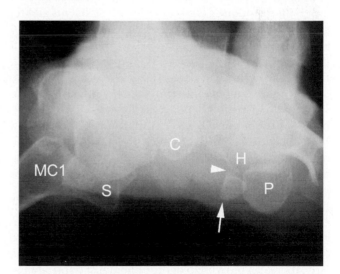

Fig. 3-123 Carpal tunnel view radiograph is obtained with the wrist dorsiflexed and the x-ray beam tangential to the wrist. P, pisiform; H, hamate; Arrow, hook of hamate; C, capitate; S, scaphoid and trapezium; MC1, thumb metacarpal. This patient has an unfused hook of the hamate (*arrowhead*). Note the straight, smooth, sclerotic margins, suggesting that this finding may be due to a developmental variant or a chronic ununited fracture.

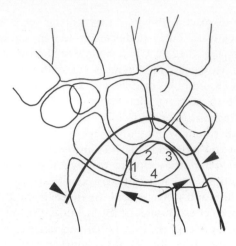

Fig. 3-124 Carpal trauma tends to concentrate disruptive forces along or close to these greater (*arrowheads*) or lesser (*arrows*) arcs. The greater arc (*arrowheads*) passes across the scaphoid waist, thus greater arc injuries are usually fracture dislocations that include a scaphoid waist fracture. The lesser arc (*arrows*) surrounds the lunate. Lesser arc injuries cause a spectrum of ligamentous injuries and dislocations that involve the lunate in a predictable pattern of increasing severity. The mildest form (stage 1) disrupts only the scapholunate ligaments, causing scapholunate dissociation (see Fig. 3-131). Stage 2 is more severe, as it also disrupts the ligamentous fixation of the lunate to the capitate. Further ligamentous disruption continues around the lunate to stage 4, resulting in lunate dislocation (see Fig. 3-126).

Lesser arc injuries, also termed *rotary subluxation of the lunate,* result from forced hyperextension (dorsiflexion) force applied to the thenar eminence. Ligamentous injury around the lunate occurs in a predictable pattern with increasing force (Figs. 3-124, 3-126). The stage 1 injury is interruption of the scapholunate ligaments and results in scapholunate dissociation (discussed below). Stage 2 injury releases the fixation between the lunate and capitate. Capitolunate instability or a perilunate dislocation are classic presentations of stage 2 rotary subluxation. Stage 3 injury continues around the circumference of the lunate with interruption of ligamentous fixation of the lunate and triquetrum. A stage 3 injury may present as a *midcarpal dislocation,* in which the lunate is tilted palmarly and the other carpal bones dislocated dorsally relative to the lunate and the radius. In stage 4 injury, there is complete disruption of the ligamentous fixation of the lunate to the radius, resulting in palmar lunate dislocation (Fig. 3-126C–E). The radiographic appearance of perilunate and midcarpal dislocations can overlap, blurring the distinction between some stage 2 and stage 3 injuries. Similarly, there can be overlap of the radiographic appearance of midcarpal and lunate dislocation, blurring the distinction between some stage 3 and stage 4 injuries. Usually the distinction is not terribly important.

Not all wrist fractures and dislocations follow the greater or lesser arc patterns. Unusual or selective application of force can fracture any bone or dislocate any joint. For example, an isolated pisiform fracture can be caused by a direct blow to the palm (Fig. 3-127). This fracture is frequently overlooked, but fortunately heals well whether or not it is recognized and treated.

Carpal Instability

Carpal instability can be a confusing and intimidating subject for the radiologist. This discussion will attempt to simplify this topic by beginning with a review of necessary terminology, followed by a simplified anatomy overview and a brief discussion of the important instability patterns.

Normal osseous carpal anatomy and motion are discussed above. *Translocation* describes a shift of the entire carpus from its normal position relative to the radius, for example *ulnar translocation. Dissociation* usually implies abnormal motion between bones within the same carpal row, often in association with interruption of the corresponding interosseous ligament, such as, *scapholunate dissociation.* Because the proximal carpal row has no tendinous attachments, its position is determined by the position of the radius and the distal carpal row. In the language of mechanical engineering, this makes the proximal carpal row an *intercalated segment.* Intercalated segment instability patterns (dorsal intercalated segment instability, DISI, and volar intercalated segment instability, VISI) refer to abnormal alignment between the carpal rows, with particular focus on alignment of the lunate and capitate. *Carpal columns* run perpendicular to the carpal rows. There are three carpal columns: central (radius–lunate–capitate), ulnar (ulna–triquetrum–hamate), and radial (radius–scaphoid–trapezoid and trapezium). The carpal columns transmit force from the hand to the forearm, primarily through the central column. Instability can be confined to one of the carpal columns. *Static carpal instability* produces abnormal carpal alignment on standard radiographs. In contrast, *dynamic* carpal instability does not, but rather requires special radiographs such as a clenched fist view or wrist fluoroscopy for detection. For example, the patient may

Key Concepts	Carpal Instability

- Most common static patterns detectable with a *properly positioned* lateral radiograph:
- Scapholunate dissociation: scapholunate angle >60°.
- DISI: lunate tilted *dorsally.* Lunocapitate angle >20°. Usually also has scapholunate dissociation, so scapholunate angle >60°.
- VISI: lunate tilted *volarly.* Lunocapitate angle >20°. Usually also has lunotriquetral dissociation, so scapholunate angle <30°.

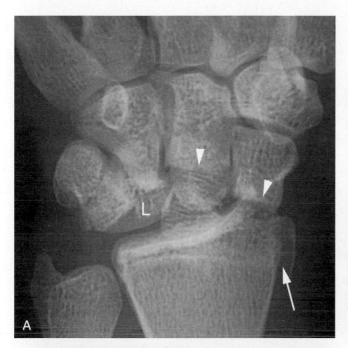

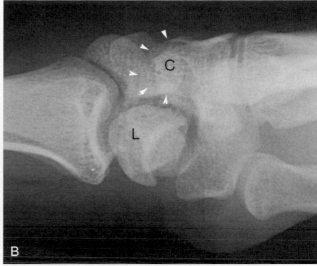

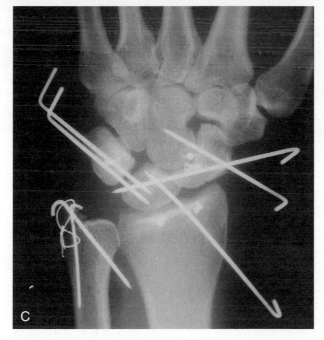

Fig. 3-125   Greater arc injury. **A, B,** Transradial, trans-scaphoid transcapitate perilunate fracture-dislocation. The PA view (**A**) shows fractures of the lateral radius (*arrow*) and the scaphoid waist and proximal capitate (*arrowheads*), with ligamentous disruption medially completing the greater arc. L marks the lunate. The lateral view (**B**) shows the lunate has normal relation with the radius, but the capitate (C) is dislocated dorsally (*arrowheads* mark the proximal capitate in **B**). This pattern is termed perilunate dislocation. **C,** Surgical reconstruction of the wrist after a trans-scaphoid perilunate fracture-dislocation in a different patient. The extensive fixation illustrates the severity of the ligamentous injuries associated with greater arc injuries.

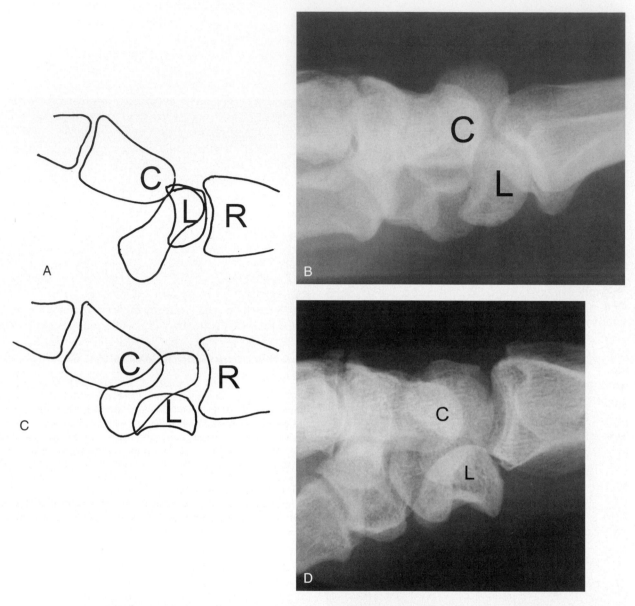

Fig. 3-126   Lesser arc injuries. **A, B,** Stage 2 lesser arc injury: perilunate dislocation. **A,** Diagram shows alignment findings in perilunate dislocation. The lunate is not displaced volarly, although it is often tilted volarly. The capitate is displaced dorsally relative to the radius. Stage 3 lesser arc injury results in midcarpal dislocation (not shown), in which the lunate is volarly subluxed but not dislocated relative to the radius and the capitate is dorsally *dislocated* relative to the lunate. **B,** Lateral radiograph shows perilunate dislocation, with alignment similar to **A.** The appearance is similar to a Stage 2 injury. (C, capitate; L, lunate.) **C–E,** Stage 4 lesser arc injury: lunate dislocation. **C,** Diagram of lunate dislocation shows the lunate (L) to be tilted and dislocated volarly. The capitate (C) is collinear with the radius (R). **D,** Lateral view shows the palmar lunate dislocation (L), with alignment similar to diagram **C.**

Continued

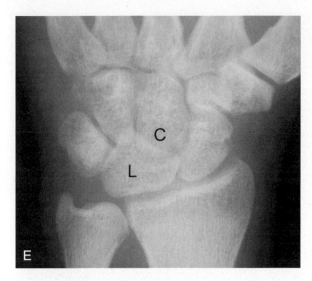

Fig. 3-126, cont'd   **E,** PA view shows disruption of the carpal arcs and abnormal contour of the lunate (L) due to the dislocation.

be able to reproduce a click or clunk with a specific maneuver, and fluoroscopy can demonstrate the corresponding abnormal carpal motion.

Instability results from ligamentous injury. Wrist ligaments are most frequently injured by trauma, but inflammatory arthritis, usually rheumatoid arthritis also may cause significant ligament damage. Ligamentous anatomy of the wrist is complex. The most important *intrinsic ligaments* are the *scapholunate* (SL) and the *lunotriquetral* (LT) interosseous ligaments located along the proximal margins of these bones (Figs. 3-115, 3-128). The SL and LT ligaments can be directly studied with arthrography and high quality MRI. Both of these ligaments have

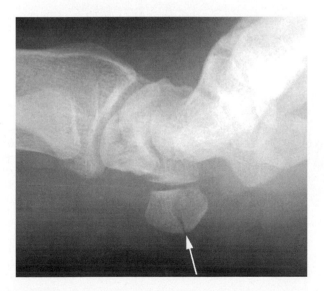

Fig. 3-127   Pisiform fracture (*arrow*), caused by a direct blow (fell on hand).

thicker, stronger dorsal and palmar components that blend into the extrinsic ligaments of the joint capsule, and thinner central portions. (It is through the thin central portion that asymptomatic age-related perforations occur. Such perforations do not indicate ligament failure, and are an important pitfall in arthrography in older patients.) Thin section MRI often reveals portions of the interosseous ligaments to be triangular in cross section. The ligaments may appear to attach onto the articular cartilage, or through the cartilage into bone. Both the LT and SL ligaments can stretch by approximately 50% to 100% of their length before tearing. Another set of interosseous ligaments unites the bones of the distal carpal row. These ligaments are rarely interrupted and are not discussed further.

The *extrinsic wrist ligaments* are a complex set of organized thickenings of the palmar and dorsal joint capsule (Fig. 3-129). These ligaments are important functionally, but are difficult to image directly. The palmar (volar) capsular ligaments are thought to be stronger and more important in maintaining wrist stability than the dorsal ligaments. Many of the capsular ligaments are named by the bones they connect. A limited enumeration of the most important capsular ligaments is included here. The main palmar ligaments include the radioscaphocapitate, radiolunotriquetral, and the ulnotriquetral and ulnar collateral ligaments. The main dorsal ligaments include the radioscaphoid, dorsal radiolunotriquetral, and a variable transverse ligament or ligaments that extend from the triquetrum laterally across the capitate to the scaphoid and trapezoid. Limited demonstration of these extrinsic ligaments is possible with thin section MR images. Much can be inferred about their functional status by assessment of carpal alignment and motion on radiographs and fluoroscopy (Figs. 3-130 to 3-133).

Scapholunate dissociation is caused by disruption of the SL interosseous ligament *and* the extrinsic ligaments that stabilize this articulation (Figs. 3-131, 3-132). Normally, the scaphoid has approximately 45° of palmar angulation (normal range 30°–60°) and the lunate is in neutral alignment. Fixation to the lunate prevents the scaphoid from further palmar angulation induced by the compressive forces across the wrist joint. In scapholunate dissociation, the scaphoid is released from the lunate and rotates in a palmar direction. The lunate may or may not roll dorsally from its normal neutral alignment. When present, rotation of the lunate alters its appearance on a PA radiograph from the normal trapezoidal configuration to a triangular shape (Fig. 3-131). A PA radiograph may also reveal widening of the scapholunate interval above its normal value of 2 mm; 4 mm is considered to be pathognomonic. A gap between the scaphoid and lunate has been called the "Terry Thomas sign" in reference to the late, gap-toothed British comedian. A more current popular reference might be the "David Letterman sign."

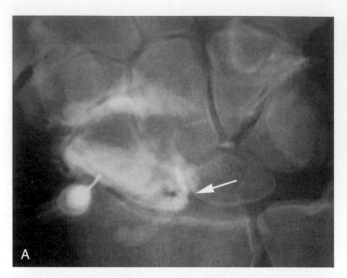

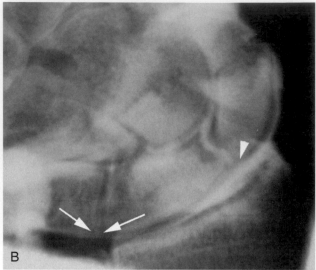

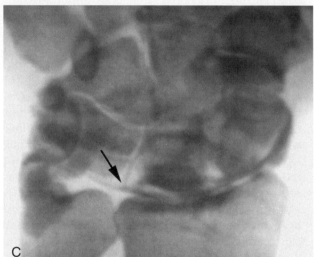

Fig. 3-128   Intrinsic ligament tears. **A,** Scapholunate ligament tear. Radiocarpal injection shows contrast passing through a scapholunate tear (*arrow*) into the midcarpal joint. **B,** Lunotriquetral ligament tear. Ulnar deviation view obtained after radiocarpal injection shows a lunotriquetral tear (*arrows*) with contrast filling the midcarpal compartment. The intact scapholunate ligament is seen as a filling defect (*arrowhead*). **C,** Lunotriquetral ligament tear. Note the contrast passing through the lunotriquetral ligament (*arrow*).

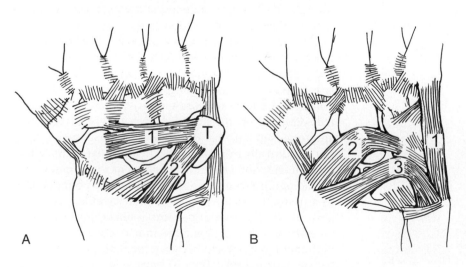

Fig. 3-129   Extrinsic (capsular) carpal ligament anatomy. **A,** Diagram of the dorsal carpal ligaments. The most important are labeled: 1, Dorsal intercarpal (transverse) ligament; 2, Dorsal radiocarpal (radioluntriquetral) ligament. Note that both insert onto the triquetrum (T). **B,** Diagram of the palmar carpal ligaments. The most important are labeled: 1, ulnar carpal complex (includes the ulnar collateral ligament); 2, distal arc (radioscaphocapitate and capitotriquetral, blends into 1); 3, proximal arc (radiolunotriquetral, also termed long radiolunate, and ulnotriquetral).

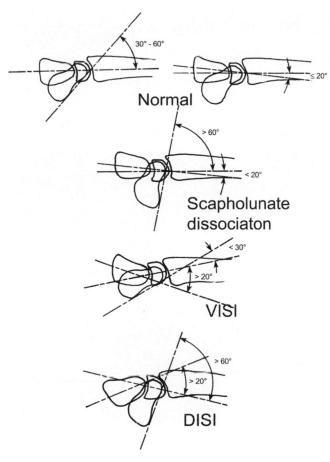

Fig. 3-130   Diagram of carpal instability patterns. All measurements require a well-positioned lateral view with the wrist in neutral alignment, not dorsiflexed.

A PA view obtained with a clenched fist or a PA view in ulnar deviation may elicit or increase this finding (Fig. 3-132). Fluoroscopy reveals the scaphoid and lunate to move independently of one another. In some cases of scapholunate dissociation, PA and lateral radiographs are normal, and the abnormality only becomes evident with fluoroscopy or a series of radiographs that reproduces the range of motion examined with fluoroscopy. Abnormal motion and distribution of forces associated with scapholunate dissociation can result in degeneration and collapse of the medial scaphoid and lateral lunate bones and radiocarpal joint, termed *scapholunate dissociation with advanced collapse* (SLAC wrist, Fig. 3-131C).

Dorsal intercalated segment instability (DISI, dorsiflexion instability) is usually but not necessarily associated with scapholunate dissociation. Like scapholunate dissociation, DISI is a derangement of the radial side of the wrist and is often associated with radial-sided symptoms. The lunate tilts *dorsally,* increasing the lunocapitate angle above 20°. The scapholunate angle is greater than 60° if scapholunate dissociation also is present, as it usually is (Fig. 3-131).

Volar intercalated segment instability (VISI, volar flexion instability) is a consequence of ulnar sided ligament derangement. The lunate is turned *volarly* and the capitolunate angle is greater than 20° (Fig. 3-133). Lunotriquetral dissociation is usually also present, so the scapholunate angle is decreased below 30°. Both lunotriquetral dissociation and VISI are associated with ulnar-sided pain. VISI is much less common than DISI. VISI may result from a fall onto the hypothenar eminence, but is also the most frequent carpal instability pattern encountered in patients with rheumatoid arthritis.

Lunotriquetral dissociation or instability results from disruption of the ligamentous fixation of the lunate and triquetrum. The condition is conceptually similar to scapholunate dissociation, but lunotriquetral instability does not typically result in LT widening. Subtle interruption of the carpal arcs may be seen, and the scapholunate angle may decrease to less than 30°. A clenched fist maneuver will roll the scaphoid and lunate into palmarflexion. Lunotriquetral instability usually occurs in association with VISI.

Capitolunate instability (capitolunate instability pattern, CLIP wrist) may occur as part of rotatory subluxation of the scaphoid, or as a dynamic instability of the central column. Manipulation of the capitate and lunate during fluoroscopy with the "CLIP maneuver," described in Appendix 1, may be needed to detect this condition.

Triquetrohamate instability is a dynamic instability of the medial column. The patients have ulnar sided pain and a reproducible click. Fluoroscopy reveals the click to correspond to the abnormal motion between the hamate and triquetrum. Normally, the proximal carpal row smoothly swings into dorsiflexion as the wrist goes into ulnar deviation. In triquetrohamate instability, the dorsiflexion is delayed until the wrist is fairly far into ulnar deviation, when the proximal carpal row abruptly flips into dorsiflexion with a painful clunk. Triquetrohamate instability is caused by forced pronation and radial deviation.

Carpal translocation can occur in any direction. Ulnar translocation of the entire carpus is associated with rheumatoid arthritis. Radial and dorsal carpal translocation is associated with a prior Colles fracture. Palmar carpal translocation is associated with a prior reverse Barton's fracture.

Miscellaneous Carpal Conditions

The tendons of the wrist can be studied with MRI, US, and injection of contrast into a tendon sheath under fluoroscopic guidance (tenography). MRI is the most widely used of these techniques. Normal tendons have very low signal intensity on all sequences; increased signal intensity may reflect degeneration, tendinitis, tearing, or fibrosis. The surrounding tendon sheath should contain only a small amount of fluid. Increased tendon sheath

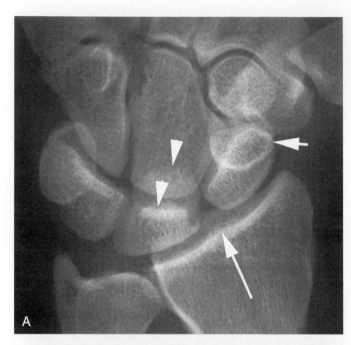

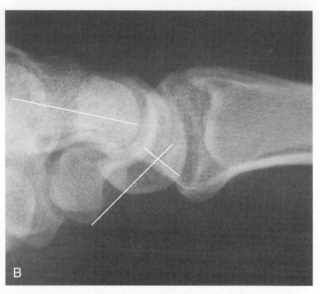

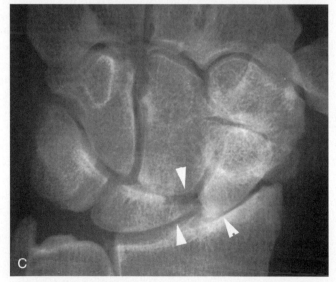

Fig. 3-131 Scapholunate dissociation and DISI. **A,** PA view shows a widened scapholunate interval (*long arrow*). The arrowheads mark the dorsal and volar margins of the distal lunate, which should be superimposed on a PA view. They do not overlap because the lunate is rotated dorsally. The scaphoid is rotated volarly, causing it to appear shortened on this PA view (*short arrow*). These findings are suggestive of scapholunate dissociation. **B,** Lateral view with lines drawn through the long axes of the lunate, scaphoid and capitate show the scapholunate angle greater than 60°, indicating scapholunate dissociation. Additionally, the capitolunate angle is greater than 20°, indicating DISI also is present. **C,** Followup PA radiograph 3 years later shows progression to SLAC wrist (*scapho*lunate *a*dvanced *c*ollapse), with collapse of the capitate into the lateral lunate and medial scaphoid (*arrowheads*).

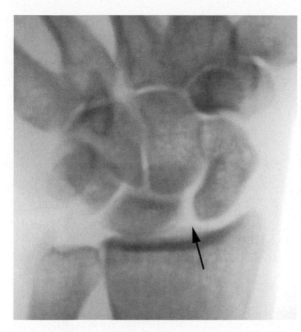

Fig. 3-132   Dynamic instability. PA and lateral radiographs (not shown) showed normal alignment. However, fluoroscopic spot view with ulnar deviation shows marked widening of the scapholunate interval (*arrow*) that was not evident on routine radiographs. (A small amount of scapholunate widening with ulnar deviation is normal). Additional fluoroscopy (not shown) showed dissociation of scaphoid and lunate motion.

fluid occurs in tenosynovitis. Rheumatoid arthritis causes pannus formation as well as fluid accumulation within the tendon sheaths. *De Quervain's disease* is stenosing tenosynovitis of the extensor pollicis brevis and abductor pollicis longus tendons.

Key Concepts   Hand Fractures

• Avulsion injuries may be subtle and are clinically important. The volar and dorsal aspects of the bases of the middle and distal phalanges, and the volar base of the thumb are the most frequent sites of important avulsion fractures.

Carpal tunnel syndrome is median nerve dysfunction caused by increased pressure within the carpal tunnel. The potential causes of carpal tunnel syndrome are many, including fracture, tenosynovitis, rheumatoid arthritis, gout, amyloid, tuberculosis, tumors, pregnancy, diabetes, and anomalous muscles. MR images may reveal edema or swelling of the median nerve. However, MRI is not a reliable method to diagnoses carpal tunnel syndrome. Most cases are diagnosed clinically, but MRI can be useful in identifying or excluding a surgically correctable cause, such as a mass lesion within the carpal tunnel (Fig. 3-134). Guyon's canal on the palmar medial wrist between the pisiform and the hook of the hamate contains the ulnar nerve and artery (Fig. 3-134). The same list of conditions that can cause median nerve impingement within the carpal tunnel can similarly afflict the ulnar nerve within Guyon's canal.

HAND

The thumb metacarpal (first MC) articulates with the trapezium constituting the first carpometacarpal joint (CMC I joint). The second MC articulates with the trape-

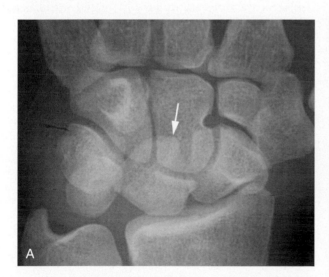
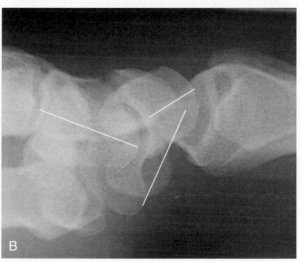

Fig. 3-133   VISI. **A,** PA view shows disruption of the carpal arcs. Note the triangular or "pie" shape of the lunate (*arrow*), indicating that it is rotated. **B,** Lateral view with lines drawn through the long axes of the lunate, scaphoid and capitate shows VISI alignment, with the scapholunate angle less than 30° and the capitolunate angle greater than 20°.

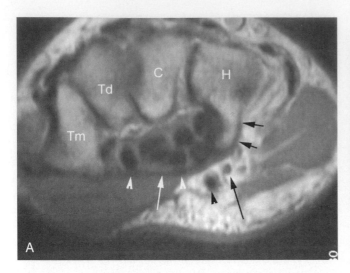
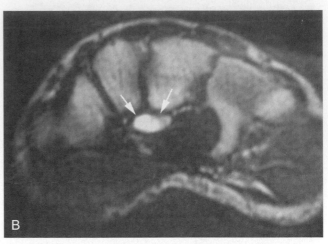

Fig. 3-134   Carpal tunnel and Guyon's canal. **A,** Axial proton density MR image shows normal anatomy of the carpal tunnel and Guyon's canal. The carpal tunnel is bounded by the trapezium (Tm), trapezoid (Td), capitate (C), hamate (H, with the hook marked by *short black arrows*), and the retinaculum (*white arrowheads*). The median nerve (*white arrow*) has intermediate signal intensity on this sequence because it contains myelin, which has signal characteristics similar to fat. A normal median nerve is difficult to identify on a fat suppressed sequence unless it is edematous. Guyon's canal is located palmar to the hook of the hamate. It contains the ulnar nerve (*long black arrow*) and the ulnar artery (*black arrowhead*). **B,** Carpal tunnel syndrome caused by a volar carpal ganglion. Axial T2-weighted MR image shows a round, sharply circumscribed mass with uniform high signal intensity in the dorsal portion of the carpal tunnel (*arrows*). These MR features are typical of a ganglion cyst. Mass effect from this cyst caused symptomatic median nerve compression. Resection of the ganglion cured the carpal tunnel syndrome.

zoid, the capitate and the third MC. The third MC also articulates with the capitate. The fourth and fifth MCs articulate with the hamate. The articulation of the second through fifth metacarpals and the distal carpal row forms a single synovial compartment, the CMC II–V joint. This compartment frequently communicates with the midcarpal joint as a normal variant. The articulations of the CMC II–V joint normally have a "zig-zag" pattern on a true PA radiograph with the palm and fingers flat against the cassette (Fig. 3-114A). Disruption of this pattern suggests that a dislocation is present (Fig. 3-135). CMC II–V dislocations are usually dorsal, may be multiple, and are often associated with small fractures. Conversely, the presence of a small fracture fragment at or adjacent to a CMC joint suggests that a dislocation is or was present.

Thumb injuries require dedicated radiographs because routine hand radiographs do not profile the thumb in true PA and lateral projection. Extraarticular fractures of the first metacarpal tend to maintain anatomic alignment because the muscle attachments along the shaft resist displacement. However, intraarticular fractures at the base of the thumb can displace and are frequently unstable. A *Bennett's fracture* is an intraarticular fracture-dislocation of the proximal first MC. The mechanism of injury is axial loading of a partially flexed first metacarpal, often sustained during a fistfight. The volar ligamentous fixation of the first MC is very strong, so a small volar bone

fragment is avulsed from the first MC and retains a normal position while the larger fragment subluxes or dislocates dorsally. A Bennett's fracture is unstable and is treated by ORIF. The unusual *Rolando's fracture* is a comminuted Bennett's fracture (Fig. 3-136). Restoration of anatomic alignment is often impossible due to the comminution, so these fractures are frequently treated with casting or traction rather than ORIF.

A *boxer's fracture* is a metacarpal fracture caused by abrupt axial loading, usually during delivery of a punch (Fig. 3-137). The neck of the fifth MC is the most frequent location, with the fourth MC similarly fractured in many cases. Apex dorsal angulation with volar comminution is common, and often results in healing with persistent angular deformity. A boxer's fracture may be complicated by an infection from the teeth of the recipient of the punch.

The metacarpophalangeal (MCP) and interphalangeal joints are stabilized against valgus stress and varus stress by ulnar (medial) and radial (lateral) collateral ligaments, respectively. Collateral ligament injuries can occur at any of these joints. The injured ligament may stretch, partially or completely tear, or avulse a small chip fragment. PA views with valgus or varus stress may be required for diagnosis of a collateral ligament injury. Comparison with the uninjured side can be helpful, as some laxity of the collateral ligaments is normal.

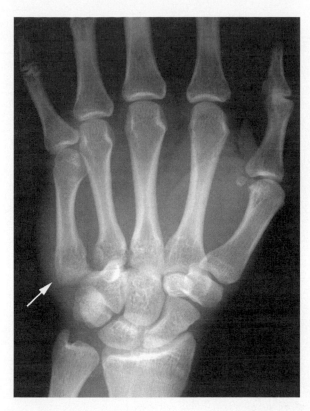

Fig. 3-135 Dislocation of the base of the fifth metacarpal. Note the lateral position of the base of the fifth metacarpal as well as the abnormal finding of a gap between the bases of the fourth and fifth metacarpals.

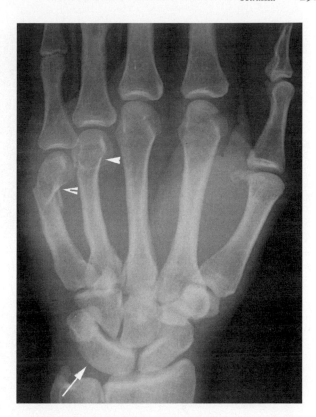

Fig. 3-137 Boxer's fractures. The fourth and fifth metacarpals show typical neck fractures with apex dorsolateral angulation (*arrowheads*). Also note the incidentally detected normal variant luno-triquetral coalition (*arrow*).

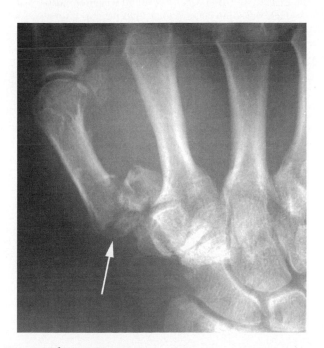

Fig. 3-136 Rolando fracture. Note the comminuted intra-articular fracture at the base of the thumb (*arrow*).

The most frequently injured collateral ligament in the hand is the ulnar collateral ligament (UCL) of the thumb MCP joint. This injury, better known as a *gamekeeper's thumb* or a *skier's thumb,* is caused by valgus stress across the thumb, often combined with hyperextension (Fig. 3-138). Gamekeeper's thumb was first recognized as an occupational hazard of British gamekeepers, whose method of killing wounded rabbits placed valgus stress across the thumb. After several years of this overuse, the gamekeeper's UCL became stretched or torn, and the consequent instability resulted in pain and disability. Today, a thumb MCP UCL injury is often sustained as an acute injury suffered while falling on an outstretched hand while holding a ski pole. The tip of the thumb extends beyond the ski pole handle into the snow as the skier's forward momentum drives the hand forward, resulting in thumb valgus and hyperextension. A faulty pole plant has also been suggested as a cause of a UCL injury in skiers. Most UCL strains and partial tears, as well as some minimally displaced complete tears or avulsions, are managed by immobilization. However, complete tears often require surgical exploration to locate and reattach the free edges of the torn UCL. In particular, the thumb adductor tendon aponeurosis can become interposed between the torn edges of the UCL, a situation

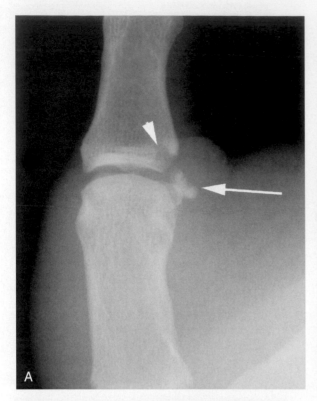

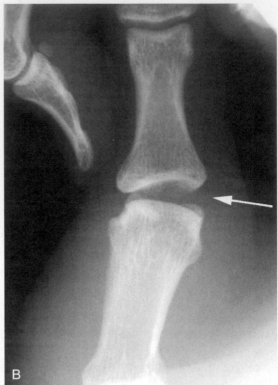

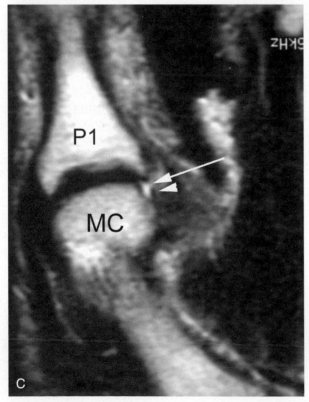

Fig. 3-138   Skier's (gamekeeper's) thumb. **A,** AP view of the thumb shows an avulsion fracture at the distal insertion of the ulnar collateral ligament (UCL). Note the small avulsion fragment (*arrow*) and the donor site on the proximal phalanx (*arrowhead*). **B,** UCL injury without avulsion fracture in a different patient. The MCP joint has widened medially with stress (*arrow*), indicating laxity or disruption of the UCL. **C,** MR diagnosis. Coronal T2-weighted image shows high signal intensity of joint fluid passing through the interruption of the UCL (*arrow*). The arrowhead marks the intact, proximal portion of the UCL. P1, proximal phalanx. MC, thumb metacarpal.

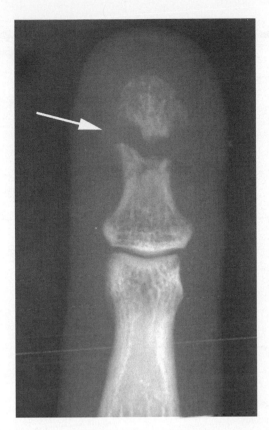

Fig. 3-145   Distal phalangeal injury (*arrow*) caused by hedge clippers.

(think hammer, car door, or table saw) (Fig. 3-145). Phalangeal shaft fractures are often dorsally angulated. Accurate assessment of fracture angulation requires a true lateral radiograph. Rotational deformity is also important, but may be assessed clinically.

REFERENCE

1. Chan KK, Muldoon KA, Yeh L, et al: Superior labral anteroposterior lesions: MR arthrography with arm traction. *AJR* 173:1117-22, 1999.

SOURCES AND SUGGESTED READINGS

Beltran J, Bncardino J, Mellad J, Rosenberg ZS, Irsh RD: MR arthrography of the shoulder: variants and pitfalls. *Radiographics* 17:1403-1412, 1977.

Beltran J, Rosenberg, ZS: Diagnosis of compressive and entrapment neuropathies of the upper extremity: value of MR imaging. *Am J Roentgenol* 163:525-31, 1994.

Gilula LA, Yin Y: *Imaging of the wrist and hand,* 1996, Philadelphia, W. B. Saunders.

Goldfarb CA, Yin Y, Gilula LA, Fisher AJ, Boyer, M: Wrist fractures: what the clinician wants to know. *Radiology* 219:11-28, 2001.

Holsbeeck MV, Introscaso JH: *Musucloskeletal Ultrasound,* ed 2, 2001, St. Louis, Mosby-Year Book.

Kaplan PA, Helms CA, Dussault R, Anderson MW, Major NM: *Musculoskeletal MRI,* 2001, Philadelphia, W.B. Saunders.

Massengill AD, Seeger LL, Yao L, et al. Labrocapuslar ligamentous complex of the shoulder: normal anatomy, anatomic variations, and pitfalls of MR imaging and MR arthrography. *Radiographics* 1994;14:1211-1223.

Manaster BJ: *Handbook of skeletal radiology,* ed 2, St. Louis, 1997, Mosby.

Oneson SR, Scales LM, Timins ME, Erickson SJ, Chamoy L: MR imaging interpretation of the Palmer classification of triangular fibrocartilage complex lesions. *Radiographics* 16:97-106, 1996.

Resnick D, Kang HS: *Internal derangements of joints* W. B. Saunders, 1997, Philadelphia

Rockwood CH, Green DP, Bucholz RW, Heckman JD, eds: *Fractures in adults,* ed 4, Philadelphia, 1996, Lippincott-Raven.

Rockwood CH, Wilkins KE, Beaty JH, eds: *Fractures in children,* ed 4, Philadelphia, 1996, Lippincott-Raven.

Smith DK. MR imaging of normal and injured wrist ligaments. *Mag Res Imaging Clin North Am* 3:229-48, 1995.

Sonin AH, Tutton SM, Fitzgerald SW, Peduto AJ: MR imaging of the adult elbow. *Radiographics* 16:1323-36, 1996.

Steinbach LS, Peterfy CG, eds: *Shoulder magnetic resonance imaging* 1998, Philadelphia, Lippincott Williams & Wilkins.

Stoller D: *Magnetic resonance imaging in orthopaedics and sports medicine,* ed 2, Lippencott-Raven, 1997, Philadelphia.

Tuite MJ, Cirillo RL, De Smet AA, Orwin JF: Superior labrum anterior-posterior (SLAP) tears: evaluation of three MR signs on T2-weighted images. *Radiology* 21:841-845, 2000.

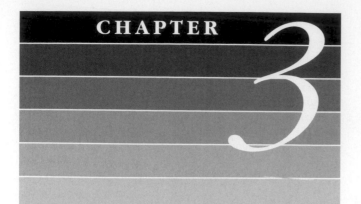

CHAPTER 3

Trauma

LOWER EXTREMITY TRAUMA

PART III

DAVID G. DISLER, M.D.

PELVIC TRAUMA

Anatomy

The pelvis is a complex anatomic region created by three bones, the two innominate bones and the sacrum. The innominate bone is formed by synostosis of the ilium, pubis, and ischium, that join at the medial wall of the acetabulum, physically recognized in childhood as the triradiate or Y cartilage of the acetabulum. In skeletally immature patients this region may be confused with fracture. Medially, the innominate bones are adjoined at the symphysis pubis, which is a synchondrosis similar embryologically and morphologically to the disks of the spine. The sacrum and ilium are adjoined at the sacroiliac joints,

Key Concepts | **Pelvic Trauma**

- Pelvic fractures may be extremely subtle. Careful attention to osseous outlines is important in radiographic assessment.
- Pelvic fractures may result from anterioposterior (AP) or PA compression, lateral compression, vertical shear, or combination forces. Stability is determined by the number of breaks in the pelvic ring, with two or more breaks being unstable.
- Acetabular fractures are classified separately from pelvic girdle fractures, although considered by some as a subtype of pelvic fractures.
- Acetabular fractures are determined by the position of the femoral head and the direction of force of the femoral head against the acetabular margin at the time of injury. There are five elementary and five combination varieties of fracture. The most common elementary fracture is a posterior wall fracture. The most common combination fracture is a transverse-posterior wall fracture.

which are a complex form of articulation consisting partly of synovial joint and of syndesmosis. The true synovial joint is in the anterior third and inferior half of the articulation whereas the strong ligamentous attachments of the syndesmosis are present in the remaining areas. The pelvis is joined with the spine at the L5–S1 disk. The pelvis is attached at the lower extremity at the hip joints, two synovial joints that act as a ball-and-socket form of articulation.

The pelvis can be considered a ringlike structure formed by two dominant arches. The major arch is posterior and superior, formed by the iliac wings and sacrum, joined at the sacroiliac joints. The smaller arch is anterior and inferior formed by the pubic and ischial bones, joined at the symphysis pubis. There are in fact three rings in the pelvis. The largest is that of the ring connecting sacrum, sacroiliac joints, iliac and pubic bones, and symphysis pubis. The other two rings are the obturator foramens consisting of pubic bones and ischia. As with any ring, a break in one portion of the ring is usually accompanied by a break in another portion of the ring. Breaks may form at bone or articulation. When isolated fractures of the pelvis occur, they are usually in the form of an iliac wing fracture or an avulsion fracture.

The pelvis is supported by extremely strong ligamentous attachments. It therefore requires enormous force to cause a fracture of the pelvis. In addition, the pelvis is rich in vascular supply and therefore prone to life-threatening hemorrhage after trauma. Neurologic injury is also possible. Injury to the smaller nerves of the pelvis are commonly affected after pelvic trauma. As an example, erectile dysfunction is a common complication after injury in males, and results from a combination of neuro-

logic and vascular injury. Furthermore, the sciatic nerve, although only rarely transected, often is affected by adjacent hematoma, edema, or posttraumatic fibrosis that results in a variable degree of transient neurologic dysfunction. Urologic injury is also common after pelvic trauma with extraperitoneal and intraperitoneal bladder ruptures and, in males, urethral disruption common sequellae.

There are five major vertically oriented radiographic lines in the innominent bone that require careful scrutiny on the AP pelvis radiograph (Fig. 3-146). The first is the *iliopectineal* (iliopubic) *line*. This runs along the inner margin of the ilium and around the superior margin of the pubis. The second is the *ilioischial line,* which runs along the inner margin of the ilium then inferiorly along the medial margin of the ischium. The third is the *teardrop,* which is a summation opacity related to the medial margin of the acetabulum and posterior acetabular wall. Finally, the fourth and fifth lines are the *anterior and posterior rims of the acetabulum.* These represent the lateral margins of the anterior and posterior walls of the acetabulum. Each of these lines should be smoothly contoured. Any interruption or irregularity of the line should be viewed with suspicion for the presence of fracture. Evaluation of the anterior and posterior acetabular rims is particularly difficult on frontal pelvis radiographs, because isolated fractures are oriented in the coronal plane and thus may be obscured on the radiograph. Usually the presence of a posterior wall fracture is inferred only by obscuration of visualization of the posterior rim.

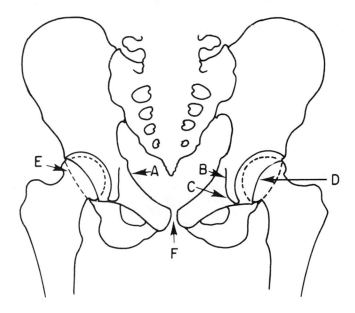

Fig. 3-146   Diagram of AP pelvis demonstrating anatomic landmarks to assess in the setting of trauma. A, Iliopubic line. B, Ilioischial line. C, Teardrop. D, Anterior acetabular rim. E, Posterior acetabular rim. F, Symphysis pubis. (From Manaster BJ. *Handbook of Skeletal Radiology,* ed 2, St. Louis, 1997, Mosby-Yearbook).

Sacral fractures can be extraordinarily subtle in appearance. The neuroformanal lines of the sacrum require careful evaluation as subtle irregularity usually indicates a fracture. The presence of a transverse process fracture at L5 suggests the presence of occult sacral fracture, as forces that produce this fracture are similar to those that produce a sacral fracture. The margins of the sacroiliac joints and symphysis pubis should be parallel and smoothly contoured. Sacroiliac joints are normally no greater than 4 mm wide in adults. Any asymmetry should be viewed with suspicion for diastasis. The symphysis pubis may be up to 5 mm in width in adults and 10 mm in skeletally immature patients. Superoinferior offset up to 2 mm is normal when evaluating the superior pubic margins. However, the inferior margins at the symphysis pubis should be symmetrically placed.

Radiography of the pelvis is limited in its sensitivity for detection of pelvic fracture. The addition of Judet views, or 45° bilateral oblique views, increases sensitivity and helps delineate fracture patterns in the pelvis. This is because the oblique views allow better evaluation of the ischium and pubis in elongated projection. The bilateral Judet views are complementary views in that although one view will show the posterior wall and anterior acetabular rim on one side, it will show the pubis and ischium on the contralateral side (Fig. 3-147). This is critical anatomy for assessment of acetabular fracture patterns. Thin section CT at 3-mm intervals is reserved for cases in which radiographically occult fracture is suspected and for preoperative planning in the setting of a fracture. Furthermore, CT allows multiplanar and 3D reformations which are helpful in preoperative planning.

Fractures

Biomechanical Classification

Fractures of the pelvis may occur in the pelvic girdle or in the acetabulum and both sites have separate classification schemes. Pelvic fractures are due to anteroposterior (or posteroanterior) compression, lateral compression, or vertical shearing forces, each with unique fracture patterns.

In *lateral compression,* the essential elemental forces result from lateral impaction injury, such as a passenger-side motor vehicle accident. The clue to lateral compression is the presence of *horizontal* fractures of the superior and inferior pubic rami (Fig. 3-148). Type I injury involves a direct blow to the acetabulum with fractures involving the medial acetabular wall without substantial associated innominate bone rotation. In a type II fracture the lateral compressive force is located more anteriorly resulting in the internal rotation of ipsilateral iliac wing, thus resulting in not only pubic and ischial fracture but also disruption of the posterior sacroiliac joint ligaments (or a fracture through the posterior iliac wing). A type III lateral compression involves a greater force in which there is internal rotation of the ipsilateral innominate bone and external rotation of the contralateral innominate bone. With the exception of type III injury, incidence of substantial arterial hemorrhage is low with lateral compression.

In *anteroposterior compression,* injury results from frontal or dorsal forces in motor vehicle accidents. With this injury pattern, the identifying fractures are the *vertical* fractures of the superior and inferior pubic rami (Fig.

Fig. 3-147 Judet (oblique) view of the pelvis. Note that the anterior (obturator) oblique view shows the anterior column and posterior acetabular rim best, whereas the posterior (iliac) oblique view shows the posterior column and anterior acetabular rim best. A, anterior column and iliopubic line. B, posterior column and ilioischial line. C, anterior acetabular rim. D, posterior acetabular rim. E, ischial spine. F, ischial tuberosity. G, obturator foramen. (From Manaster BJ. *Handbook of Skeletal Radiology,* ed 2, St. Louis, 1997, Mosby-Yearbook).

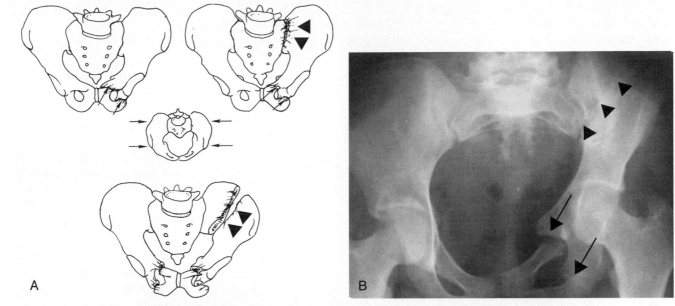

Fig. 3-148   Diagram illustrating lateral compression injury. Central figure with arrow demonstrates direction of force. Note that signature fracture pattern is horizontal fractures of the superior and inferior pubic rami (*arrows*). Note that greater degrees of force result in ipsilateral iliac wing internal rotation with sacroiliac joint disruption or iliac wing fracture (*arrowheads*). **A,** Greater force will result in contralateral innominate bone external rotation. **B,** Radiograph demonstrating features of lateral compression with horizontal fractures of superior and inferior pubic rami (*arrows*). Iliac wing fracture (*arrowheads*) and internal rotation of ipsilateral innominate bone.

3-149). Depending on the location of impact, variable fracture patterns are shown. For example, impact directly to the symphysis pubis may result in bilateral superior and inferior pubic rami fractures called a "*straddle*" fracture. Impact posteriorly can result in an "open-book" pattern, in which either sacroiliac joint and symphysis pubis diastasis are shown or vertically oriented fractures adjacent to these articulations occur. This results in disruption of both the anterior and posterior pelvis, with disruption of the anterior and posterior sacroiliac joint ligaments as well as variable disruption of the sacrospinous and sacrotuberus ligaments. As the femoral head often impacts the acetabulum with anteroposterior compression, there is a high incidence of posterior acetabular fractures with this form of injury. A type I fracture shows vertical pubic ramus fractures, a type II fracture is an "open-book" type fracture with symphysis pubis diastasis and disruption of the anterior sacroiliac ligaments, and a type III fracture is a "sprung pelvis" and involves diastasis of the symphysis pubis and sacroiliac joints, with disruption of the anterior and posterior sacroiliac joint ligaments. Variations occur, such as the "bucket handle" fracture, in which ipsilateral vertical fractures of the superior and inferior pubic rami are associated with contralateral sacroiliac joint diastasis versus adjacent fracture. Type II and III fractures have a higher likelihood of associated arterial hemorrhage.

In *vertical shear,* superior–inferior forces predominate resulting in *vertical displacement* of a portion of the pelvis (Fig. 3-150). The appearance of ipsilateral rami and sacroiliac disruptions is termed a *Malgaigne* fracture. The site of displacement may be at the symphysis pubis and sacroiliac joint or adjacent pubic ramus, sacrum, and ilium. This injury is an unstable injury with the highest association with arterial hemorrhage.

Management of pelvic fractures in the acute setting is the control of life-threatening hemorrhage. Hemorrhage is most highly associated with type III lateral compression, types II and III anteroposterior compression and vertical shear injuries. Initial orthopedic management is to stabilize the pelvis, most commonly with the placement of external fixation pins in the iliac wings. This is usually performed in the emergency department. Sacroiliac joint diastasis or sacral distraction can be treated with placement of percutaneous transverse lag screws. Symphysis pubis, pubic ramus, and iliac wing fractures are usually reduced intraoperatively with malleable plates. The adoption of percutaneous external fixation has resulted in reduced bleeding complications and has diminished the need for arteriographic embolization. Hemodynamically unstable patients, however, require immediate arteriography and embolization.

Pelvic ring classification   Pelvic fractures can also be classified by the degree of disruption of the pelvic

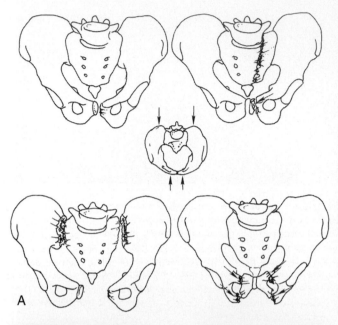

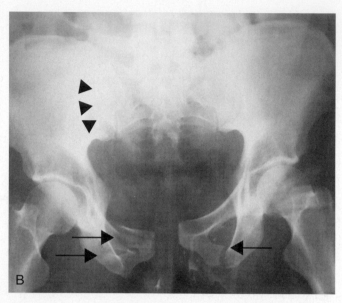

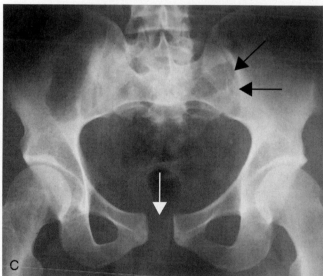

Fig. 3-149   Anteroposterior compression. **A,** Diagram demonstrates features of anteroposterior compression. Central figure demonstrates direction of forces. Signature fracture pattern is vertically oriented fractures of superior and inferior pubic rami (*arrows*) or symphysis pubis diastasis. With increasing force there is variable sacroiliac diastasis or sacral fracture. **B,** Radiograph demonstrates features of anteroposterior compression with vertically oriented fractures of superior and inferior pubic rami (*arrows*), symphysis pubis diastasis, and right sacroiliac joint diastasis (*arrowheads*). **C,** Radiograph demonstrating features of anteroposterior force with symphysis pubis and left sacroiliac joint diastasis (*arrows*).

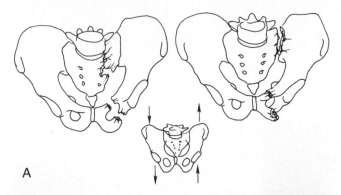

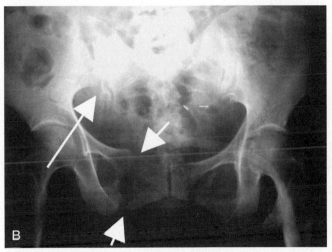

Fig. 3-150 Vertical shear. **A,** Diagram demonstrating features of vertical shear. Central lower figure demonstrates direction of forces. Signature feature is that of vertical malalignment of pelvis. **B,** Radiograph demonstrates Malgaigne fracture. This pelvic fracture demonstrates ipsilateral fractures of the inferior and superior pubic rami as well as the iliac wing adjacent to the SI joint (*arrows*). Note that there is superior displacement of the right innominate bone relative to the sacrum and left side. This is an unstable fracture.

ring. Class I fractures (Fig. 3-151) are isolated fractures that do not disrupt the pelvic ring. Class II fractures disrupt the ring in one location (Fig. 3-152). Class III fractures disrupt the ring in at least two locations and Class IV fractures disrupt the acetabulum.

Class I and Class II Fractures: Apophyseal avulsion injuries are one form of Class I fractures (Fig. 3-151). There are five apophyses that appear by puberty and fuse by the mid-third decade. These are at the iliac crest, the anterior-superior iliac spine (the origin of the sartorius muscle), the anterior-inferior iliac spine (the origin of the rectus femoris muscle), the iscial tuberosity (the origin of the hamstring muscles), and the inferior pubic ramus (the origin of the adductor muscles). Avulsions may be subtle in the skeletally immature patient, because they are in fact Salter-Harris growth plate injuries. Subtle asymmetry in the width of the growth plates may be apparent initially; however, such injuries usually become evident only during healing when amorphous bone formation between the pelvis and the avulsed fragment becomes apparent. In early stages of healing, immature bone formation may be confused with osteosarcoma. Such avulsions are particularly confusing at the ischial tuberosity and the inferior pubic ramus with the occasional appearance of osseous enlargement and sclerosis further confusing the correct diagnosis. Other forms of Class I fracture

are iliac wing fractures, isolated sacral fractures and isolated ischial or pubic rami fractures. Sacral fractures may occur acutely because of direct blows and are usually transverse. Occasionally insufficiency fractures may occur in the sacrum (Fig. 3-153), most often in the setting of osteoporosis or after radiation therapy and are seen as vertical areas of mixed lucency and density along the sacral wings, often with a horizontal portion through the mid S2 or S3 levels. More commonly they are radiographically occult and are detected at CT, MRI, or bone scan imaging. An isolated pubic ramus fracture may also occur from a direct blow, and like the sacrum, is also prone to insufficiency fracture among osteoporotic patients and patients post-radiation therapy. These fractures may assume bizarre appearances with bone expansion and aggressive appearing new bone formation mimicking osteosarcoma. The pubic bones are also common locations for pseudofractures of osteomalacia (Looser's zones). Among patients with normal bone mineralization, pubic stress fractures are most common at the junction of the pubis and ischium, especially among long distance runners. This is also the location of the ischiopubic synchondrosis which in the skeletally immature patient can produce difficulty with diagnosis.

Class III fractures: Class III fractures are unstable fractures and represent one-third of cases of pelvic

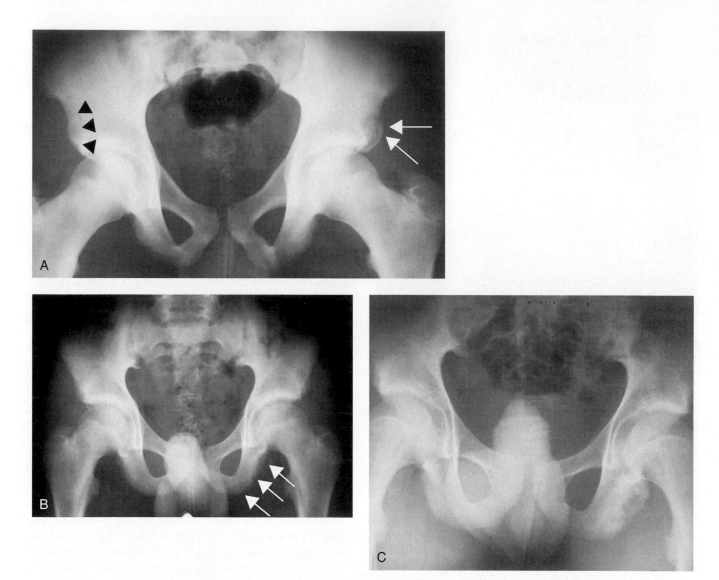

Fig. 3-151   Examples of class I fracture. **A,** Frontal radiograph of pelvis demonstrates avulsion of left anterior inferior iliac spine (*arrows*). Fracture occurred at growth plate. Note open growth plate on contralateral side (*arrowheads*). **B,** AP radiograph demonstrates avulsion of left ischial tuberosity (*arrows*). Note follow-up film, **C,** with proliferative bone formation mimicking osteosarcoma. Follow-up radiograph was obtained 13 months after the first study.

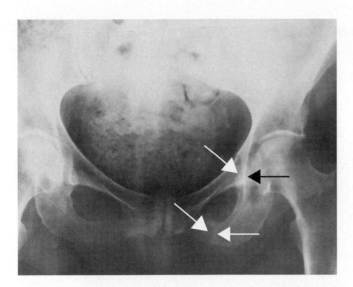

Fig. 3-152 AP radiograph demonstrating Class II fracture. There are fractures isolated to the left superior and inferior pubic rami (*arrows*).

trauma. These involve pelvic disruption in two or more locations and can assume any of the patterns as described under the biomechanics section. These are unstable fractures due to the presence of extensive ligamentous injury and are associated with significant risk for visceral injury and internal hemorrhage.

Class IV fractures: Class IV fractures, or acetabular fractures, occur in the setting of forces directed to the acetabulum through the femoral head. Depending on the direction of forces and the position of the femoral head at the time of injury a variety of fracture patterns may be found (Fig. 3-154). The most commonly used classification system is that of Letournet and Judet. This classification system is based on an understanding of the anterior and posterior column anatomical description of load bearing. The *anterior column* is the anterior portion of the pelvis that allows load bearing from the spine to the lower extremity. The *posterior column* is the posterior portion of the pelvis that allows load bearing from the spine to the lower extremity. The anterior and posterior columns are not the anterior and posterior walls. Instead, they are the entire load-bearing portion of the hemipelvis anteriorly and posteriorly. Thus the posterior column consists of the sciatic notch region of the hemipelvis, the posterior acetabular wall, and the ischium. The anterior column consists of the iliopectineal line, the anterior acetabular wall, and the superior and inferior pubic rami.

There are five primary or elemental fracture patterns of the acetabulum. These are anterior wall, posterior wall, transverse, anterior column, and posterior column fractures. The most common primary fracture of the acetabulum is a *posterior wall* fracture, occurring in 17% of all acetabular fractures (Fig. 3-155). Wall fractures refer to fracture lines in the nonweight bearing lips or rims of

the anterior and posterior acetabulum. Column fractures refer to separation of the anterior or posterior weight bearing portions of the pelvis from the remainder of the pelvis. For example, in the *posterior column* fracture, the fracture line extends from the sciatic notch through the medial wall of the acetabulum, the acetabular floor, and the ischiopubic junction. Thus the ischium, posterior acetabulum, and sciatic notch region are separated from the remainder of the hemipelvis. *Anterior column* fractures appear as fracture lines extending through the iliac wing, the medial wall of the acetabulum, the acetabular floor, and the ischiopubic junction. Thus anterior column fracture separates the anterior weight-bearing portion of the hemipelvis from the remainder of the hemipelvis. A *transverse* fracture (Fig. 3-156) separates the upper hemipelvis from the lower hemipelvis and can occur above, at, or inferior to the roof of the acetabulum. Transverse fractures occur in 10% of acetabular fractures.

Associated, or combination, fractures are those in which more than one elementary fracture is present. The five major associated fracture patterns are transverse-posterior wall (Fig. 3-157), T-shaped (Fig. 3-158), both column, posterior column-posterior wall, and anterior wall-posterior hemitransverse fractures. Of these associated fracture patterns, the *transverse-posterior wall* fracture is most common, occurring in 19% of acetabular fractures.

Judet views are extremely useful in evaluating acetabular fractures because the oblique views give assessment of the cortical margins both anteriorly and posteriorly at the acetabulum. A fracture line extending anteroposteriorly involving iliopectineal and ilioischial lines must be a transverse fracture. Vertical fractures arising from the sciatic notch must be posterior column fractures. Vertically oriented fractures through the iliac wing and acetabulum must be anterior column fractures. Fractures isolated to the rims of the acetabulum must be anterior or posterior wall fractures. If the obturator ring is disrupted, the acetabular fracture must be either a T-shaped fracture or a column fracture. If there is a "spur" sign, representing a spur of bone, located superior and posterior to the acetabulum on the obturator oblique view, there must be a posterior column or both column fracture. CT imaging is also extremely useful in evaluation of the acetabulum because fracture lines are more clearly demonstrated, and multi-planar and 3-D reformations are possible, thus aiding preoperative planning. On CT, if an acetabular fracture plane is sagittal (directed anteroposteriorly) it is a transverse fracture. If it is coronal and through the medial wall it is either an anterior or posterior column fracture. Sagittally oriented or oblique fractures isolated to the anterior or posterior rim are wall fractures.

MR Imaging

MR imaging has two distinct advantages over the other forms of imaging. First it is capable of superb soft tissue

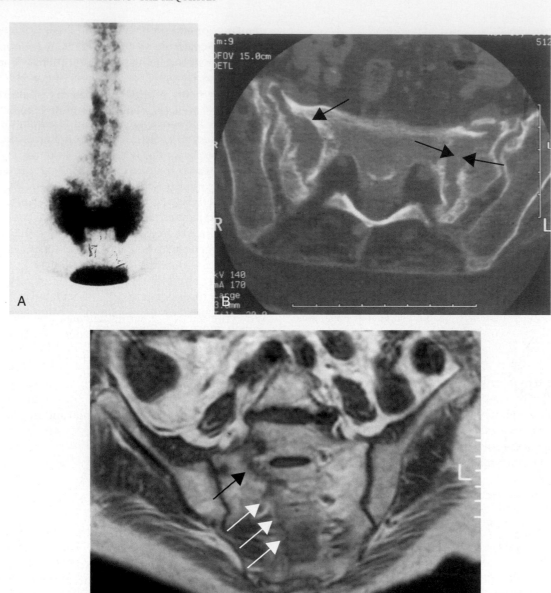

Fig. 3-153   Stress fracture of the sacrum. **A,** Radionuclide bone scan image demonstrates intense H-shaped uptake in sacrum. This pattern is typical of sacral insufficiency fracture. **B,** Axial CT image of same patient demonstrates chronic fracture lines in both sacral wings (*arrows*). Sclerotic opposing margins indicate chronic nature of insufficiency fracture. **C,** Oblique coronal T1-weighted spin echo image (600/15; TR msec/TE msec) demonstrating insufficiency fracture line in right sacral wing (*arrows*).

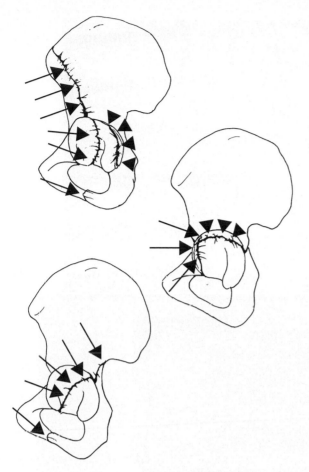

Fig. 3-154 Diagram demonstrating fracture patterns of the acetabulum. Top diagram shows anterior column (*arrows*) and posterior wall (*arrowheads*) patterns. Middle diagram demonstrates anterior wall (*arrows*) and transverse (*arrowheads*) patterns. Bottom image demonstrates posterior column (*arrows*) pattern.

contrast, thus allowing assessment for extensive soft tissue injury. Secondly, it allows excellent marrow contrast permitting high sensitivity and specificity in the detection of radiographically occult fracture. MR imaging thus has a particularly useful role in the assessment of radiographically occult fracture, stress fracture (especially sacral stress fracture), and muscle strain. It is useful in studying patients with substantial pelvic pain in the absence of radiographic or CT findings, and can explain patient symptoms thus directing further therapy.

HIP TRAUMA

Anatomy

The hip is a ball and socket joint. The joint is invested by a strong capsule and is supported by the iliofemoral, pubofemoral, and ischiofemoral ligaments, with further support from the acetabular labrum, the transverse acetabular ligament, and the ligament of the head of the femur (ligamentum teres). The vascular supply to the femoral head is tenuous. Although there is contribution to the vascular supply of the femoral head by the artery of the ligamentum teres, the majority of arterial supply is from the medial and lateral circumflex femoral arteries, which are primary branches of the common femoral artery. In the frontal plane, the normal angle between the femoral neck and shaft averages 135° with a range of 115–140°. On a groin lateral (true lateral) radiograph, femoral neck-shaft ankle is 125–130°. The femoral neck is also *anteverted* (anteriorly rotated) relative to the femoral shaft by approximately 15°. The greater trochanter and lesser trochanter are both *posterior* structures. The lesser trochanter is posteromedial in location and the greater trochanter posterolateral. Thus, when the femur is internally located, the greater trochanter is shown in profile and the lesser trochanter is hidden from view. When the femur is externally rotated, the lesser trochanter is in profile and the greater trochanter is hidden from view. This anatomic relationship plays an important role in assessment of hip dislocations, which will be described later in the chapter. Furthermore, the posterior positions of the greater and lesser trochanters obscure visualization of the femoral neck on both frontal and frog-lateral radiographic views of the hip. These two views also foreshorten the radiographic appearance of the femoral neck. Because of these limitations, assessment of trauma to the hip requires the groin lateral (true lateral) view. This view profiles the femoral neck without superimposition of the trochanters (Fig. 3-159).

There are three fat planes evident on a hip radiograph. These are the iliopsoas, gluteal, and obturator internus fat planes. They are occasionally useful for assessing the presence of hip effusion, because in the presence of hip effusions, these fat planes may bulge away from the hip joint. As one may expect, assessment of fat planes at the hip lacks sensitivity and specificity for the assessment of effusion. A more reliable indicator may be measurement of the distance between the teardrop of the acetabulum and the medial femoral head with asymmetric increase indicating the side of effusion.

Dislocation

Dislocation is an unusual complication of trauma, often overlooked because of its common association with femoral shaft fractures that dominate the clinical evaluation. Approximately 90% of dislocations are posterior. Posterior dislocations are especially common after motor vehicle accidents in which the flexed knee strikes the dashboard. Because the femoral head is driven posteriorly, posterior hip dislocation is commonly associated with fracture of the posterior acetabular wall. With posterior dislocation, the femoral head is typically not only

Text continued on p. 310

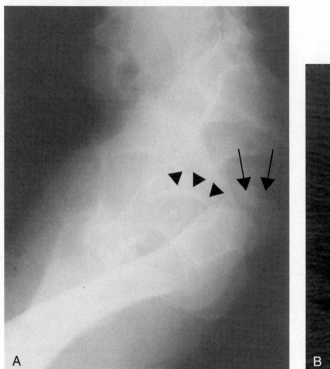
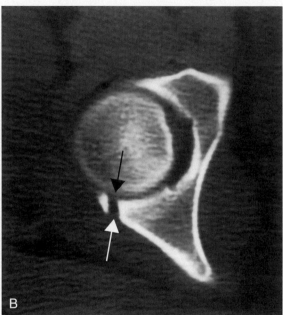

Fig. 3-155   Posterior wall fracture in setting of posterior dislocation. **A,** Lateral radiograph demonstrates posterior dislocation of femoral head (*arrows*). Note empty acetabular fossa (*arrowheads*). **B,** Axial CT image obtained after hip relocation demonstrates fracture of posterior wall (*arrows*) with only minimal displacement.

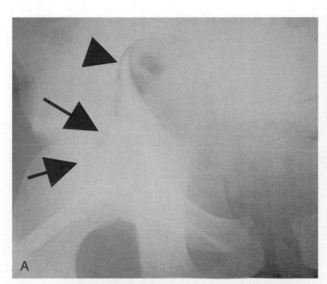

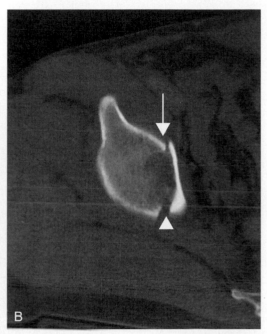

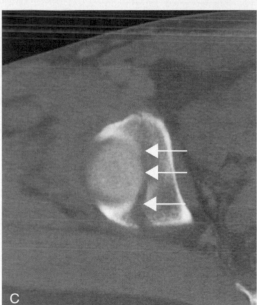

Fig. 3-156 Transverse fracture of acetabulum. **A,** Frontal radiograph demonstrates fracture line through the acetabulum with involvement of ilioischial line (*arrowhead*). Note transverse orientation of fracture line through the acetabulum (*arrows*). **B,** Axial CT image demonstrates transverse fracture line. Note sagittal orientation of fracture with involvement of anterior (*arrow*) and posterior (*arrowhead*) walls. **C,** Axial CT image (caudal to **B**) demonstrates transverse fracture line (*arrows*) as it courses laterally through the acetabulum.

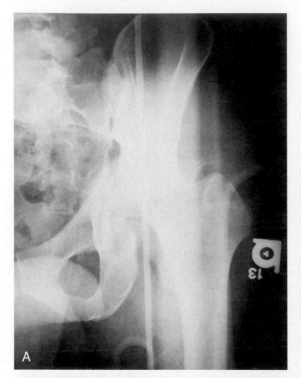

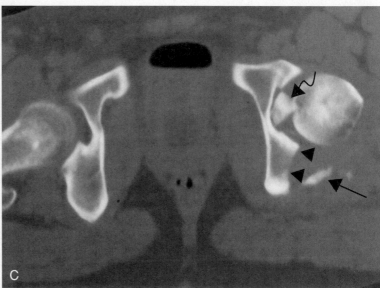

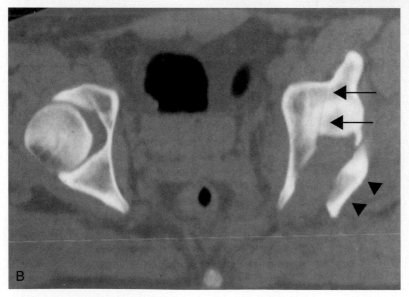

Fig. 3-157   Transverse-posterior wall associated fractures. **A,** Frontal radiograph demonstrates posterior dislocation or hip and complex fracture pattern at acetabulum. **B,** Axial CT image after hip relocation demonstrates transverse fracture line (*arrows*) and displaced posterior wall fragments (*arrowheads*). **C,** Axial CT image caudal to (**B**) demonstrates posterior wall fracture (*arrow*) with blunted posterior wall margin (*arrowheads*) and displaced intraarticular fracture fragment (curved arrow) preventing complete femoral head reduction.

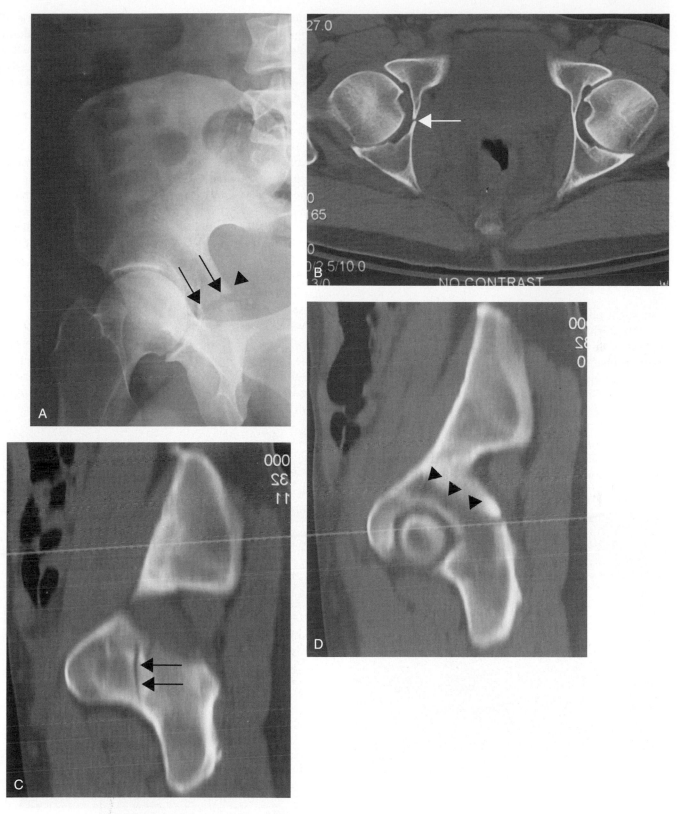

Fig. 3-158   T-shaped fracture. **A,** Iliac Judet view demonstrates transverse fracture line (*arrows*) extending to ilioischial line (*arrowhead*). **B,** axial CT image demonstrates a vertical component of T-shaped fracture in medial wall of acetabulum (*arrow*). **C** and **D,** sagittal reformations of acetabulum demonstrating vertical (*arrows*) and transverse (*arrowheads*) components of T-shaped fracture in medial wall and roof of acetabulum.

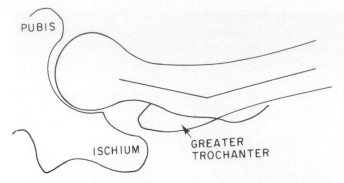

Fig. 3-159   Groin lateral view of hip, demonstrating the normal anatomy and normal neck-shaft angle. Note that the trochanters project posterior to the femoral neck, allowing radiographic assessment of femoral neck fracture without superimposition of the trochanters. (From Manaster BJ. *Handbook of Skeletal Radiology,* ed 2, St. Louis, 1997, Mosby-Yearbook).

posteriorly positioned relative to the acetabulum, but also superiorly positioned, and the femur is in internal rotation with the greater trochanter in profile and the lesser trochanter obscured (Fig. 3-160). Clinically, the lower extremity appears adducted, extended, and internally rotated, and is shortened because of superior femoral head displacement. Radiographically, dislocations are easy to recognize if the femoral head is superior in position relative to the acetabulum. However, the degree of superior displacement may be minimal. In these situations dislocation may be difficult to recognize on the frontal film. In such subtle cases there may be lack of congruence of the femoral head and the acetabulum. Additionally, a dislocated femoral head appears smaller than the contralateral femoral head because the dislocated femoral head is posterior in position and closer to the film, thus less magnified.

Anterior dislocations are rare, and occur in the externally rotated and abducted thigh. They may occur with the femur in either a flexed or extended position. In a flexed position the dislocation is known as an obturator anterior dislocation because the femoral head is positioned medially and inferiorly, overlying the obturator foramen (Fig. 3-161). In the extended thigh, anterior dislocation is superior to the acetabulum, much like a posterior dislocation. However, this form of anterior dislocation, known as iliac dislocation can be discriminated from a posterior dislocation because the femur is in external rotation with the lesser trochanter in profile and the greater trochanter obscured.

With both anterior and posterior dislocations, there is risk of fracture of the femoral head. This can result from impaction injury with compression of a portion of the femoral head, not unlike the Hill-Sachs and trough fractures associated with shoulder dislocations. Another form of femur fracture dislocation is shear fracture of

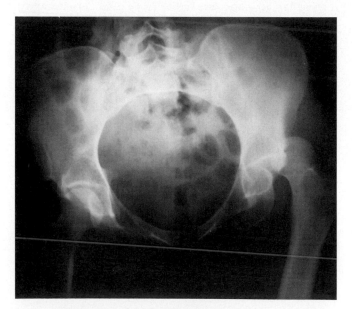

Fig. 3-160   Frontal (AP) pelvis radiograph demonstrating left posterior hip dislocation. Note superior position of the femoral head and internal rotation of the femur. Note also the smaller appearance of the left femoral head. This is due to the closer positioning of the femoral head to the xray cassette, and thus less radiographic magnification, compared with the contralateral side.

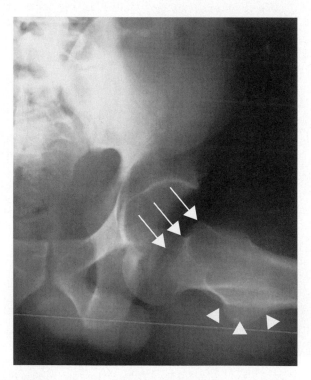

Fig. 3-161   Frontal radiograph demonstrates anterior dislocation of the hip. This is an example of an obturator anterior dislocation with inferomedial displacement of the femoral head. Note external rotation of the femur with obscuration of greater trochanter (*arrows*) and profile view of lesser trochanter (*arrowheads*).

the femoral head (Fig. 3-162). Intraarticular fragments may result from such fractures. Fragments may also result from acetabular fracture fragments. Avulsion fractures related to tension of ligamentum teres insertion in on the femur are a third cause of intraarticular loose bodies. Intraarticular loose bodies can be suspected with demonstration of widening and incongruence of the femoral head and acetabulum, and can be measured by increased distance between the acetabular teardrop and the medial femoral head. Another common complication after hip dislocation is AVN, which markedly increases in likelihood if a dislocation is not reduced within 24 hours. Approximately 50% of hip reductions delayed after 24 hours undergo subsequent AVN.

Snapping Hip

The sensation of snapping can be due to one of three causes. These are: (1) tendon snapping over the greater trochanter by the iliotibial band or the anterior margin of the gluteus maximus; (2) tendon snapping over the pubic tubercle by the iliopsoas tendon; and (3) a local detachment of the acetabular labrum. The tendinous causes of snapping can be diagnosed clinically and confirmed with ultrasonography. The iliopsoas variety can be diagnosed with iliopsoas bursography, although ultrasound has also been found to show the tendon snapping on dynamic examination. Detachment of the acetabular

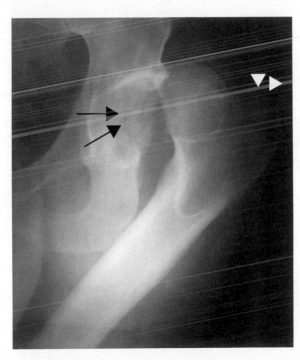

Fig. 3-162 Frontal radiograph of left hip demonstrates posterior dislocation with shear fracture of femoral head (*arrows*). Note internal rotation of femur with obscuration of lesser trochanter and profile view of greater trochanter (*arrowheads*).

labrum is diagnosed with MR-arthrography, which demonstrates contrast undermining a portion of the acetabular labrum. The location of labral attachment is variable though usually anterosuperior.

FEMUR TRAUMA

Femoral Neck Fractures

Fractures of the femur are divided into those involving the femoral head, the femoral neck, the intertrochanteric region, the shaft, and the condyles. As noted above, femoral head fractures occur during dislocations and appear as impaction or shearing injuries. Such fractures have high risk for nonunion and AVN. CT imaging is useful to search for intraarticular fracture fragments, which require surgical removal.

Femoral neck and intertrochanteric fractures are rare in young adults and middle-aged patients but extremely common in the elderly population. This high prevalence corresponds to the high prevalence of osteoporosis in the elderly. By age 80, 10% of Caucasian females and 5% of Caucasian males sustain a hip fracture. By age 90, the rates increase to 20% and 10%, respectively. Falls resulting in femoral neck fractures are highly associated with fractures of the distal radius and proximal humerus.

Femoral neck fractures are divided into subcapital, midcervical, and basicervical types. In general, the more proximal the fracture line and the more displaced the fracture, the higher the risk for AVN and nonunion. Basicervical and midcervical fractures are rare. The subcapital fracture is common. The *Garden classification* categorizes subcapital fractures into four stages. Stage I fractures are considered incomplete fractures with lateral impaction and valgus of the femoral head (Fig. 3-163). This is identified by the valgus orientation of the femoral head trabeculae relative to the acetabular trabeculae. Stage II fractures are complete subcapital fractures without displacement. In this stage, there is anatomic positioning of the femoral shaft, and the femoral head shows mild varus or anatomic position. Stage III fractures are complete fractures with partial displacement. The femoral shaft is externally rotated, and the femoral head is medi-

---

Key Concepts | **Femoral Neck Fracture**

- The more proximal the location of a femoral neck fracture, the more likely there is to be nonunion and/or AVN.
- Capital and subcapital fractures have the highest risk for avascular necrosis, particularly if displaced.
- Treatment can first be attempted with percutaneous pinning, with placement of bipolar prosthesis reserved for treatment failure.

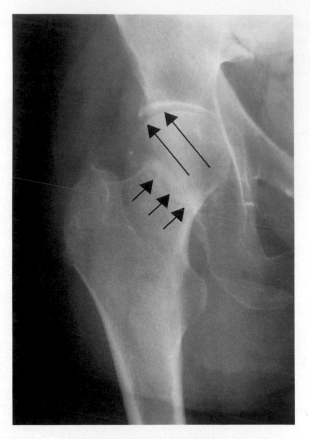

Fig. 3-163   Frontal radiograph of femur demonstrating Garden stage I subcapital fracture. Note fracture line (*short arrows*) and lateralized direction of femoral head trabecular lines. Thin long arrows indicate the direction of the femoral head trabecular lines.

ally rotated and in mild varus (Fig. 3-164). Stage IV fractures are complete fractures with full displacement, in which the femoral shaft is not only externally rotated but telescoped. However, the femoral head is in anatomic alignment relative to the acetabulum (Fig. 3-165). *Noting the femoral head position is useful in the assessment of subcapital fracture; valgus of the femoral head indicates a stage I fracture, varus of the femoral head stage II or III fracture, and anatomic position of the femoral head stage IV fracture.*

The Garden staging system is useful because it indicates the higher degree of complication with higher stage fractures. Major complications after subcapital fracture are nonunion and AVN. The occurrence of both complications increases substantially with higher stages. Among stage IV fractures there is a greater than 40% nonunion rate and a 30% rate of AVN.

The detection of subcapital fractures may be extremely difficult. Detection may be limited to a subtle area of disruption along the lateral femoral neck or to a line of increased density due to overlying bone fragments or impaction. Femoral ring osteophytes in a setting of OA may yield a similar appearance to fracture and give a false impression of fracture. In situations where the

diagnosis is unclear, radionuclide bone scan imaging (Fig. 3-166) is useful, but insensitive for fracture detection in the first 72 hours among the elderly. With MR imaging, accuracy is extremely high and is not affected by patient age or osteoporosis. Thus, diagnosis with MR imaging can be made in the acute setting. Furthermore, the evaluation can be abbreviated to T1-weighted spin echo and inversion recovery sequences.

The treatment for subcapital fracture is somewhat controversial and partly dependent on patient age. Garden stage I fractures have a generally better prognosis and can be adequately treated with percutaneous Knowles pin fixation. Stage IV fractures might also be initially treated with Knowles pin fixation, particularly if the patient is in poor health, as percutaneous fixation requires shorter anesthesia time and thus lessens the surgical risk for the patient. However, because of the higher risk of nonunion and AVN with stage IV fractures, primary bipolar hip replacement is preferred.

Intertrochanteric Fractures

These fractures occur in an older age group than subcapital fractures and have half the incidence as that of subcapital fractures. They are classified by the number

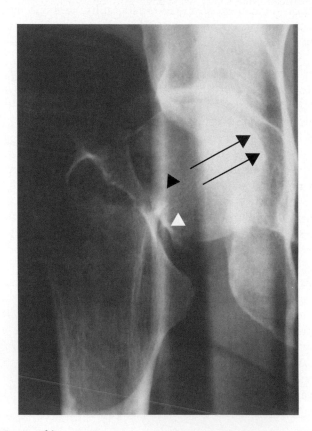

Fig. 3-164   Garden stage III subcapital femoral fracture. Note medial direction of trabecular lines. Long thin arrows indicate the direction of trabecular lines. Note partial superior displacement of medial femoral neck margin (*black arrowhead*) compared with medial femoral head margin (*white arrowhead*).

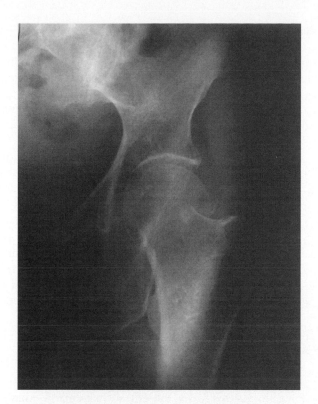

Fig. 3-165   Garden stage IV fracture. Femoral neck is completely displaced. Note substantial shortening of femoral neck and anatomic femoral head alignment.

of fracture parts as two-, three-, or four-part fractures, depending on involvement of lesser and greater trochanters. The dominant fracture is usually obliquely oriented along a line joining the greater and lesser trochanter (Fig. 3-167). Opposite obliquity is rare and unstable. Generally, intertrochanteric fractures have a good prognosis without compromise of blood supply. AVN or nonunion as a result of such fractures is uncommon.

Treatment is usually with internal fixation using a dynamic hip screw (Fig. 3-168). This device consists of a femoral diaphyseal cortical plate with a superior hollow cylindrical shaft that is placed over a femoral head screw. There are no threads where the screw contacts the cylinder. Thus the screw is restricted from transverse displacement but is free to undergo compression when the patient stands. This form of fixation allows settling with impaction which accelerates healing. Occasionally there may be excessive settling, and the femoral head screw can back out of the hollow cylinder. This most commonly occurs in the setting of collapse of the fixation into a varus configuration.

Avulsion Fracture of the Lesser Trochanter

This is an occasional type of fracture in children and adolescents resulting from avulsion of the iliopsoas at the lesser trochanteric apophysis. In adults it is an unusual injury, most commonly due to underlying pathology, particularly metastatic disease.

Slipped Capital Femoral Epiphysis (SCFE)

This disorder is seen during periods of rapid skeletal growth, at 10–16 years of age, during the period of time in which the femoral neck configuration changes from valgus to varus. This results in increased loading on the capital femoral physis and predisposes the child to Salter I fracture with displacement; the injury is felt to relate to minor repetitive trauma. SCFE is seen more commonly in males, Blacks, and obese individuals. The disorder may be seen bilaterally in 20% of children though is usually asymmetric in appearance. The capital epiphysis is shown to displace posteromedially resulting in a radiographic appearance in which the physis appears wider and with indistinct margins (Fig. 3-169). The most helpful sign of SCFE is demonstrated by drawing a line tangent to the lateral margin of the femoral neck. Ordinarily, this line should intersect a portion of the capital epiphysis. In SCFE, however, the tangent line is found to be lateral to the capital epiphysis. Frog lateral and groin lateral views are especially useful for revealing the posteromedial displacement of the epiphysis. SCFE is treated with 3-point pinning without reduction. This results in varus deformity with a short and broad femoral neck. The disorder is commonly complicated by OA in adulthood, usually occurring after 30 years of age. In addition, AVN occurs in 10% of individuals, especially after attempts at epiphyseal reduction. Rarely, *acute chondrolysis* can occur, which is the sudden diffuse uniform loss of articular cartilage. The cause for the sudden loss of articular cartilage is unclear. The loss of articular cartilage may relate to changes to cyclic load bearing at the joint because cyclic load bearing is essential for diffusion of nutrients across the cartilage tissue. Articular cartilage is avascular and dependent upon joint fluid for its nutrition. Interference with nutrient diffusion will result in cell death. The appearance of acute chondrolysis can be confused with infection, which is identical in uniform articular cartilage thinning and joint space narrowing. Acute chondrolysis may also be seen idiopathically and among immobilized individuals.

Femoral Shaft Fracture

These fractures may be seen in isolation or in combination with other femoral fractures, including femoral neck fractures and condylar fractures. They are often comminuted with butterfly or segmental fragments. Reduction is usually with an intramedullary rod. The surgeon must check for rotational deformity so that appropriate reduction may be achieved. CT imaging can help assess for the degree of rotation (version) by obtaining only a few CT-sections at the femoral neck and at the femoral con-

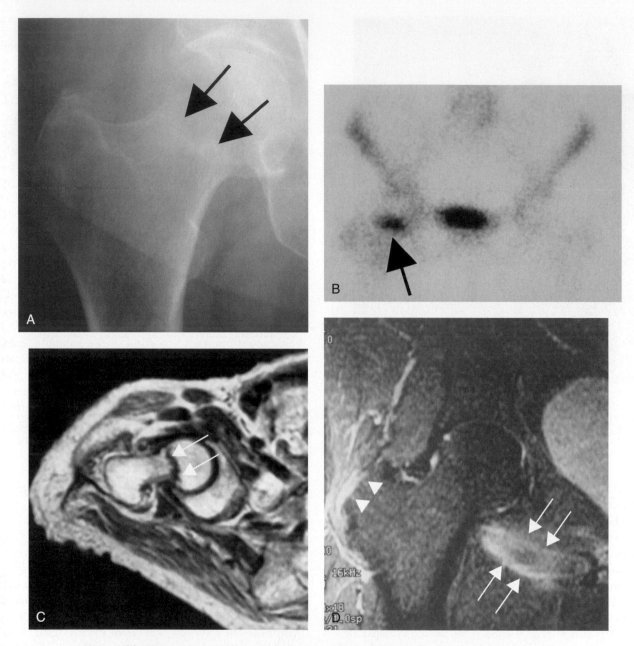

Fig. 3-166   The utility of radionuclide bone scan imaging and MR imaging for evaluating hip trauma. **A,** Radiograph demonstrates subtle, sclerotic line in subcapital femoral neck (*arrows*). **B,** Radionuclide bone scan demonstrates intense radionuclide uptake (*arrow*) in femoral neck indicating fracture. **C,** Axial T1-weighted image (600/16; TR msec/TE msec) demonstrates subcapital low intensity line (*arrows*) diagnostic of fracture. **D,** Coronal inversion recovery image (4000/20; inversion time 100 msec) in a different patient shows use of MR imaging for the exclusion of fracture and demonstration of the cause of the patient's symptoms. Note high signal in obturator externus (*arrows*) indicating strain, and similar findings at insertion of gluteus medius muscle (*arrowheads*), also indicating strain.

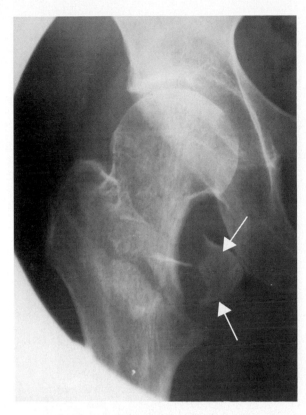

Fig. 3-167 Frontal radiograph demonstrates three part intertrochanteric fracture with displaced lesser trochanter fragment (*arrows*).

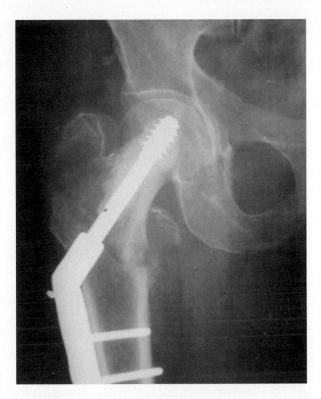

Fig. 3-168 Dynamic hip screw. This patient with an intertrochanteric fracture has been stabilized with a dynamic screw and plate system, which allows settling at the fracture site without the screw cutting-out through the osteoporotic bone of the femoral head.

dyles. The degree of version can be measured by summing the angles of the femoral neck and condyles. This is done at each location by drawing a line parallel to the bottom edge of the film, a second line drawn through the middle of the femoral neck, and another line at the knee drawn tangent to the posterior margin of the femoral condyles. The two angles are summed and can be compared with the contralateral side, which should be within 5° of the fractured side.

Intramedullary rods are usually placed with proximal and distal locking screws to prevent translocation, rotation, and shortening of the fracture (Fig. 3-170). Occasionally the locking screws at one or both ends are removed if delayed union or malunion ensues. This will allow the fracture fragments to come into greater compression, in order to stimulate osteoinduction and osteoconduction.

Stress Fractures of the Femur

The femur is susceptible to stress fracture, particularly involving the medial cortex in the proximal and midshaft regions, and at the posterior cortex in the distal shaft. They may also occur along the medial femoral neck proximal to the lesser trochanter; such patients usually present

with vague hip or groin pain. Radiographs may reveal linear sclerosis with occasional central linear lucency or solid periosteal new bone formation, but findings may be equivocal or even normal. In such cases MR imaging

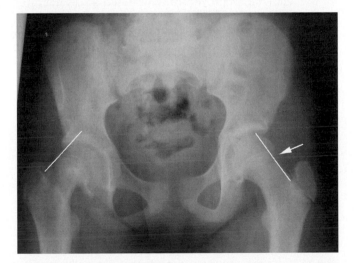

Fig. 3-169 AP pelvis in child with slipped capital femoral epiphysis. Line drawn along lateral femoral neck of affected side fails to intersect femoral capital epiphysis. Note intersection of line with normal femoral head on contralateral side (*arrow*). (Courtesy of L. Das Narla, Richmond, VA.)

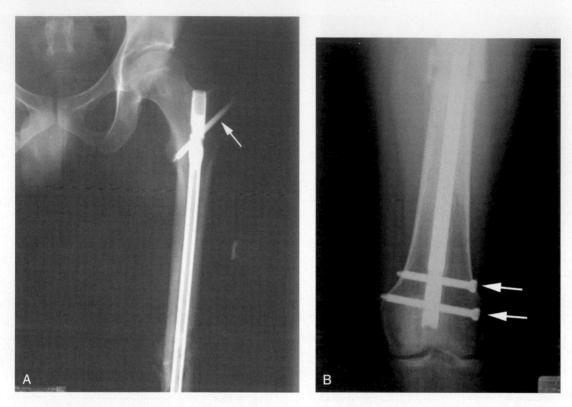

Fig. 3-170   Frontal radiograph of proximal (**A**) and distal (**B**) femur demonstrates intramedullary rod. Note interlocking screws (*arrows*), which prevent rotation after reduction.

is useful for diagnosis of stress fracture, because of its remarkable marrow contrast (Fig. 3-171). Stress fractures that are not treated with non-weightbearing can result in a complete fracture requiring internal fixation. Stress fractures are usually transversely oriented to the length of the shaft, although vertically oriented stress fractures rarely occur. Vertical stress fractures are extremely subtle on radiographs and can produce a confusing marrow edema pattern on MRI. CT is often helpful in these situations because reformatted images reveal a vertical thin sclerotic line.

KNEE TRAUMA

Intercondylar Fractures

Transcondylar fractures usually involve metaphyseal and condylar components (Fig. 3-172). The metaphyseal component is usually transverse in orientation. The condylar component may be in sagittal or coronal planes. Coronal intraarticular fractures place the patient at risk for AVN of the condylar components. Coronally oriented intraarticular condylar fractures have a worse prognosis than sagittal fractures because of the risk of displacement when the patient begins weight bearing after reduction and fixation.

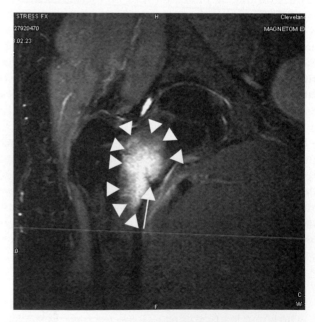

Fig. 3-171   Stress fracture of femoral neck. Coronal inversion recovery MR image (4449/22, TRmsec/TE msec, inversion time 140 msec) demonstrates linear fracture line at medial femoral neck cortex (*arrow*) with surrounding bone marrow edema (*arrowheads*). (Courtsey of Michael Recht, M.D., Cleveland, OH.)

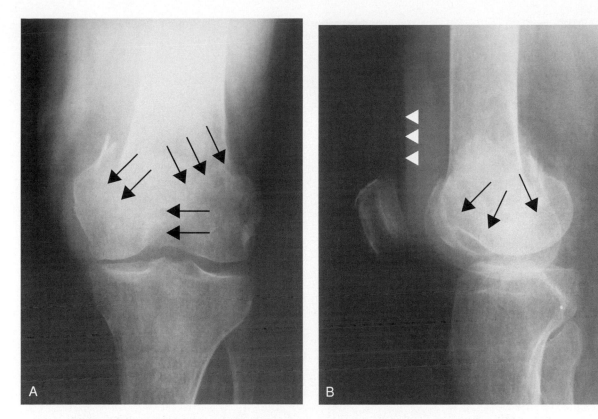

Fig. 3-172   **A,** Frontal radiograph of femur demonstrates comminuted intercondylar fracture of femur (*arrows*). **B,** Lateral view demonstrates fracture line (*arrows*) and hemarthrosis (*arrowheads*).

Osteochondritis Dissecans

The etiology of osteochondritis dissecans is uncertain but likely due to repeated minor trauma during an age when the epiphysis reaches skeletal maturation. It is therefore a disease of children and teenagers. The knee is a common site for osteochondritis dissecans especially at the lateral aspect of the medial femoral chondral (Fig. 3-173). Osteochondritis dissecans can be graded based on the stability of the osteochondral fragment. Grade I lesions are considered subchondral bone bruises with intact overlying articular cartilage. Grade II lesions have subchondral fracture lines with intact overlying articular cartilage. Grade III lesions are partially attached osteochondral fractures in which the osteochondral fragment is attached at one margin by its articular cartilage but can be easily displaced at arthroscopy with a probe. Grade IV lesions are *in situ* loose fragments in which the overlying articular cartilage is completely disrupted, and grade V lesions are those in which the osteocondral fragment is displaced as a loose body in the joint. Lesions with at least partial articular cartilage disruption, namely the grade III, IV, and V lesions, are unstable because of their propensity to displace. Although stable lesions are treated with non-

weight bearing and have a good prognosis, higher grade lesions require surgery. Partially displaceable lesions are treated with subchondral pin fixation. *In situ* fragments may be treated with pin fixation if the overlying articular cartilage is largely intact, but otherwise require removal of the fragment with debridement of the crater. Grade V lesions are treated with debridement and removal of the loose body. With the advent of new surgeries aimed at restoring articular surfaces, there is potential to restore articular congruence of osteochondral defects. One such treatment is with osteochondral autologous transplantation (OATS), in which osteochondral plugs from nonweightbearing parts of the joint are transplanted to the site of an osteochondral defect. Another method of treatment is with autologous chondrocyte implantation (ACI), in which cartilage tissue is harvested and chondrocytes from this tissue grow ex vivo, after which a second surgery is performed and the new cells implanted into a site of articular defect under a periosteal flap. Both techniques show great potential though they have been used mainly in purely articular defects rather than osteochondral defects, and predominately in adult populations.

The best means of imaging osteochondritis dissecans is with MR imaging and MR arthrography. The goal is to detect articular cartilage disruption of the overlying

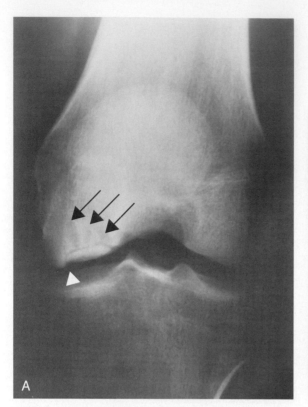
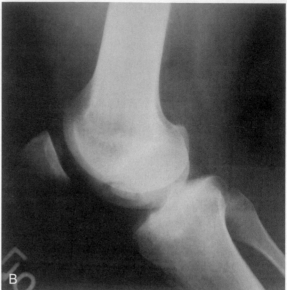

Fig. 3-173 Osteochondritis dissecans. AP (**A**) and lateral (**B**) knee radiographs demonstrate typical location of osteochondritis dissecans along lateral aspect of medial femoral condyle. Note osteochondral fragment and linear lucency separating fragment from underlying bone. Note also adjacent bone lucencies (*arrows*), which suggest instability of bone fragments. Incongruence of osteochondral fragment and underlying bone (*arrowhead*) also suggests instability of fragment.

osteochondral defect (Figs. 3-174, 3-175). This can be performed with cartilage-sensitive sequences such as fat-suppressed three dimensional spoiled gradient-echo imaging and proton density fast spin echo imaging. Another means to determine stability of an osteochondral fragment is by detecting separation of the subchondral fracture line from the underlying bone. This can be with the demonstration of fluid signal at the margin between the lesion and underlying bone at T2-weighted spin-echo or fast spin-echo imaging. It can also be shown with MR-arthrography, by demonstrating contrast extension into the margin between the lesion and adjacent bone.

Osteochondritis dissecans occurs in the skeletally immature. Because of this, normal variation in epiphyseal bone growth can be confused with osteochondritis dissecans. Irregularity of the condylar epiphysis is common in 3–6-year-olds especially in the medial epiphysis. Among 10–13-year-olds femoral condylar irregularity is shown in both condyles posteriorly. Bilateral symmetry of these findings is helpful in clarifying whether findings represent normal growth variation or an osteochondral lesion. In unclear cases, MR imaging provides the answer by demonstrating normal bone marrow signal and normal articular cartilage.

Because osteochondritis dissecans is a posttraumatic lesion, it should be no surprise that osteochondral lesions can also occur in adults. Osteochondral defects in adults have a more variable localization than the osteochondritis dissecans of children. However, the orthopedic treatment principals and the imaging algorithms are the same. The goal is to demonstrate stability of the lesion and to treat unstable lesions. Osteochondral defects of adults likely fall into the spectrum of articular shear injuries.

Tibial Plateau Fracture

Tibia plateau fractures are usually seen in pedestrian-automobile accidents because the plateau is at the level of car bumpers. The vast majority (80%) are localized to the lateral tibial plateau as most fractures result from a valgus load due to impaction at the lateral tibial condyle. Tibial plateau fractures are intraarticular fractures that typically produce large hemarthroses and are classified by the occurrence of cleavage planes, articular depres-

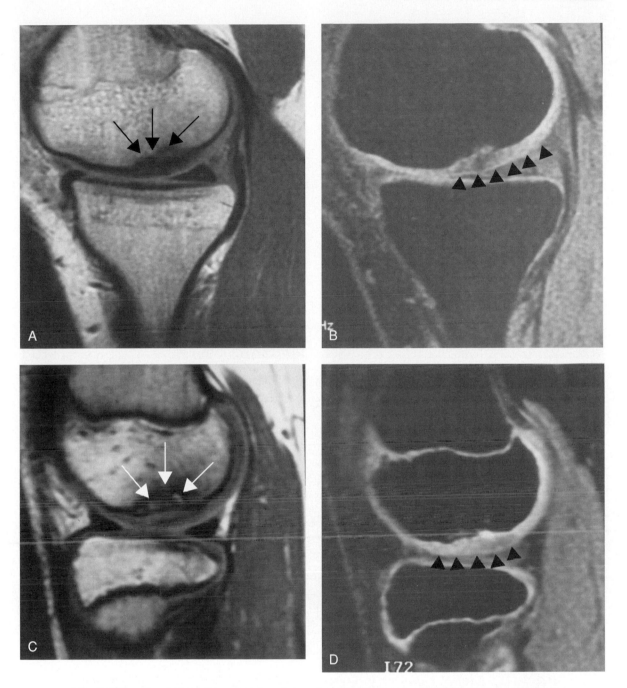

Fig. 3-174   Two MR imaging examples of osteochondritis dissecans with intact overlying articular cartilage. **A** and **C** are T1-weighted spin echo images (700/14; TR msec/TE mscc) from two separate patients with their corresponding (**B** and **D**) fat-suppressed 3-D spoiled gradient-echo images (60/5; flip angle 40 degrees). T1-weighted images demonstrate the osteochondral fracture lines (*arrows*). Note how the overlying articular cartilage is intact on **B** and **D** (*arrowheads*). (Fig. 3-174B adapted and reproduced, with permission, from Disler DG. Fat-suppressed 3-D spoiled gradient-recalled MR imaging: assessment of articular and physeal hyaline cartilage. *AJR* 169:1117-1123, 1997.)

sion, and metaphyseal extension. Though not a reflection of the severity of injury, the Schatzker classification is useful in surgical planning (Fig. 3-176). The classification is as follows: A type I fracture is a cleavage fracture of the lateral tibial plateau. A type II fracture is a combined cleavage and depressed fracture of the lateral tibial pla-

teau. A type III fracture is a purely depressed fracture of the lateral tibial plateau. A type IV fracture is a lateral condylar tibial cleavage fracture that extends to the medial tibial condyle. A type V fracture is a bicondylar fracture, and a type VI fracture is any fracture with a transmetaphyseal component.

Text continued on p. 322

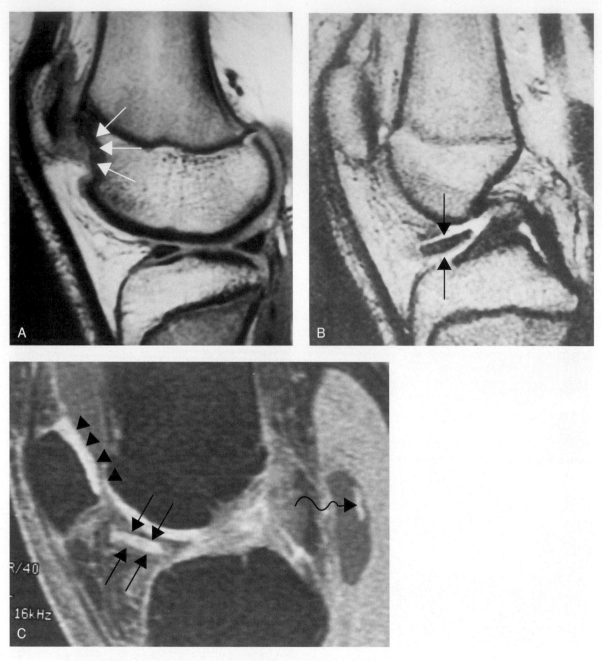

Fig. 3-175   Grade V osteochondritis dissecans. **A,** sagittal T1-weighted image (TR/TE; 600 msec/ 18 msec) demonstrates osteochondral defect (*arrows*) without osseus fragment at site of defect. **B,** T2-weighted image (3000/80) demonstrates displaced fragment (*arrows*). **C,** Sagittal fat-suppressed 3-D spoiled gradient-echo image (60/5; flip angle, 40°) demonstrates fragment (*arrows*) of signal intensity similar to that of articular cartilage (*arrowheads*) indicating it to be of chondral origin. Note additional cartilaginous fragment in popliteal bursa (*curved arrow*). (Fig. 3-175C adapted and reproduced, with permission, from Disler DG. Fat-suppressed three-dimensional spoiled gradient-recalled MR imaging: assessment of articular and physeal hyaline cartilage. *AJR* 169: 1117-1123, 1997.)

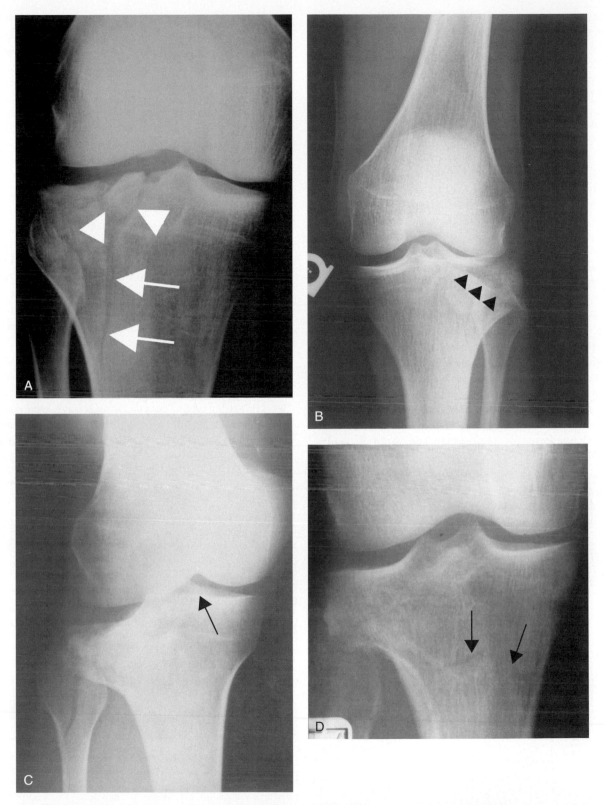

Fig. 3-176   Examples of tibial plateau fracture. **A,** Schatzker II fracture demonstrating cleavage line (*arrows*) and depressed lateral plateau fracture (*arrowheads*). **B,** Schatzker III fracture demonstrating depressed lateral tibial plateau (*arrowheads*). **C,** Schatzker IV fracture. Note extension of fracture to medial tibial plateau (*arrow*). **D,** Schatzker VI fracture. Note metaphyseal fracture line (*arrows*).

Imaging is important in the assessment of tibial plateau fractures because the goal of surgery is restoration of congruence of the articular margin, in order to decrease the risk of eventual posttraumatic OA. Radiographs can be confusing because the lateral tibial plateau is normally sloped 10–20° posteriorly and thus its margins are not tangential to the knee joint on AP radiographs. Depressed fragments are easily overlooked anteriorly and exaggerated posteriorly. The cleavage fracture line is often in an oblique plane; therefore, an AP view may completely miss a tibial plateau fracture whereas the oblique view will show the fracture. Both MRI (Figure 3-177) and CT imaging are useful in the evaluation of these fractures for presurgical planning, although CT is particularly helpful in showing osseous margins. CT multiplanar reformations can demonstrate the degree of fracture depression and displacement. The threshold of depression or displacement at which surgery is indicated is controversial. Many centers are adopting a "zero tolerance" approach to articular depression and the need for surgical reduction. Generally, however, depression greater than 3 mm or distraction greater than 3 mm requires internal fixation. Various forms of fixation are used in tibial plateau fractures. Cleavage fractures typically are treated with lateromedial lag screws, whereas combination depressed and cleavage fractures usually require a lateral buttress plate. Depressed fractures usually require elevation of the articular fragment with placement of subarticular bone graft. Bicondy-lar fractures require both medial and lateral pinning. Bicondylar fractures and fractures with metaphyseal components often require the addition of external fixation.

Patellar Fractures

Patellar fractures (Fig. 3-178) may be due either to direct impaction (falling on the patella) resulting in a comminuted fracture, or to sudden tension of the extensor mechanism of the thigh, resulting in transverse and often distracted fractures. Sixty percent of patellar fractures result from the latter and the degree of distraction depends upon the integrity of the medial and lateral patellar retinacula. A patellar sleeve fracture is a nonarticular fracture at the inferior margin of the patella, at the origin of the patellar tendon. It is also a result of sudden tension of the extensor mechanism of the thigh, typically in the skeletally immature. Osteochondral fractures of the patella may occur as well. These are usually located at the medial patellar facet and are associated with transient patellar dislocation (see below).

Patellar fractures may be confused with normal variants of the patella. Bipartite and multipartite patellae represent fragments of bone that are found at the superolateral border of the patella though have well corticated margins and at MR imaging normal adjacent articular cartilage (Fig. 3-179). They are often bilateral and their

Text continued on p. 325

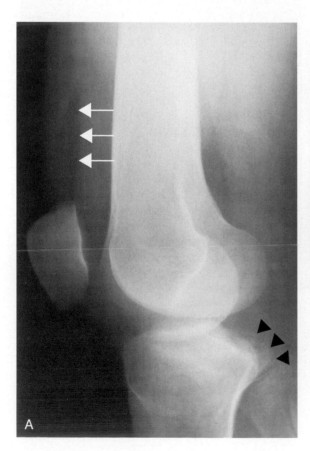

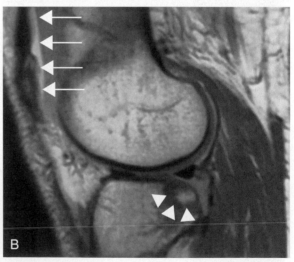

Fig. 3-177   Utility of MR imaging for assessment of tibial plateau fracture. **A,** Lateral radiograph demonstrates lipohemarthrosis (*arrows*) with subtle irregularity of posterior tibial articular margin (*arrowheads*). **B,** Sagittal T1-weighted spin echo MR image (TR/TE; 700 msec/18 msec) demonstrates lipohemarthrosis (*arrows*) and fracture of posterior lateral tibial condyle (*arrowheads*).

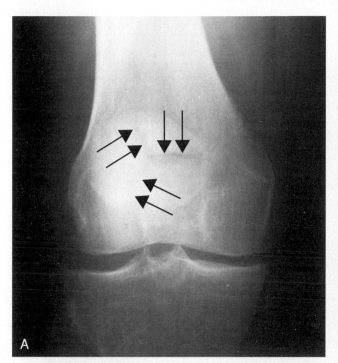

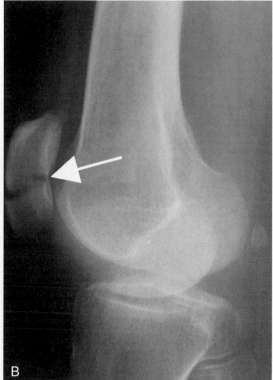

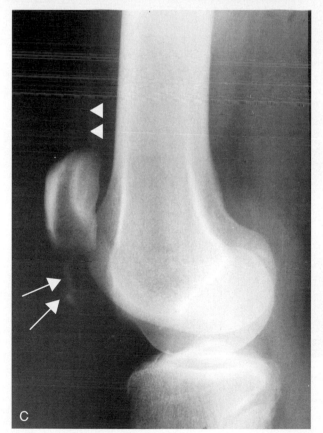

Fig. 3-178   Patellar fracture. **A,** Frontal radiograph demonstrates stellate patellar fracture (*arrows*) from direct impaction injury. **B,** Lateral radiograph demonstrates transverse fracture of mid pole of patella (*arrow*), due to sudden quadriceps contraction. **C,** Patellar sleeve fracture (*arrows*). These fractures are often extraarticular. Note absence of hemarthrosis (*arrowheads*).

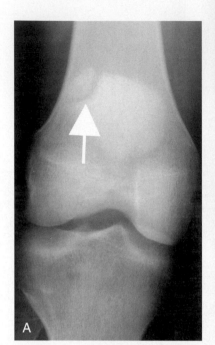

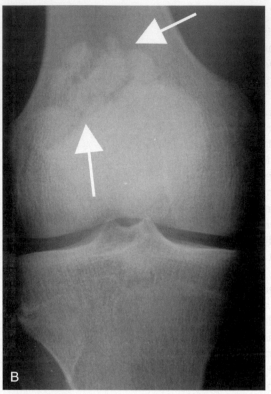

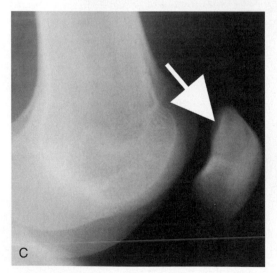

Fig. 3-179 **A,** Bipartite patella (*arrow*). Note superolateral location of fragment. **B,** Multipartite patella (*arrows*). **C,** Dorsal defect of the patella (*arrow*).

location is a clue to its nontraumatic etiology. Dorsal defect of the patella is a rounded lucency at the superolateral dorsal (articular) margin of the patella. It is also a normal variant.

Patellar Dislocation

Patellar dislocation is almost always transient in nature and is a commonly overlooked injury. In *transient patellar dislocation,* the patella briefly dislocates laterally and then relocates. Dislocations are almost always lateral because of the weaker mechanical properties of the medial patellar retinaculum and vastus medialis. In the process of relocating, impaction occurs between the medial pole of the patella and the anterolateral margin of the lateral femoral condyle. The medial patellar retinaculum becomes stretched or torn. Bone bruises occur at the sites of impaction at the medial patella and the lateral femoral condyle. Hemarthrosis is usually present. As noted above, there is often an osteochondral fracture arising from the medial patella as a result of shearing injury at the site of impaction at the lateral femoral condyle during relocation (Fig. 3-180). The osteochondral fracture will either be present at the site of impact adjacent to the lateral femoral condyle, or adjacent to the medial facet of the relocated patella. MR imaging is the ideal modality to evaluate transient patellar dislocation (Fig. 3-181). At MR imaging a large hemarthrosis is evident as are the bone bruises of the medial patella and lateral femoral condyle. The disruption of the medial patellar retinaculum is clearly evident, and usually occurs at the medial patellofemoral ligament at either the femoral or patellar attachments. The osteochondral fragment is also readily demonstrated.

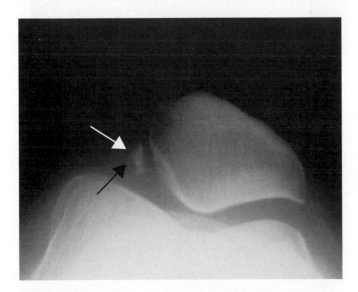

Fig. 3-180   Axial view of patella demonstrates medial pole patellar fracture (*arrows*) due to transient dislocation.

The relocated patella usually demonstrates residual lateral patellar tilt or subluxation.

Being a sesmoid bone with a large cranial caudal excursion, the patella is prone to tracking abnormalities as it courses through the trochlear groove of the femur. Tracking abnormalities are usually laterally oriented with lateral patellar tilt and subluxation. Trochlear dysplasia is one predisposing factor for tracking abnormalities and is shown on radiographs and MR images as an abnormally shallow trochlear groove or a shelf-like prominence of the proximal trochlea on the lateral radiograph or sagittal MR image (Fig. 3-182). Tracking abnormalities and recurring subluxations are also associated with the patella alta, which is a result of an elongated patellar tendon. This can be diagnosed on a lateral view with flexion of 20–30° (Fig. 3-183). The ratio of the patellar tendon length (as measured from the inferior pole of the patella to the anterior tubial tubericle) to the length of the patella should yield a ratio of 1.0 ± 0.2. A ratio greater than 1.2 of tendon to patella represents patella alta.

There are many orthopedic measurements of lateral patellar tilt and subluxation. These measures are obtained from studying an axial (Merchant) radiographic view obtained with the knee flexed only 20°. If greater flexion is used for obtaining this view the patella becomes engaged in the trochlear groove, precluding assessment for patellar alignment abnormalities. Ordinarily the lateral patellar facet is somewhat longer than the medial patellar facet and the lateral facet is parallel to the lateral trochlea. Lateral tilt is present when the margins between lateral patella and lateral trochlea are no longer parallel but narrower laterally. Another angle that is useful for determining trochlear dysplasia is the *sulcus angle,* which is the angle formed by connecting the two highest points of the medial and lateral femoral trochlea with the deepest portion of the trochlear groove. This is normally 138°. A third measure is the *congruence angle.* This is formed by drawing two lines to the sulcus of the trochlear groove. The first line extends to the groove from the anterior apex of the patella. The second line to the base of the trochlear groove is drawn from the posterior apex of the patella. The line formed by the posterior apex should always be medial to that formed by the anterior apex. If lateral, it suggests lateral subluxation, particularly if the angle is greater than 16°.

Avulsion Injuries

There are numerous avulsion sites at the knee (Fig. 3-184). Common locations include the anterior cruciate ligament insertion on the intercondylar eminence of the tibia (Fig. 3-185), the posterior cruciate ligament insertion at the posterior tibia, and the lateral joint capsule at the lateral margin of the tibia (this is also termed a *Segond fracture,* and is highly associated with anterior cruciate liga-

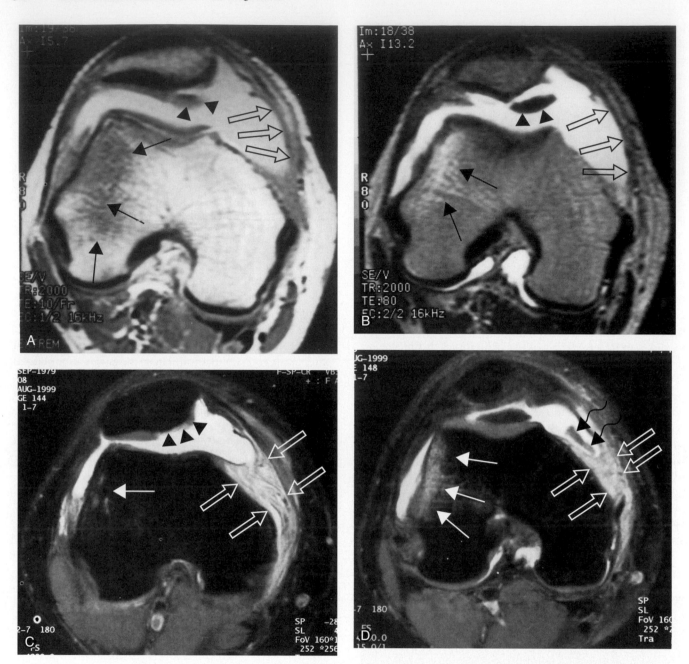

Fig. 3-181   MR imaging of transient dislocation of the patella. **A,** Axial proton density weighted spin echo image (2000/10; TR msec/TE msec) demonstrates bone bruises of anterolateral femoral condyle (*closed arrows*), osteochondral fragment of medial pole of patella (*arrowheads*) and medial patellar retinaculum tear (*open arrows*). **B,** Axial T2-weighted spin echo image (2000/80) showing lateral femoral bone bruise (*arrows*), medial patellar osteochondral fracture (*arrowheads*) and medial patellar retinaculum tear (*open arrows*). **C** and **D,** Two contiguous axial fat-suppressed fast spin echo (4000/15) images in another patient showing lateral femoral bone bruise (*arrows*), chondral defect at medial pole of patella (*arrowheads*), and medial patellar retinaculum tear with substantial edema (*open arrows*). Note chondral loose body (*curved arrows*).

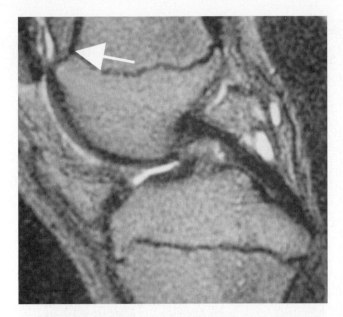

Fig. 3-182 Sagittal T2-weighted spin echo image (2000/80; TR msec/TE msec) demonstrates shelflike prominence of midtrochlear groove at superior margin (*arrow*) in patient with trochlear dysplasia.

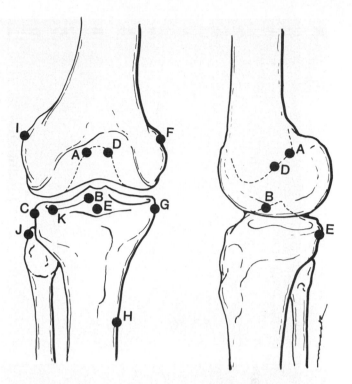

Fig. 3-184 Avulsion sites around the knee: (A) ACL origin. (B) ACL insertion. (C) lateral capsular attachment. (D) PCL origin. (E) PCL insertion. (F) MCL origin. (G) MCL deep fiber (manisco-tibial) insertion. (H) MCL superficial fibers insertion. (I) LCL origin. (J) Common insertion of LCL and biceps femoris, (K) Gerdy's tubercle, insertion of iliotibial band. (From Manaster BJ. *Handbook of Skeletal Radiology,* ed 2, St. Louis, 1997, Mosby-Yearbook.)

ment injury). Other avulsions include the anterior lateral tibial margin (Gerdy's tubercle) at the site of the iliotibial band insertion, the lateral collateral ligament insertion at the proximal fibia (which is also the biceps femoris insertion), and the medial collateral ligament origin and insertion at the medial femoral and tibial condyles, respectively. The anterior tibial tubercle is another site prone to tension injury of the patellar tendon, which is commonly seen in children and young adolescents. With repetitive stress, the tubercle may become fragmented, and if associated with tenderness and swelling, the disorder is termed *Osgood-Schlatter disease* (Fig. 3-186).

Physeal Injury

Growth plate injuries at the knee are uncommon though highly associated with complications, particularly that of growth plate arrest and malunion (Figs. 3-187, 3–188). Salter-Harris II fractures predominate, occurring in 70% of injuries with the next most common pattern being Salter-Harris III fractures occurring in 15% of children. Most Salter III fractures at the knee involve the medial femoral condyle and are due to valgus stress. They are usually without displacement and are occult radio-

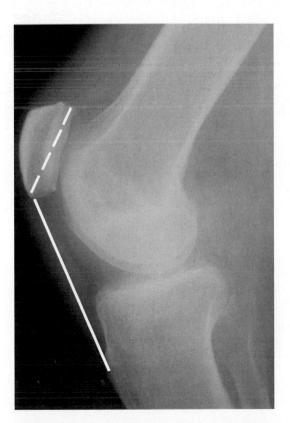

Fig. 3-183 Lateral radiograph in patient with patella alta. Note substantially greater length of patellar tendon (*solid line*) compared with length of patella (*dashed line*).

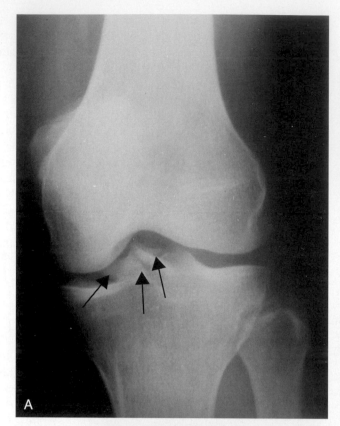

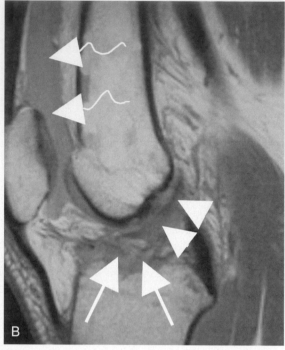

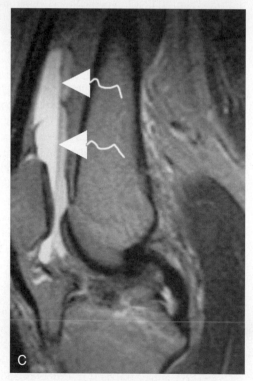

Fig. 3-185   Avulsion of insertion of anterior cruciate ligament. **A,** Frontal radiograph demonstrates fracture at tibial intercondylar eminence (*arrows*). **B** and **C,** Sagittal proton density and T2-weight spin echo images (2000/20, 80; TR msec/TE first echo, TE second echo msec) demonstrates avulsion fracture fragment (*arrows*), bone bruise at fracture donor site, intact anterior cruciate ligament (*arrowheads*), and hemarthrosis (*curved arrows*).

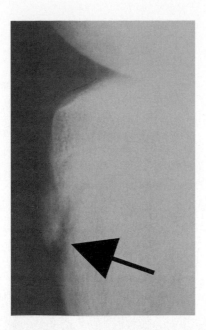

Fig. 3-186 Lateral radiograph of proximal tibia demonstrates osseus irregularity at patellar tendon insertion (*arrow*) in patient with Osgood-Schlatter disease.

graphically yet can be demonstrated at MR imaging. The knee is the most common site for Salter-Harris V fractures, which occur at the proximal tibia and are complicated by localized growth plate arrest with angular deformity or limb length shortening.

Stress Fracture

Stress fractures are common in the tibia and appear similar to stress fractures elsewhere, with early faint trans-verse or oblique lucency followed by sclerosis involving the same distribution in the overlying cortex (Fig. 3-189). Most occur within the posterior cortex of the proximal tibial shaft, discriminated from "shin-splints" that occur anteriorly. Some sports such as basketball and ballet are associated with stress fractures in the anterior cortex of the mid-tibia. Stress fractures are usually multiple and ra-diographically can be detected by numerous small trans-verse partial fractures at various stages of healing. Because the radiographic detection of stress fracture lags several weeks behind clinical findings, MR imaging and nuclear bone scan imaging play an important role in the early de-tection of these injuries. Bone scan images will show ec-centric cortically based increased activity on the side of symptoms. MR imaging demonstrates the localized mar-row abnormality with a linear low signal intensity line cen-trally within the area of bone marrow edema (Fig. 3-190).

Knee Dislocation

Articular Knee Injury Knee dislocations can occur in any direction though anterior dislocation is most com-mon. A large minority of patients with knee dislocation (30%) have associated arterial injury, due to the close proximity of the popliteal artery, which is fixed proxi-mally in the adductor canal and distally at its bifurcation near the tibiofibular syndesmosis. Patients with knee dis-location are assessed for distal pulses and hue at the time of injury. Any question of arterial injury requires arteriography for detection of intimal arterial disruption or pseudoaneurysm (Fig. 3-191). Other soft tissue injury is common in the setting of knee dislocation. These include tears of the cruciate ligaments, the collateral ligaments,

Text continued on p. 333

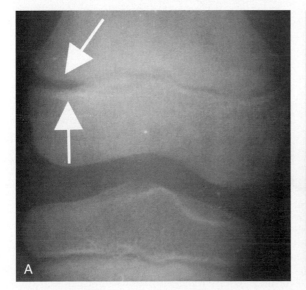 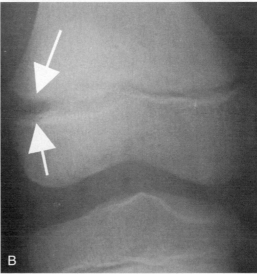

Fig. 3-187 Salter-Harris I fracture of distal femur. **A,** Note slight widening of lateral distal femoral physis (*arrows*). **B,** Varus stress view demonstrates exaggerated widening of lateral physis (*arrows*).

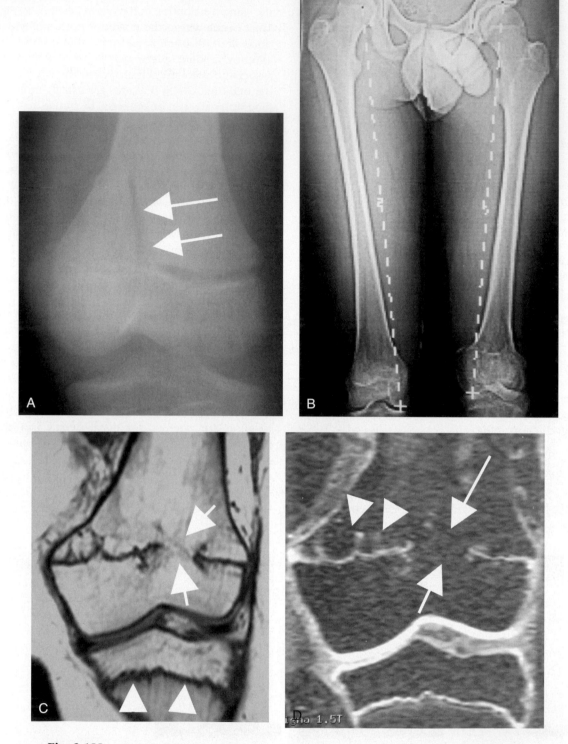

Fig. 3-188   Growth plate arrest after physeal fracture. **A,** Frontal radiograph at time of injury demonstrates Salter-Harris II fracture of femur. Note metaphyseal component (*arrows*). **B,** CT scanogram obtained 3 years later demonstrates shortening of left femur, the site of previous fracture. Dashed lines of each femur indicate degree of left-sided shortening. **C,** Coronal T1-weighted MR image (600/14; TR msec/TE msec) show substantial irregularity of distal femoral physis and focal absence of growth plate (*arrows*). Note smooth contour of proximal tibial physis (*arrowheads*). **D,** Coronal fat-suppressed 3-D spoiled gradient-echo MR image (60/5; flip angle 40°) shows cartilaginous irregularities of medial aspect of distal femoral physis (*arrowheads*) and focal absence of growth plate cartilage (*arrows*). Note smooth contour of proximal tibial physis. (Fig. 3-188D adapted and reproduced, with permission, from Disler DG. Fat-suppressed three-dimensional spoiled gradient-recalled MR imaging: assessment of articular and physeal hyaline cartilage, *AJR* 169:1117-1123, 1997.)

Key Concepts | Articular Knee Injury

- Most knee injuries involve soft tissues; Radiographs may show only an effusion as a sign of serious underlying injury. Occasionally, hemarthrosis is demonstrated with a fluid-fluid level (in the suprapatellar recess) on the cross table radiograph.
- Hemarthrosis is usually due to one of three injuries: intraarticular fracture, large bone bruise, or anterior cruciate ligament rupture.
- MR imaging is particularly suited to the evaluation of the soft tissues at the knee. MR imaging of the knee is the most commonly ordered MR examination of the musculoskeletal system.
- An orderly approach to the evaluation of the knee is useful with attention paid specifically to bone marrow edema patterns, meniscal contours, ligaments and tendons, and hyaline cartilage.
- Meniscal tear is diagnosed on proton density or T1-weighted MR images if increased signal in the meniscus is shown to extend to either a superior or inferior articular margin, if the free margin of the meniscus is blunted, or if linear fluidlike signal is found within the meniscus.

- Bucket handle tears of the meniscus are easily overlooked. One must search the femoral notch for meniscal signal in continuity with the anterior or posterior horns of the meniscus, particularly if the native meniscus is small. Also, one must search for a meniscal horn that appears too large as this may represent a meniscal displacement to another horn rather than to the intercondylar notch.
- The anterior cruciate ligament is the most commonly injured knee ligament. The four primary signs of any ligament tear at MR imaging are swelling, increased signal, fiber discontinuity, and an abnormal geographic position, which in the setting of ACL tear is a horizontal lie.
- Articular cartilage defects are very easily overlooked particularly if imaging is limited to spin-echo and T2* gradient-echo images. Articular cartilage defects are found with the highest sensitivity using fat-suppressed 3-D spoiled gradient-echo or proton-density fast spin-echo images.

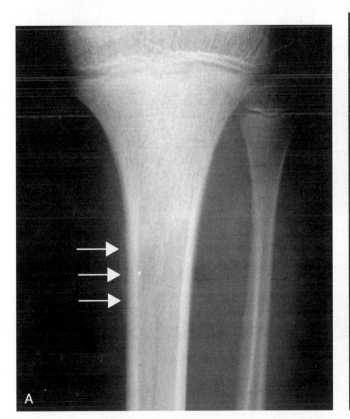 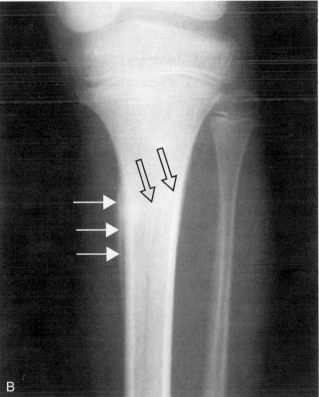

Fig. 3-189 Stress fracture of proximal tibia. **A,** Radiograph shows ill-defined lamellar periosteal bone formation in proximal tibial diaphysis. **B,** Frontal tibial radiograph 3 weeks later demonstrates progressive formation of medial periosteal new bone formation (*arrows*) and appearance of linear sclerosis at stress fracture site (*arrowheads*).

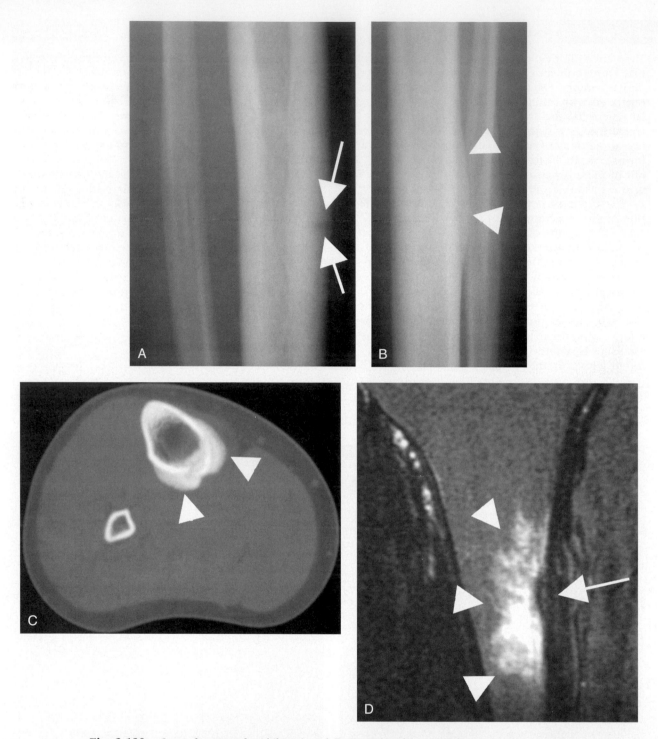

Fig. 3-190   Stress fracture of midtibia. **A** and **B,** Frontal and lateral radiographs show typical posteromedial location of stress fracture as indicated by fracture line (*arrows*) and periosteal new bone formation (*arrowheads*). **C,** Axial CT image shows prominent posteromedial solid periosteal new bone formation (*arrowheads*). **D,** Coronal inversion recovery MR image (4000/30; TR msec/ TE msec; inversion time, 140 msec) shows fracture (*arrow*) and substantial surrounding bone marrow edema (*arrowheads*).

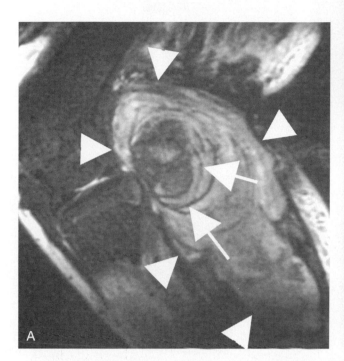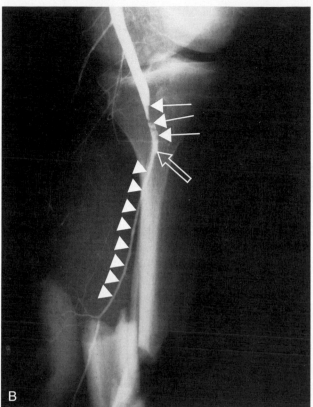

Fig. 3-191   A, Sagittal inversion recovery image (4000/30, TR msec/TE msec; inversion time, 140 msec) demonstrates large popliteal pseudoaneurysm (*arrowheads*). Note concentric rings of clot (*arrows*). **B,** Frontal radiograph during angiogram in patient with comminuted tibial fracture and knee dislocation (after reduction) demonstrates popliteal artery intimal injury with in situ thrombosis (*arrows*) and occlusion at popliteal trifurcation (*open arrow*). There is still flow within peroneal artery (*arrowheads*).

the joint capsule, and often the articular cartilage. Peroneal nerve injury is also common in dislocation, owing to its tenuous course at the knee where it runs close to the margin of the fibular head.

Meniscal Tears

The menisci of the knee are semicircular bands of fibrocartilage that line the peripheral aspects of the medial and lateral compartments and function to increase the tibiofemoral contact area, thus allowing for a more evenly distributed load across the knee joint. Because the medial tibial plateau is larger, the medial meniscus is larger than the lateral meniscus, and thus the medial meniscus is slightly more C-shaped than is the more circular lateral meniscus. The menisci taper from a height of 3–5 mm at the periphery to a thin, sharp central free margin. Therefore, the menisci appear triangular in shape on coronal and sagittal MR images (Fig. 3-192). The anterior and posterior horns of the lateral meniscus are similar in size; however, the posterior horn of the medial meniscus is larger than its anterior horn. On sagittal imaging, the lateral meniscus shows a bowtie configuration with

closely apposed anterior and posterior horns. Because the medial meniscus is larger, the horns are more separated from one another and the bowtie appearance is not present (Fig. 3-193).

The menisci function not only as shock absorbers but as passive stabilizers for the knee. The menisci are firmly attached to the tibia at anterior and posterior tibial insertion sites. In addition, there are meniscofemoral ligaments that course from the posterior horn of the lateral meniscus to the medial femoral condyle. These ligaments are variably present. If anterior to the posterior cruciate ligament, it is called the meniscofemoral ligament of Humphry, and if posterior to the posterior cruciate ligament, it is called the meniscofemoral ligament of Wrisberg (Fig. 3-194). There is also a variable presence of oblique intermeniscal ligaments that course from the posterior horn of one meniscus to the anterior horn of the other meniscus. The menisci are firmly attached to the joint capsule and are mobile except at the anterior and posterior tibial insertion sites. The lateral meniscus is less intimately attached to the joint capsule than is the medial meniscus, because the lateral meniscus must be loosely attached at its body and posterior horn to allow passage

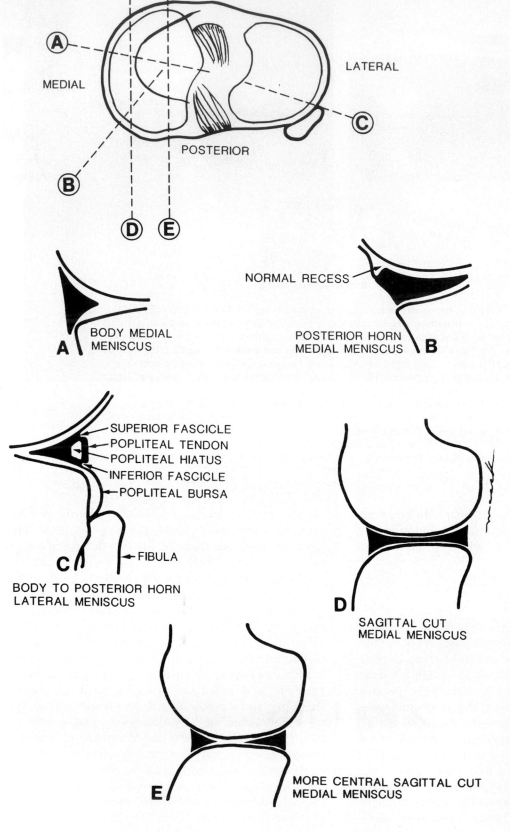

ANTERIOR

MEDIAL

LATERAL

POSTERIOR

NORMAL RECESS

A BODY MEDIAL MENISCUS

B POSTERIOR HORN MEDIAL MENISCUS

SUPERIOR FASCICLE
POPLITEAL TENDON
POPLITEAL HIATUS
INFERIOR FASCICLE
POPLITEAL BURSA

FIBULA

C BODY TO POSTERIOR HORN LATERAL MENISCUS

D SAGITTAL CUT MEDIAL MENISCUS

E MORE CENTRAL SAGITTAL CUT MEDIAL MENISCUS

Fig. 3-192   Top: Diagram of the medial and lateral menisci, looking down on the tibial plateau. The labeled lines represent the various planes in which MR sequences are commonly obtained. **A** and **B,** represent radial planes through the body and posterior horns, respectively, of the medial meniscus. **C,** represents radial cuts through the body and posterior horn of the lateral meniscus. **D** and **E,** are sagittal cuts through the medial meniscus at different distances from the periphery. (From Manaster BJ. *Handbook of Skeletal Radiology,* ed 2, St. Louis, 1997, Mosby-Yearbook.)

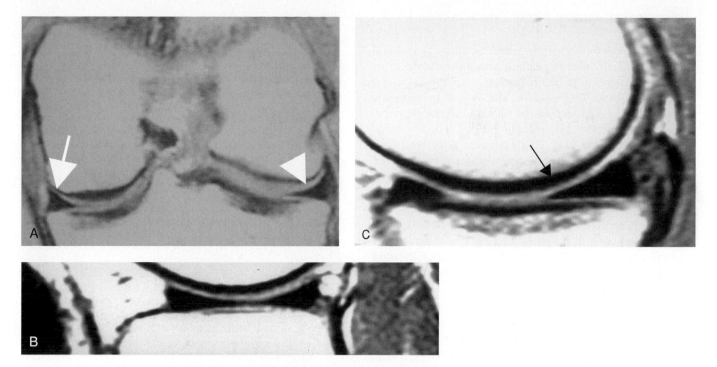

Fig. 3-193 MR images demonstrating normal meniscal morphology. **A,** Coronal MR image (600/14; TR msec/TE msec) demonstrates triangular appearance of medial (*arrow*) and lateral (*arrowhead*) menisci. Note that height is greatest peripherally and that height tapers to a sharp central free margin. **B** and **C,** Sagittal MR images (2200/14) of lateral (**B**) and medial (**C**) menisci demonstrate uniform dark signal intensity. Note equal size of anterior and posterior horns of lateral meniscus in **B** compared with larger size of posterior horn of medial meniscus in **C.** Arrow indicates larger posterior horn of medial meniscus.

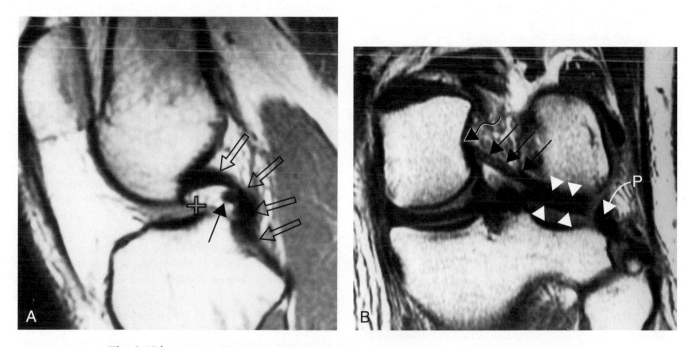

Fig. 3-194 Sagittal (**A**) and coronal (**B**) MR images (2200/20; TR msec/TE msec) demonstrate the meniscofemoral ligament of Humphry (*arrows*). Note ligament is anterior to posterior cruciate ligament (*open arrows*). Note course of ligament from posterior horn of lateral meniscus (*arrowheads*) to lateral margin of medial femoral condyle (*curved arrow*). Note popliteus tendon (P) along periphery of lateral meniscus. Increased signal between tendon and peripheral margin of meniscus can be confused with meniscal tear. Knowledge of anatomy allows discrimination between popliteus tendon and meniscal tear.

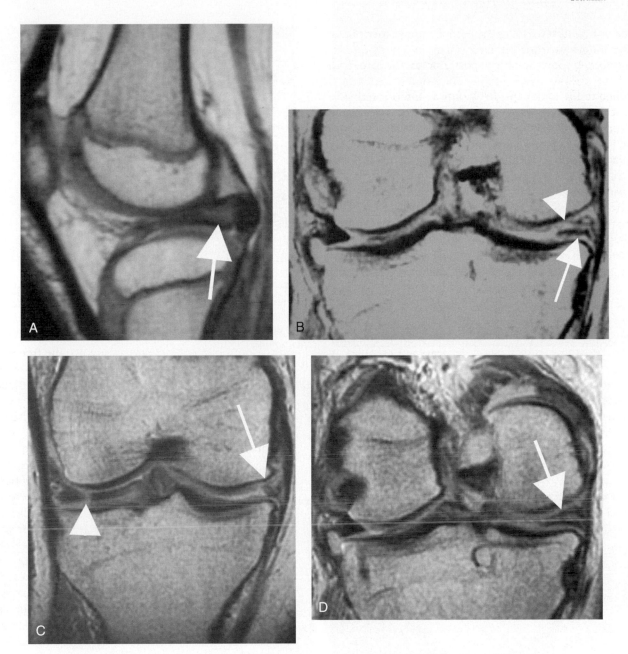

of the popliteus tendon, as the tendon courses peripheral to the meniscus from the lateral femoral condyle to its musculotendonous junction posterior to the proximal tibial metaphysis (Fig. 3-195). The lateral meniscus is attached to the joint capsule by only an inferior retinaculum at the body, by superior and inferior retinaculum at the junction of the body and posterior horn, and by a superior retinaculum at the posterior horn. Because the medial meniscus is less mobile, is at greater risk for tear. Microscopic anatomy also places both medial and lateral meniscus at risk for tear. Microscopically, menisci consist of circumferential horizontal bundles of collagen fibers interspersed with fibers extending radially from the periphery toward the free margin. This allows stabilization of fibers with centripetal loading, which is the most common form of loading of the knee. However, this orientation yields a relative weakness in the meniscus to loads in the horizontal and vertical planes.

Disruptions of menisci are called meniscal tears and these tears can occur in various configurations (Fig. 3-196). Most commonly, meniscal tears are complex in nature meaning that they attain multiple orientations. A *vertical-radial* meniscal tear occurs in a vertical plane extending from the periphery of the meniscus to the free margin of the meniscus, thus radially splitting a meniscus. A *horizontal cleavage* tear consists of a tear in a plane splitting the meniscus into superior and inferior portions. A *vertical-longitudinal* tear is a circumferential tear perpendicular to the tibial plateau that extends from the superior to inferior meniscal margin and propagates around the circumference of the meniscus. These tears

Fig. 3-195 Sagittal MR image (2200/15; TR msec/TE msec) shows course of popliteal tendon (*arrows*) adjacent to periphery of posterior horn of lateral meniscus (*open arrows*). The popliteal hiatus is an intraarticular structure that may contain synovial fluid. Localized increased signal from fluid between tendon and meniscus (*curved arrow*) may mimic a peripheral meniscal tear. Note portion of superior meniscal retinaculum (*arrowhead*).

Fig. 3-196 Frontal fluoroscopic image obtained during a knee arthrogram demonstrates articular air within a horizontal tear of the body of the medial meniscus (*arrows*).

may be peripheral in location, or involve the free margin as a *parrot-beak* tear. Bucket-handle tears are vertical-longitudinal tears that are so extensive that the central portion displaces.

MR imaging criteria for meniscal tears have been extensively studied, and T1-weighted and proton density-weighted spin-echo MR images have been found to have the highest acccuracy in detecting meniscal tears. Fast spin-echo imaging with proton density weighting has also been shown to be accurate in meniscal tear detection. Although the exact appearance of a meniscal tear at imaging may not closely correlate with what is found at surgery, there is high accuracy for the detection of meniscal tear as well as the determination of its location (Fig. 3-197). Evaluation of menisci in both sagittal and coronal planes is essential as the coronal plane evaluates the body of the meniscus and the sagittal plane evaluates the anterior and posterior horns. The signal within normal meniscus should be uniformly diminished in intensity. Lobular areas of increased signal within the central portion of the meniscus as demonstrated on sagittal or coronal proton density or T1-weighted spin-echo images are named Grade I signal abnormalities and have no clinical significance as they do not correlate with meniscal disruption. Grade II signal abnormalities represent linear increased signal in the central portion of the meniscus, which does not reach an articular surface. Grade II signal has a low association with meniscal tear. However, extensive areas of Grade II signal or large globular areas of internal signal change have a higher association with meniscal tear. Patients with extensive intrameniscal signal are found to have a 10%–20% incidence of meniscal tear at arthroscopy. Grade III signal is increased signal within the meniscus that comes in contact with either the superior or inferior articular surface. This represents

Fig. 3-197   Meniscal pathology in four different patients. **A,** Sagittal MR image (2200/14; TR msec/T msec) in child with discoid meniscus demonstrates prominent intrameniscal signal (*arrow*). Note that signal does not extend to an articular margin (grade II). **B,** Coronal MR image (600/14) shows abnormal medial meniscus (*arrow*) with intrameniscal signal extending to superior articular margin (*arrowhead*). This finding constitutes grade III signal. **C,** Coronal MR image (600/14) shows complex tear of body of medial meniscus (*arrow*). Note small meniscal body and blunted free margin. In the lateral meniscus there is vertical signal (*arrowheads*) related to a radial tear. **D,** Coronal MR images (600/14) demonstrates horizontal grade III signal within medial meniscus (*arrow*).

direct MR imaging evidence of meniscal tear and has a sensitivity and specificity exceeding 90%. It is noteworthy that meniscal tears are largely inapparent on T2-weighted images unless there is fluidlike signal within the linear defects (Fig. 3-198). Rarely, intrameniscal cysts can occur, which can be confused with meniscal tear.

However, intrameniscal cysts are rare compared with the extremely common occurrence of meniscal tears.

Menisci can also be evaluated for indirect evidence of meniscal tear (Fig. 3-199). Indirect evidence is primarily shown morphologically. As noted above, the menisci should appear triangular in shape. The anterior and poste-

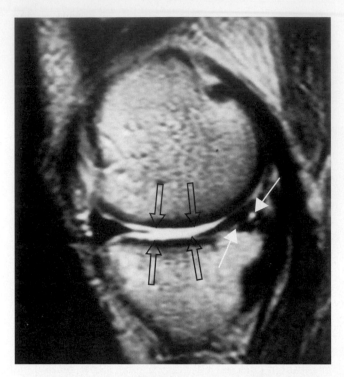

Fig. 3-198 Sagittal T2-weighted spin echo image (2200/80; TR msec/TE msec) demonstrates linear fluid signal (*arrows*) within the posterior horn of the medial meniscus, indicating meniscal tear. Note signal within meniscus is similar to fluid elsewhere in the joint (*open arrows*).

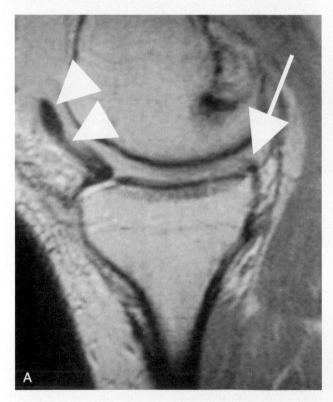

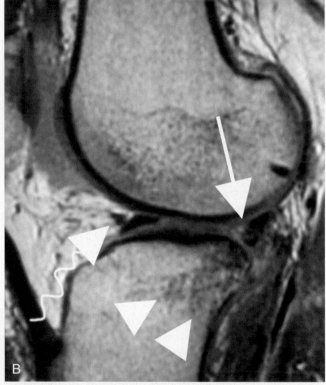

Fig. 3-199 Indirect evidence for meniscal tear. **A,** Sagittal MR image (2200/14; TR msec/TE msec) demonstrates small posterior horn of medial meniscus (*arrow*). This patient had a large peripheral meniscal tear involving all three horns of meniscus. Note displaced meniscal fragment (*arrowheads*) at anterior horn. **B,** Sagittal MR image (2200/14) in another patient demonstrates blunted posterior margin of lateral meniscus (*arrow*) indicating meniscal tear. Note transverse meniscal ligament (*curved arrow*), which because of its location adjacent to periphery of anterior horn can mimic meniscal tear. Also note indirect evidence of anterior cruciate ligament tear (discussed later in text) with posterior lateral tibial bone bruise (*arrowheads*) and substantial anterior tibial subluxation.

rior horns of the lateral meniscus are symmetric in size, whereas the posterior horn of the medial meniscus is larger and more elongated in appearance compared with the anterior horn of the medial meniscus. Therefore the appearance of a similar size in the posterior horn of the medial meniscus as the anterior horn is abnormal, and diagnostic of a meniscal tear. Also, a blunted appearance of the triangular free margin of a meniscus also indicates a tear. Finally, menisci should be uniformly diminished in signal intensity on all sequential imaging slices. If an intervening slice fails to demonstrate a meniscus or shows a meniscus of substantially higher diffuse signal, this suggests the presence of a radial tear (a tear in the plane of imaging). A radial tear would be supported by the finding of ipsilateral meniscal peripheral displacement beyond the margin of the corresponding cortical margin of the tibial plateau.

A *bucket handle* meniscal tear is a vertical-longitudinal tear that involves all three horns of the meniscus. The meniscus is displaced but remains attached at at least one of the two-tibial insertion sites. The displacement may extend to the intercondylar notch or to an adjacent meniscal horn. Bucket handle tears must be carefully sought at MR imaging because the sensitivity of their detection is low, around 60%, and detection will be missed unless conscious search is made for them (Fig. 3-200). On MR images in which there is intercondylar meniscal displacement, one should be able to follow the signal of meniscus along its displaced course in the intercondylar notch in a continuous fashion, connecting to the anterior and posterior horns. This must be associated with a small meniscal body and a posterior horn of proportionately diminished size. Because the displaced fragment is apposed adjacent to the posterior cruciate ligament, it can give the appearance of a second posterior cruciate ligament. When there is displacement adjacent to another meniscal horn, the donor meniscal site appears too small, whereas the site of displacement appears too large.

Discoid meniscus is a variant in which the meniscus is more disc-shaped than semicircular shaped and in which a portion of meniscus extends to the central portion of the tibial plateau (Fig. 3-201). This is far more common in the lateral meniscus and is clinically significant for two reasons. First, a discoid meniscus itself may be symptomatic, giving patients symptoms of locking and joint line pain. Second, a discoid meniscus is prone to tear because of its aberrant morphology and suboptimal biomechanical properties. Discoid meniscus is suspected when children and young adolescents present with signs of meniscal tear. Discoid meniscus is demonstrated on coronal MR images when the horizontal measurement between the free margin and periphery of the body of the meniscus is more than 1.4 cm. In addition, on sagittal

images obtained at 3–4 mm slice thickness with 1 mm interslice sections, the body of the meniscus should not be shown on more than two to three sequential images. If shown on more than three images, discoid meniscus is diagnosed.

There are pitfalls at MR imaging in diagnosing meniscal tears. These are due to the presence of normal structures that are in close proximity to the periphery of the meniscus causing signal that can be confused with Grade III meniscal signal. One example is the popliteus tendon within the popliteal hiatus. Higher signal from fluid within the hiatus, located between the tendon and the periphery of the lateral meniscus, may produce signal mimicking meniscal tear. The meniscofemoral ligaments also may produce an appearance mimicking meniscal tear, because they course posterior to the posterior horn of the lateral meniscus. The transverse meniscal ligament is a ligament connecting the anterior horns of the medial and lateral menisci. Like the meniscofemoral ligaments, this ligament may extend peripheral to the anterior horn of either meniscus with intervening signal mimicking that of meniscal tear. The oblique meniscal ligaments, which are found occasionally, and which connect the anterior horn of one meniscus with posterior horn of the other meniscus, can be confused with bucket handle tears as this ligament is identified coursing through the intercondylar notch. Finally, the normal fibrofatty meniscocapsular junction can be confused with meniscal tear due to its high signal (Fig. 3-202).

Parameniscal cysts are occasionally found at MR imaging and have a high association with meniscal tear. These are located at the peripheral margin of the meniscus and are occasionally intrameniscal. They are usually located along the anterolateral margin of the meniscus and are more common in the lateral meniscus (Fig. 3-203). When a parameniscal cyst is found, a careful search for the presence of a meniscal tear must be made because the likelihood of meniscal tear is greatly increased. Occasionally, parameniscal cysts are ganglion cysts or synovial cysts whose appearance is identical except for the lack of a coincident meniscal tear.

In a postoperative situation in which there has been previous meniscal repair or partial resection, MR imaging is unreliable. This is primarily because Grade III signal persists in the meniscus after primary repair and cannot be discriminated from a meniscal re-tear. The more extensive the meniscal surgery the less accurate meniscal evaluation is at postoperative MR imaging. However, in such postoperative situations, accuracy for detection of re-tears is greatly enhanced with MR-arthrography. The goal at MR-arthrography is to demonstrate contrast material within the meniscus. MR-arthrography has a high accuracy in the diagnosis of a re-tear, approaching 90%.

Text continued on p. 342

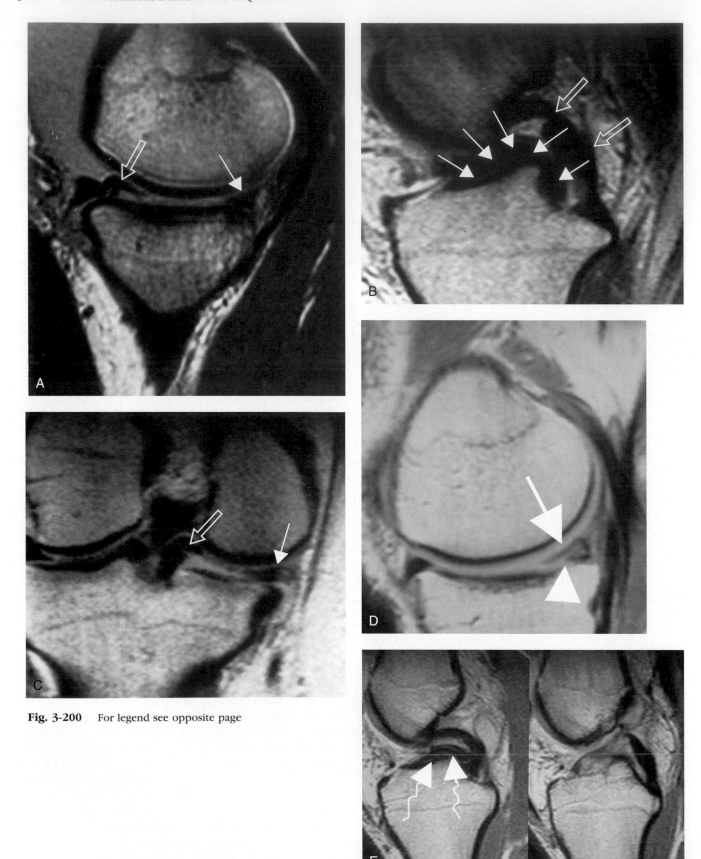

Fig. 3-200   For legend see opposite page

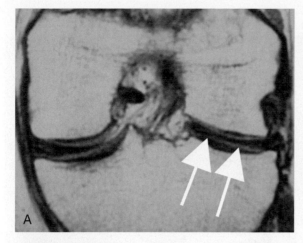

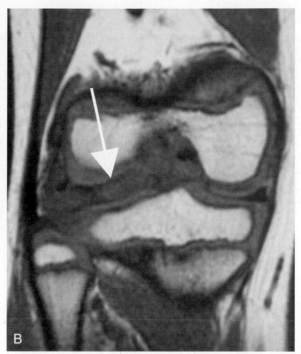

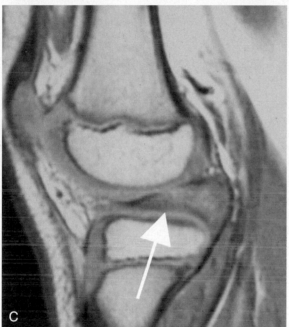

Fig. 3-201 Examples of discoid meniscus. **A,** Coronal MR image (600/14; TR msec/TE msec) shows meniscal signal (*arrows*) crossing entire intercondylar region of lateral compartment. **B** and **C,** Coronal (600/14) and sagittal (2200/14) MR images demonstrate discoid lateral meniscus (*arrows*) in another child with extremely prominent intrameniscal grade II signal. Meniscus was found to be degenerated and torn at arthroscopy.

Fig. 3-200 Examples of bucket handle meniscal tear. **A,** Sagittal MR image (200/14; TR msec/TE msec) demonstrates small posterior horn of medial meniscus (*arrow*) and displaced attached meniscal fragment (*open arrow*) at anterior horn. **B,** Sagittal MR image (2000/14) lateral to **A** demonstrates displaced meniscal fragment (*arrows*) within intercondylar notch region. This finding is called the "double PCL" sign because of its intercondylar notch location and similar shape as posterior cruciate ligament (*open arrows*). **C,** Coronal MR image (600/14) in same patient demonstrates small meniscal body (*arrow*) and intercondylar notch fragment (*open arrow*). **D** and **E,** Sagittal MR images (2200/14) in another patient demonstrate small posterior horn of medial meniscus (*arrow*) with grade III signal (*arrowhead*) and double PCL sign (*curved arrows*). The normal intercondylar notch region should only contain the anterior cruciate ligament and posterior cruciate ligament. The displaced meniscal fragment (*curved arrows*) represents a third intercondylar region structure, and thus is a clue to the presence of bucket handle meniscal tear.

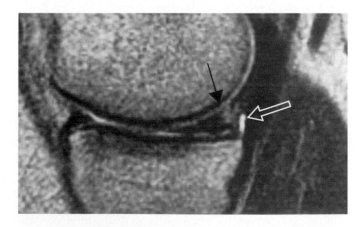

Fig. 3-202 Sagittal MR image (2200/14; TR msec/TE msec) shows fibrofatty signal (*arrow*) peripheral to posterior horn of medial meniscus mimicking a tear. Note the presence of fluid (*open arrow*) at joint periphery. This parameniscal cyst was not associated with a meniscal tear at arthroscopy.

341

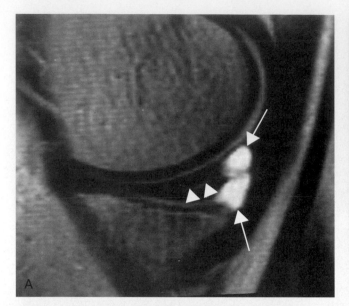

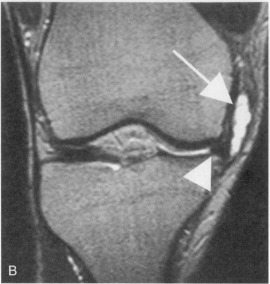

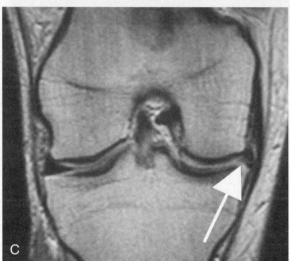

Fig. 3-203   Parameniscal cysts. **A,** Sagittal T2-weighted MR image (2800/80; TR msec/TE msec) demonstrates meniscal cyst (*arrows*). Intrameniscal signal (*arrowheads*) was shown on other images to represent a horizontal tear of the body and posterior horn of the medial meniscus. **B,** Coronal T2-weighted image (2800/80) in another patient demonstrates meniscal cyst (*arrow*) in patient with meniscal tear. Note small meniscal body (*arrowhead*) with blunted free margin. **C,** Proton density weighted MR image (2800/16) in same patient as **B** shows medial meniscus with small meniscal body and grade III intrameniscal signal (*arrow*).

Cruciate Ligament Injury

The cruciate ligaments are crossing ligaments that are intracapsular yet extrasynovial in location. With the medial and lateral collateral ligaments, the cruciate ligaments form the major stabilizers of the knee joint. The anterior cruciate ligament (ACL) is the primary stabilizer of the knee against anterior tibial subluxation. It originates from the medial margin of the lateral femoral condyle at the intercondylar notch and courses anteriorly, medially, and inferiorly to insert at the anterior aspect of the intercondylar eminence (Fig. 3-204). The posterior cruciate ligament is the primary restraint against posterior subluxation of the tibia and it originates from the lateral margin of the medial femoral condyle at the intercondylar notch

to course in a posterior, lateral, and inferior direction to insert in a depression behind the intercondylar region of the tibia (Fig. 3-205). The anterior cruciate ligament appears thin and taut on the MR images with the knee in extension, the posterior cruciate ligament appears thick and curved with its apex posterior in its mid portion.

The anterior cruciate ligament is the most commonly torn ligament at the knee. This occurs typically in the setting either of a clipping injury in which the knee is placed in valgus, or a pivot-shift injury, in which the femur laterally rotates on the planted leg. Thus valgus and anterolateral rotatory subluxation of the knee can lead to ACL injury. *There are four primary signs of a ligament tear.* These signs apply for any ligament, and for the assessment of the anterior cruciate ligament they

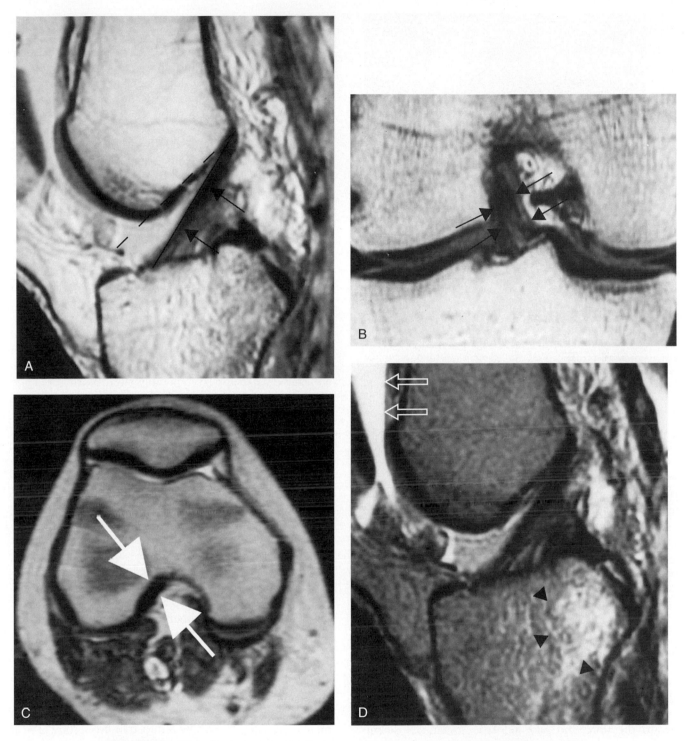

Fig. 3-204 Normal anterior cruciate ligament. **A,** Sagittal proton density weighted spin echo image (2200/14; TR msec/TE msec) demonstrates uniform low signal intensity of anterior cruciate ligament (*arrows*). Note normal course of ligament: lines drawn along ligament (*solid line*) and roof of intercondylar notch (*dashed line*) form an angle whose apex projects posteriorly. **B,** Coronal T1-weighted image (600/14) shows normal fanlike appearance of anterior cruciate ligament (*arrows*) with linear bands of dark signal interspersed with fibrofatty bands of intermediate signal. **C,** Axial T2-weighted MR image (2200/80) shows normal ACL (*arrows*) at origin along medial margin of lateral femoral notch. **D,** Sagittal T2-weighted MR image (2800/80) in another patient shows intact ACL signal and course in patient with large knee joint effusion (*open arrows*) and extensive tibial bone bruise (*arrowheads*). This patient had an isolated posterior cruciate ligament injury (not shown).

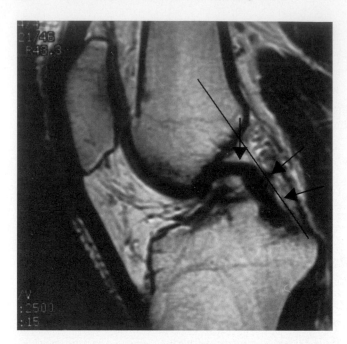

Fig. 3-205 Sagittal MR image (2500/15; TR msec/TE msec) demonstrates normal posterior cruciate ligament (*arrows*). Note that a line drawn tangent to the posterior margin of the descending limb (*solid line*) intersects distal femur. This is an indirect sign of an intact anterior cruciate ligament.

are highly accurate. These signs are *swelling, increased signal, fiber discontinuity,* and *change in the expected ligament course* (Fig. 3-206). For ACL evaluation, these primary signs have an accuracy in excess of 90%. Lines drawn along the course of the normal anterior cruciate ligament and the roof of the femoral notch form an angle whose apex points posteriorly. In the setting of anterior cruciate ligament disruption, the ligament fibers flatten to a horizontal position, and the angle formed by the torn ligament and the roof of the intercondylar notch has an apex that points anteriorly. It should be noted that ligament rupture is by far more common than ligament avulsion. The location of rupture is usually near the femoral origin. The MR imaging plane most useful for evaluation of the anterior cruciate ligament is the sagittal imaging plane. This allows demonstration of fiber continuity, ACL swelling and signal changes, and ACL course. However, because the ACL is a thin and fanlike ligament, spreading transversely as it extends inferiorly toward the tibia, the sagittal plane sometimes poorly demonstrates the anterior cruciate ligament, even though it is not torn. In this situation, coronal and axial imaging planes are extremely useful, because these planes show the ACL in cross section. The demonstration of a normal anterior cruciate ligament without swelling or edema-like signal in these imaging planes excludes ACL tear. The most useful type of imaging sequence for the evaluation of the ACL are the T2- weighted spin-echo, and the fat suppressed proton density or T2-weighted fast spin-echo sequences. This allows the best demonstration of

edema-like signal while still allowing clear visualization of soft tissue anatomy. Inversion recovery images are sensitive to the detection of edema but anatomic resolution is diminished owing to lower signal-to-noise-ratio.

There are several secondary signs of anterior cruciate ligament tear that independently show high accuracy in assessment of ACL disruption (Fig. 3-207). However, none of these signs augment the accuracy of the four primary signs. Some of these associations are of soft tissue origin, others are of osseous origin. First, hemarthrosis is commonly associated with ACL rupture. In fact, as many as 75% of acute hemarthroses are due to ACL rupture. Other causes for hemarthrosis in the setting of trauma are large bone bruises and intraarticular fractures. Bone bruises are commonly associated with anterior cruciate ligament ruptures, particularly posterior-lateral tibial bone bruises and anterior-lateral femoral bone bruises. The presence of a posterior-lateral tibial bone bruise itself has a high predictive value for ACL tear. An exception to this association is with pediatric patients in whom a bone bruise in this location may occur in the absence of ACL tear. This is due to greater laxity of the ACL in children. In the setting of ACL injury, the posterior cruciate ligament can appear hyperangulated. Normally, a line drawn tangent to the posterior margin of the PCL should intersect the distal 4-6 cm of the femur. When this line fails to intersect the distal femur there is implied ACL tear. Another sign is known as the "anterior drawer sign." This is shown when the tibia subluxes relative to the femur. If lines are drawn vertical to the posterior margins of the lateral tibial and femoral condyles in the mid lateral compartment, and the tibia is more than 7 mm anteriorly subluxed, this is considered a sign of a complete ACL rupture. A related finding is when the posterior horn of the lateral meniscus is posteriorly subluxed relative to the posterior cortical margin of the lateral tibial condyle. Any posterior meniscal displacement is associated with anterior cruciate ligament tear.

Anterior cruciate ligament injury can be associated with medial collateral ligament injury and medial meniscal tear. This association is termed *O'Donoghue's terrible triad.* In truth, however, the lateral meniscus is more commonly torn in the setting of ACL injury because of lateral impaction that occurs with clipping and pivot-shift injuries. However, sensitivity of detecting lateral meniscal tears is drastically reduced in the setting of ACL tear. Another associated injury pattern is the occurrence of posterolateral corner injury with ACL tear. Posterolateral corner structures include the lateral collateral ligament, lateral capsule, popliteus tendon, and several smaller ligaments that are poorly seen with MR imaging, such as the arcuate ligament, the fabellofibular ligament, and the ligament of Winslow. The occurrence of lateral corner injuries at MR imaging implies anterior cruciate ligament tear. Injuries at this location are only now being studied, and are considered an indication for early surgi-

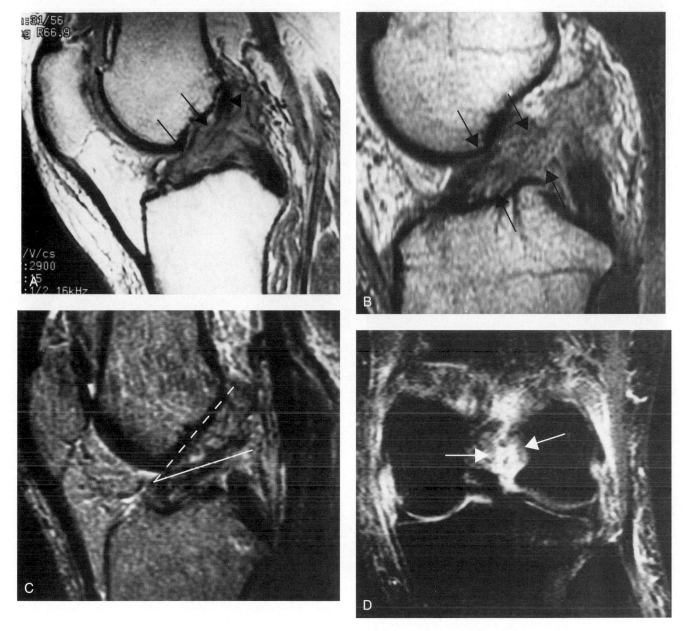

Fig. 3-206   Anterior cruciate ligament tear. **A,** Sagittal proton density-weighted spin echo image (2900/15; TR msec/TE msec) shows fiber discontinuity, swelling, and increased signal of torn anterior cruciate ligament (*arrows*). Note intact origin (*arrowhead*). **B,** T2-weight spin echo image (2900/80) shows amorphous globular increased signal (*arrows*) along expected course of anterior cruciate ligament. **C,** Sagittal T2-weighted image (2800/80) in another patient shows abnormal course of anterior cruciate ligament. Line drawn through torn ACL (*solid line*) and line drawn through roof of acetabulum (*dashed line*) form an angle whose apex points anteriorly, not posteriorly. **D,** Coronal inversion recovery image (3000/30; inversion time 140 msec) shows localized increased signal (*arrows*) in lateral intercondylar notch at expected location of anterior cruciate ligament origin, indicating tear.

cal repair owing to concern for delayed instability if the posterolateral corner is not repaired. Other signs of posterolateral corner injury are the Segond fracture, which is a lateral capsule avulsion fracture at the lateral tibial plateau, and avulsion at the fibular head. Although impaction injuries at the posterior rim of the lateral tibial plateau, and avulsions at Gerdy's tubercle where the ilio-

tibial band inserts are associated with ACL tear, they are not associated with posterolateral corner injury.

ACL reconstruction can be performed arthroscopically with either tendon autografts or with cadaver or synthetic allografts. Autografts are the most common, with patellar bone-tendon-bone autografts the most common. The tendon is placed along the course of the ACL and secured

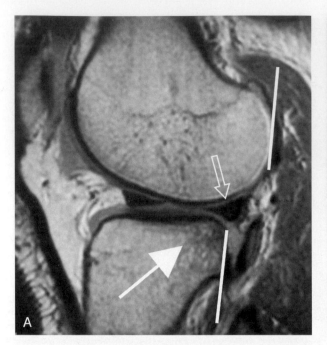
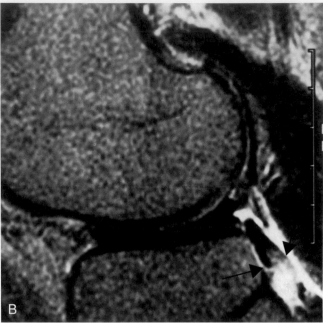

Fig. 3-207 Secondary signs of anterior cruciate ligament tear. **A,** Sagittal proton density spin echo image (2700/15; TR msec/TE msec) demonstrates posterolateral tibial condyle bone bruise (*arrow*). Note that vertical lines drawn along posterior margin of the lateral femoral and tibial condyles demonstrate substantial anterior tibial subluxation. Note also posterior subluxation of posterior horn of lateral meniscus (*open arrow*). **B,** Sagittal T2-weighted spin echo image (2800/80) in another patient demonstrates complete tear of popliteus tendon at musculotendinous junction (*arrows*). Posterolateral corner injury such as this has high association with anterior cruciate ligament tear.

within posterolateral femoral and anteromedial tunnels using the bone graft as a wedge between the edge of the tunnel and an interference screw (Fig. 3-208). Normal placement of the tibial tunnel should be posterior to the line extended from the roof of the intercondylar notch in the extended knee position. Failure of this tunnel placement will limit terminal extension of the knee. Additional complications after ACL repair include bone plug migration, graft rupture, and fibrous proliferation anterior to the graft known as a *cyclops lesion,* which interferes with terminal extension. In addition, fibrous proliferation within the lateral femoral notch can occur, interfering with graft mobility, which is often avoided by performance of a "notch-plasty" (surgical enlargement of the notch along its lateral margins). Rarely, the patella can fracture at the bone graft harvest site. MR imaging after ACL graft repair is useful for evaluating the integrity of the graft. Fiber continuity and anatomic alignment should be expected. Graft failure is diagnosed in a similar fashion as primary ACL rupture. Cyclops lesions are demonstrated as a rounded area of diminished signal in T2 weighted images anterior to the mid and distal portions of the ACL graft.

Posterior cruciate ligament ruptures are uncommon due to the large size and strength of the PCL. Usually PCL rupture occurs with ACL rupture and usually after severe injury such as posterior dislocation of the knee. Isolated PCL injury can also occur, often after blunt trauma to the anterior proximal tibia with the knee in flexion (dashboard injury). Criteria for PCL rupture are the same as for other ligaments and include swelling, increased signal intensity, fiber discontinuity, and abnormal course of the PCL (Fig. 3-209). Normally, in the extended knee position, the PCL is slightly curved with its apex posteriorly directed and is easily shown on at least two contiguous sagittal cuts. Sharp bowing of the PCL indicates laxity of the tendon either from a tear of the PCL or as a secondary sign of ACL disruption. Avulsions of the PCL rarely occur and are located either at the medial femoral origin or at the posterior tibial insertion. Posterior cruciate ligament reconstructions are controversial. At many centers, PCL ruptures are not repaired as isolated PCL injury is not felt to be associated with substantial instability. One rarely encounters knees in which PCL repair has been performed. Complications and imaging are as for the anterior cruciate ligament.

Collateral Ligament Injury

The medial and lateral collateral ligaments are the primary restraints to valgus and varus loads, respectively. The medial collateral ligament (MCL) is a large, complex

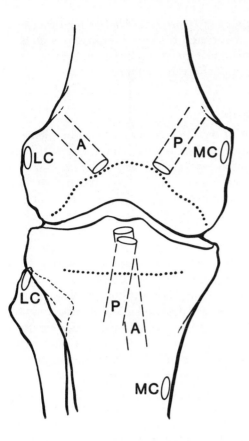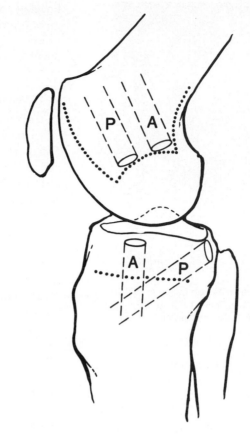

Fig. 3-208 Diagrams show anatomic sites for ACL and PCL reconstructions (A and P, respectively), as well as isometric points for attachments of the LCL and MCL. Tunnel positioning or ligament attachment should roughly parallel the sites shown on these diagrams. (From Manaster BJ. *Handbook of Skeletal Radiology,* ed 2, St. Louis, 1997, Mosby-Yearbook.)

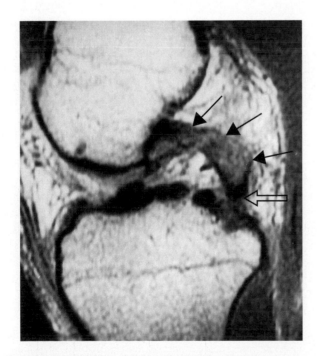

Fig. 3-209 Sagittal MR image (2400/15; TR msec/TE msec) shows increased size and signal within the posterior cruciate ligament (*arrows*). Note discontinuity of distal ligament (*open arrow*).

structure. There are three layers to the medial collateral ligament. The most superficial layer is the superficial fascia. The middle layer is the true ligament, which originates just distal to the adductor tubercle of the femur, coursing inferiorly to the medial tibial tubercle, inserting at a level 5 cm below the joint line (Fig. 3-210). The deep layer of the medial collateral ligament is actually the joint capsule and is intimately associated with the medial meniscus, originating and inserting on the margins of the joint.

The lateral collateral ligament (LCL) is part of the posterolateral complex of the knee and originates in a sulcus along the lateral femoral condyle, extending distally and posteriorly to insert as a conjoint insertion with the biceps femoris tendon on the fibular head. It is a major contributor to posterolateral stability.

Injuries of the MCL and LCL usually occur in combination with other injuries. MCL rupture is commonly associated with anterior cruciate ligament tears and meniscal tears. MCL ruptures are associated with valgus injuries and, like other ligament injuries, range from partial ligament disruptions, in which edema and hemorrhage predominate, to complete ligament disruptions, in which fiber discontinuity is evident (Fig. 3-211). Osseous abnormalities can be associated with MCL injury and include bone bruises in the opposing lateral margins of the lateral

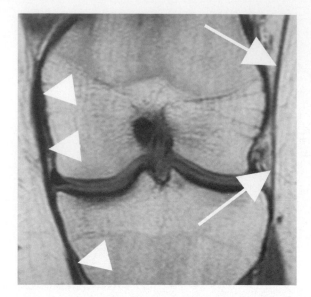

Fig. 3-210 Coronal T1-weighted spin echo image (450/14 ; TR msec/TE msec) demonstrates normal medial collateral ligament (*arrowheads*). Note iliotibial band (*arrows*) laterally.

tibial and femoral condyles at the site of impaction during valgus injury. *Pellegrini-Stieda* disease represents posttraumatic calcification around the MCL origin related to previous trauma. LCL ruptures are uncommon and rarely isolated. They are associated not only with ACL injury but with posterolateral corner instability. They can also be associated with peroneal nerve injury owing to the nerve's proximity to the fibular head and LCL insertion.

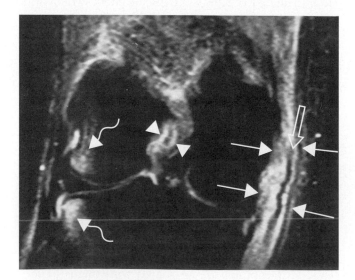

Fig. 3-211 Coronal inversion recovery image (300/40; TR msec/TE msec; inversion time 140 msec) demonstrates increased signal medial to knee (*arrows*) and discontinuity of medial collateral ligament (*open arrow*). Also note bone bruises in lateral femoral and tibial condyles (*curved arrows*), indicating valgus injury. Bright signal in lateral intercondylar notch (*arrowheads*) is due to tear of ACL origin.

Imaging criteria of LCL disruption are as for other ligament injuries. Associated osseous abnormalities include avulsion of the fibular head. Medial bone bruises may occur as a result of the varus injury pattern.

Tendon Injury

The tendons of the knee are important to evaluate as injury of the knee may be isolated to tendon pathology. The most common tendons affected at the knee are the extensor tendons (quadriceps tendon and patellar tendon), the pes anserinus (sartorius, gracilis, and semitendinosus insertions at the medial aspect of the proximal tibia), and the popliteus musculotendinous junction.

On axial images of the knee, it can be difficult to determine medial and lateral landmarks. Helpful landmarks include the patella, whose lateral facet is longer than the medial facet. Furthermore, consideration of muscle anatomy allows easy determination of geography because in the popliteal fossa, excluding the gastrocnemius muscles, there is only one muscle group laterally (the biceps femoris), yet four medially (semimembranosus, semitendinosus, sartorius, and gracilis) (Fig. 3-212). Anteriorly, the quadriceps muscles (rectus femoris, vastus lateralis, vastus intermedius, vastus medialis) join to form the quadriceps tendon in multiple layers, usually three, as noted on sagittal MR images, with the superficial layer being the rectus femoris, the middle layer being the conjoint vastus lateralis and medialis, and the deep layer being the vastus intermedius. Fascial extensions of the

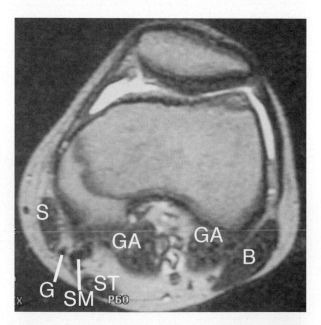

Fig. 3-212 Axial T2-weighted fast spin echo image (4000/80; TR msec/TE msec) shows normal muscle anatomy of popliteal fossa. GA, Gastrocnemius muscles. B, Biceps femoris muscle. S, Sartorius muscle. SM, Semimembranosus tendon. ST, Semitendinosus tendon. G, Gracilis tendon.

quadriceps aponeurosis form a hood over the anterior half of the knee, known as the flexor retinaculum. It is the medial retinaculum that can stretch and tear during transient patellar dislocation.

All tendon tears are graded in a similar fashion. Grade 1 tendinosis represents a tendon that is thickened, resulting from multiple repetitive tears and repairs. With grade 1 tendinosis, a tendon may be of homogeneously diminished signal on T1-weighted and T2-weighted images if repair predominates over injury. A heterogeneous pattern indicates the presence of mucoid degeneration or interstitial tendon tears (tears that are longitudinally oriented along the course of the tendon). Grade 2 tendinosis represents a tendon that is abnormally thin. This results from a tendon that is partially ruptured, with diminished transverse dimension. Grade 3 tendinosis represents tendon discontinuity. On MR imaging, tendon tears, like ligament tears, may manifest with swelling, increased signal, fiber discontinuity, and abnormal course (Fig. 3-213). However, tendons are also prone to overuse injuries, particularly the patellar tendon at the knee. This occurs with athletes whose activities include repetitive jumping, such as basketball. The condition is known as *jumper's knee.* In jumper's knee, findings predominate in the proximal patellar tendon and appear at MR imaging as increased transverse dimension and increased signal on T2-weighted images, particularly in the posterior midline fibers.

Repetitive stress injury in the skeletally immature may occur at the knee. Earlier, Osgood-Schlatter disease was discussed. Another overuse injury at the knee is the *cortical desmoid,* in which bony irregularity may occur in the posteromedial aspect of the distal femoral diametaphysis, the site of insertion of the adductor magnus muscle and origin of the medial gastrocnemius muscle. Chronic injury at this location produces a cortical defect that can mimic osseous neoplasia. However, neoplasia is excluded by MR imaging, which shows a marrow edema pattern.

Patients may present with pain at the pes anserinus insertion related to a bursitis, which can be documented at MR imaging with the demonstration of a fluid collection surrounding the tendons as they insert on the medial aspect of the proximal tibia. Other sites of bursal fluid accumulation in the knee include the gastrocnemius-semimembranosus bursa (Baker's cyst), the prepatellar bursa, and the superficial and deep infrapatellar bursae. A final

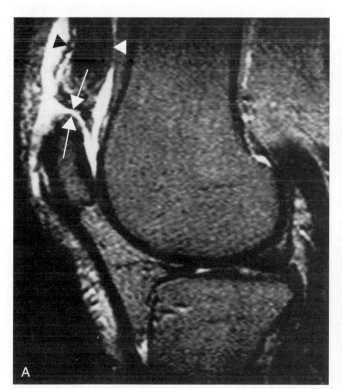
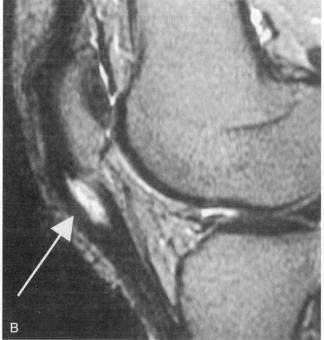

Fig. 3-213   Tendon tears. **A,** Sagittal T2-weighted spin echo image (2800/80; TR msec/TE msec) demonstrates distal quadriceps tendon rupture. Note tendon discontinuity (*arrows*) at tendon insertion and marked tendon thickening (*arrowheads*). **B,** Jumper's knee. This sagittal T2 MR (2350/80) demonstrates high signal within the posterior proximal patellar tendon adjacent to the patella (*arrow*).

area of tendon and bursal pain occurs around the insertion of the iliotibial band with symptoms anterolaterally at the knee. At MR imaging, altered signal in the fat deep to the iliotibial band is shown, and represents the occurrence of an adventitial bursal fluid collection.

Hyaline Cartilage Injury

There has been little interest until recently in the evaluation of articular cartilage. Recent interest has been generated by the development of new surgical therapies for articular cartilage derangement, which has sparked a need by orthopedic surgeons to evaluate articular cartilage both preoperatively and postoperatively. Articular cartilage is an avascular tissue that relies on the diffusion of nutrients from synovial fluid and, to a lesser extent, the extracellular space of subchondral bone. The cell of articular cartilage is the chondrocyte, which produces an abundant extracellular matrix rich in water, with solid components primarily consisting of type II collagen and proteoglycan aggregate. The result is a tissue that permits a uniform distribution of loads to the subchondral bone, and an extremely low coefficient of friction for smooth gliding.

Articular cartilage is one of the few tissues of the body that is incapable of regeneration. Limited repair of tissue only occurs if subchondral bone is breached by injury, so

that the subchondral blood supply can elicit a cytokine-generated repair response. However, the repair tissue does not maintain the same mechanical properties as native hyaline cartilage and is of limited durability. The eventual response is OA. OA is the most common disability in the United States and is associated with enormous direct and indirect costs to society, not only from a treatment standpoint, but from economic loss of productivity.

The goal of MR imaging is to accurately detect and stage articular cartilage defects. The ideal sequences for imaging articular cartilage defects are rapidly evolving but currently the most useful sequences are fat-suppressed 3-D spoiled gradient-echo and proton-density or T2-weighted fast spin-echo images (Fig. 3-214). These sequences allow high sensitivity in the detection of morphologic articular cartilage defects. There are several grading schemes that are used by orthopedic surgeons in the evaluation of articular cartilage. This assessment is done at arthroscopy and involves not only a search for visually apparent morphologic defects but for palpable defects as well. Articular cartilage is normally smooth, firm, and glistening. The earliest surgically detectable form of cartilage derangement is the detection of cartilage softness to a metal probe at arthroscopy. This is classified as a grade 1 articular cartilage defect. The remaining grades are morphologic grades. Grade 2 defects are defects less than 50% thickness of articular cartilage or

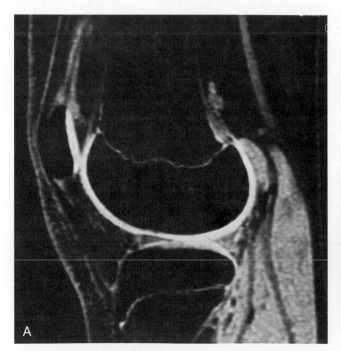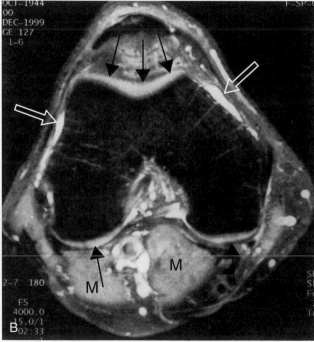

Fig. 3-214   **A,** Sagittal fat-suppressed 3-D spoiled gradient-echo MR image (60/5; TR msec/TE msec; flip angle 40°) shows normal articular cartilage at knee. Also note normal signal of distal femoral and proximal tibial growth plates. Hyaline cartilage is bright on this imaging sequence. **B,** Axial fat-suppressed proton density fast spin echo image (4000/15) shows articular cartilage (*arrows*) as intermediate signal between that of muscle (M) and joint fluid (*open arrows*).

localized areas of swelling of articular cartilage. Grade 3 defects are greater than 50% thickness. Grade 4 defects are full thickness defects, often with underlying bone sclerosis. MR imaging grades reflect the arthroscopic grades and are based on depth detection and signal change in the underlying bone. The surfaces of the joint must be carefully searched for contour defects and signal abnormality (Fig. 3-215). Lesions can be subtle owing to the thinness of articular cartilage, which is maximally only 6 mm at the patella. Defects are most common at the medial femoral and the patellar surfaces.

Injuries to articular cartilage range from chondral to osteochondral injury and associated injuries are common. In particular, there is association of articular cartilage injury with meniscal tears. These associated injuries are usually in close proximity to one another. *If a meniscal tear is found, a careful search for associated articular cartilage tear should be undertaken.*

ANKLE TRAUMA

Anatomy

The ankle joint is formed by the tibia, the fibula, and the talus, creating a hinge joint. The tibial articular margin is called the tibial plafond (ceiling). The lateral malleolus is positioned 1 cm distal and posterior to that of the medial malleolus. The medial and lateral articular margins of the ankle joint are formed by the talus and medial malleolus, and by the talus and lateral malleolus, which are obliquely oriented such that a 15°–20° internal

---

Key Concepts   Ankle Trauma

- Ankle fractures are classified according to the mechanism of injury. Understanding the sequence of injury for each mechanism allows for prediction of severity of injury and thus treatment.
- The most common mechanism of injury at the ankle is supination-external rotation. With this injury, the lateral malleolus is the most commonly fractured bone. The fracture may only be evident on the lateral view because the fracture is in the coronal plane.
- Maisonneuve fractures involve disruption of the tibiofibular syndesmosis and a proximal fibular fracture. Proximal fibular fracture should be suspected if an ankle radiograph demonstrates swelling over the medial malleolus and posterior malleolar fracture. In this situation one must search the entire leg for fibular fracture proximal to the level of the ankle. The significance is not the fibular fracture itself, but the implied instability of the ankle.

---

oblique view (mortise view) allows visualization of the articular margins in profile. The talus is a dome shaped structure. It fits snugly within the articulation formed by the tibia and fibula such that there is a symmetric 3–4 mm margin between the entire talar surface and the apposing plafond and malleolar margins.

The ankle is supported by a complex array of ligaments (Fig. 3-216). A syndesmosis is present between the tibia and fibula, the distal aspect of which forms the anterior and posterior distal tibiofibular ligaments. The anterior and posterior distal tibiofibular ligaments are the most superior set of ankle ligaments, seen on axial MR images immediately above the ankle joint. These appear as uniform thin low signal structures on all imaging sequences, passing between anterior and posterior margins of the tibia and the apposing fibula. The medial margin of the fibula is convex or straight at this level. Below the anterior and posterior distal tibiofibular ligaments, the lateral collateral ligaments are found. This ligament complex is composed of three structures (Fig. 3-217). The anterior talofibular ligament extends from the anterior fibula to the lateral talar neck, shown best on the axial plane at the level where the medial aspect of the fibula is concave. The anterior talofibular ligament is the most frequently torn ankle ligament. The posterior talofibular ligament is a large fan-shaped ligament extending from the distal aspect of the lateral malleolar fossa to the lateral tubercle of the posterior talar process. The ligament is seen at the same level on axial MR images as the anterior talofibular ligament but appears more inhomogeneous because of the fan-shaped ligament fibers. The third ligament of the lateral collateral ligaments is the calcaneofibular ligament, which extends from the tip of the lateral malleolus to the lateral aspect of the calcaneus. This is the most difficult of the lateral ankle ligaments to see at MR imaging, shown partially on either coronal or axial images, but best shown on oblique axial images with the foot in plantar flexion. The medial collateral ligament is also known as the deltoid ligament and consists of five components. The medial collateral ligament is a much stronger ligament complex than the lateral collateral ligament and is less commonly torn. Located deep to the flexor tendons, the deltoid ligament consists of superficial and deep components. The superficial ligaments are the tibiocalcaneal, tibiospring, and tibionavicular ligaments, which course from the tibia to the calcaneus, spring ligament, and navicular bone. The deep ligaments are the anterior and posterior tibiotalar ligaments. Of all the deltoid ligaments, the tibionavicular ligament is the weakest.

The largest of the tendons found at the ankle is the Achilles tendon, which is the tendon formed by the gastrocnemius and soleus muscles that merge to form a thick tendon that inserts on the posterior calcaneus. The flexor tendons of the ankle are found posteromedially at the ankle and are, from medial to lateral, the tibialis posterior,

Text continued on p. 355

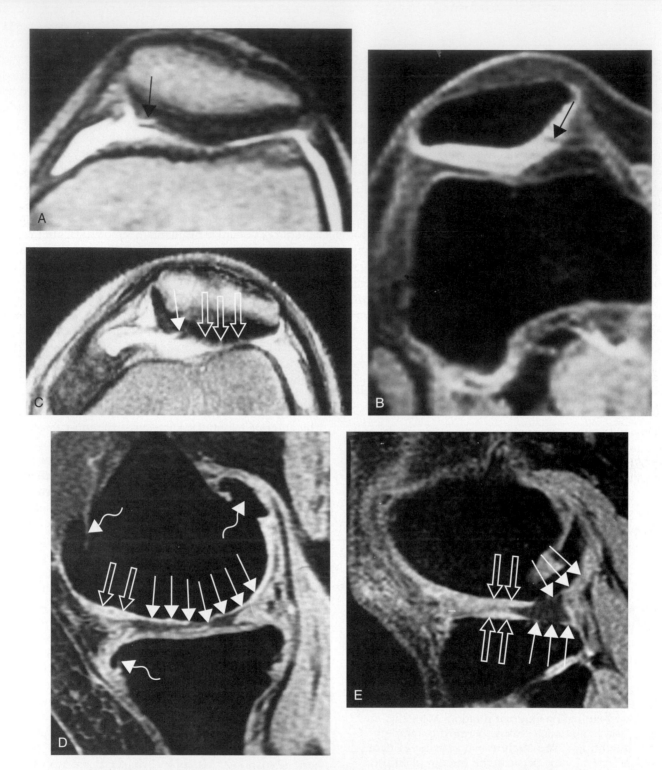

Fig. 3-215 Examples of articular cartilage injury. **A,** Axial fast spin echo image (4000/80; TR msec/TE msec) shows linear flap tear (*arrow*) at medial facet of patella. **B,** axial fat-suppressed 3-D spoiled gradient-echo (60/5; flip angle 40°) in another patient shows flap tear (*arrow*) at medial facet of patella. Note the intermediate depth of the articular defects in both **A** and **B. C,** Axial T2-weighted fast spin echo image (4000/80) in another patient shows more extensive partial thickness tear of patellar articular cartilage as surface fissuring (*arrow*) and fibrillation (*open arrows*). **D,** Sagittal fat-suppressed 3-D spoiled gradient-echo image (60/5; flip angle 40°) in a patient with OA shows extensive near-complete articular cartilage thinning of the weight bearing portion of the medial femoral condyle (*arrows*). Note smooth transition into normal thickness articular cartilage (*open arrows*). Note also marginal osteophytes (*curved arrows*) on the femur and tibia. **E,** Sagittal fat-suppressed 3-D spoiled gradient-echo image (60/5; flip angle 40°) in another patient with OA demonstrates apposing areas of full thickness cartilage thinning (*arrows*) in medial femoral and tibial condyles with smooth transition to normal thickness cartilage (*open arrows*). (Fig. 3-215E adapted and reproduced, with permission, from Disler DG. Clinical magnetic resonance imaging of articular cartilage, *Topics Magn Reson Imaging* 9:360-376, 1998.)

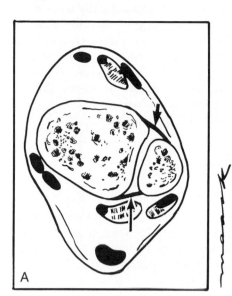
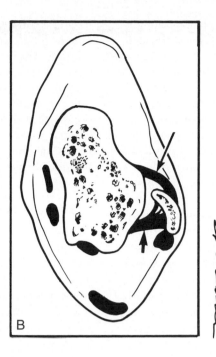

Fig. 3-216 Lateral ligaments at the ankle. **A,** Axial diagram immediately superior to the ankle joint, demonstrating the anterior and posterior tibiofibular ligaments (*short and long arrows* respectively). Note the convex medial fibular shape at this level. **B,** Axial diagram demonstrating the anterior talofibular (*long arrow*) and posterior talofibular (*short arrow*) ligaments. Note that the fibular shape is concave at its medial aspect at this level. (From Manaster BJ. *Handbook of Skeletal Radiology,* ed 2, St. Louis, 1997, Mosby-Yearbook.)

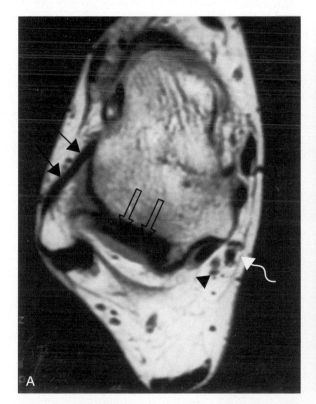
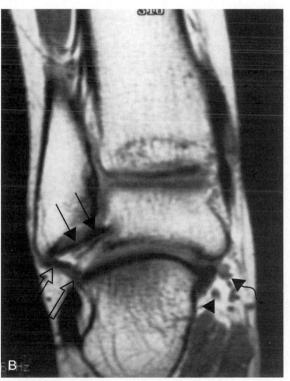

Fig. 3-217 Lateral collateral ligament complex. **A,** Axial proton density fast spin echo image (4000/15; TR msec/TE msec) demonstrates anterior talofibular ligament (*arrows*) and posterior talofibular ligament (*open arrows*). **B,** Coronal T1-weighted spin echo image (600/14) shows anterior talofibular ligament (*arrows*) and calcaneofibular ligament (*open arrows*). In **A** and **B** note the medial (*curved arrow*) and lateral (*arrowhead*) plantar arteries, veins, and nerves. These represent the distal extension of the tibial nerve and the posterior tibial artery and veins.

the flexor digitorum longus and the flexor hallucis longus tendons (Fig. 3-218). These three tendons course through the tarsal tunnel, which is a space confined by the flexor retinaculum, in which is also found the medial and lateral plantar nerves, arteries, veins, and lymphatics. The posterior tibial tendon is found in a groove along the medial malleolus, and continues through the tarsal tunnel to insert on the navicular bone with continuation of the tendon to the plantar aspect of the medial and middle cuneiform bones and the second through fourth metatarsal bases. It is the principle inverter of the foot and helps maintain the longitudinal arch. As a rule of thumb, the normal posterior tibial tendon should be no greater than twice the diameter of the other tendons at the ankle with the exception of the Achilles tendon. The flexor digitorum longus tendon also courses in the groove found in the medial malleolus, and acts as a pulley continuing through the tarsal tunnel to insert on the second to fifth distal phalanges. The flexor hallucis longus passes beneath the sustentaculum tali of the calcaneus using its groove as a pulley and continues between the two sesamoid bones of the hallux to insert on the base of the first distal phalanx. The muscle and musculotendinous junction of the flexor hallucis longus is found more distally than the other flexor tendons, and can usually be found at the level of the ankle joint line. The peroneal tendons are found posterolaterally at the ankle. The peroneus longus is found posteromedial to the peroneus brevis, and both pass behind the lateral malleolus within a groove. The tendons are confined by a retinaculum, with the peroneus brevis inserting on the fifth metatarsal base and the peroneus longus extending beneath the midfoot to insert on the first metatarsal base. The extensor tendons are found anteriorly at the ankle, and from medial

to lateral consist of the tibialis anterior, extensor hallucis longus, extensor digitorum longus, and peroneus tertius tendons. These tendons are confined by the anterior extensor retinaculum. The tibialis anterior inserts on the medial and inferomedial base of the first metatarsal bone. The extensor hallucis longus inserts on the dorsal base of the distal phalanx of the hallux. The extensor digitorum longus inserts on the dorsal bases of the second through fifth distal phalanges, and the peroneus tertius inserts on the dorsal base of the fifth metatarsal bone.

Trauma Patterns

Ankle injuries are extremely common and the most common cause for trauma-associated radiographic evaluation in emergency departments in the United States. In general, the presence of an ankle joint effusion or soft tissue swelling should prompt for search of underlying fracture, particularly if the patient is unable to bear weight. In the ankle, effusion is seen on the lateral film as an anteriorly convex soft-tissue density at the ankle joint (Fig. 3-219). Soft-tissue swelling may be evident over the medial and lateral malleoli as well as in the fat posterior to the ankle. This posterior fat is known as the pre-Achilles triangle and is usually sharply circumscribed at its margin with the Achilles tendon. Obscuration of the margins of the fat triangle in the setting of trauma indicates soft-tissue swelling.

There are two classifications used in the assessment of ankle fractures. The first to be discussed is the *Lauge-Hansen classification,* which is a classification based on the mechanism of forces that result in fractures at the ankle. This consideration is useful because an understanding of the forces producing injury indicates the direction

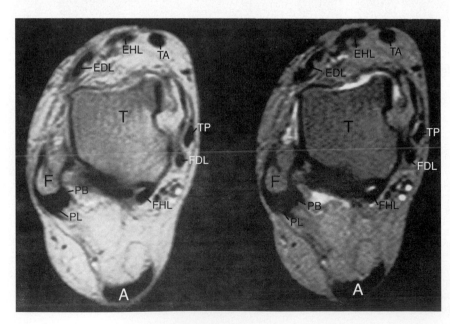

Fig. 3-218   Axial proton density (2300/14; TR msec/TE msec) and T2-weighted (2300/80) spin echo MR images of ankle demonstrate the tibialis posterior (TP), flexor digitorum longus (FDL), and flexor hallucis longus (FHL) tendons of the posterior compartment. The anterior compartment tendons are the tibialis anterior (TA), extensor hallucis longus (EHL), and extensor digitorum longus (EDL) tendons. Note also peroneus brevis (PB) and peroneus longus (PL) tendons and Achilles tendon (A). T, talus; F, fibula.

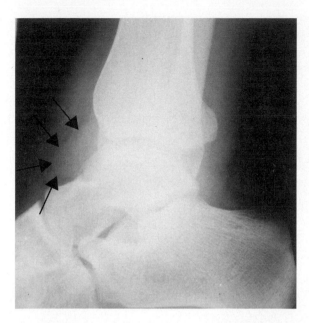

Fig. 3-219   Lateral radiography shows soft tissue density in shape of teardrop (*arrows*) anterior to ankle joint indicating an ankle effusion.

of forces required for fracture reduction (reverse of the mechanism of injury). There are five basic patterns of ankle fracture: axial loading, supination, supination-external rotation, pronation, and pronation-external rotation. Supination refers to plantar flexion of the ankle, inversion of the hindfoot, and adduction of the foot, whereas pronation refers to dorsiflexion of the ankle, eversion of the hindfoot, and abduction of the foot. Either supination or pronation may be isolated or associated with external rotation. It is useful to be mindful of the *fracture pattern in the fibula* in each of these four injury patterns because the fibular fracture pattern in each injury will be unique. For each fracture pattern, the ankle mortise is carefully assessed for any evidence of loss of parallel margins, because this implies extensive ligament and osseus disruption resulting in ankle instability. In considering the Lauge-Hansen classification, injury stages are sequential with lowest stage injury patterns being found among the higher stage injuries; with a higher stage of injury, there is increasing severity and instability.

Axial loading results in intraarticular fractures of the tibial plafond. These are called *pilon* fractures. Axial forces result in severe distal tibial comminution, while the malleoli usually maintain an anatomic relationship with the talus. Talar fractures may coexist. Pylon fractures are classified as type 1 (nondisplaced), type 2 (moderately displaced), and type 3 (severely displaced and impacted).

In pure *supination*, tension is placed on the fibula resulting in either a tear of the lateral collateral ligament or a low transverse avulsion fracture of the lateral malleo-

lus (Fig. 3-220). This is considered a stage 1 injury. Stage 2 injury includes the findings at stage 1 injury with the addition of a vertically oriented fracture of the medial malleolus.

Supination-external rotation is the most common injury pattern at the ankle accounting for nearly three-fourths of all ankle injuries. In supination-external rotation, the lateral wall of the distal talar pole impacts the anterior wall of the lateral malleolus, driving it posteriorly. This results in an oblique fracture oriented in the coronal plane that is best seen on the lateral view of the ankle (Fig. 3-221). Stage 1 supination-external rotation injury represents disruption of the anterior distal tibiofibular ligament. Stage 2 injury includes stage 1 findings plus the distal fibular fracture. Stage 3 findings include findings from stages 1 and 2 plus a tear of the posterior distal tibiofibular ligament versus posterior malleolar fracture (avulsion of posterior distal tibiofibular ligament insertion). Stage 4 injury represents findings at stages 1–3 plus transverse fracture of the medial malleolus.

In *pronation,* the lateral wall of the proximal talar pole impacts the medial wall of the lateral malleolus, driving it laterally. This results in an oblique fracture of the lateral malleolus oriented in the sagittal plane, that is best shown on the frontal view of the ankle (Fig. 3-222). There are three stages of pronation injury. The first stage is that of an avulsion of the medial malleo-

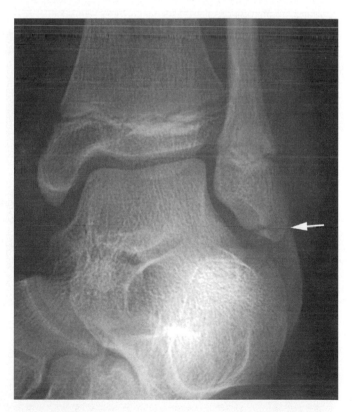

Fig. 3-220   Supination ankle injury results in a low transverse fracture (*arrow*) through the lateral malleolus.

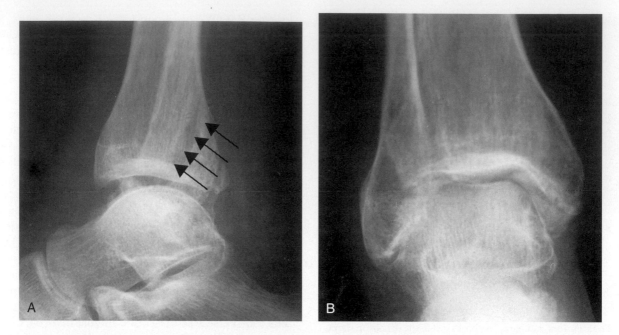

Fig. 3-221   Supination-external rotation injury at ankle. **A,** Lateral view demonstrates coronally oriented oblique fracture of distal fibula. Note absence of visualization of fracture on frontal view (**B**).

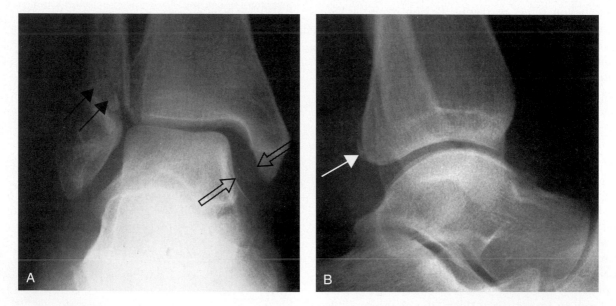

Fig. 3-222   Pronation injury. **A,** Frontal view of ankle demonstrates sagittally oriented oblique fracture (*arrows*) in distal fibula. Note widened ankle joint at medial mortise (*open arrows*) indicating deltoid ligament tear. **B,** Lateral view demonstrates avulsion fracture at posterior malleolus (*arrow*).

lus versus a tear of the deltoid ligaments. Stage 2 represents stage 1 findings plus rupture of the anterior and posterior distal tibiofibular ligaments. Stage 3 represents stage 1 and 2 findings plus the fibular fracture. Thus, demonstration of a sagittally oriented oblique fracture of the fibula indicates the most severe form of pronation injury.

In *pronation-external rotation,* impaction at both lateral and anterior surfaces on the lateral malleolus results in a spiraling force through the tibiofibular syndesmosis with forces exiting through the fibula at a point more proximal to the ankle joint (Fig. 3-223). There are four stages of pronation-external rotation injury. Stage 1 injury involves avulsion of the medial malleolus or a deltoid ligament tear. Stage 2 represents stage 1 findings plus tear of the anterior distal tibiofibular ligament and the tibiofibular syndesmosis. Stage 3 represents stage 1 and 2 findings plus the fibular fracture. Stage 4 injury represents the findings from stages 1–3 plus tear of the posterior distal tibiofibular ligament versus posterior malleolar fracture. Therefore, if medial malleolar swelling is demonstrated and there is posterior malleolar fracture, absence of visualization of a fibular fracture on an ankle film implies a more proximal fibular fracture prompting search with leg radiographs.

The *Weber (AO) classification* is a more useful classification because it is simpler to use and because it correlates well with treatment and prognosis. It is based on determining the level of fibular fracture to deduce the injury to the tibiofibular ligaments. A Weber A injury corresponds to supination injury by the Lauge-Hansen criteria, and represents transverse avulsion fracture of the lateral malleolus at or distal to the ankle joint. There may be associated fracture of the medial malleolus. If the fibula is intact, the lateral collateral ligament is disrupted. In type A injury, the tibiofibular ligaments and syndesmosis are intact. Weber B injury represents oblique fractures of the lateral malleolus beginning at the level of the ankle joint. This injury corresponds to Lauge-Hansen classification of supination-external rotation or pronation. The important point with type B injury is that there is partial disruption of the tibiofibular ligaments. These injuries may be associated with fractures of the medial malleolus below the ankle joint or with deltoid ligament rupture. Weber C injury represents fibular fracture proximal to the level of the ankle joint. This involves tear of the tibiofibular ligaments and tibiofibular syndesmosis. This injury corresponds to Lauge-Hansen pronation-external rotation. A proximal fibular fracture indicates a *Maisonneuve fracture* with syndesmosis tear to the level of the fracture.

In the skeletally immature, fusion of the distal tibial epiphysis begins at 12–13 years of age, beginning anterocentrally, and proceeding medial and laterally.

Children in this age range are prone to growth plate injury. One type of injury is known as the *juvenile Tillaux fracture,* which is a Salter-Harris III fracture of the lateral portion of the distal tibial epiphysis, sparing the fused medial portion of the epiphysis (Fig. 3-224). It relates to avulsion of the anterior and posterior distal tibiofibular ligaments. Fracture displacement of more than 2 mm or articular incongruance indicate the need for surgical intervention. A *triplane fracture* is the other growth plate fracture at the ankle, and involves the lateral half of the distal tibial epiphysis and a posterior triangular metaphyseal fragment. The term "triplane" indicates the three planes of the fracture, coronal-oblique through the posterior distal metaphysis, horizontal through the growth plate, and sagittal through the epiphysis (Fig. 3-225). There are two types. If a triplane fracture occurs after the medial portion of the epiphysis has fused, the medial malleolus remains intact and a two-fragment triplane fracture results. If the triplane fracture occurs before the epiphysis begins to fuse, there may be a three-fragment fracture. With either type, the appearance of a triplane fracture consists of a combination of a juvenile Tillaux fracture and Salter-Harris II fracture. Other growth plate injury patterns at the ankle occur, including Salter-Harris II and Salter-Harris IV fractures of the distal tibia and fibula (Fig. 3-226). Salter-Harris V fractures are uncommon and a result of axial loading.

It is important to include the base of the fifth metatarsal on images of the ankle because metatarsal fractures may clinically mimick ankle fractures (Fig. 3-227). Fractures at the base of the fifth metatarsal are due to avulsion of the insertion of the peroneus brevis tendon. There is variable distraction of the avulsed fracture fragment with retraction occasionally extending to the level of ankle with lateral ankle pain. Lateral and frontal views are both useful for detection of fifth metatarsal base fracture.

Fatigue fractures may occur at the ankle, especially among skeletal immature runners, seen as irregularity and widening of the distal fibular growth plate (Fig. 3-228), or as linear bands of lucency or sclerosis (depending upon the age of healing) in the fibula 3–7 cm from the tip of the lateral malleolus (Fig. 3-229). Insufficiency fractures also occur and may be simultaneous in the distal tibia and fibula and are usually located 3–4 cm proximal to the level of the tibial plafond.

Instability is a common complication of ankle injury. Stress films with varus and valgus force applied to the calcaneus and anterior drawer stress (which is anterior force applied to the calcaneal tuberosity) are useful for determining laxity in the ankle joint (Fig. 3-230). Medial talar tilt (varus) is normally 10°–12° and anterior drawer is usually less than 1 cm. However, it is important to compare with the contralateral side as occasional

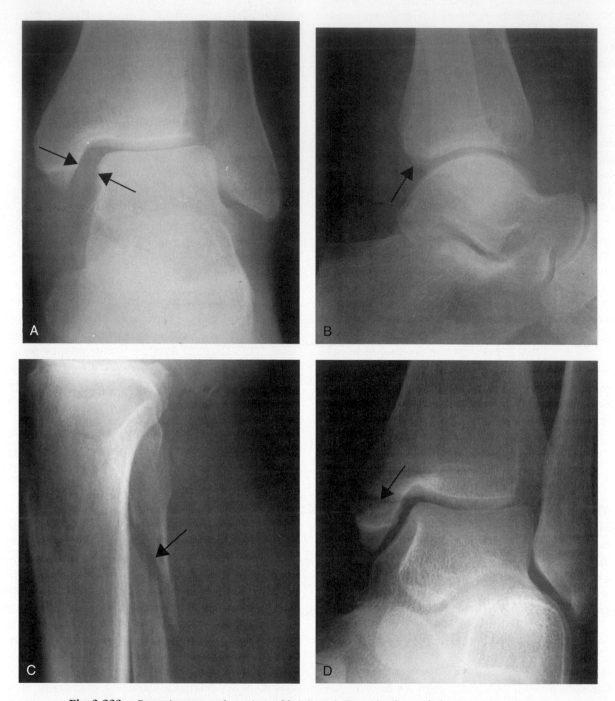

Fig. 3-223   Pronation-external rotation ankle injury. **A,** Frontal radiograph demonstrates widening of ankle joint space at medial ankle mortise (*arrows*) indicating deltoid ligament tear. **B,** Lateral view demonstrates avulsion fracture at posterior malleolus (*arrow*). **C,** Lateral view of proximal leg demonstrates oblique fracture of proximal fibular diametaphysis (*arrow*). Fractures of the proximal fibula in the setting of ankle injury are known as Maisonneuve fractures.

Continued

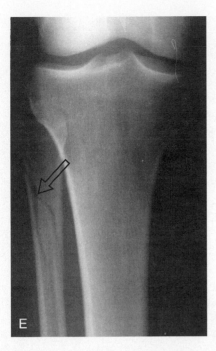

Fig. 3-223, cont'd   **D** and **E,** Frontal views in another patient demonstrate transverse fracture of medial malleolus (*arrow*) and proximal fibular fracture (*open arrow*) in another Maisonneuve fracture.

congenital laxity is present. In general, varus greater than 15° strongly suggests lateral collateral ligament injury and anterior talar displacement greater than 1 cm indicates injury to the anterior talofibular ligament. Although rarely used, arthrography is helpful for detecting ligament injury.

Ordinarily, contrast opacifies the ankle joint, the posterior subtalar joint, and occasionally the tendon sheath of the flexor hallucis longus. If contrast extends around the tip of the fibula, a tear of the anterior talofibular ligament is present. Filling of the peroneal tendon sheath indicates a tear of the calcaneofibular ligament. If contrast is found in the tibiofibular syndesmosis above the level of the ankle joint, a tear of the anterior distal tibiofibular ligament is suggested. It should be noted that anterior talofibular ligament tears precede other lateral collateral ligament injuries in supination-external rotation and supination.

A final fracture of the ankle to consider is osteochondral injury. Osteochondral injury may involve the medial or lateral talar dome. As discussed for the knee, the critical diagnostic consideration with such fractures is the grade of injury and the stability of the osteochondral fragment. This is assessed by determining the integrity of the overlying articular cartilage, which can be performed with sequences sensitive to imaging articular cartilage or with MR-arthrography (Fig. 3-231).

Tendon Injury

Tendon abnormalities at the ankle and hindfoot are primarily degenerative disorders of multifactorial origin. Age, chronic repetitive overuse injury, and certain congenital predispositions such as anomalous muscle insertions and bone dysplasias each play a role. With repetitive injury and repair tendons undergo mucoid degeneration and hyalinization, which eventually can result in tendon rupture. All tendon tears are graded in a similar fashion.

Text continued on p. 366

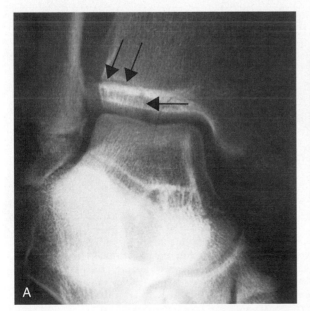
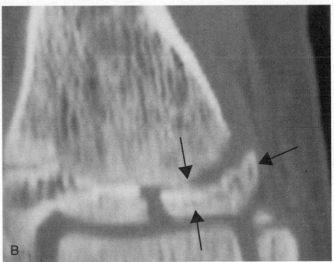

Fig. 3-224   Tillaux fracture. **A,** Frontal radiograph demonstrates epiphyseal fracture of lateral tibial plafond (*arrows*). **B,** Coronally reformatted CT image (right and left reversed from A) shows same fracture (*arrows*).

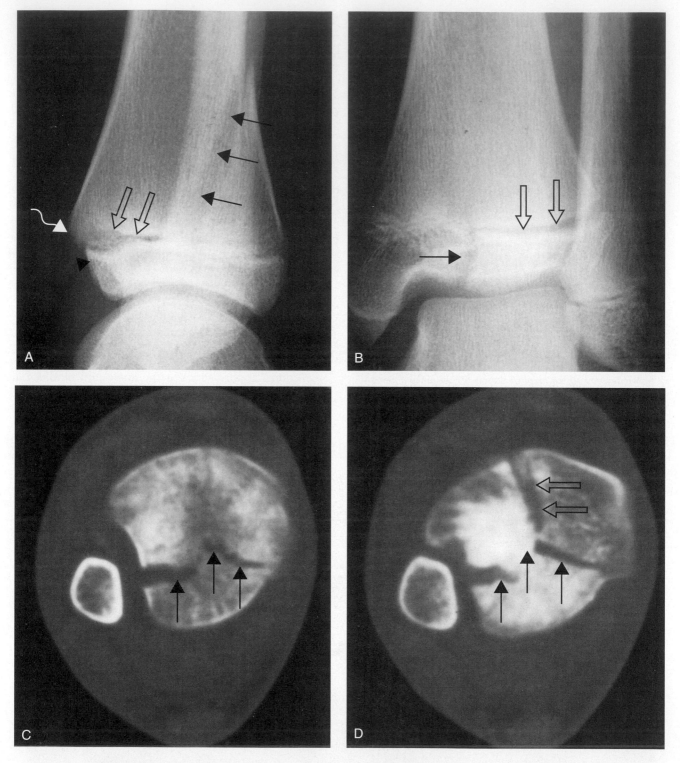

Fig. 3-225   Triplane fracture. **A,** Lateral ankle view demonstrates oblique fracture of posterior aspect of distal tibial metaphysis (*arrows*) and transverse fracture through anterior growth plate (*open arrows*). Note posterior offset anteriorly of distal tibial metaphysis (*curved arrow*) and epiphysis (*arrowhead*). **B,** Frontal radiograph demonstrates sagittally oriented epiphyseal fracture (*arrow*) and transversely oriented physeal fracture (*open arrows*). **C,** Axial CT image shows coronally oriented fracture through distal tibial metaphysis (*arrows*). **D,** Axial CT image more distal to **C** shows coronally oriented metaphyseal fracture (*arrows*) and sagittally oriented epiphyseal fracture (*open arrows*).   *Continued*

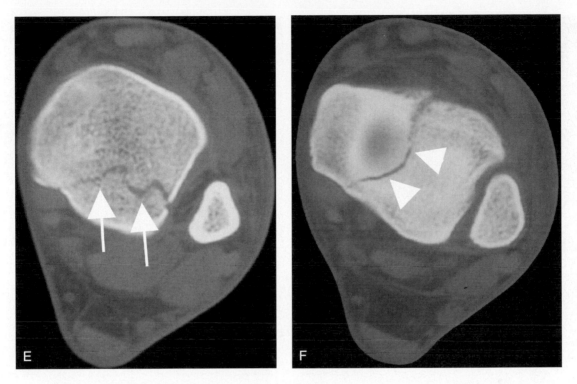

Fig. 3-225, cont'd   E and F, Axial CT images in another patient demonstrate coronally oriented metaphyseal fracture (*arrows*) and sagittally oriented epiphyseal fracture (*arrowheads*). Note that slice (F) is more distal to that of (E)

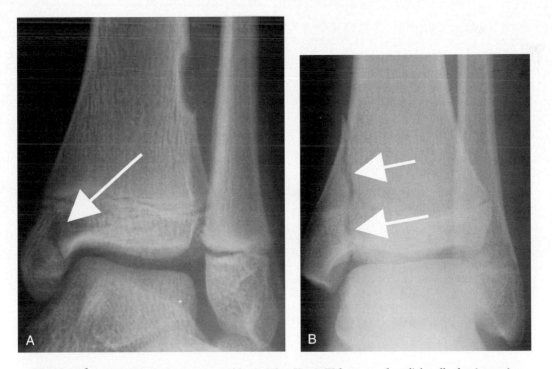

Fig. 3-226   Salter-Harris fractures at ankle. **A,** Salter-Harris III fracture of medial malleolus (*arrow*). **B,** Salter-Harris IV fracture of distal tibial metaphysis and epiphysis (*arrows*).

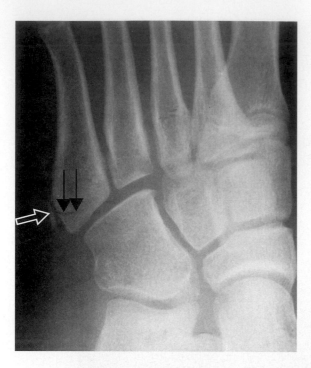

Fig. 3-227   Oblique foot radiograph demonstrates fracture at base of fifth metatarsal bone (*arrows*). Note apophysis (*open arrow*).

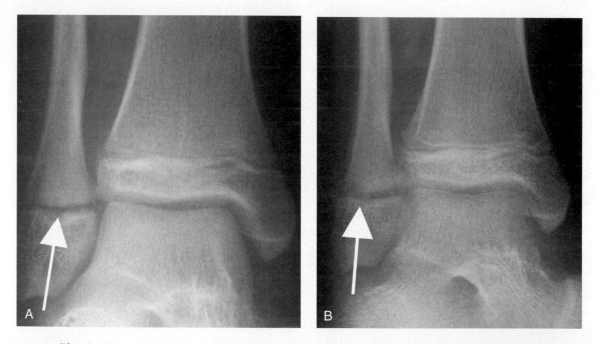

Fig. 3-228   Stress fracture of distal fibular physis. **A,** Radiograph obtained at time of injury demonstrates only minimal irregularity of distal fibular growth plate (*arrow*). **B,** Radiograph obtained 3 weeks later demonstrates interval widening and irregularity of growth plate of distal fibula (*arrow*), indicating partial healing. Note periosteal new bone along distal fibular shaft.

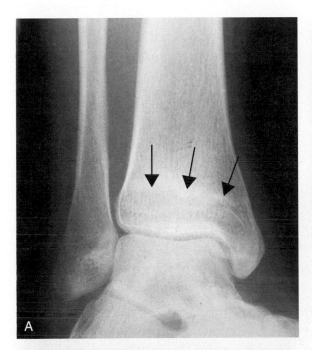

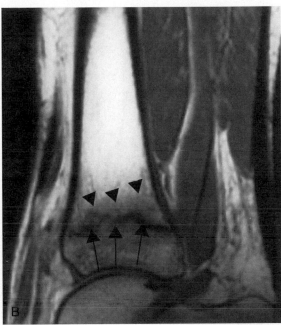

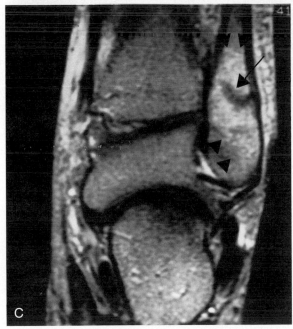

Fig. 3-229 Stress fractures. **A,** Oblique radiograph of ankle demonstrates linear sclerotic band (*arrows*) related to healing stress fracture. **B,** Sagittal T1 weighted spin echo image (600/16; TR msec/TE msec) demonstrates linear band of low signal intensity representing fracture line, surrounded by poorly defined zone of low signal intensity edema (*arrowheads*). **C,** Coronal T2-weighted spin echo MR image in another patient demonstrates stress fracture of the fibula with incomplete line of low signal intensity (*arrow*) surrounded by large and ill-defined zone of high signal intensity edema (*arrowheads*). (Fig. 3-229B adapted and reproduced, with permission, from Aerts P, Disler DG. Abnormalities of the foot and ankle: MR imaging findings. *AJR* 165:119-124, 1995.)

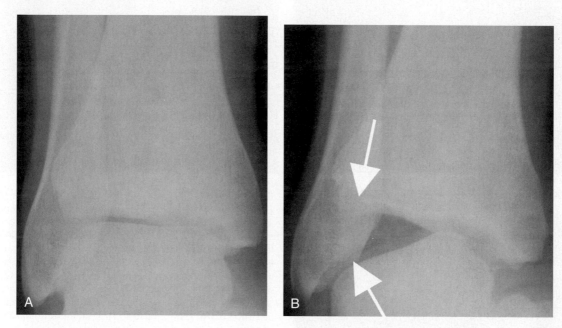

Fig. 3-230   Instability of the ankle related to chronic lateral collateral ligament tears. **A,** Frontal radiograph of ankle is normal. **B,** With varus stress at calcaneus, there is substantial widening of the lateral ankle mortise (*arrows*).

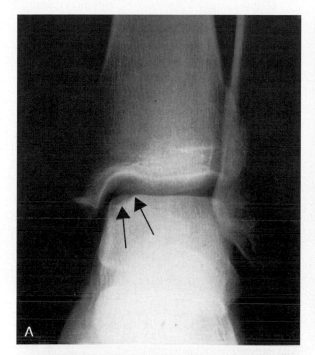

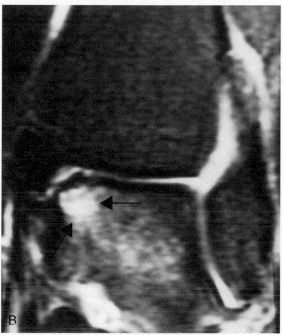

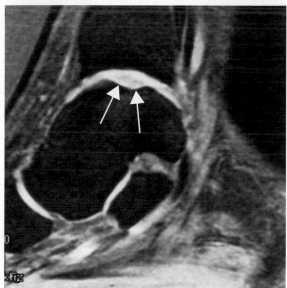

Fig. 3-231   Osteochondral fracture of medial talar dome. **A,** Frontal radiograph demonstrates defect at medial talar dome (*arrows*), with mildly sclerotic margin. **B,** Coronal T2-weighted spin echo image (2300/80; TR msec/ TE msec) shows substantial edema (*arrows*) adjacent to radiographically apparent osteochondral lesion as noted in **A. C,** Sagittal fat-suppressed 3-D spoiled gradient-echo image (60/5; flip angle 40°) shows osteochondral lesion (*arrows*).

Grade 1 tendinosis represents a tendon that is thickened, resulting from multiple repetitive tears and repairs. With grade 1 tendinosis, a tendon may be of homogeneously diminished signal on T1-weighted and T2-weighted images if repair predominates over injury. A heterogeneous pattern indicates the presence of mucoid degeneration or interstitial tendon tears (tears that are longitudinally oriented along the course of the tendon). Grade 2 tendinosis represents a tendon that is abnormally thin. This results from a tendon that is partially ruptured, with diminished transverse dimension. Grade 3 tendinosis represents tendon discontinuity. As is implied by the grading scheme, tendinosis is a chronic mechanical failure of the tendon that evolves from recurrent bouts of tendinitis and repair. Clearly, not all pathology that involve tendons is a result of repetitive microtrauma. For example, tenosynovitis may be of inflammatory origin, infectious etiology, or even a result of impingement.

The Achilles tendon is the most commonly injured tendon at the ankle. Normally, its anteroposterior dimension is no more than 8-mm thick and anterior margins are concave or flat. Achilles tendinitis is common among runners and jumpers. Acutely, the tendon margins are inflamed resulting in blurring on radiography between the anterior Achilles tendon margin and the adjacent pre-Achilles fat. At MR imaging, peritendinitis is shown by fluidlike signal in the peritendinous region (Fig. 3-232). Recurrent bouts of tendinitis and peritendinitis result in enlargement of the tendon (Fig. 3-233). Acute ruptures are superimposed upon chronic tendinopathy, occurring most commonly in middle aged males who are involved in sporadic exercise (the weekend warrior), or sports involving running or jumping (Fig. 3-234). Rupture may also be seen in individuals with weakened tendons as a result of systemic diseases such as RA, renal disease, and diabetes, or as a result of chronic steroid use. The most typical location of partial or complete Achilles tendon rupture is 2–6 cm proximal to the calcaneal insertion. This is a relatively avascular zone. Partial ruptures may be either within the substance or marginal in location, and may be either transverse or longitudinal in orientation. The plantaris tendon, which originates from the lateral femoral condyle, and which inserts anterior to the Achilles tendon on the calcaneal tuberosity, is important to know about for two reasons. First, an intact plantaris tendon may mimic a partially intact Achilles tendon on both clinical and radiologic grounds. Clinically, with an intact plantaris tendon the patient may still be able to plantar flex the ankle suggesting a partially intact Achilles tendon. Radiologically, the plantaris tendon may mimic the Achilles tendon by its similar anatomic course, although the anteromedial location of the plantoris tendon at the calcaneus should provide a clue to its origin. Nontraumatic causes of thickening of the Achilles tendon may also occur. An accessory soleus muscle may mimic

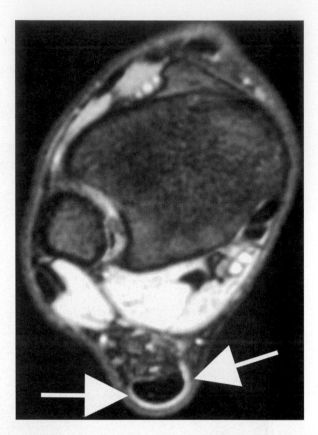

Fig. 3-232 Axial fat-suppressed T2-weighted fast spin echo MR image (4800/100; TR msec/TE msec) demonstrates acute Achilles peritendinitis with ill-defined ring of increased signal intensity (*arrows*) surrounding Achilles tendon.

Achilles tendon thickening, although the signal at MR imaging of the accessory soleus is that of muscle and not of tendon. Postsurgically, the Achilles tendon may appear thickened and retain areas of high signal. A thickened Achilles tendon may also be seen with xanthomas, which occur in the setting of familial hyperlipidemias. The appearance is of marked tendon enlargement, heterogeneously mixed low and intermediate signal masses, and stippled, linear areas of central low signal intensity. Multiple tendons may be affected, though the Achilles is the most common. Finally, edema and bursitis at the distal Achilles is seen in Haglund's disease (Fig. 3-235).

The second most common site of ankle tendinosis is the posterior tibial tendon. Posterior tibial tendinopathy is most common among women over the age of 50 years, usually with a clinical picture of an acute painful flatfoot that progressively worsens. As with other tendinopathies, predisposing conditions include RA, renal failure, diabetes, and steroid use. Anomalies of the navicular insertion site also predispose to posterior tibial tendinosis. These include the presence of an *os naviculare*. An os naviculare is a large ossicle closely apposed to the medial pole of the navicular bone. With os naviculare, the posterior tibial tendon often inserts solely on the ossicle without

Text continued on p. 369

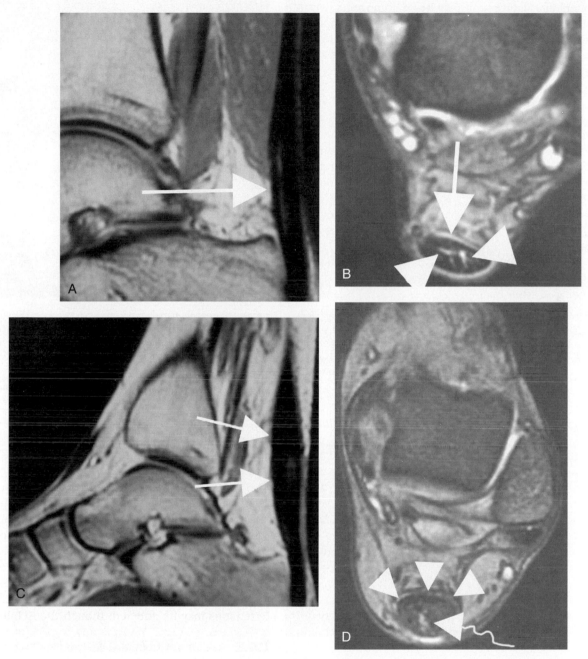

Fig. 3-233   Chronic tendinosis of Achilles tendon. **A,** sagittal T1-weighted spin echo image (600/
14; TR msec/TE msec) demonstrates anteroposterior thickening of Achilles tendon (*arrow*) with
central vertically oriented increased signal indicating longitudinal interstitial tear. **B,** Axial gradient-
echo image (450/40; flip angle 15°) shows convex anterior margin of Achilles tendon with mild
peritendinous increased signal (*arrow*) and central tendinous increased signal (*arrowheads*) related
to interstitial tear. **C** and **D,** Another patient with chronic tendinosis of the Achilles tendon showing
substantial thickening of the tendon (*arrows*), convex anterior margin of tendon (*arrowheads*) and
substantial intratendinous signal (*curved arrow*). (Figs. 3-233 **C** and **D** adapted and reproduced,
with permission, from Aerts P, Disler DG. Abnormalities of the foot and ankle: MR imaging findings,
AJR 165:119-124, 1995.)

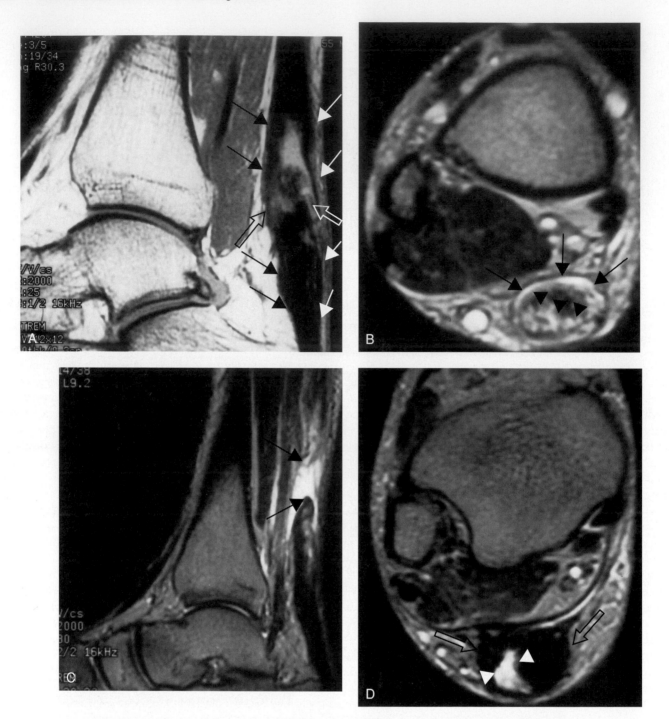

Fig. 3-234 Achilles tendon rupture. **A,** Sagittal proton density weighted spin echo image (2000/ 25; TR msec/TE msec) demonstrates marked thickening of Achilles tendon (*arrows*) and tendon discontinuity at level of distal tibial metaphysis (*open arrows*). **B,** Axial T2-weighted spin echo image (2000/80) shows marked tendon thickening, substantial peritendinous fluid (*arrows*) and intratendinous fluid (*arrowheads*). **C** and **D,** Sagittal and axial T2-weighted spin echo images (2000/ 80) in another patient demonstrates tears at the musculotendinous junction of the Achilles. Note wide gap due to retraction of the distal muscle fibers (*arrows*). Marked tendon thickening (*open arrows*) and fluid within tendon (*arrowheads*) is shown.

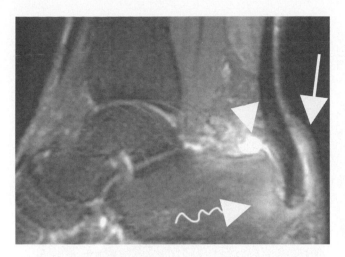

Fig. 3-235   Sagittal inversion recovery image (4000/30; TR msec/ TE msec; inversion time 140 msec) in patient with Haglund's disease, a disorder related to wearing high heeled shoes, shows edema surrounding distal Achilles tendon (*arrow*), calcaneal bone marrow edema (*curved arrow*), and retrocalcaneal bursal fluid (*arrowhead*).

continuing distally to insert on the plantar surfaces of the cuneiforms and the metatarsal bases. The normal posterior tibial tendon should be no greater than twice the diameter of other tendons at the ankle (with the exception of the Achilles tendon), and should be no more than the combined thicknesses of the peroneus longus and brevis tendons. A greater degree of thickening indicates grade 1 tendinosis (Fig. 3-236). An exception is the normal appearance of the posterior tibial tendon insertion, where the tendon broadens and may give the appearance of appearing larger than normal. Furthermore, T2-weighted images should always be checked in cases of apparent tendon thickening on T1 and proton density weighted MR images, because apparent enlargement on the sequences may be due to tendon sheath fluid and not true tendon thickening (Fig. 3-237). Finally, heterogeneous signal within tendons should be viewed with caution at the locations where the tendon is aligned at approximately 55° relative to the main magnetic field. One example is where the tendons curve around the malleoli at the ankle. Increased signal within tendons at this location may not be due to tendinopathy but rather to a phenomenon known as the *magic angle effect*. This artifact is a result of a slight lengthening of T2 relaxation, at 55° to the main magnetic field, in highly anisotropic structures (structures that have a directional orientation such as tendons and ligaments). The effect on T2 relaxation is small and thus only noticeable on short echo sequences such as T1 and proton density weighted spin-echo images. Therefore, a sequence with a longer TE such as a T2-weighted spin-echo sequence is helpful because the increased signal is not apparent at the longer echo time, as the effect is too small to be demonstrated on images obtained with longer echo-times. Thus, when

one is unsure of magic angle effect versus tendinopathy on a T1-weighted or a proton density-weighted spin-echo sequence, review of the T2-weighted sequence should be performed.

Among the other flexors at the ankle and among the extensors at the ankle, injury is rare with the exception of the flexor hallucis longus where occasionally injury may be seen in ballet dancers related to the repetitive push-off from the forefoot or from impingement against the os trigonum (Fig. 3-238). Fluid within the tendon sheath of the flexor hallucis longus does not necessarily indicate the presence to tenosynovitis, because in 20% of the population there is normally free communication of joint fluid between the ankle joint and the flexor hallucis longus tendon sheath. However, disproportionately increased fluid within the tendon sheath helps make the diagnosis. Extensor tendon injury is quite rare; the anterior tibial tendon is occasionally injured in downhill runners and hikers but rarely progresses to complete rupture.

The peroneal tendons are the third most commonly injured tendons at the ankle. The peroneus quartus is an occasionally demonstrated accessory muscle that originates from the muscular portion of the peroneus brevis, the peroneus longus, or the fibula, and inserts on the peroneal tubercle of the calcaneus, which is located laterally along the calcaneal tuberosity. Tendinopathy is more common in the peroneus brevis, and is most commonly affected with a pattern known as *split peroneus brevis syndrome*. With this disorder, the peroneus brevis, which is the more anteriorly located tendon, is impinged between the peroneus longus and the fibula (Fig. 3-239). This may be on account of several factors, among them a tight compartment as a result of an accessory muscle, an abnormally distal position of the peroneus longus or brevis muscle bellies, dysplasia of the adjacent fibula, or peroneal subluxation. Normally, the posterior margin of the fibula is concave where it contacts the peroneal tendons. If the posterior margin is convex, the tendons are prone to sublux laterally during plantar flexion of the ankle. Occasionally, a hook may be seen posterolaterally in the fibula, which further predisposes to split peroneus brevis. The overlying peroneal retinaculum may avulse during forced plantar flexion further leading to tendon subluxation or dislocation. What is meant by split peroneus brevis is that in this disorder there is a longitudinal tear within the tendon at the level of the retromalleolar groove, which may extend over a variable course. The tendon may assume a boomerang shape, being thin and draped over the peroneus longus similar to the shape of a boomerang, or indeed split in two along its longitudinal course around the malleolus.

The peroneal tendons are prone to stenosing tenosynovitis, which is difficult to diagnose radiologically unless tendon sheath contrast is administered. In this disorder, contrast within the tendon sheath appears cut off or beaded rather than continuous. It is important to recog-

Text continued on p. 372

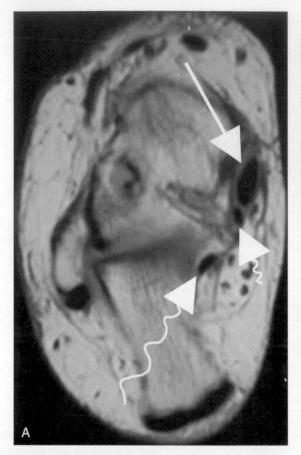

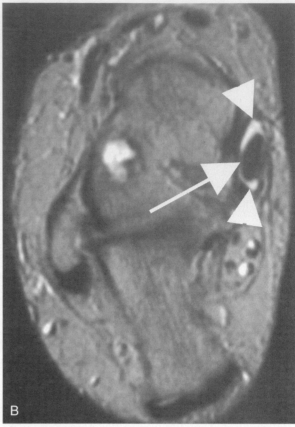

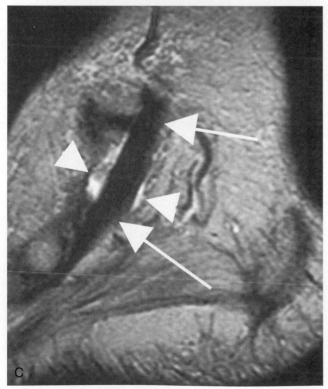

Fig. 3-236   Grade I tendinosis of posterior tibialis tendon. **A** and **B,** Axial proton density (**A**) and T2-weighted (**B**) spin echo MR images (2300/20, 80; TR msec/first echo TE msec, second echo TE msec) show enlargement of inframalleolar posterior tibial tendon (*arrow*) and tendon sheath fluid (*arrowheads*). Note the substantial degree of enlargement of the posterior tibialis tendon relative to other tendons at the ankle. Curved long arrow points to flexor hallucis longus tendon, and curved short arrow points to flexor digitorum longus tendon. **C,** Sagittal T2-weighted spin echo image (2600/80) shows thickened posterior tibialis tendon (*arrows*) and tendon sheath fluid (*arrowheads*). (Fig. 3-236 **A** and **C** adapted and reproduced, with permission, from Aerts P, Disler DG. Abnormalities of the foot and ankle: MR imaging findings, *AJR* 165:119-124, 1995.)

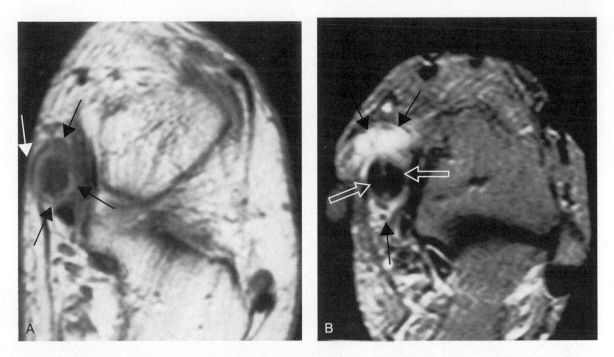

Fig. 3-237   Posterior tibialis tendinosis. **A,** Axial proton density spin echo MR image (2000/20; TR msec/TE msec) demonstrates marked thickening of tendon (*arrows*). **B,** T2-weighted spin echo image (2000/80) shows that a great deal of the appearance of tendon thickening is due to tendon sheath fluid (*arrows*). However, substantial tendon thickening (*open arrows*) is still shown.

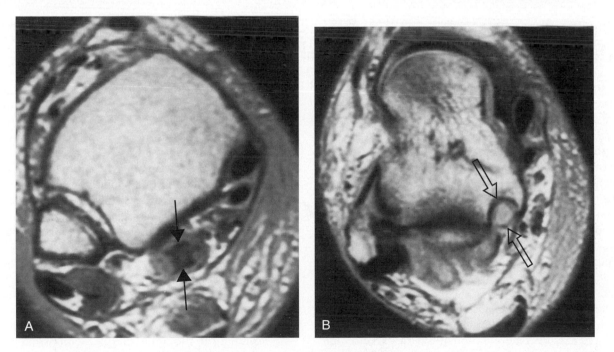

Fig. 3-238   Flexor hallucis longus tendon tear. **A** and **B,** Axial proton density spin echo MR images (2000/20; TR msec/TE msec) demonstrate marked tendon thickening at level of distal tibial epiphysis (*arrows*) and absence of tendon in expected groove (*open arrows*) more distally at level of talus. Findings constitute grade III tendinosis (tendon rupture).

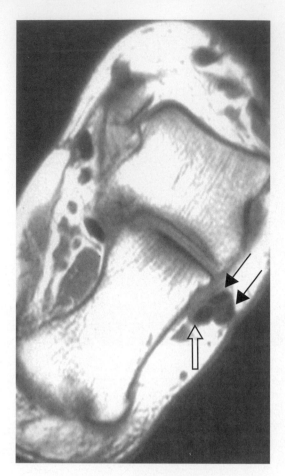
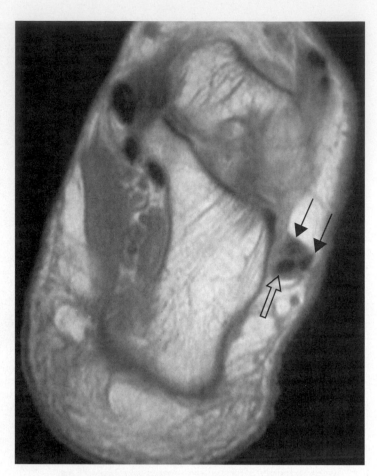

Fig. 3-239   Split peroneus brevis tendon. Two contiguous proton density fast spin-echo MR images (4400/14, TRmsec/TEmsec) show split peroneus brevis tendon (*arrows*) anterior to peroneus longus (*open arrows*). (Courtesey of Michael Recht, M.D., Cleveland, OH.)

nize the occasional presence of the peroneus quartus muscle. This muscle and tendon can give an appearance suggesting a peroneus tendon longitudinal tear because fat is present between the accessory structure and the adjacent normal peroneus tendons. It can be recognized by following the course of the accessory tendon to the insertion at the peroneus tubercle of the calcaneal tuberosity rather than continuing into the midfoot as do the peroneus longus and brevis. The peroneus quartus may be responsible for peroneus longus and brevis tendinopathy because the accessory muscle and tendon causes impingement. Accessory muscles at the ankle are very common, occurring in 8% of the population. They are important to recognize because they may mimic tendinopathy, occasionally cause impingement within compartments, and may become symptomatic with exercise due to tenuous blood supply.

Ligament Injury

Ligament injury is far more common than tendon injury, and is typically a result of acute ankle trauma,

unlike tendon injury, which is usually chronic in nature. Ligament injuries were extensively discussed under the Lauge-Hansen classification of ankle trauma, but a few points will be discussed here. First, as supination-external rotation is the most common injury at the ankle, the most commonly injured ligaments are the lateral collateral ligaments. Among the lateral collateral ligaments, the anterior talofibular ligament is most commonly torn. In fact, if the anterior talofibular ligament appears intact, then no lateral collateral ligament injury has occurred. Ligament sprains are graded on a 3-point scale. A first degree sprain represents ligament swelling. A second degree sprain represents partial ligament discontinuity. A third degree sprain indicates complete ligament discontinuity. It should be noted that while the ligaments at the ankle can be demonstrated at MR imaging, there have been no studies that have proven the accuracy of MR imaging in diagnosing ligament tears at the ankle. Fortunately, the anterior talofibular ligament is perhaps the best shown ligament on MR images. Nonvisualization of this ligament on MR images usually indicates the presence of ligament sprain, partic-

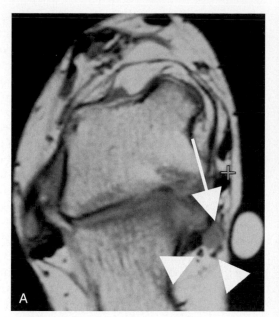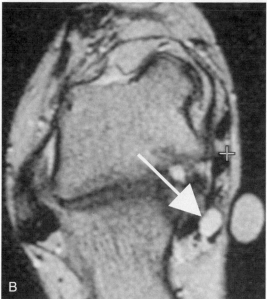

Fig. 3-240   Tarsal tunnel syndrome. **A** and **B**, Axial proton density weighted (2000/14; TR msec/ TE msec) and T2-weighted (2000/80) spin echo MR images show ganglion cyst (*arrow*) in tarsal tunnel. Note adjacent medial and lateral plantar vessels and nerves (*arrowheads*). High signal intensity skin marker is present.

ularly if in the acute situation there are supporting findings of injury such as ankle effusion, lateral edema, and swelling. The spring ligament is perhaps the most important ligament in the hindfoot because it supports the longitudinal arch. It is located between the talus, calcaneus, and navicular bone. However, there is yet to be published any study that evaluates the accuracy of MR imaging for diagnosing disruption of this ligament.

Miscellaneous Soft Tissue Injuries

Tarsal tunnel syndrome   The tarsal tunnel represents the soft tissues invested by the flexor retinaculum at the ankle. The flexor tendons, fat, lymphatic tissues, and the medial and lateral plantar arteries, veins, and nerves lie within the tarsal tunnel. The medial margin of the tunnel is the flexor retinaculum whereas the lateral margin consists of the talus and calcaneus. Pressure on the nerve results in the syndrome that is analogous to carpal tunnel syndrome, and consists of tingling, pain and burning in the sole and the medial toes. Fully half of the cases of tarsal tunnel syndrome will not have a morphologic abnormality identified on MR images. However, abnormalities that can be shown are space occupying lesions that produce mass effect on the medial and lateral plantar nerves. Abnormalities include such common pathologies as flexor tendon tenosynovitis, an abnormally distal extent of the abductor hallucis muscle, thickening of the flexor retinaculum, and ganglion cysts

(Fig. 3-240). Uncommon causes include neurogenic tumors, lymphangiomas or hemangiomas, or other masses.

Sinus tarsi syndrome   Another anatomic compartent at the ankle and hindfoot is the sinus tarsi, which is the central and lateral space between the mid pole of the talus and the anterior process of the calcaneus, located between the posterior subtalar joint and the talocalcaneonavicular joint. The space is occupied by fat and talocalcaneal ligaments. In addition, a small neurovascular bundle crosses the space. The syndrome occurs as a result of inflammation or hemorrhage within this site and results in lateral foot pain. On MR images, the abnormal sinus tarsi does not show signal compatible with fat (Fig. 3-241). It may show signal consistent with edema, fibrosis, and synovial cysts arising from the adjacent posterior subtalar and talocalcaneonavicular joints. Although subtalar ligament tears may be present, they are not shown reliably with MR imaging. As this disorder usually arises after supination injury, many patients have lateral collateral ligament tears of the ankle.

FOOT TRAUMA

Anatomy

There are at least 28 bones in the foot and perhaps more, depending upon the number of accessory ossicles

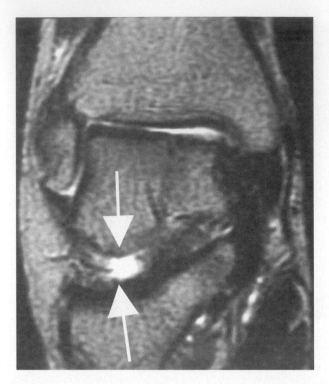

Fig. 3-241   Coronal T2-weighted spin echo image (2600/80; TR msec/TE msec) demonstrates fluid-like signal (*arrows*) in sinus tarsi in patient with sinus tarsi syndrome. (Adapted and reproduced, with permission, from Aerts P, Disler DG. Abnormalities of the foot and ankle: MR imaging findings. *AJR* 165:119-124, 1995.)

present. Accessory ossicles are extremely common and are often bilateral in occurrence. They are corticated and smoothly contoured, which helps differentiate them from fractures. The most common accessory ossicles are the os trigonum (shown posterior to the talus on the lateral view of the foot), os peroneum (adjacent to the cuboid), and os tibiale externum (adjacent to the navicular bone on the frontal foot film). Radiologists usually refer to atlases of normal variants, and a good source is the *Atlas of Normal Roentgen Variants that May Simulate Disease,* by Theodore Keats.

The calcaneus is the largest bone of the foot and is a tent-shaped bone consisting of a nonarticulating tuberosity and an articulating anterior process. The talus articulates with the calcaneus at the posterior, middle, and anterior subtalar joints. The cuboid articulates with the calcaneus at the calcaneocuboid joint. The cuboid spans the midfoot between two rows of tarsals. The first row consists of the navicular bone and the second row consists of the medial, middle, and lateral cuneiform bones. The cuboid articulates with the fourth and fifth metatarsals whereas the medial, middle, and lateral cuneiforms articulate with the first, second, and third metatarsals, respectively. The foot then terminates with the phalanges. The hindfoot consists of the talus and calcaneus. The midfoot consists of the navicular, cuboid, and cunei-

forms, and the forefoot of all ossifications at and distal to the metatarsals. It is extremely important to study the tarsal-metatarsal articulations carefully on frontal, oblique, and lateral radiographic images because subtle malalignment may indicate the presence of midfoot (Lisfranc) fracture-dislocation, which is discussed later. The frontal film will show the lateral border of the first metatarsal aligning with lateral border of the medial cuneiform, and will also show the medial border of the second metatarsal aligning with the medial margin of the middle cuneiform (Fig. 3-242). The oblique radiograph will show the alignment of the lateral margins of the lateral cuneiform and third metatarsal and the medial margins of the fourth metatarsal and the cuboid. The fifth metatarsal should be parallel in alignment proximally with its articulation with the distal-lateral margin of the cuboid. The lateral margins of the cuboid and fifth metatarsal do not align because the lateral margin of the fifth metatarsal base extends proximally and laterally relative to the cuboid bone. The second metatarsal base lies proximal and dorsal to the bases of the other metatarsal bones. It functions similar to a keystone of a Roman arch. Its anatomic position assures the proper position of the other metatarsal bones. The second metatarsal base is supported by a strong ligament, named the *Lisfranc ligament,* connecting the lateral-distal margin of the medial cuneiform with the adjacent medial-proximal margin of the second metatarsal bone.

In the skeletally immature, there are two secondary centers of ossification to be aware of. The first is at the apophysis of the calcaneal tuberosity. In the skeletally immature the apophysis is normally dense and fragmented. This is a normal appearance and does not represent AVN or fracture. The second ossification center to

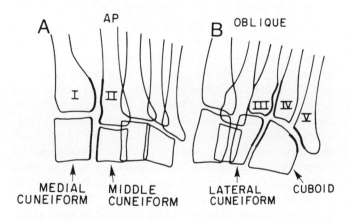

Fig. 3-242   Normal alignment of the tarsometatarsal joints. The first and second are evaluated on the AP film. The third, fourth, and fifth are evaluated on the oblique film. The bold lines indicate which surfaces of the tarsals and metatarsals must align with one another on each view. The alignment must be precise. (From Manaster BJ. *Handbook of Skeletal Radiology,* ed 2, St. Louis, 1997, Mosby-Yearbook.)

be aware of is the apophysis at the lateral base of the fifth metatarsal, which is longitudinally oriented (Fig. 3-243). This must not be mistaken for an avulsion fracture. Avulsion fractures are transverse in orientation.

Calcaneus Fracture

Calcaneus fractures usually occur after falls from heights and are therefore associated with thoracolumbar fractures. These are known as "lover's" fractures or "Don Juan" fractures. In patients with calcaneus fracture, with a history of falling from a height, evaluation of the thoracic and lumbar spine is indicated, to assess for associated spine fracture (Fig. 3-244). Ten percent of calcaneus fractures are bilateral. The most commonly employed classification scheme is the Rowe classification scheme. Type I fractures occur in 21% of cases and are fractures of the calcaneal tuberosity, sustintaculum tali, or anterior process. Type II fractures occur in approximately 4% of cases, and are horizontal fractures of the calcaneal tuberosity. Type III fractures occur in approximately 20% of the cases and are oblique fractures without extension to the subtalar joint. Type IV fractures occur in approximately 25% of cases and are fractures that extend to the subtalar joints. Type V fractures occur in 31% of cases and are intraarticular fractures with depression of the posterior subtalar joint or substantial comminution. In assessing radiographs of the calcaneus, the degree of the osseous depression is important to ascertain. Boehler's angle is measured from two lines off the lateral film (Fig 3-245). One line connects the superior margin of the

anterior process and the posterior margin of the posterior articular facet of the calcaneus. The other line connects the posterior margin of the posterior articular facet of the calcaneus and the postero-superior margin of the calcaneal tuberosity. The angles subtended by these two lines should be between 28° and 48°. With depression of the posterior articular facet in type V fractures, the angle can diminish substantially. Not only is articular depression important to evaluate on radiographs but the degree of comminution of the lateral margin of the calcaneus is important to assess, as plate fixation is usually placed along the lateral calcaneus. Excessive comminution of the lateral calcaneus limits placement of hardware plates (Fig. 3-246). CT assessment is extremely useful for evaluation of calcaneal fractures. Both coronal and axial imaging planes are useful as are sagittal reformations in determining the degree of comminution of the lateral margin of the calcaneus and the degree of depression of the posterior calcaneal facet.

Stress fractures of the calcaneus are often seen within the calcaneal tuberosity, which occur by 10–14 days after the onset of symptoms. They usually run perpendicular to the major trabeculae of the calcaneal tuberosity and are also seen as vertically oriented linear densities on the lateral radiographic view. An avulsion at the Achilles insertion can occur as an insufficiency fracture especially among diabetics. MR imaging and bone scan imaging are useful in assessing for radiographically or clinically suspected calcaneal stress fractures.

Avulsion of the extensor digitorum brevis origin is an uncommon injury. The origin of this muscle is at the anterolateral calcaneus. It is best shown on the frontal view of the ankle with the fragment located adjacent to the lateral margin of the calcaneus, 2 cm distal to the lateral malleous. It may also be seen on the frontal foot film lateral to the anterior calcaneus.

Talus Fracture

Talus fractures are less common than calcaneal fractures. Three-fourths of fractures occur in the neck and body of the talus. The remainder are avulsion fractures or chip fractures. Talar neck fractures may be associated with talar dislocations (Fig. 3-247). Owing to the precarious vascular supply of the proximal talar pole, fractures at and proximal to the mid-pole of the talus are highly susceptible to AVN within the proximal pole (Fig. 3-248). Avulsion fractures are most common in the anterior-superior surface of the mid-talar neck, which is the ankle capsule attachment site. Other avulsion fractures are seen along the lateral process of the talus, and along the superomedial margin of the talus. Osteochondral fractures of the talus are injuries involving the talar dome and are similar in etiology, appearance, and treatment as discussed extensively under knee injuries. Osteo-

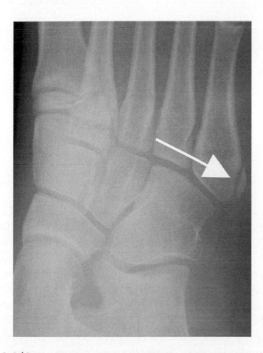

Fig. 3-243   Oblique foot radiograph demonstrates normal apophysis at base of fifth metatarsal (*arrow*).

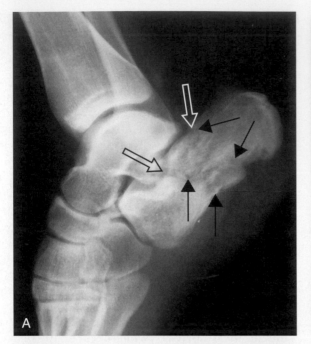

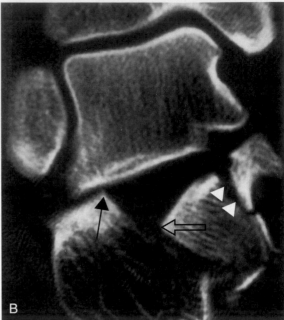

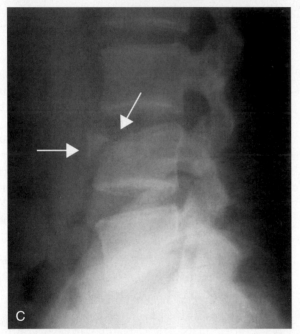

Fig. 3-244 Calcaneus fracture. **A,** Lateral radiograph demonstrates marked comminution of calcaneus (*arrows*). Note fracture extension to posterior subtalar joint (*open arrows*). **B,** Coronal CT image at level of posterior subtalar joint demonstrates intraarticular fracture margin at posterior subtalar joint (*arrow*) with marked depression of medial fragment (*open arrow*). Note fracture also extends to base of sustentaculum tali (*arrowheads*). **C,** Lateral view of lumbar spine in same patient shows compression fracture at superior endplate margin (*arrows*).

chondral fractures may occur laterally or medially. The medial lesions are found posteriorly along the talar dome whereas the lateral lesions are found mostly in the mid portion.

The os trigonum may be symptomatic, a condition known as os trigonum syndrome. The os trigonum is usually attached to the underlying talus through a synchondrosis. During skeletal growth the apophysis usually fuses with the talus but in approximately 10%–14% of individuals remains as a separate ossicle. Its appearance may simulate or may be a result of ununited fracture.

Occasionally, the area may be painful as a result of repetitive microtrauma especially after forced plantar flexion of the foot or after activities associated with extreme plantar flexion such as ballet dancing. The flexor hallucis longus tendon lies medial to the os trigonum. Tenosynovitis of the flexor hallucis longus may thus produce symptoms in this region. Posterior ankle impingement pain may be due to a large os trigonum or posterolateral process of the talus, which is compressed between the calcaneus and posterior tibia in extreme plantar flexion. Bone scan imaging is useful in demonstrating intensely in-

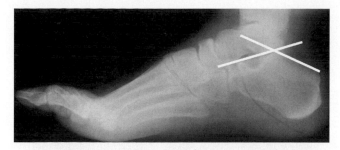

Fig. 3-245 Lateral radiograph of normal foot demonstrates Boehler's angle with line drawn along superior-anterior margin of anterior process and superior-posterior margin of posterior facet, and line drawn between posterior-superior margin of posterior facet and posterior-superior margin of calcaneal tuberosity. Angle subtended by these two lines should be between 28° and 48°.

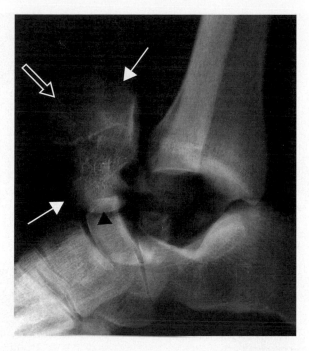

Fig. 3-247 Lateral radiograph demonstrates anterior talar dislocation (*arrows*). Talar dome is denoted by open arrow and navicular articular margin by arrowhead.

creased activity in the posterolateral talus with the syndrome. MR imaging provides greater anatomic detail and demonstrates abnormal signal consistent with edema within the os trigonum and underlying talus. The appearance may mimic a fracture, although a fracture line is linear and sharply marginated, unlike an os trigonum, which shows smooth and well-corticated margins. CT may be useful in difficult cases to discriminate between margins of an os trigonum and a fracture line.

Navicular Bone Fracture

Stress fractures of the navicular bone are uncommon but may occur in joggers and basketball players. Patients present with pain that is usually poorly localized in the medial arch of the foot. Fractures are usually sagitally oriented at the junction of the middle and lateral thirds of the navicular bone (Fig. 3-249). Although they are usually occult on radiographs, these are well shown on

MR images in the true axial and coronal planes. Bone scan imaging will show localized activity in the navicular bone and is thus sensitive but nonspecific. AVN of the lateral fragment is a potential complication of complete navicular fracture. Avulsion fractures of the navicular bone also occur. These occur at the talonavicular capsule insertion and present as a dorsal bone fragment at the proximal navicular margin. Rarely, fractures of the medial tuberosity of the navicular bone may occur at the insertion site of the posterior tibialis tendon and the tibionavi-

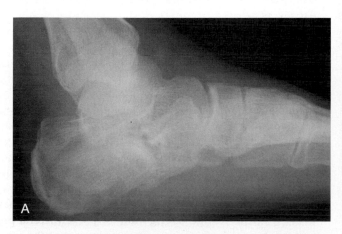
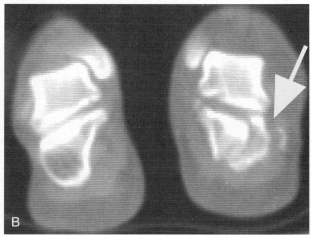

Fig. 3-246 Comminuted calcaneal fracture. **A,** Lateral radiograph demonstrates comminuted fracture with loss of Boehler's angle and depression of posterior calcaneal facet. **B,** Substantial comminution of lateral calcaneal wall (*arrow*) is demonstrated on CT.

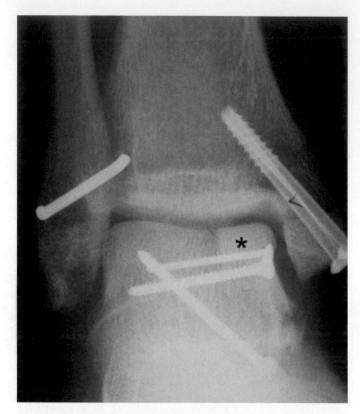

Fig. 3-248 Frontal radiograph of ankle shows medial malleolar, lateral malleolar, and talar fixation. AVN of medial talar bone fragment (*asterisk*) is shown as increased density, related to lack of hyperemic healing response.

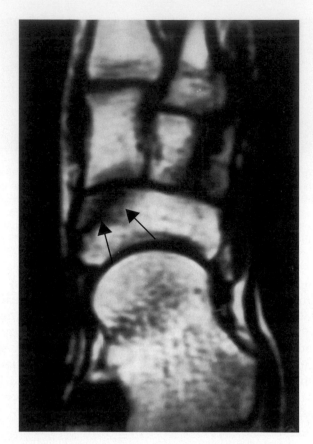

Fig. 3-249 Axial T1-weighted spin echo image (600/14; TR msec/TE msec) demonstrates stress fracture of medial pole of navicular bone (*arrows*).

cular ligament of the deltoid ligament complex. Os naviculare may be symptomatic. Patients with os naviculare often have an anomalous insertion of the posterior tibialis tendon solely on the os naviculare without continuation to cuneiform and metatarsal based insertions. These patients are prone to flatfoot deformity and hindfoot valgus. MR imaging will show edema-like signal within the ossicle and adjacent navicular bone.

Lisfranc Fracture-Dislocation

This injury typically occurs in the setting of axial loading of the plantar-flexed foot. This can occur with minimal trauma such as misstepping when coming down stairs, foot entrapment on an automobile break pedal, and as a sports injury when an opponent falls on the heel of a plantar flexed foot. These injuries involve rupture of the major supporting ligaments of the tarsal-metatarsal articulations, especially the Lisfranc ligament. Alternatively, the Lisfranc ligament may remain intact although an avulsion occurs at either the medial cuneiform or second metatarsal base insertions. With this injury, stability of the tarsal-metatarsal articulations is disrupted and lateral subluxation of the second through fifth metatarsals ensues (Fig. 3-250). There is usually dorsal subluxation or dislocation of the tarsal-

metatarsal joints, which may appear quite subtle on the lateral views (Fig. 3-251). Two types of subluxation occur. One is the *homolateral* subluxation in which all five metatarsal bones are subluxed laterally (Fig. 3-252). The other is *divergent* subluxation in which there is lateral subluxation of the second through fifth metatarsals and variable medial subluxation of the first metatarsal (Fig. 3-253). There are usually associated fractures of the metatarsal bones, although these may be radiographically occult. The degree of subluxation may be extremely subtle and in suspected cases CT or MR imaging will prove useful for detecting radiographically occult fracture and subluxation at the tarsal-metatarsal articulations. Slight widening of the interspace between the first and second metatarsals may be the only clue to the appropriate diagnosis on radiographs and should prompt additional imaging with CT or MRI. Lisfranc fracture-dislocations are also common complications of diabetic neuropathic arthropathy. However the findings in the setting of neuropathic arthropathy are usually not subtle and usually do not carry the same urgency for surgical intervention as do those of traumatic etiology. Lisfranc fracture-dislocations have a poor prognosis. The likelihood of eventual OA is high. For this reason, subluxation and intraarticular fractures which demonstrate any

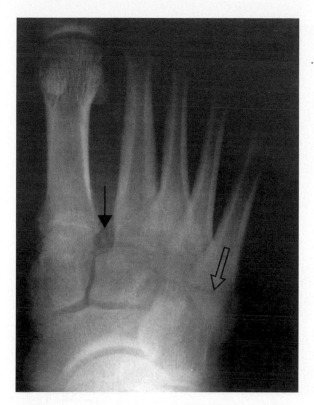

Fig. 3-250 Oblique foot radiograph demonstrates Lisfranc fracture-dislocation. Note widening of interspace between first and second metatarsals associated with lateral subluxation of second metatarsal base, with avulsion fracture (*arrow*) between metatarsal bases. A fracture in the base of the fifth metatarsal bone is shown (*open arrow*).

degree of displacement undergo surgical reduction and fixation.

Jones' Fracture

These are fractures located at the base of the fifth metatarsal 1.5–2 cm distal to the tuberosity (Fig. 3-254).

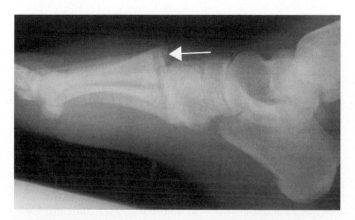

Fig. 3-251 Lateral view of patient with Lisfranc fracture-dislocation demonstrates superior subluxation at tarsometatarsal joints (*arrow*).

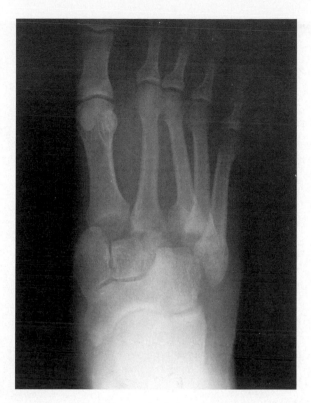

Fig. 3-252 AP (anteroposterior) foot radiograph demonstrates homolateral Lisfranc fracture-dislocation. Note lateral offset of all five metatarsal bones, including first metatarsal.

The Jones' fracture is a different fracture than avulsion of the proximal articular margin of the fifth metatarsal bone (see Fig. 3-227). The articular fracture results from tension of the peroneous brevis tendon insertion, whereas the Jones' fracture is an impaction injury, which usually develops as a stress fracture. The differentiation is important because articular avulsion fractures usually heal easily whereas the Jones' fracture is prone to delayed union and nonunion.

Metatarsal Stress Fracture (March Fracture)

Metatarsal stress fractures are common stress fractures that occur usually in the second or third metatarsal shafts. They are usually nondisplaced and become radiographically apparent 7–10 days after onset of symptoms, with the appearance of ill-defined periosteal new bone formation at the site of fracture (Fig. 3-255). Eventually a sclerotic healed fracture line will appear.

Stubbing one's toe is a common injury. These may be occasionally associated with nail bed injuries or with fractures of the distal phalangeal tuft. In the skeletally immature, Salter-Harris I or II fractures may result from a stubbed toe because the nail bed of the toe is attached to the periosteum of the distal phalanx at the level of the proximal metaphysis. Because the nail bed is often disrupted, patients are prone to osteomyelitis.

Text continued on p. 382

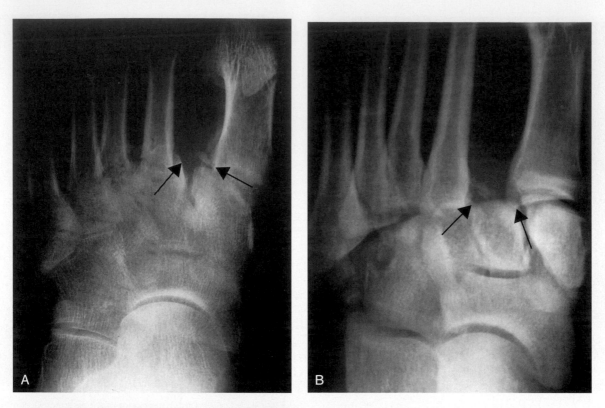

Fig. 3-253   Divergent Lisfranc fracture-dislocation. **A** and **B,** Two different patients with divergent fracture-dislocation. Note widening of space between first and second metatarsals (*arrows*).

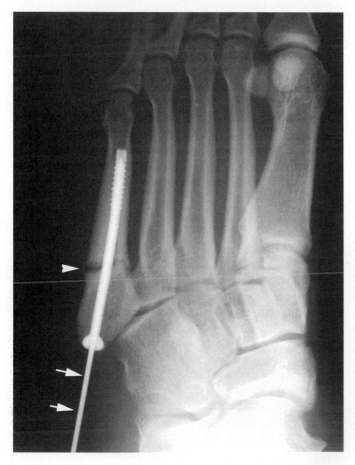

Fig. 3-254   Oblique radiograph of foot shows Jones fracture (*arrowhead*) in a colleagiate basketball player. Note cannulated screw placed over a guide pin (*arrows*) in this intraoperative film.

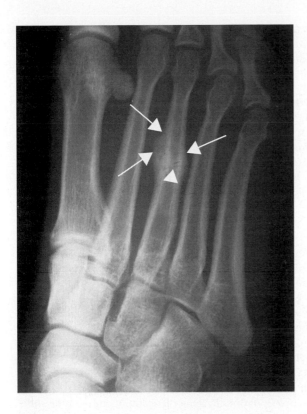

Fig. 3-255   Oblique foot radiograph demonstrates stress fracture of mid third metatarsal bone. Note prominent mature callus (*arrows*) and ill-defined fracture line (*arrowhead*).

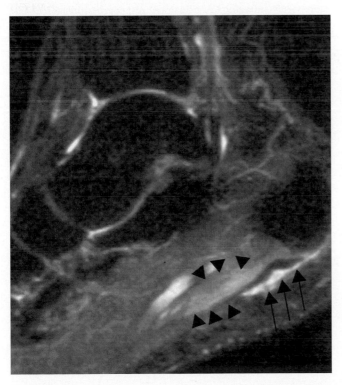

Fig. 3-256   Sagittal inversion recovery image (4480/22); TR msec/ TE msec; inversion time 150 msec) in patient with plantar fasciitis shows increased signal and thickening of medial cord of plantar aponeurosis (*arrows*) and increased signal from acute atrophy in the flexor digitorum brevis muscle (*arrowheads*). (Courtesy of Michael Recht, M.D., Cleveland, OH.)

Soft Tissue Injury

Plantar Fasciitis

The plantar fascia arises from two cords at the plantar aspect of the calcaneal tuberosity. The medial cord is the flexor digitorum brevis and the lateral cord is the abductor digiti minimi. Chronic repetitive trauma may result in tendinopathy and inflammation of the origin of the plantar aponeurosis, resulting in extreme tenderness as well as pain with ambulation at the plantar calcaneal tuberosity. At MR imaging (Fig. 3-256) one may see heterogeneous signal in the origin of the plantar aponeurosis and adjacent subtle bone marrow signal changes. There is variable thickening of the plantar aponeurosis. Occasionally, one may see atrophy with fatty infiltration in either the flexor digitorum brevis or abductor digiti minimi. Heel spurs may result from plantar fasciitis but are entirely nonspecific, as traction at the origin of the plantar aponeurosis similarly may produce heel spurs. Furthermore, heel spurs may result from inflammatory enthesitis, which is commonly at the origin of the plantar apponeurosis in the setting of Reiter's syndrome or psoriatic arthropathy.

SOURCES AND SUGGESTED READINGS

Affram P: An epidemiologic study of cervical and trochanteric fractures of the femur in an urban population. Analysis of 1664 cases with special reference to etiologic factors, *Acta Orthop Scand Suppl* 64:11, 1964.

Allen W, Cope R: Coxa saltans: the snapping hip revisited, *J Am Acad Orthop Surg* 3:303-308, 1995.

Applegate GR, Flannigan BD, Fox T, Del Pizzo W: MR diagnosis of recurrent tears of the knee: Value of intraarticular contrast material, *AJR* 161:821-825, 1993.

Bayliss A, Davidson J: Traumatic osteonecrosis of the femoral head following intracapsular fracture. Incidence and earliest radiological features, *Clin Radiol* 28:407, 1997.

Ben-Menachem Y, Coldwell D, Young J, Burgess A: Hemorrhage associated with pelvic fractures: causes, diagnosis, and emergent management, *AJR* 157:1005-1014, 1991.

DeSmet A, Fisher D, Burnstein M, Graf B, Lange R: Value of MR imaging in staging osteochondral lesions of the talus (osterochondritis dissicans): results in 14 patients, *AJR* 154:555-558, 1990.

Deutsch A, Mink J, Fox F, et al: Peripheral meniscal tears: MR findings after conservative treatment or arthroscopic repair, *Radiology* 176:485-488, 1990.

Deutsch A, Mink J, Fox J, et al: The posteroperative knee, *Mag Reson O* 8:23-54, 1992.

Dussault R, Kaplan P, Roederer G: MR imaging of Achilles tendon in patients with familial hyperlipidemia, *AJR* 164:403-407, 1995.

Fisher S, Fox J, Del Pizzo W, et al: Accuracy of diagnoses from magnetic resonance imaging of the knee, *J Bone Joint Surg* 73A(1):2-10, 1991.

Garden RS: Stability and union of subcapital fractures of the femour, *J Bone Joint Surg* 46b:630-712, 1964.

Gill K, Bucholy R: The role of CT scanning in the evaluation of major pelvic fractures, *J Bone Joint Surg Am* 66A:34, 1984.

Holder J, Yu J, Goodwin D, Haghighi P, Trudall D, Resnick D: MR arthrography of the hip: improved imaging of the acetabular labrum with histologic correlation in cadavers, *AJR* 165:887-891, 1995.

Judet R, Judet J, Letournel E: Fractures of the acetabulum: Classification and surgical approaches to reduction, *J Bone Joint Surg* 46a:1615-1646, 1964.

Karasick D, Schweitzer M: The os trigonum syndrome: imaging features. *AJR* 166:125-129, 1996.

Lauge-Hansen N: Fractures of the ankle: Genetic roentgenologic diagnosis of fractures of the ankle, *AJR* 71:456, 1954.

Laurin C, Dussault R, Levesque H: The tangential x-ray investigation of the patellofemoral joint, *Clin Orthop* 144:16, 1979.

Mainwaring B, Daffner R, Reiner B: Pylon fractures of the ankle: a distinct clinical and radiographic entity, *Radiology* 168:215-218, 1998.

Manaster BJ: Imaging knee ligament reconstructions. *RSNA Categorical course in Musculoskeletal Radiology* 211-218, 1993.

Resnick C, Stackhouse D, Shanmuganathan K, Young J: Diagnosis of pelvic fractures with acute pelvic trauma: efficacy of plain radiographs, *AJR* 158:109-112, 1992.

Rowe CR, Sakellarides HT, Freeman PA, Sorbie C: Fractures of the os calcis: a long term follow-up study of 146 patients. *JAMA* 184:920, 1963.

Schwappach J, Murphey M, Kokmayer S, Rosenthal H, Simmons M, Huntrakoon M: Subcapital fractures of the femoral neck: prevalence and cause of radiographic appearance simulating pathologic fractures, *AJR* 162:651-654, 1994.

Smith D: Imaging of sports injuries of the ankle and foot, *Operative Techniques in Sports Medicine* 3:47-70, 1995.

Smith D, May D, Phillips P: MR imaging of the anterior cruciate ligament: frequency of discordant findings on sagittal-oblique images and correlations with arthroscopic findings, *AJR* 166:411-413, 1996.

Steinbach L, Tirmon P: MRI of the ankle, *The Radiologist* 2:111-124, 1995.

CHAPTER 3

Trauma

SPINE TRAUMA

PART IV

B.J. MANASTER, M.D., Ph.D., and DAVID A. MAY, M.D.

INTRODUCTION

An essential concept in spine trauma is the *three column model* of spine stability. The *anterior column* consists of the anterior longitudinal ligament and the anterior half of the vertebral bodies, intervertebral discs, and supporting soft tissues. The *middle column* consists of the posterior longitudinal ligament and the posterior half of the vertebral bodies, intervertebral discs, and supporting soft tissues. The *posterior column* consists of the posterior elements, the facet joints, and the numerous associ-

ated ligaments. Disruption of only one column generally does not result in instability. Disruption of two or three columns results in spine instability. Because a column disruption may involve only the soft tissues, spine instability may be present even in the absence of a fracture. Lateral flexion-extension films can be valuable to exclude ligamentous instability. If there is concern on the radiographic series relating to fracture, CT with sagittal and coronal reformation can further define osseous injury. Finally, additional critical soft-tissue injuries may accompany spine trauma, such as epidural hematoma or injury to the spinal cord, vertebral arteries, conus medullaris, or nerve roots. MR imaging may be needed to search for these lesions.

The same basic forces that cause fractures in the appendicular skeleton cause spine fractures: compression, tension, and shear. Rotational forces, which combine the basic forces, are a frequent factor in spine trauma.

Key Concepts | Spine Trauma

- Assessment of the traumatized spine requires high quality radiographs and careful assessment for patterns of injury, some of which can be very subtle.
- Flexion-extension radiographs, when appropriate, can reveal or exclude significant ligamentous injury.
- CT and sometimes MRI are needed to fully characterize a spine injury.
- The three column model predicts whether a spine injury is stable or unstable.

CERVICAL SPINE

Cervical spine injuries can be extremely subtle radiographically, yet clinically devastating. Radiographic assessment of the traumatized cervical spine must include high quality AP, lateral, and open mouth odontoid views. Many trauma centers also include oblique views in adults. An alternative approach that can be useful in large patients is combining lateral radiographs with axial CT of the entire spine. The following discussion pertains to radiographs.

Familiarity with normal anatomy and subtle signs of injury is essential. Most of the relevant information can be found on the lateral radiograph. The lateral radiograph must show the anatomy from the clivus to the top of the T1 vertebral body. A swimmer's view is often necessary to demonstrate the lower cervical spine. The following items must be evaluated:

1. The prevertebral soft tissues should be normal in width. In adults, the normal measurement is ≤5 mm at the level of C3 and C4, increasing to ≤22 mm at C6. In children, the prevertebral soft tissues should measure no more than two-thirds the width of the C2 body at the level of C3 and C4 and no more than 14 mm at C6.

2. Normal cervical alignment is lordosis. However, it should be remembered that loss of lordosis is expected in patients on a backboard or in a cervical collar. Loss of lordosis may also represent muscle spasm or can even be attributed to patient positioning, as lordosis of the cervical spine is absent in 70% of normal patients if the chin is depressed by 1 inch.

3. Four continuous curves (Fig. 3-257) describe the normal position of the bony elements, including the anterior vertebral body line, posterior vertebral body line, spinal laminar line, and the posterior spinous process line. The spinal laminar line should form a continuous line, regardless of the degree of flexion or extension. The exception of

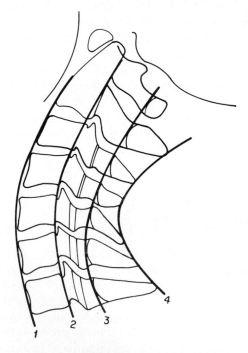

Fig. 3-257   Diagram of the lateral cervical spine, with the 4 lines which should be evaluated for following a continuous curve. 1, anterior vertebral line; 2, posterior vertebral line; 3, spinal laminar line; 4, posterior spinous line. (From Manaster, *Handbook of Skeletal Radiology,* Mosby, 1997).

the continuous alignment of the three other curves is found in children, where there is often a physiologic off-set of 2–3 mm at the C2-3 and C3-4 levels with flexion and extension.

4. In the absence of degenerative disk disease, the distance between adjacent posterior vertebral bodies is uniform at all levels. A gap at one level suggests posterior ligamentous injury, a finding that can be supported by distraction of the associated spinous processes. Note that the normal "fanning" of the spinous processes is normally not uniform, as it is greater for the proximal and distal cervical elements than for the middle elements.

5. On a perfectly positioned lateral view, the right and left facet joints are superimposed. A slightly off-lateral radiograph will show partial overlap of the right and left facet joints. In the absence of rotation, the degree of overlap should be uniform at all levels in the cervical spine. An abrupt change in the amount of overlap in adjacent levels indicates abnormal rotation along the longitudinal axis of the spine. Therefore the degree of overlap at each level must be evaluated. Furthermore, the articular surfaces of each facet must be congruent. Absence of such congruence indicates a subluxed, perched, or dislocated facet.

6. The odontoid process normally is tilted posteriorly on the body of C2. If this posterior tilt is not seen, you should consider that there may be a fracture of the odontoid at its waist, with anterior subluxation of the odontoid process. This can be confirmed by spinal laminar line disruption.

7. The atlantoaxial distance is measured at the base of the dens between the anterior cortex of the dens and the posterior cortex of the atlas' anterior arch. In adults, this distance is not more than 2.5 mm and does not change with flexion. In children, the distance may be as great as 5 mm and may change by 1–2 mm with flexion.

8. Radiographic signs of instability include abnormal spinous process fanning, widening of the intervertebral disk space, horizontal displacement of one body on another more than 3.5 mm, angulation greater than 11°, disruption of facets, or severe injury, such as multiple fractures at one segment (Fig. 3-258).

9. On an AP radiograph, the spinous processes should form a fairly continuous, although often slightly irregular line. A fractured spinous process may be obviously displaced from this line, or what appears to be two spinous processes may be seen, one representing the nondisplaced base of the fractured process, and the other representing the displaced fragment.

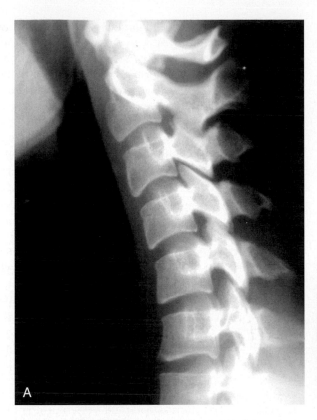 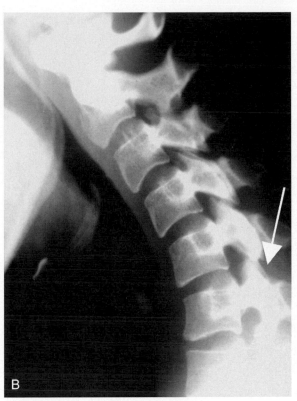

Fig. 3-258 Cervical spine instability. **A,** is a lateral view in the patient's neutral position. It demonstrates a mild kyphosis of the cervical spine, centered at the C5–6 level. There is however, no subluxation and only minimal uncovering of the posterior facets at C5–6. The lateral flexion view (**B**) demonstrates that this is indeed an unstable spine, with C5–6 showing significant posterior gapping at the spinous processes, and near complete uncoverage of the facets (*arrow*). Even in flexion, facets should remain normally covered, as at the other levels in this spine.

10. The open-mouth odontoid view is used to detect odontoid process fractures and the integrity of the ring of C1. In neutral position, there is alignment of the lateral margins of the lateral masses of C1 and C2. With rotation, the atlas normally moves as a unit with lateral facet offset on one side and medial offset on the contralateral side. Bilateral-lateral offset of the lateral margins of the lateral masses of C1 indicates a C1 ring fracture in adults. In children, bilateral offset is a normal variant due to discrepant growth of C1 and C2.
11. Oblique radiographs may be used to evaluate the posterior elements for fracture and to confirm the normal alignment of the facets. On the oblique view, facets line up like roof shingles, with each more superior facet placed posterior to the facet below.

Cervical Spine Normal Variants

Several developmental variants can simulate an upper cervical spine fracture. *Occipitalization of the atlas* is lack of segmentation at the atlanto-occipital junction.

This presents radiographically with atlantoaxial subluxation, which can simulate a traumatic disruption (Fig. 3-259). In this situation, there is an abnormally large gap between the spinous processes of C1 and C2, with the atlas located unusually close to the occiput. The diagnosis is established by a flexion radiograph, which demonstrates fixation of the atlas to the occiput. In addition, the odontoid often has a bizarre shape. CT may also be used to establish the diagnosis.

Normal variant absence or lack of fusion of ossification centers can be especially confusing at C1 and C2. At C1 the body is occasionally bifid. The neural arches of C1 and C2 may have focal defects or absence of the normal synchondrosis between the arch and the body. In C2, there are four ossification centers: one for each neural arch, one for the body, which occasionally may be bifid, and one for the odontoid process. The body/neural arch synchondroses fuse asymmetrically between the ages of 3 and 6 years. The body/odontoid synchondrosis also fuses at this time. A *persistent lucent synchondrosis* may persist into adult life, located well below the level of the apparent "base" of the odontoid, seen as a thin, straight well-defined transverse lucency in the body of C2 below

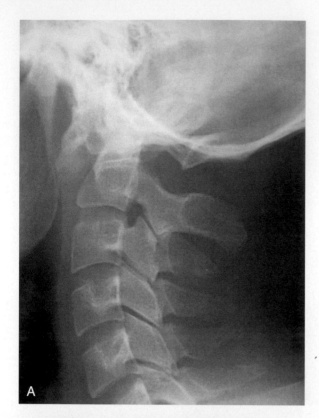

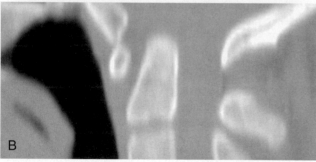

Fig. 3-259   Occipitalization of the atlas. **A,** is a lateral radiograph demonstrating no significant separation between the occiput and the atlas. The CT demonstrates that the anterior arch as well as the hypoplastic posterior arch of the atlas are fused to the occiput (**B**). The odontoid moves independently of the occipitalized atlas; hence the abnormal atlantoaxial distance.

the base of the dens. This must be differentiated from an odontoid fracture, which usually occurs at the true base of the odontoid (Fig. 3-260). A transverse dens fracture may also be simulated by a Mach line from the superimposed bottom of the teeth incisors or the arch of the atlas.

The os terminale is an ossification center located at the superior tip of the odontoid process. Before it ossifies, the tip of the dens is V-shaped on radiographs. The os terminale normally fuses by age 12, but may persist unfused, simulating a fracture of the odontoid tip.

The *os odontoideum* is an anatomic variant, large ossicle that occupies the space normally occupied by

the odontoid process. This ossicle is separated from the hypoplastic odontoid by a wide gap. It is fixed to the arch of the atlas, and moves with C1 on flexion and extension. It may appear quite bizarre and may simulate a fracture (Fig. 3-261). The etiology of os odontoideum is controversial. An old ununited fracture may cause this finding, and previous trauma accounts for many of these lesions. However, a large os terminale may enlarge to form an os odontoideum in the setting of a hypoplastic odontoid process.

Cervical Spine Fractures

Cervical spine injuries usually occur in predictable patterns based on the mechanism of injury. Knowledge of these patterns can help the radiologist to avoid missing an important injury.

Fracture of the occipital condyle is more common than was previously understood, and often requires CT for diagnosis. These fractures may involve the hypoglossal canal or jugular foramen, so clinical features of injury to cranial nerves IX–XII may be found (Fig. 3-262).

Occipital vertebral dissociation (craniocervical dissociation) can be a surprisingly easy injury to miss radiographically. The normal occipital vertebral relationship is maintained by ligaments extending from the axis to the clivus. In patients with injuries resulting in severe facial trauma, trauma to this portion of the neck may also occur. A true dislocation is often fatal and obvious on the lateral film (Fig. 3-263). Subluxation is rare and may not have a neurologic deficit or obvious radiographic findings. In such a case, a line drawn from the interior tip of the clivus (the basion), to a line drawn along the posterior body of C2, should show a distance of less than 12 mm. Also, a line from the basion to the top of the odontoid process should be less than 12 mm.

Axial loading can cause bilateral vertical fractures through the neural arch of the atlas. This must be differentiated from congenital defects of the atlas. A *Jefferson fracture* is a C1 ring fracture that involves both the anterior and posterior arches. The normal angulation of the C1 facets tends to spread the C1 fragments laterally. Surprisingly, this may be a stable fracture with minimal fragment displacement and no neurologic deficit unless there is also disruption of the transverse atlantal ligaments which normally fixes the odontoid to the anterior arch of the atlas. CT or MRI can be helpful in diagnosing and characterizing this fracture and associated soft-tissue injuries (Fig. 3-264).

Atlantoaxial rotatory displacement is rotation injury with locking of the facets of C1 and C2, usually seen in childhood and presenting as torticollis. Radiographs of this condition can be difficult to interpret owing to the alteration of familiar landmarks by the cervical rotation. On the open-mouthed view, one lateral mass of C1 ap-

Text continued on p. 389

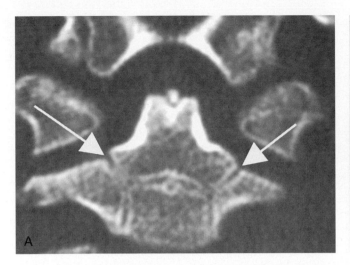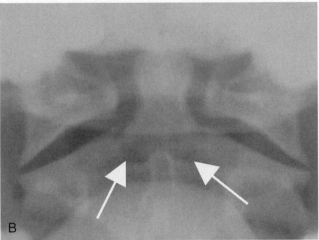

Fig. 3-260   Normal synchronoses of C2. **A,** A coronal CT demonstrating the multiple synchondroses of C2. The body of C2 is seen with the adjacent ossification centers of the posterior arches. The odontoid is a large structure, which extends below the level of the apparent "base of the odontoid." This synchondrosis (*arrows*) may remain unfused throughout life, but normally fuses between the ages of 3 and 6 years. Finally, there is a small os terminali, which is located at the superior tip of the odontoid process. Before its ossification, the tip may be seen as a V-shaped defect. The os terminali normally fuses by age 12, but may also persist unfused, simulating a tip of odontoid fracture. The open mouth odontoid on a different patient, **B,** shows an unfused synchondrosis between the odontoid and the body that simulates a fracture of the odontoid (*arrows*). (Reprinted with permission from the ACR learning file.)

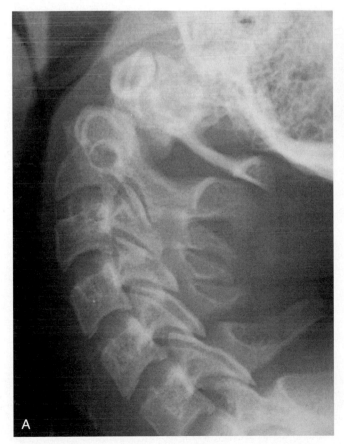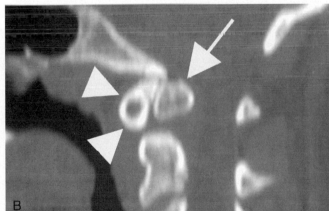

Fig. 3-261   Os odontoideum. **A,** is a lateral radiograph of the cervical spine held in extension. It demonstrates that C1 is posteriorly displaced relative to C2, with the enlarged anterior arch of C1 appearing to be in the expected position of the odontoid relative to the body of C2. The odontoid is not well seen. This simulates a fracture of the odontoid and there quite clearly is abnormal motion of C1 relative to C2. This represents a variant termed os odontoideum, where the actual odontoid is hypoplastic. **B,** The sagittal reconstructed CT clearly shows the hypoplastic odontoid which is fused to the body of C2, the overgrown os terminali (*arrow*), and the overgrown anterior arch of the atlas (*arrowheads*). The os terminali moves with the atlas, and independent of C2.

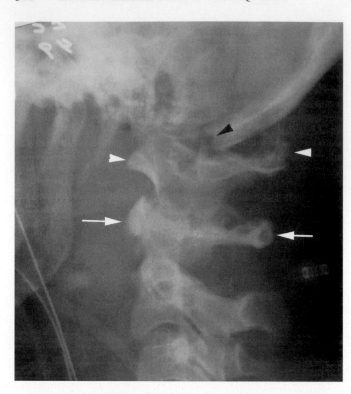

Fig. 3-262 Occipital condyle fractures. Condylar fragments (*white arowheads*) are inferiorly and posteriorly displaced. Note the fracture margin at the skull base (*black arrowhead*). Arrows mark C1. (Courtesy of William Howard, M.D., Richmond, VA.)

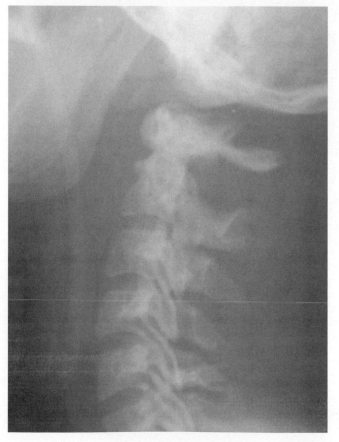

Fig. 3-263 Occipital atlas dissociation. This lateral radiograph demonstrates a critical injury. There is tremendous prevertebral soft tissue swelling, and complete dissociation of the occiput from the atlas.

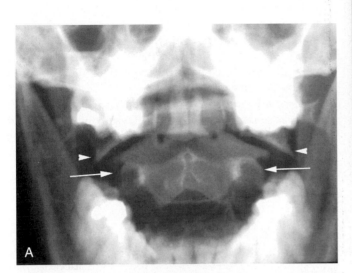

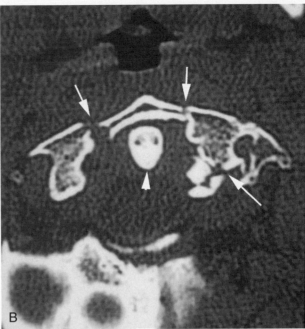

Fig. 3-264   Jefferson fracture of C1. **A,** Open mouth odontoid view shows lateral translocation of the lateral masses of C1 (*arrowheads*) relative to C2 (*arrows*). **B,** Axial CT image shows multiple breaks in the ring of C1 (*arrows*). The arrowhead marks the dens. (Courtesy of W. Smoker, M.D., Richmond, VA.)

pears wider and closer to the midline with the opposite appearing narrower and laterally offset. Overlapping osseous and soft tissue structures may obscure the facets. CT with reconstruction may be extremely helpful in diagnosing this condition (Fig. 3-265).

Odontoid fractures are the most commonly missed significant cervical spine fracture. Odontoid fractures may be classified by the location of the fracture. Type 1 dens fractures involve only the tip. These usually but not always are stable injuries. Type 2 dens fractures are through the waist or base. This is the most common pattern, with the base of the dens the most frequent site. Type 3 dens fractures extend below the base of the dens through the body of C2. Type 2 and 3 dens fractures

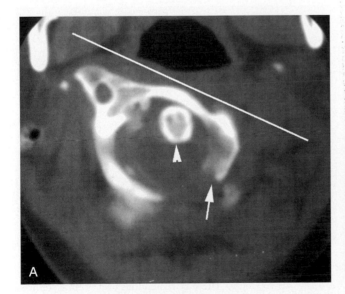

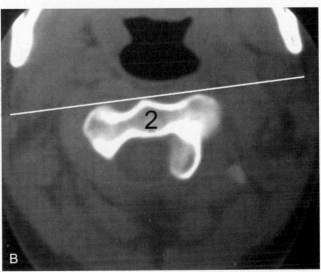

Fig. 3-265   Rotatory subluxation of C1 on C2. Axial CT images through the ring of C1 and the body of C2 show rotation of C1 (**A**) relative to C2 (**B**). Also note the fracture of C1 (*arrow* in **A**). Arrowhead marks the dens in **A.** (Courtesy of W. Smoker, M.D., Richmond, VA.)

are unstable injuries. Transverse dens fractures can be difficult to detect with CT because the CT beam is parallel to the fracture line. Thus attention to the odontoid view and the spinal laminar alignment on the lateral view are critical to diagnose these fractures. However, if the fracture has an oblique extension into the vertebral body anteriorly, it may not be seen on the open-mouth view (Fig. 3-266), but CT will detect the fracture.

The *Hangman's fracture* (or more appropriately, "hanged man") is most frequently seen at C2, but can be seen at other levels. This most frequently occurs from a hyperextension injury that results in bilateral neural arch fractures (traumatic spondylolysis). Interruption of the spinal laminar line is the radiographic hallmark of

this injury (Fig. 3-267). The odontoid and its attachments are usually intact and cord damage is uncommon owing to the width of the cervical canal at this level. Most Hangman fractures are type I, involving the posterior part of the body of C2 or any part of the ring without displacement or angulation and leaving the C2-3 disk intact. If there is greater than 3 mm displacement of C2 on C3 or a 15° angulation at this level, the C2-3 disk is likely disrupted, leading to a type II or III designation and implied instability.

Flexion injuries may range from the innocuous *anterior wedge compression* to the devastating *flexion teardrop* (*burst*) fracture. Anterior wedge compression generally affects only the anterior column and thus is a stable

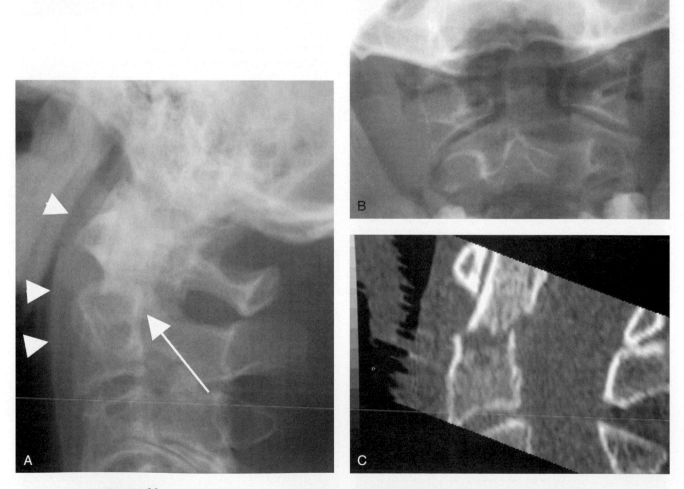

Fig. 3-266   Odontoid fracture. **A,** This lateral radiograph shows that this patient has only mild prevertebral swelling, but the focus is at the odontoid (*arrowheads*). There is offset of the odontoid relative to the C2 body (*arrow*). **B,** the open-mouth odontoid radiograph, appears normal. Even though a distinct fracture line is not seen on either the lateral or the open-mouth odontoid the offset and abnormal tilt of the odontoid process relative to the body of C2 must be diagnosed as a fracture. **C,** This is confirmed on sagittal reconstruction of the CT.

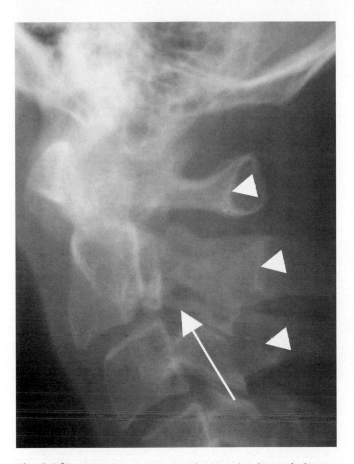

Fig. 3-267   Hangman's fracture. The lateral radiograph demonstrates the bilateral neural arch fractures at C2 that constitute a hangman's fracture (*arrow*). The fracture extends into the posterior body of C2 and there is anterior subluxation of C2 on C3, making this a type III injury. Note the disruption of the spinal laminar line (*arrowheads* at C1, C2, and C3).

anterior-inferior border of the vertebral body. The posterior body is displaced into the spinal canal, with a high probability of neural damage. The extent of injury is often underestimated on radiographs but is well demonstrated on CT. Cord and ligamentous injury, and epidural hematoma are best shown by MRI (Fig. 3-269).

A *unilateral locked facet,* or more precisely, *unilateral interfacetal dislocation,* results from flexion, distraction, and rotation. Radiographically, there is an abrupt change in the amount of facet overlap seen on the lateral image (Fig. 3-270). The most common location for a unilateral locked facet is C4-5 or C5-6. Thirty-five percent of these cases are associated with fracture, most frequently of the facet. With a unilateral locked facet there need not be significant subluxation of the vertebral body. *Bilateral locked facets (bilateral interfacetal dislocation)* are also due to flexion, but with enough distraction for the facets to become disarticulated. With a bilateral lock the vertebral body is displaced, usually 50% of the body length as seen on the lateral radiograph (Fig. 3-271). Both lateral and oblique films show the "jumped" and locked facets. There is a high incidence of cord injury with bilateral locked facets.

Extension injuries may have extremely subtle radiographic signs. With extension injuries, there may be a tear or stretch of the anterior longitudinal ligament and disruption of the anterior annulus fibrosis. This may result in avulsion of the adjacent anterior vertebral body endplate. More severe extension injuries may also involve the middle and posterior columns and result in profound instability. Despite the serious soft-tissue disruptions, these injuries can spontaneously reduce, so radiographs may not reveal the true extent of injury. Prevertebral soft-tissue swelling is an important clue. There may be posterior body displacement or a widened intervertebral disk space, especially anteriorly. A vacuum phenomenon at the annulus fibrosis is highly suggestive of an extension injury. When present, anteroinferior vertebral body avulsion usually is found at C2 or C3 may suggest the diagnosis of hyperextension injury (Fig. 3-272). Facet compression fractures can result from hyperextension with rotation but are subtle injuries to diagnose, even with CT. Facet compression fractures may result in nerve root compression. Hyperextension injuries can cause spinal cord injury even without fracture or dislocation. When hyperextension injury is suspected, MR should be performed to delineate the soft-tissue injury and to determine the likelihood of instability. With MR, the spinal cord, any disk herniation, and epidural hematoma are directly visualized (Fig. 3-273). Vertebral artery injury must be suspected in patients with facet fractures or instability.

A *clay shoveler's* fracture is an avulsion of the C7 or T1 spinous process. It is caused by abrupt contraction of the trapezius and other muscles that attach to these spinous processes.

injury. However, if the posterior ligamentous complex is disrupted, then there is a potentially unstable, two column injury. Severe flexion injuries often disrupt the posterior longitudinal ligament, in which case there is localized increased height of the intervertebral disk space, associated with fanning of spinous processes and a local kyphotic angulation. These findings are accentuated on flexion films and may allow facet subluxation or even locking. However, cervical stability may be maintained, at least temporarily, by surrounding soft tissues and muscle spasm. Delayed instability is found in 20% of these patients (Fig. 3-268). The *teardrop burst* (flexion teardrop) fracture is the most severe flexion injury compatible with life, with 80% of patients sustaining neurologic injury. The mechanism of a teardrop burst fracture is combined flexion and compression, with diving and motor vehicle accidents being most frequent. In these cases there are coronal and sagittal comminuted vertebral body fractures with a triangular fragment found at the

Text continued on p. 397

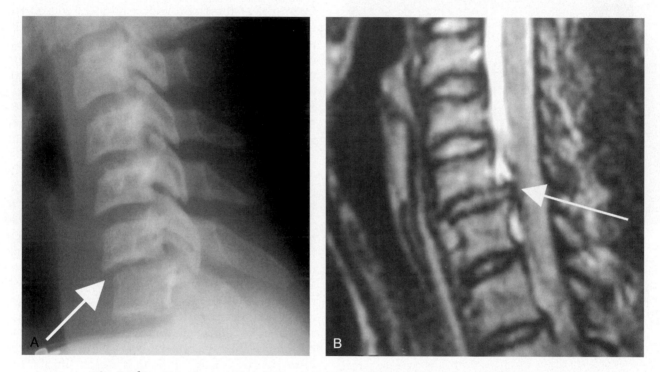

Fig. 3-268 Hyperflexion injury. **A,** is a lateral flexion view of the cervical spine in this patient who suffered neck injury in a motor vehicle accident. Although the neutral view (not shown) showed no abnormality, the flexion view shows anterolysthesis of C6 on C7 (*arrow*) as well as narrowing of the disk space. This is not normal in a 14-year-old. **B,** T2-weighted sagittal MR (3200/ 102) demonstrates the anterolisthesis of C6 on C7, along with the disk herniation and posterior longitudinal ligament disruption (*arrow*).

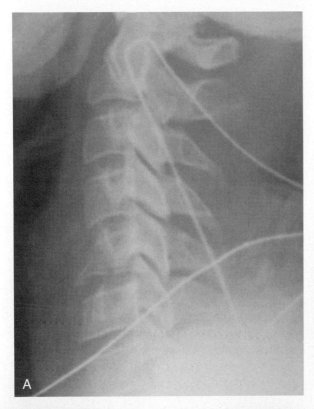

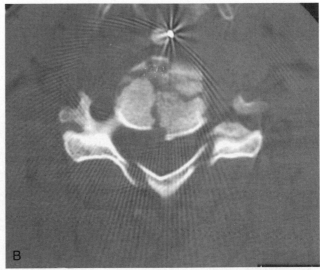

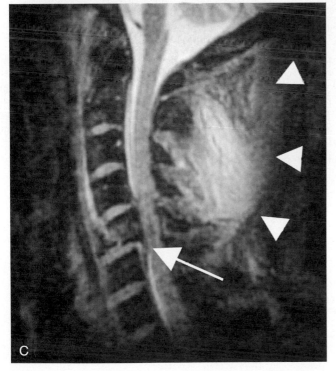

Fig. 3-269   Flexion teardrop burst fracture. **A,** A lateral radiograph that shows a "teardrop" type fracture at the anterior-inferior aspect of the body of C5. There is no obvious retropulsed fragment, and the extent of this injury is easily underestimated on this radiograph. **B,** The CT allows an understanding of the severity of the injury, showing 3-column disruption. **C,** Gradient echo MR shows not only the fracture, but also the diffuse high signal in the posterior ligamentous structures (*arrowheads*), the retropulsion of the vertebral body, and cord contusion (*arrows*).

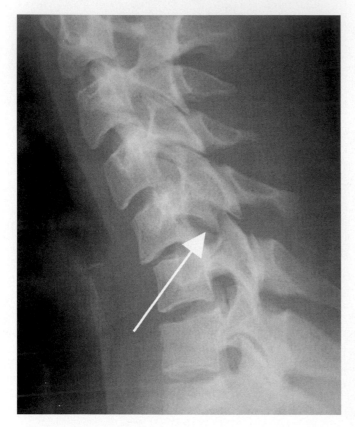

Fig. 3-270   Unilateral locked facet. Lateral radiograph demonstrates the abrupt transition of the cervical spine at the C5-6 level, where there is mild anterolisthesis of C5 on C6, splaying of the spinous processes, and a change in alignment of the facets (*arrow*). The facets at C3, C4, and C5 are in a bow-tie configuration, whereas they are in a pure lateral configuration at C6 and C7. There is a lock of the more anterior-inferior C5 facet on the superior facet of C6.

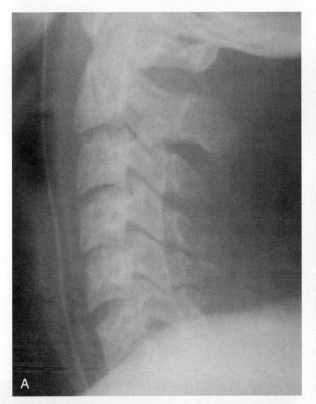

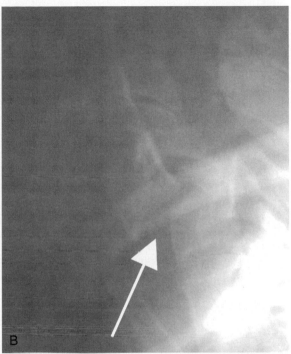

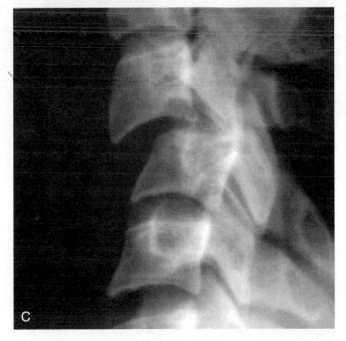

Fig. 3-271 Bilateral locked facets. This lateral radiograph demonstrates the necessity of seeing to the level of T1. **A,** The initial lateral shows a normal appearing cervical spine to the level of C6. However, the swimmer's view (**B**) shows a bilateral locked facet of C6 with near complete anterolisthesis of C6 on C7 (*arrow*). **C,** A more easily diagnosed bilateral locked facet is seen in a different patient at the level of C3-4.

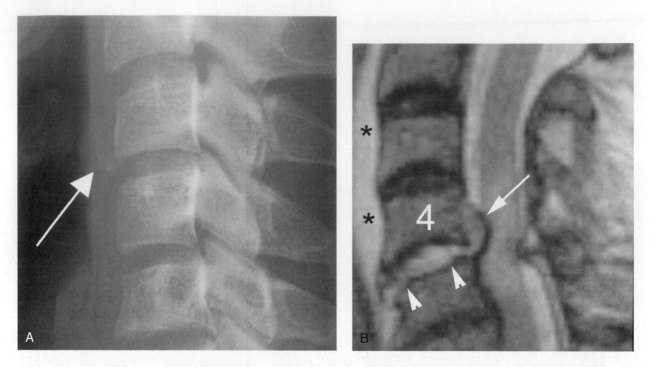

Fig. 3-272 Hyperextension injury. **A,** This patient has no prevertebral soft tissue swelling. However, there is a subtle avulsion fracture of the anteroinferior vertebral body endplate (*arrow*). This is an indicator of a hyperextension injury, and MRI should be obtained for evaluation of possible spinal cord injury. **B,** T2-weighted MRI of a different patient with hyperextension injury shows disruption of the C4–5 disc (*arrowheads*) and epidural (*arrow*) hematomas. (Courtesy of W. Smoker, M.D., Richmond, VA.)

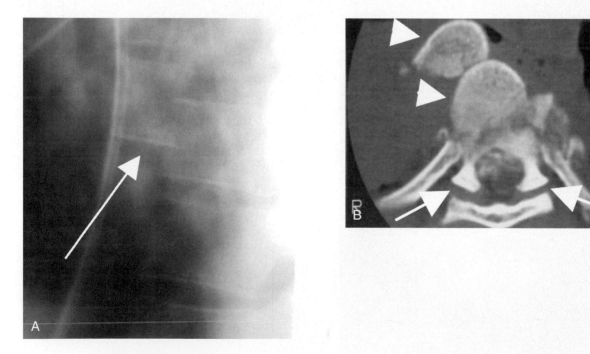

Fig. 3-273 Unstable upper thoracic spine injury. **A,** The lateral radiograph shows offset of the thoracic spine at its mid-portion (*arrows*). This implies sternal and likely multiple rib fractures as well to allow this degree of instability. **B,** The CT shows the two vertebral bodies as they overlap in this unstable position (*arrowheads*), as well as the retropulsed fragments at the canal, and the diastasis of the facets (*arrows*). (Reprinted with permission of the ACR learning file.)

THORACIC AND LUMBAR SPINE

Traumatic injury to the thoracic and lumbar spine is easier to understand than the cervical spine because the anatomy is less complex. The thoracic and lumbar spine also differ from the cervical spine because of the generally larger, stronger discs, supporting ligaments, and muscles.

In addition, the rib cage and the orientation of the thoracic facets above T11 help to stabilize the thoracic spine, and the exceptionally strong ligaments and muscular support help to stabilize the lower lumbar spine. As a result, forces acting on the thoracic and lumbar spine are focused at the thoracolumbar junction, with 60% of fractures occurring at the T12–L2 levels and 90% at T11 through L4.

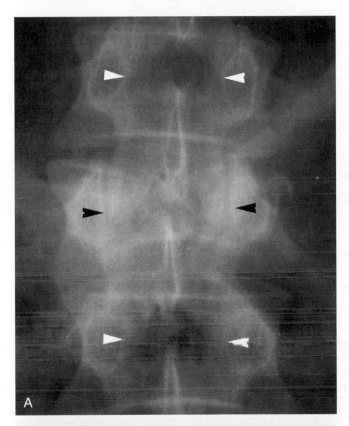

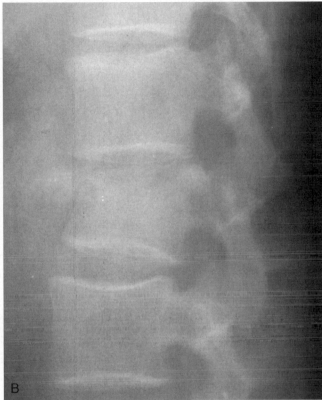

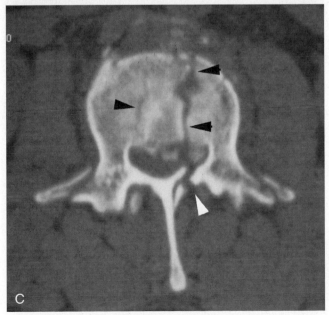

Fig. 3-274   Burst fracture. **A,** An AP radiograph demonstrating widened interpediculate distance at L-2 (*arrowheads*). This indicates the "burst" nature of the fracture. **B,** lateral, shows both anterior body compression and posterior body retropulsion. **C,** CT confirms the involvement of all these columns (*arrows*).

Routine radiographs of the traumatized thoracic and lumbar spine should include AP and lateral views. Suspected thoracolumbar region injuries may require dedicated views of this region. On the AP radiograph, careful attention should be given to the interpediculate distance, because widening at a single level suggests a burst fracture. Widening of the paraspinous soft tissues may be caused by a hematoma. A mid or upper thoracic fracture is more likely to be unstable if multiple rib fractures or a sternal fracture is present (Fig. 3-273).

The normal appearance of the lumbar spine includes a gradual widening of the interpediculate distance from L1 to L5 as seen on the AP radiograph. On the lateral view, the disk spaces gradually increase in height from the L1-2 level to L4-5, with L5-S1 being slightly narrower.

A limbus vertebrae is considered to be a normal variant. It is an unfused ring apophysis seen in an adult secondary to anterior disk herniation, and appears as a lucent line at a superior or inferior corner of a vertebral body anteriorly. This could simulate a fracture.

The presence of a calcaneus fracture after a fall from a height is associated with a significantly increased risk of a thoracic or lumbar spine fracture (and vice versa). Thus, if a calcaneus fracture is found, thoracic and lumbar radiographs are required.

Thoracic and Lumbar Fractures

As with the cervical spine, thoracic and lumbar injuries usually occur in predictable patterns based on the mechanism of injury.

Compression and flexion injuries tend to overlap in the thoracic and lumbar spine, as the strong posterior and middle columns can convert flexion force into vertebral body compression in a nutcracker-like mechanism. Compression and flexion account for 75% of injuries. Most are vertebral body *compression fractures* with anterior wedging or depression of the superior endplate but intact posterior elements. This is a one column injury and hence is stable. However, 20% of lumbar injuries are fracture dislocations, involving the posterior elements as well. Most of these are *burst fractures* and require CT to evaluate for bony fragments in the spinal canal and to guide therapy and surgical approach. With burst fractures the facets may be fractured, subluxed, perched, dislocated, or locked (Fig. 3-274). The presence of a burst fracture is associated with a 40% chance that another spine fracture is present. Thus, if a burst fracture is found, the entire spine must be radiographed.

Chance fractures (*seat belt fractures*) are less frequent and may be subtle because of spontaneous reduc-

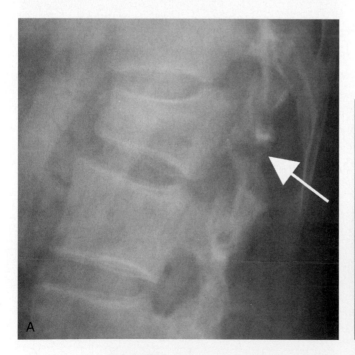
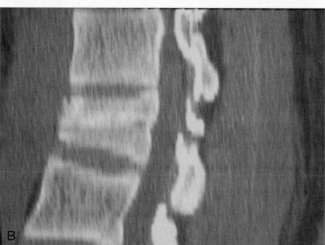

Fig. 3-275   Chance fracture. **A,** An L1 fracture extending across the vertebral body, with compression of the vertebral body. If you look carefully, there is also a fracture through the pars intraarticularas (*arrow*). The AP radiograph added no additional information. **B,** The sagittal reconstruction of the CT confirms that this is a transverse fracture across both anterior and posterior portions of the vertebral body, as well as a pars fracture, qualifying as a Chance-type injury.

tion. In this injury, fixation at the waist by a lap-type seat belt acts as a fulcrum during rapid decelleration during a motor vehicle crash, resulting in distraction of the mid and lower lumber spine. A transverse fracture extending through the posterior elements and the vertebral body or disk space with little or no vertebral body compression may be seen (Fig. 3-275). There may be an associated abdominal wall hematoma or intraabdominal injury. The introduction of shoulder belts has reduced the frequency of Chance fractures. These injuries are now most frequently seen after a fall from a height, with hyperflexion occurring as the victim's feet strike the ground while flexed at the waist.

The current use of a lap *and* shoulder belt concentrates forces in a motor vehicle crash at the cervicothoracic junction, often with a twisting component as only one shoulder is braced by the shoulder belt. Cervicothoracic transverse process fractures may be seen.

A *lateral compression fracture* is caused by lateral flexion. An AP radiograph reveals a vertebral body compression that is asymmetrically greater on the right or left side, often with associated scoliosis.

Hyperextension injuries of the thoracic and lumbar spine are unusual, but can disrupt the anterior longitudinal ligament and cause posterior element and facet compression injuries.

Transverse process fractures can occur as an isolated finding or as part of a more extensive spine injury. A finding of multiple lumbar transverse process fractures on radiographs is associated with an increased risk of significant intraabdominal injury.

Spondylolysis is interruption of the pars intrarticularis. This is generally considered to be a stress fracture variant rather than a consequence of an acute traumatic injury. Spondylolysis is discussed further in Chapter 5.

Metabolic Bone Diseases

DAVID G. DISLER, M.D.

DISORDERS OF CALCIUM HOMEOSTASIS

Understanding the means by which the body maintains calcium and phosphate homeostasis is key to understanding the metabolic bone diseases of the musculoskeletal system. Calcium and phosphate balance, and sodium/phosphate balance are critical in cellular electrolyte equilibrium and maintenance of numerous energy dependent

Key Concepts	Disorders of Calcium Homeostasis

- Parathyroid hormone and vitamin D are the two main regulators of calcium and phosphate homeostasis
- Parathyroid hormone acts on bone and kidney to increase serum calcium while maintaining phosphate levels constant
- Vitamin D depends on dietary intake and normal function in small bowel, liver, and kidney
- Vitamin D acts on bone and gut to calibrate serum calcium and phosphate levels. Phosphate balance is the target

cellular transactions, not the least of which is the integrity of ATP production. Not only is bone important structurally, but it provides a large reserve for calcium and phosphate.

Serum calcium and phosphate levels are constant. Normal levels are maintained by gut absorption of electrolytes, use of mobile bone reserves, and kidney tubular action. The hormones responsible for interacting with these targets are parathyroid hormone, vitamin D, and calcitonin.

Parathyroid hormone is produced by the four parathyroid glands. Low serum levels of calcium induce the glands to produce the hormone. Parathyroid hormone acts on several sites to increase calcium levels in the serum. For example, in the kidney, the hormone acts on the proximal tubules to enhance phosphate excretion and calcium reabsorption through calcium-phosphate pumps. At the bone surface, parathyroid hormone stimulates osteoclast-mediated bone resorption, which results in hydroxyapatite dissolution and thus increases calcium and phosphate levels in the blood. The net effect from action of the hormone in bone and kidney is increased calcium and stable phosphate levels. Finally, parathyroid hormone acts in the kidney as a cofactor to enhance the synthesis of 1,25-hydroxyvitamin D and in the action of vitamin D in bone and gut, thus indirectly increasing calcium levels through vitamin D action.

The endogenous form of vitamin D (vitamin D_3) is derived from cholesterol and synthesized in the skin after exposure to ultraviolet light. Most vitamin D, however, comes from dietary supplementation as vitamin D_2. Exogenous forms of vitamin D are absorbed through the gut and are converted in the liver to 25-hydroxy-vitamin D. However, the active form of the vitamin is produced in the kidney, where it is 1-hydroxylated. The 1,25-hydoxylated form is the active form of the hormone; it acts on bone, gut, kidney, parathyroid glands, and other tissues including the skin. In bone, the vitamin binds with intranuclear receptors and causes transcription of osteocalcin, osteopontin, and alkaline phosphastase. This action results in mobilization of calcium and phosphorus, and also promotes maturation and mineralization of organic matrix. For this activity, vitamin D requires the presence of parathyroid hormone as a cofactor. In gut, 1,25-hydroxyvitamin D causes the production of calcium binding protein and thus increased intestinal calcium transport, with passive absorption of phosphate. This action of vitamin D requires parathyroid hormone as a cofactor. It also acts to increase phosphate resorption in the proximal renal tubules, also requiring the presence of parathyroid hormone. The active form of vitamin D inhibits the release of parathyroid hormone from the parathryroid glands, enhances parathyroid hormone action in the kidney, and is a cofactor of action of parathyroid hormone in bone. Thus, vitamin D acts to increase calcium and phosphate levels in the blood. Activation of vitamin D through 1-hyroxylation in the kidney is increased in the setting of hypophosphatemia and hypocalcemia. Vitamin D is self-regulated as well: renal 1-hydroxylation decreases in the setting of increased levels of 1,25-hydroxyvitamin D.

Calcitonin is a hormone produced by the cortex of the adrenal gland from cells of neural crest origin and, while not critically important in humans, is a physiologic antagonist to parathyroid hormone. The hormone is under the direct control of blood calcium levels such that increased blood levels of calcium results in increased levels of calcitonin. The hormone's action is to inhibit osteoclast-mediated bone resorption, and to stimulate renal calcium clearance.

Hyperparathyroidism

This disease can take three forms, named primary, secondary, and tertiary hyperparathryroidism. Primary hyperparathyroidism occurs in the setting of a parathyroid gland adenoma in most cases (60%–90% of cases),

though occasionally parathyroid gland hyperplasia, or rarely glandular adenocarcinoma, is a cause. In about 10% of cases, adenomas can be multiple. There are familial forms that are associated with the multiple endocrine neoplasia (MEN) syndromes including MEN I in 95% of cases and II in 33% of cases. In primary hyperparathyroidism, serum levels of calcium are elevated whereas serum levels of phosphate are decreased. Patients usually present clinically with generalized weakness, urolithiasis, peptic ulcer disease, pancreatitis, and bone and joint pain and tenderness. Secondary hyperparathryroidism implies elevated hormone levels due not to disease of the parathyroid glands themselves but rather to other causes with resultant physiologic activation of the parathyroid glands to produce increased amounts of hormone. The most common cause of secondary hyperparathyroidism is renal failure. In renal failure there is tubular dysfunction and diminished capacity to excrete phosphate. Elevated serum phosphate levels result in calcium-phosphate binding and nonmeasurable diminished serum calcium, which in turn promotes parathryoid hormone synthesis. The result is the maintenance of normal serum calcium levels at the expense of elevated parathyroid hormone levels. Tertiary hyperparathyroidism, which occurs in situations of longstanding secondary hyperparathyroidism, refers to a condition in which the cause for secondary hyperparathyroidism has been corrected but the parathyroid glands function autonomously, producing hormone despite a lack of calcium imbalance to induce hormone synthesis.

Radiographic Features of Hyperparathyroidism The effect of increased parathyroid hormone levels in bone is crystal dissolution. As the hormonal effect is generalized, the bone loss is diffuse and most apparent at sites of greatest surface area. Generalized bone dimineralization is therefore a uniform feature of this disease (Fig. 4-1A). Bone loss in the skull can yield a "salt-and-pepper" appearance (Fig. 4-1B). In addition, bone resorption can be seen in typical sites of high bone surface area including subperiosteal, intracortical, endosteal, trabecular, subchondral, and subligamentous locations (Fig. 4-1C–E). This nonpreferential loss of bone is an important feature of the disease, and can appear extremely aggres-

---

Key Concepts | **Hyperparathyroidism**

- Primary hyperparathyroidism is most commonly due to adenomas. Primary hyperparathyroidism is associated with the multiple endocrine neoplasias.
- Bone demineralization is key radiologic feature. Diagnostic sites to look for demineralization are the radial aspects of the second and third middle phalanges of the hand
- Secondary hyperparathyroidism is due to renal disease that causes physiologic activation of the hormone
- In hyperparathyroidism, the proportion of mineralized bone to osteoid is normal

---

Key Concepts | **Radiographic Features of Hyperparathyroidism**

- Bone demineralization—primary and secondary
- Calcium pyrophosphate dihydrate deposition disease—primary > secondary
- Brown tumors—primary > secondary
- Soft tissue calcification—secondary > primary
- Bone sclerosis—secondary > primary
- Periostitis—secondary > primary

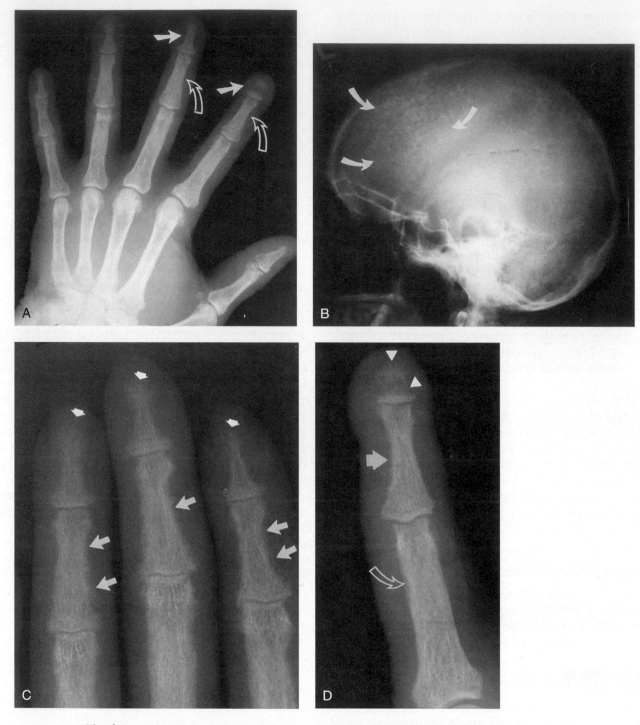

Fig. 4-1   Radiographic features of hyperparathyroidism. **A,** PA radiograph of hand reveals diffuse bone demineralization. Note the presence of localized resorption of bone at the distal phalangeal tufts (*closed arrows*) and along the radial margins of the second and third middle phalanges (*open arrows*). **B,** Lateral radiograph of skull shows salt-and-pepper appearance (*arrows*). **C,** Magnified PA radiograph of fingers demonstrating subperiosteal bone resorption in phalanges (*arrows*) and subcortical tuft resorption (*arrowheads*). **D,** Magnified PA radiograph of finger demonstrates subperiosteal (*closed arrow*), intracortical (*open arrow*) and tuftal (*arrowheads*) bone resorption.

Continued

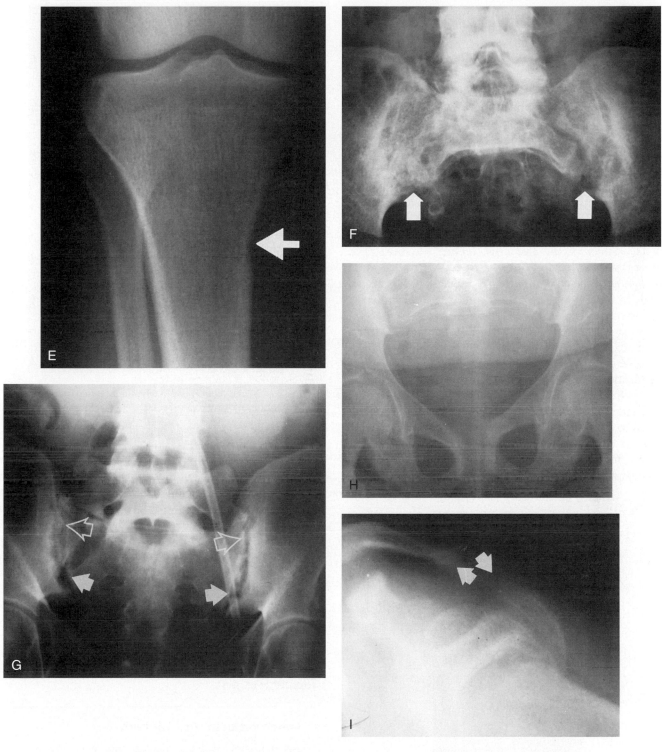

Fig. 4-1, cont'd   **E,** AP radiograph of proximal tibia demonstrates subperiosteal bone resorption at the medial aspect of the proximal tibial metaphysis (*arrow*). **F,** AP radiograph of sacroiliac joints shows bilateral subarticular bone resorption (*arrows*) mimicking inflammatory arthropathy. **G,** AP radiograph of sacroiliac joints shows subarticular (*closed arrows*) and subligamentous (*open arrows*) bone resorption of both sacroiliac joints. Recall that the true synovial articulation of the sacroiliac joints are located at the inferior two-thirds and the anterior third of the sacroiliac interspace. The remainder of the interspace is a syndesmosis. **H,** AP radiograph of the pelvis shows subarticular bone resorption of the symphysis pubis and, to a lesser extent, the sacroiliac joints. **I,** Angled radiograph of the acromioclavicular joint shows subchondral bone resorption (*arrows*) mimicking inflammatory arthropathy.

sive. Subchondral bone loss can mimic inflammatory arthropathy and is especially seen in the sacroiliac, acromioclavicular, sternoclavicular, and temperomandibular joints, and at the symphysis pubis (Fig. 4-1F–I). Subligamentous bone resorption is most common at the trochanters, ischial tuberosities, the inferior surface of the calcaneus and distal clavicle, and the elbow. Intracortical and subperiosteal changes can mimic highly aggressive neoplasia, and endosteal bone resorption can mimic endosteal erosion that is seen in marrow dyscrasias such as multiple myeloma (Fig. 4-2). Important areas to look for bone resorption that is specific for hyperparathyroidism include the superiosteal locations of the radial aspects of the second and third middle phalanges (Fig. 4-1C,D). Other sites of subperiosteal bone resorption include the medial aspect of the humerus, femur, and tibia (Fig. 4-1E), the superior and inferior aspects of the ribs and the lamina dura of the teeth. Hyperparathyroidism can produce tuftal bone resorption similar in appearance to acroosteolysis (Fig. 4-1C,D). Weakened bone due to osteopenia risks the occurrence of insufficiency fracture.

Other radiographic features of hyperparathyroidism can give clues to its diagnosis. These include soft tissue calcification, periostitis (Fig. 4-3), brown tumors (Fig. 4-4), calcium pyrophosphate dihydrate (CPPD) deposition, and bone sclerosis (Fig. 4-5). Soft tissue calcification, periostitis, and osteosclerosis are more frequently seen in secondary hyperparathyroidism. CPPD deposition, and brown tumors are more frequent in primary hyperparathyroidism. CPPD deposition can occur in up to 40%

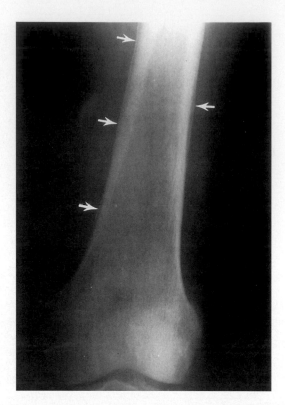

Fig. 4-3   AP radiograph of distal femur in patient with secondary hyperparathyroidism shows solid periosteal new bone formation (*arrows*).

of patients with primary hyperparathyroidism. Brown tumors, which are accumulations of osteoclasts and fibrous tissue, can be multiple and tend to heal after treatment of the underlying disorder. They appear as eccentric, occasionally intracortical lytic, and often expansive lesions that can be confused radiographically with giant cell tumor and fibrous dysplasia. Brown tumors can also be seen in secondary hyperparathyroidism, and in fact, account for more cases of brown tumors even though their incidence is greater in primary hyperparathyroidism. This is because the prevalence of secondary hyperparathyroidism is far greater than that of primary hyperparathyroidism. Finally, patients with hyperparathyroidism are prone to tendon and ligament laxity and rupture (Fig. 4-6).

Osteomalacia and Rickets

Any pathophysiologic process that interferes with the production of vitamin D will result in osteomalacia. In the absence of vitamin D, bone mineral is not laid down, although osteoid production is normal. Understanding how the hormone is produced allows one to determine a differential of potential causes. These include lack of dietary intake and diminished gut absorption of the vitamin or of calcium, as can occur in malabsorption syndromes including Crohn's disease or small bowel resec-

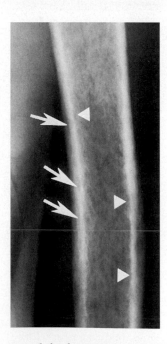

Fig. 4-2   AP view of the humerus in patient with secondary hyperparathyroidism shows numerous intracortical lucencies (*closed arrows*) and endosteal bone resorption (*open arrows*) mimicking aggressive neoplasia.

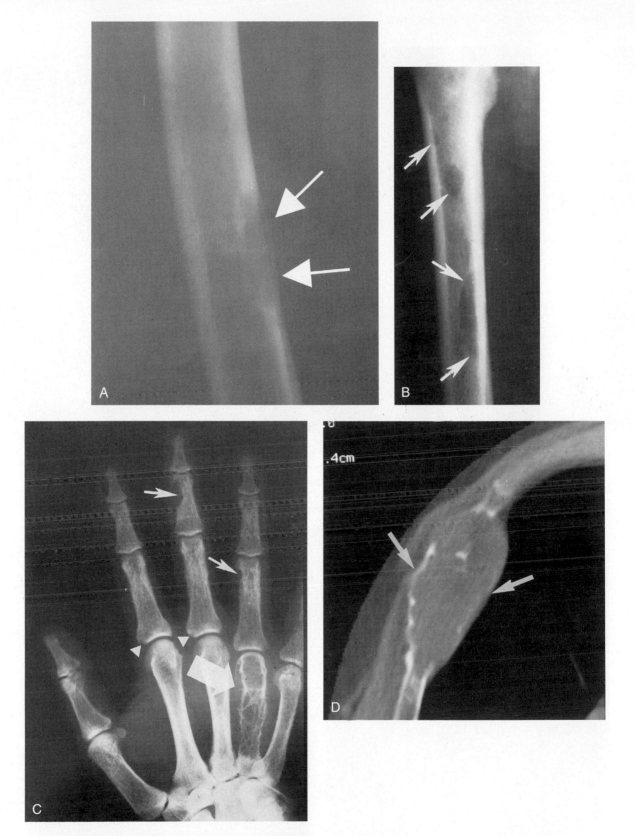

Fig. 4-4 Brown tumors of hyperparathyroidism. **A,** AP view of femur shows mildly expansile intracortical lytic mass (*arrows*). **B,** AP view of femur shows multiple brown tumors (*arrows*). **C,** PA view of hand shows brown tumor in fourth metacarpal bone (*large arrow*). Typical features of hyperparathyroidism are also shown with diffuse bone demineralization, subperiosteal bone resorption and marginal subarticular bone resorption (*arrowheads*). Two additional brown tumors are shown in the third middle phalanx and the fourth proximal phalanx (*small arrows*). **D,** Axial CT image of a right rib shows typical brown tumor as expansile lytic mass (*arrows*).

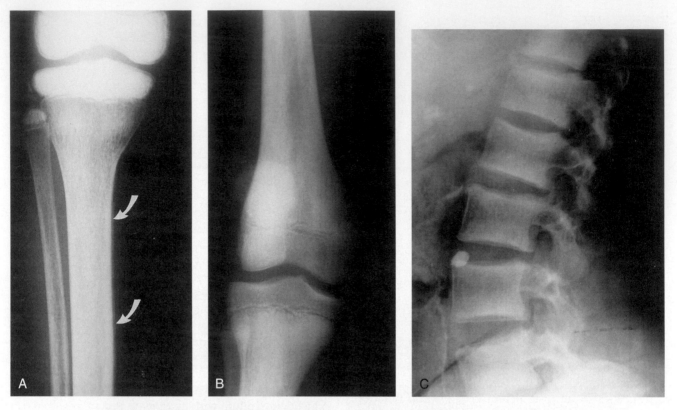

Fig. 4-5   Secondary hyperparathryroidism and bone sclerosis. **A,** AP radiograph of proximal tibia shows epiphyseal bone sclerosis and tibial diaphyseal solid periosteal new bone (*arrows*). **B,** AP radiograph of knee shows generalized increased bone density. Note increased thickness of cortical bone. **C,** Lateral radiograph of lumbar spine shows typical features of rugger jersey spine with alternating bands of density and lucency. The denser bone is located in the subendplate regions.

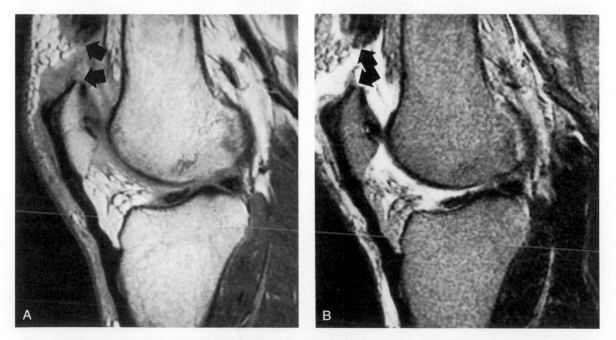

Fig. 4-6   Sagittal proton density (2200/18; TR ms/TE ms) **(A)** and T2-weighted (2200/80) **(B)** MR images of knee in patient with primary hyperparathyroidism show acute rupture of quadriceps tendon at patellar insertion (*arrows*).

Key Concepts **Osteomalacia and Rickets**

- Multiple causes, reflecting the pathway of synthesis of the active form of vitamin D.
- Proportion of mineral to osteoid matrix diminished, resulting in distinct pathologic features.
- Radiographic features include diminished bone density and pseudofractures (Looser zones).

tion. Liver (both biliary and hepatocellular) and renal diseases will also interfere with hormone production. Biliary diseases will result in problems with gut absorption of vitamin D, wheareas hepatocellular disease will interfere with 25-hydroxylation of vitamin D. Renal disease similarly has two causes for osteomalacia. First, renal failure can interfere with 1-hydroxylation of 25-vitamin D. Second, renal tubular disorders (vitamin D resistant rickets), such as X-linked hypophosphatemia and cystinosis, result in abnormally increased clearance of inorganic phosphorus (hypophosphatemia) and thus diminished ability to mineralize osteoid. In these disorders there is also an intrinsic defect in osteoblast function, as normally hypophosphatemia stimulates production of 1,25-hydroxyvitamin D. However in the X-linked form of disease there is a failure to stimulate the hydroxylase; thus vitamin D levels are abnormally low for the level of phosphate depletion. Another cause for osteomalacia is rare receptor resistance to vitamin D action, which can also interfere with mineralization of osteoid. Certain drugs such as dilantin and phenobarbital can interfere with vitamin D hydroxylation and thus function. Finally, there is a rare oncogenic form of osteomalacia due to hormone production by tumors that interfere with tubular resorption of phosphate. Often, these tumors are very small, benign, and asymptomatic, and curiously are found in bone. Such lesions include hemangioma, nonossifying fibroma, and giant cell tumor of bone. In this setting the osteomalacia is cured by resection of the lesion. Diagnosis is helped by lab analysis, which is similar to that found with renal tubular disorders, with high levels of urine phosphate.

Generalized bone demineralization is a major feature of osteomalacia, as it is in hyperparathyroidism. However, unlike the proportionate loss of mineral and cartilaginous osteoid matrix that is seen histologically in hyperparathyroidism, there is disproportionately decreased mineral relative to osteoid matrix found in osteomalacia. This occurs in osteomalacia because of the loss of osteoblastic capacity to deposit hydroxyapatite crystals on the cartilaginous matrix. Thus osteomalacia is a pathologically distinct disease. Radiographs reflect the underlying histology: osteomalacic bone appears lucent, coarsened

and smudgy (Fig. 4-7), which is probably due to a mixture of decreased bone density and possibly radiographic density contributed by nonmineralized osteoid. A highly specific feature of osteomalacia is the appearance of *Looser zones,* or pseudofractures, which are linear foci of undermineralized osteoid at sites of mechanical loading (Fig. 4-8). Often bilateral and symmetric, these appear as linear lucencies perpendicularly oriented to the cortex of the bone, with incomplete penetration of the bony width. They usually occur along the concave (compressive) margins of the curvature of the bone, unlike fatigue fractures that typically occur along the convex (tensile) margins of curves. Characteristic locations include the medial aspects of the proximal femurs, the pubic bones, the dorsal aspect of the proximal ulnae, the distal parts of the scapulae and the ribs.

Rickets   In the immature skeleton, features of rickets will predominate. These include undermineralization of osteoid at metabolically active sites, namely the metaphyseal zones of provisional calcification. The disease is especially well demonstrated at sites of rapid bone growth such as the proximal and distal femur, the proximal tibia, the proximal humerus, and the distal radius. The appearance is that of widened and irregularly shaped physeal lucencies, often with flaring of the metaphyses (Fig. 4-9A). In the ribs, a rachitic rosary will appear (Fig. 4-9B), owing to the same physeal pathophysiology at multiple costochondral junctions. The bones are soft, sometimes resulting in bizarre deformities after the onset of weight bearing, which results from repeated insufficiency fractures (Fig. 4-9C). Patients are also at substantial risk of displaced Salter-Harris I fractures (slipped epiphyses), which occur most commonly bilaterally at the hips. Cor-

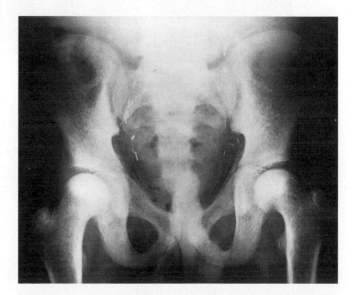

Fig. 4-7   AP radiograph of the pelvis in patient with osteomalacia shows diffuse bone demineralization and coarsened appearance of bone typical for osteomalacia.

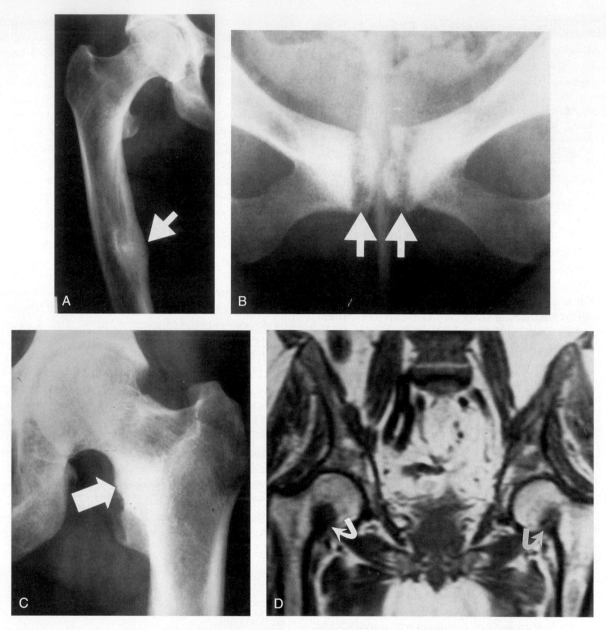

Fig. 4-8   Pseudofractures (Looser zones). **A,** AP radiograph of femur shows typical appearance of pseudofracture as incomplete linear penetration along concave, or weight-bearing, aspect of the femur (*arrow*). **B,** AP radiograph of pelvis shows bilateral symmetric linear lucencies in os pubi (*arrows*) consistent with pseudofractures. **C,** AP radiograph of the left femur shows ill-defined linear lucency at weight-bearing, medial margin of the basicervical femoral neck with surrounding sclerosis (*arrow*). **D,** Coronal T1-weighted MR image (800/14; TR ms/TE ms) of hips in same patient as (**C**) shows bilateral pseudofractures, symmetric in nature, in the femoral necks. The broad zones of diminished signal (*arrows*) correlate with sclerosis on the radiographs.

Key Concepts	Rickets

- Rickets is the manifestation of osteomalacia in children.
- Undermineralization of osteoid at growth plates is distinct feature radiographically.
- Differential diagnosis: metaphyseal dysplasia (type Schmid) and hypophosphatasia.

recting the metabolic deficiency will reverse the findings at the growth plates, although bone deformities will persist (Fig. 4-10). There are two important differential diagnoses to consider for rickets. The first is metaphyseal dysplasia (type Schmid) that looks similar to osteomalacia with growth plate widening, but this disease is due to an inborn error in enchondral ossification and laboratory values and bone mineralization are normal. The other is hypophosphatasia in which bone is severely osteopenic,

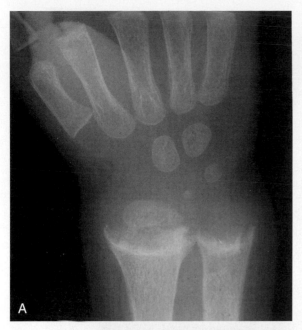

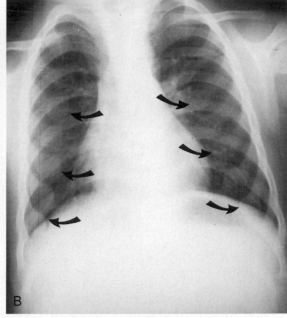

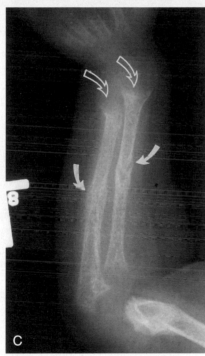

Fig. 4-9 Radiographic features of rickets. **A,** PA radiograph of wrist shows widened physes, irregular zones of provisional calcification, and flaring of the metaphyses in distal radius and ulna. Note diffuse osteopenia and coarsened appearance of trabecular bone. **B,** AP radiograph of chest shows rachitic rosary with diffuse bilateral costochondral enlargement (*arrows*). **C,** AP radiograph of the forearm shows radial and ulnar insufficiency fractures (*closed arrows*) associated with typical features of rickets. Note diffuse bone demineralization, coarsened trabeculae, flared metaphyses, and irregular margin of zones of provisional calcification (*open arrows*).

growth plates wide, and multiple fractures are seen. However, in this disease serum alkaline phosphatase is low, unlike other causes of rickets in which the enzyme is elevated.

Renal Osteodystrophy

Renal osteodystrophy represents the clinical, pathologic, and radiologic manifestations of osteomalacia combined with secondary hyperparathyroidism that occur in chronic renal failure. Renal failure results in hyperphos-

phatemia and thus increased synthesis of parathyroid hormone. In addition, renal failure results in decreased 1,25-vitamin D production in the kidney. Furthermore, diminished gut calcium absorption as a result of diminished vitamin D production activates parathyroid hormone synthesis. Thus, these patients will manifest features of both metabolic disorders (Fig. 4-11). In truth, the mechanisms of action are quite complicated; for example, there is skeletal resistance to parathyroid hormone action because vitamin D is a cofactor of parathyroid hormone action in bone. In addition, patients with

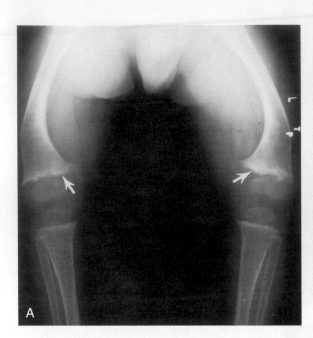

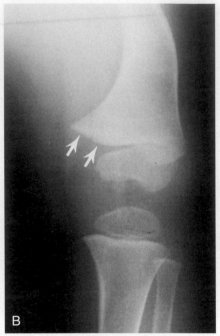

Fig. 4-10   Rickets before and after treatment. **A,** AP radiograph of knees shows irregular contour of femoral metaphyseal zones of provisional calcification (*arrows*), metaphyseal flaring, and varus deformity of distal femurs. **B,** After treatment, AP radiograph of left knee shows narrowing of physes, restored smooth contour of distal femoral metaphyseal zones of provisional calcification (*arrows*), and diminished metaphyseal flaring. Femoral varus deformity persists.

renal failure are often on dialysis, and aluminum in the dialysate, that is present to bind phosphate, can lead to bone toxicity mimicking osteomalacia. Amyloidosis also can be seen in patients on dialysis leading to findings in joints and spinal disc spaces that can appear similar to infection. Further compounding these patients' skeletal findings are the risk for osteomyelitis and septic arthritis because of chronic immune suppression, and the risk for avascular necrosis due to long-term steroid therapy and traumatic subchondral bone collapse in osteopenic bone (Fig. 4-12).

Patients with renal osteodystrophy can show areas of decreased bone density and osteosclerosis, with sclerosis often predominating at the endplate regions of the spine (rugger jersey spine), although occasionally diffuse osteosclerosis can be found (Fig. 4-5). In addition, profuse soft tissue calcifications can be seen, including vascular calcifications and paraarticular accumulations of calcium-phosphate precipitates, which can occasionally take on

Key Concepts	Renal Osteodystrophy

- Renal osteodystrophy occurs in patients with long-standing renal failure
- Features of hyperparathyroidsm and osteomalacia are seen

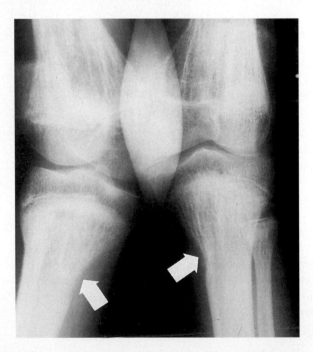

Fig. 4-11   AP radiograph of knees in boy with renal osteodystrophy shows combined features of osteomalacia and hyperparathyroidism. Note coarsened trabecular appearance typical of osteomalacia, and subperiosteal bone resorption in proximal tibias (*arrows*) typical of hyperparathyroidism. Genu valgum, as shown in this case, is often found in children with hyperparathryoidism.

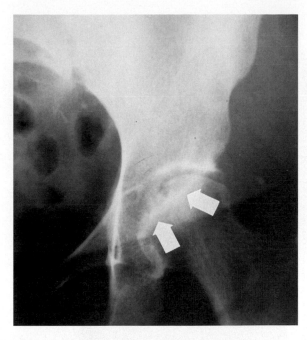

Fig. 4-12 AP radiograph of hip in patient with renal osteodystrophy and long-term steroid use demonstrates avascular necrosis of the left femoral head (*arrows*) with increased density and subchondral lucency.

a liquid form as milk of calcium; these accumulations can be massive and are referred to as *tumoral calcinosis* (Fig. 4-13). Insufficiency fractures and Looser zones can be found in addition to the classic features of hyperparathyroidism.

OSTEOPOROSIS

Generalized Osteoporosis

Osteoporosis is a major health issue in the United States and the world because of its high prevalence in elderly women and thus its enormous impact on morbidity, mortality, and societal cost. Osteoporosis is a disease of diminished bone mass. Pathologically, there is evidence of cortical thinning and dropout of trabecular bone, but the ratio of nonmineralized to mineralized bone is normal. Any given bone spicule is normal histologically, but its mass is diminished. In osteoporosis, lab values that are markers for bone and bone turnover are found to be normal. Although the exact cause for osteoporosis is not known, there are numerous associations including postmenopausal diminished estrogen levels in women; thus contributing factors include amenorrhea and low body weight. Other contributing factors include low levels of weight-bearing exercise, a family history for osteoporosis, poor nutrition, smoking, alcohol abuse, and hypogonadism. In fact, 30%–50% of women over the age of 60 years old show evidence of significant bone loss.

Key Concepts Generalized Osteoporosis

- Osteoporosis is a major health problem wordwide.
- Risk of fracture (in spine, hip, and forearm) is major complication.
- Radiography is insensitive in the detection of osteoporosis. Features include decreased bone density, cortical bone thinning, accentuated trabecular bone contrast, and increased contrast between cortical and medullary bone.
- DEXA scans identify patients at risk for fracture by comparing bone density values to normal ranges of values in healthy, young patients.
- Common causes of generalized osteoporosis:
Senile osteoporosis
Alcoholism
Poor nutrition
Smoking
Diffuse marrow replacement (metastatic disease, myeloma, Gaucher disease)
Hypogonadism, hyperthyroidism, hyperparathyroidism, Cushing's disease
Drugs: heparin, dilantin, corticosteroids
Congenital diseases (osteogenesis imperfecta) and inborn errors of metabolism

Bone is found to progressively diminish in mass throughout life in both men and women, though the rate of bone loss is greater in women. Among women, the incidence of osteoporosis is greater among whites and Asians than it is among blacks. The loss of bone mass results in an increased risk of fracture, with the most common locations being the spine, the hip, the proximal humerus, and the distal forearm.

Besides senile osteoporosis, other causes of osteoporosis should be considered. Other major causes include: hypercorticism (steroid therapy or Cushing disease); effects of other drugs especially heparin, dilantin, and phenobarbital (Table 4-1); alcoholism; smoking; congenital diseases such as osteogenesis imperfecta; and inborn errors of metabolism such as homocystinuria and ochronosis. Other less common etiologies for generalized osteoporosis include amyloidosis, hyperthyroidism, mastocytosis, and rare idiopathic juvenile forms of osteoporosis.

There are effective treatments for osteoporosis, and these include calcium supplementation, estrogen therapy, and bisphosphonate drugs such as etridronate. These drugs are so effective that the rate of bone loss can be reversed. The role of the radiologist is to identify patients at risk and to monitor progression of disease after the initiation of treatment.

Radiographs can reveal osteoporosis by several means, but it should be remembered that radiographs are insensitive to the detection of diminished bone density. This is because approximately 50% bone loss is required before

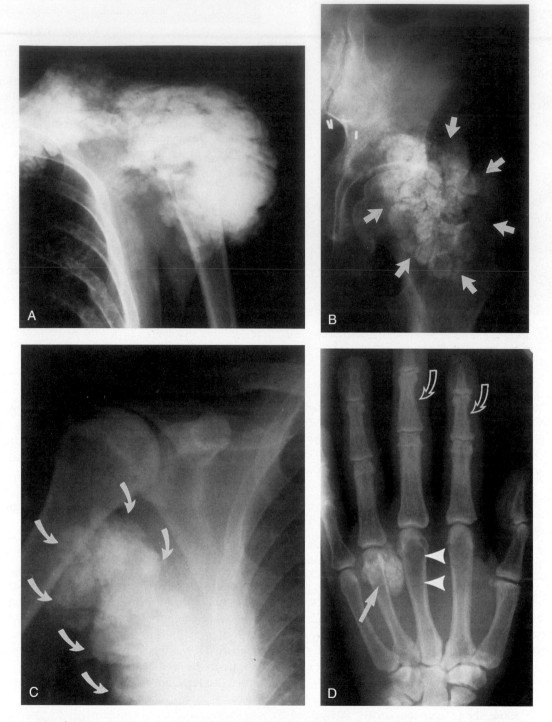

Fig. 4-13   Examples of tumoral calcinosis. **A,** AP radiograph of the left shoulder demonstrates massive paraarticular soft tissue calcification due to tumoral calcinosis. Note the diffuse demineralization of bone and multiple left rib fractures. **B,** AP radiograph of left hip, shows multiple paraarticular calcifications (*arrows*) due to tumoral calcinosis. **C,** AP radiograph of the right shoulder shows massive tumoral calcinosis (*arrows*). **D,** PA radiograph of the right hand shows soft tissue deposit of tumoral calcinosis (*closed arrow*) as well as features of hyperparathroidism with diffuse demineralization of bone, subperiosteal bone resorption (*open arrows*), and third metacarpal brown tumor (*arrowheads*).

Continued

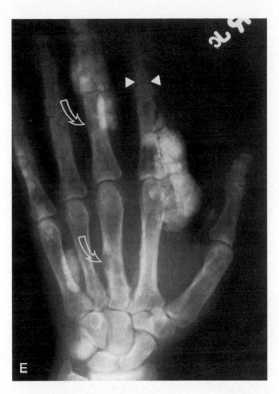

Fig. 4-13, cont'd   E, PA radiograph of the right hand shows multiple deposits of tumoral calcinosis, diffuse bone demineralization, third metacarpal and phalangeal brown tumors (*open arrows*), and Looser zone in second middle phalanx (*arrowheads*).

it can be detected subjectively on radiographs. The most obvious radiographic finding is the appearance of diminished bone density, though this is insensitive because variation in radiographic technique can interfere with the detection of osteoporosis or may falsely suggest disease. A better way to determine the presence of diminished bone density is to compare cortical width to that of the shaft of a long bone, because osteoporosis is associ-

ated with cortical bone thinning. A specific location to look for this finding is in the second and third metacarpal bones, where middiaphyseal cortical width should account for at least 50% of bone width in individuals with normal bone density. However, it should be noted that bone loss in osteoporosis is greater in trabecular bone than in cortical bone, and thus looking at trabecular bone for osteoporosis will be more rewarding. For example, in the vertebral body, trabecular bone loss in osteoporosis is manifested as exaggerated contrast between endplate and central density, and often the endplates will appear thinned (Fig. 4-14A). Compression fractures might be seen, which can take the shape of anterior wedging, biconcavity of endplates, or generalized loss of height. In addition, osteoporosis can be manifested with increased conspicuity of vertically-oriented trabecular bone in the spine, because of generalized dropout of horizontally oriented trabeculae. A similar finding is shown in the femur with progressive loss of the least important trabecular lines of force, starting with the secondary tensile trabeculae, followed by the primary tensile trabeculae, then the secondary compressive followed by the primary compressive trabeculae (Fig. 4-14B). The diminished bone density of osteoporosis is not radiographically specific, and thus other major important causes for diffuse bone demineralization should be included in the differential diagnosis. These include hyperparathyroidism, osteomalacia, and multiple myeloma.

The major complication of osteoporosis is fracture. The degree of demineralization in osteoporosis can be quantified, thus allowing assessment of fracture risk. The World Health Organization has established guidelines for diagnosis using dual x-ray absorptiometry (DEXA), allowing patient categorization as normal, osteopenic, and osteoporotic. DEXA works by comparing a patient's bone density with normal ranges of bone density in age-matched and young populations. One can compare a bone density value for the patient with the mean density of an age-matched reference population (standard deviation known as Z-score) and with the mean bone mineral density of a normal young adult population (standard deviation known as *T*-score). *T*-scores are more useful because they give an indication of the fracture risk. *T*-scores between 1 and 2 standard deviations below the mean density are defined as osteopenic, whereas scores below 2 standard deviations are defined as osteoporotic. Although it is still not clear when is the optimal time to intervene with drug therapy in patients with osteoporosis, or at risk for osteoporosis, most women regardless of bone mass are advised to undergo dietary supplementation with calcium and are advised to undergo exercise programs. In postmenopausal women, estrogen therapy is encouraged, and osteoporotic women are treated aggressively with a combination of calcium supplements, estrogen, and bisphosphonates.

Table 4-1   Drug-Induced Changes in Bone
Heparin: Osteoporosis (dose-related)
Dilantin and phenobarbital: osteomalacia
Corticosteroids: osteoporosis, avascular necrosis
Coumadin: embryopathy with stippled epiphyses
Lead and other heavy metals (e.g. bismuth): osteoclast poison, dense metaphyseal bands and undertubulation of metaphyses
Vitamin A: painful periostitis
Vitamin D: increased bone density, periostitis, soft tissue calcifications
Fluorosis: increased bone density, periostitis, ligament ossification, stress fractures
Alcohol: fetal alcohol syndrome, osteoporosis, avascular necrosis
Prostaglandins: periostitis in infants

From Manaster BJ, *Handbook of Skeletal Radiology,* 2nd ed. St. Louis, Mosby, 1997.

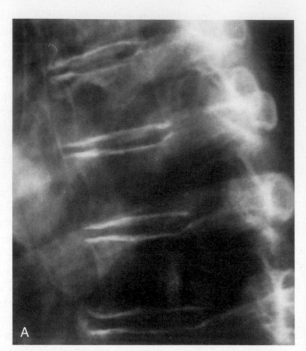
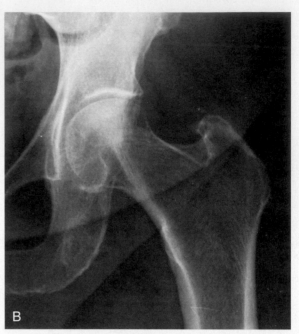

Fig. 4-14   Osteoporosis. **A,** Lateral radiograph of spine shows exaggerated contrast between the endplates and the medullary bone. **B,** AP view of hip shows exaggerated trabecular pattern in primary compressive lines of force. The tensile lines of force are largely absent indicating advanced osteoporosis.

In evaluating DEXA scans the radiologist's role is to assure proper placement of regions of interest for bone density measurement and to assure absence of radiographic abnormalities that might interfere with measurement. Such confounders include osteophytes in the spine, compression fractures, and soft tissue calcification (diffuse idiopathic skeletal hyperostosis, aortic calcification), each of which can erroneously increase a DEXA bone density value. Usually measurements at four lumbar levels are averaged and a measure of the proximal femur and occasionally the wrist are obtained. Measurements at each site of risk are more predictive of fracture risk at that site than a measurement from a remote site. Thus, the risk for hip fracture is best made from a bone density measurement of the hip. Measurements at two or three sites are routine in patients undergoing DEXA scans.

Other tests of bone density include CT densitometry, which is more accurate and precise than DEXA scans. This is because the cross-sectional nature of data acquisition allows evaluation limited to trabecular bone where generalized osteoporosis is most greatly manifested. CT densitometry may be more accurate for assessing bone density than DEXA scans in patients with diffuse idiopathic skeletal hyperostosis, aortic calcification, spine fracture, and excessive degenerative osteophyte formation. CT densitometry is less popular because of higher cost and slightly higher radiation dose. A novel and prom-

ising means to assess osteoporosis may occur with MRI or fractal analysis of radiographs or CT. These forms of analysis are not measures of bone mass per se but rather measures of bone morphology and trabecular arrangement. This may prove valuable because fracture risk may in part relate to structural orientation of trabecular bone such as trabecular bone thickness, trabecular connectivity, and the volume of space between trabeculae. These parameters have been shown to correlate with fracture risk at least as well as bone density measurements.

Regional Osteoporosis

There are regional forms of osteoporosis that are of unclear cause, the best known being transient osteoporosis of the hip (TOH) and regional migratory osteoporosis.

Key Concepts	Regional Osteoporosis

Causes for regional osteoporosis:
- Transient osteoporosis of the hip
- Regional migratory osteoporosis
- Reflex sympathetic dystrophy
- Hyperemic states—healing fracture, tumor, infection
- Diminished weight bearing

It is unclear whether these diagnoses are unique or related, and whether they are related to transient forms of avascular necrosis (AVN). Transient osteoporosis of the hip is seen most commonly among middle aged men (either hip) and pregnant women (usually left hip), and often occur in patients with no known risk factors for AVN. Patients present with sudden onset of severe hip pain. Asymmetric diminished bone density is seen radiographically in the affected hip and MR imaging reveals striking edema in the proximal femur, often associated with a joint effusion. MR imaging shows diminished signal on T1-weighted images (Fig. 4-15), increased signal on T2-weighted MR images, and contrast enhancement throughout the femoral head and neck. As implied by its name, TOH is self limited, usually reversing after a several month course. No treatment other than conservative therapy is warranted.

Regional migratory osteoporosis is usually seen in men in the fourth and fifth decades of life and is similar to TOH at imaging, but unlike TOH, multiple consecutive joints become affected with bone marrow edema, usually in the lower extremities at and distal to the knee. Treatment and natural history is otherwise the same as TOH.

Regional osteoporosis is also to be expected in the setting of hyperemia because hyperemia induces osteoclast activation and thus bone resorption. Thus, inflammatory arthropathy, hypervascular tumors, reflex sympathetic dystrophy, and healing fractures are associated with regional osteoporosis. Disuse of a limb is also associated with localized diminished bone density, because bone mass is directly proportional to the forces acting across the bone. Regional forms of osteoporosis can appear aggressive owing to active remodeling of bone, with evidence of intracortical lucencies (cortical tunneling), metaphyseal bandlike lucencies, and subcortical/subchondral resorption of bone. Reflex sympathetic dystrophy is felt to be mediated by the sympathetic nervous system. Its cause is unknown but associated with trau-

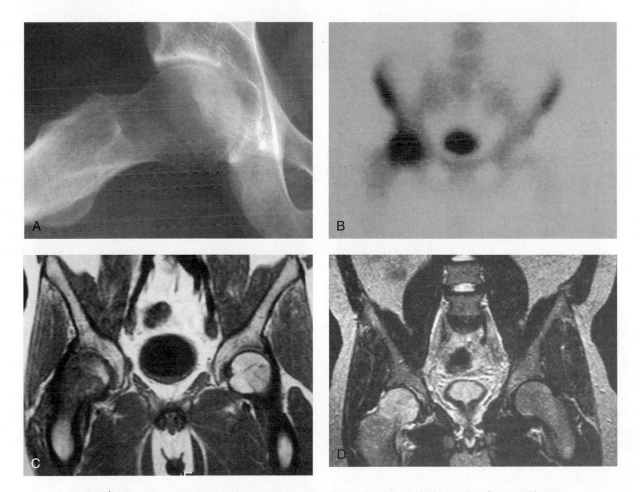

Fig. 4-15 Transient regional osteoporosis. AP radiograph of the right hip in this 45-year-old man shows osteoporosis (**A**). Radionuclide bone scan (**B**) shows increased uptake in the same region. T1-weighted (**C**, 600/20) and T2-weighted MR images (**D**, 2000/80) show diffuse low signal and high signal intensity, respectively.

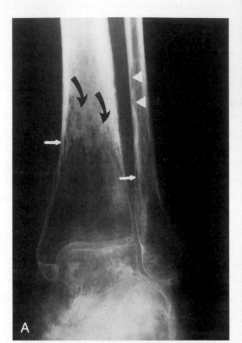
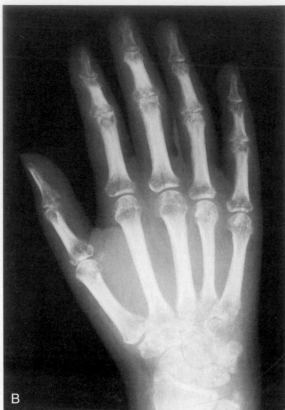

Fig. 4-16   Reflex sympathetic dystrophy. **A,** AP view of the ankle shows pronounced bone demineralization in the distal leg and hindfoot with aggressive features including intracortical lucency (*straight arrows*), endosteal resorption of bone (*arrowheads*), and broad zone of transition (*curved arrows*) to more normal appearing proximal tibial and fibular diaphyses. **B,** PA radiograph of the hand of another patient shows pronounced periarticular osteopenia and diffuse soft-tissue swelling in the wrist and hand.

matic, neurologic, or vascular events. It is associated not only with severely diminished bone density but with soft tissue trophic changes (Fig. 4-16) including swelling and hyperesthesia followed by atrophy and contracture of an entire extremity at and distal to the affected site.

PAGET'S DISEASE

Paget's disease is discussed in this chapter not because it is a metabolic disease *per se* but rather because it is a disease of disturbed osteoblast and osteoclast

Key Concepts	Paget's Disease

- Paget's disease is a disease of activated osteoclasts.
- Radiographic triad—bone expansion, cortical bone thickening, trabecular bone thickening
- Three sequential phases—lytic, mixed lytic and sclerotic, and sclerotic.

equilibrium. Paget's disease was described as "osteitis deformans" by Sir James Paget in 1877. It is a chronic progressive skeletal disorder that is expressed initially as bone resorption and can be localized to one or more bones. Although its exact cause is not known, an environmental cause is thought likely, due to its higher occurrence in extreme latitudes and low incidence in Asia and Africa. It is a disease that can cross joints. An infectious etiology is suggested by the discovery of paramyxovirus inclusion bodies in osteoclasts of patients with Paget's disease. In the United States, Paget's disease is rare before the age of 40 years, occurs in 3% of people over 40 years old, and occurs in 10% of people over 80 years old, with a 2:1 male to female occurrence. Most patients are asymptomatic with greatest sites of bone involvement being the skull, spine, pelvis, and femur.

Paget's disease is a disease of osteoclasts. Osteoclasts are activated with resultant osteolysis, followed by an osteoblastic response until a new equilibrium is established between bone production and bone lysis. The rapid, disordered bone resorption and production results in a mosaic-like appearance of osteoid histologically. Serum phosphorus and calcium levels are normal, but serum alkaline phosphatase is markedly elevated. In addition serum and urine hydroxyproline are elevated and parallel the course of disease.

There are three sequential, though often coexistent, stages described for Paget's disease. Stage I is the lytic phase. Stage II is the mixed lytic and blastic phase, and corresponds to the onset of osteoblastic activation in response to osteoclastic bone resorption. Stage III is the sclerotic phase. In the long bones the disease begins at the ends of bones and extends in a progressive fashion toward the diaphysis with a sharp margin, a feature highly uncharacteristic of neoplasia (Fig. 4-17). In the tibia, however, Paget's disease can occasionally be first found in the diaphysis. At the leading edge of the lytic component, names are used such as "osteoporosis circumscripta," which describes acutely marginated bone demineralization during the lytic phase of disease in the skull (Fig. 4-18), and "blade of grass" and "flame-shaped margin," which describes acutely marginated demineralization in the long bones (Fig. 4-19). "Picture frame vertebra" is a term that describes the mixed lytic and sclerotic phase

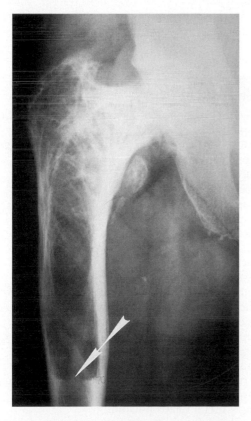

Fig. 4-17   AP radiograph of patient with Paget's disease shows sharp linear transition between Pagetic and normal bone (*arrow*). This finding is highly uncharacteristic of neoplasm. Moderate bone expansion, increased cortical thickness and trabecular bone thickening assures the diagnosis of Paget's disease.

in the spine (Fig. 4-20), and "cotton wool" describes the mixed lytic and sclerotic phase in the skull (Fig. 4-21). *The pathognomonic triad of findings in Paget's disease is bone expansion, cortical bone thickening, and trabecular bone thickening* (Fig. 4-22). These findings reflect the pathophysiology of the disease and indicate accelerated bone turnover including bone deposition and bone expansion. An often quoted classic clinical presentation involves the story of a man who is asked by his doctor whether his hat size has increased, and the man responds, with hand to ear, and says, "eh?" The cause for deafness can be from otosclerosis related to enlargement and diminished function of the middle ear ossicles or expansion of surrounding bone in the inner ear (Fig. 4-23).

There are several complications that occur in the setting of Paget's disease. First, there are complications that relate to disorganized and fragile bone production. One is osteoarthritis, which is felt to relate to effects on cartilage of weakened subchondral bone (Figs. 4-22 and 4-24). Osteoarthritis occurs in 50%–96% of patients with Paget's disease. Basilar skull invagination is common (Fig. 4-23), occurring in one-third of patients, as are insufficiency fractures (Fig. 4-24), protrusio acetabuli and proximal femoral varus deformity (Fig. 4-24), due to chronically weakened osseous matrix. Neurologic complications related to osseous expansion include sensorineural and conductional hearing loss and spinal stenosis. Neoplastic transformation, most commonly osteosarcoma, occurs in 1% of patients with Paget's disease (Fig. 4-25), although in the skull, giant cell tumor is the most common form of neoplastic transformation. New onset pain in a patient with Paget's disease should alert the clinician to the possibility of sarcomatous transformation, which has a 1% survival at 2 years. Osteomyelitis is more common in patients with Paget's disease, and is felt to relate to the hypervascularity and subsequent increased risk of organisms such as *Staphylococcus aureus* seeding affected bones. Crystal deposition diseases including monosodium urate and calcium pyrophosphate dihydrate occur, possibly due to increased calcium mobilization in patients with Paget's disease. High output cardiac failure is a rare complication of the disease, but anemia can occur because of the increase in plasma volume associated with high output failure. Occasional occurrence of metastasis in pagetic bone may relate to increased vascularity as well. Another occasional complication of increased bone turnover in these patients is the possibility of rapid osteolysis that may occur when equilibrium between bone production and lysis is disrupted in situations in which patients become non-weightbearing (Fig. 4-26).

Treatment with bisphosphonates that inhibit osteoclast mediated bone resorption can be helpful in patients with severe manifestations of Paget's disease. Calcitonin is occasionally used for treatment.

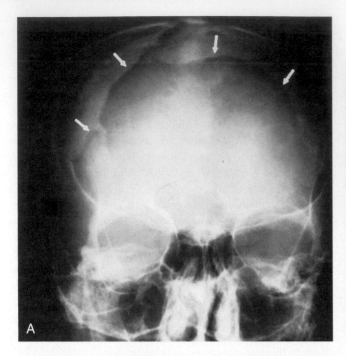
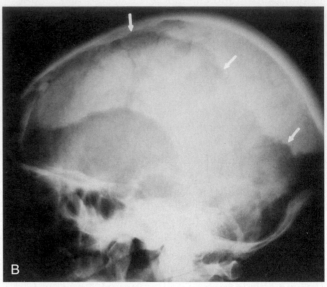

Fig. 4-18   AP (**A**) and lateral (**B**) skull films show osteoporosis circumscripta with sharp margins (*arrows*) between pagetic and normal bone in the acute, lytic phase of disease.

MISCELLANEOUS

There are a few other metabolic conditions that need to be discussed, though this discussion is far from exhaustive.

Fluorosis, vitamin A toxicity, and hypervitaminosis D each tend to cause increased bone density and periostitis due to metastatic deposition of calcium salts. Fluorosis and vitamin A toxicity can cause flowing ossification of the anterior longitudinal ligament of the spine that is so pronounced it can mimic diffuse idiopathic skeletal hyperostosis and seronegative spondyloarthropathy. Similarly, thyroid acropachy, which is rarely seen after treatment for thyrotoxicosis, can also manifest as prominent, fluffy solid periosteal new bone deposition, particularly in the metacarpals/tarsals and phalanges in the hands and feet (Fig. 4-27). Clubbing can be seen in this disease, and soft tissue swelling is found, such as in the orbits (exopthalmos) and lower extremities (myxedema). Lead is an osteoclast poison that results in increased bone density and undertubulation in the metaphyses due to unopposed osteoblast action. Dense metaphyseal bands are also seen physiologically in growing children, though their presence in the proximal fibula and distal ulna are diagnostic for lead poisoning (Fig. 4-28).

Key Concepts

Differential diagnosis of ligamentous ossification (in the spine):
- Diffuse idiopathic skeletal hyperostosis (diagnosis of exclusion)
- Ankylosing spondylitis
- Severe spondylosis
- Vitamin A toxicity
- Fluorosis

Differential diagnosis of diffuse increased bone density (3MsPROF):
- Myelofibrosis
- Mastocytosis
- Metastatic disease, rarely myeloma
- Sickle cell anemia
- Paget's disease, Pyknodysostosis
- Renal Osteodystrophy
- Osteopetrosis
- Fluorosis

Differential diagnosis of dense metaphyseal bands:
- Normal variant
- Heavy metal (lead) poisoning
- Hypervitaminosis D
- Metaphyseal stress lines
- Rickets (after treatment)
- Scurvy (rare)

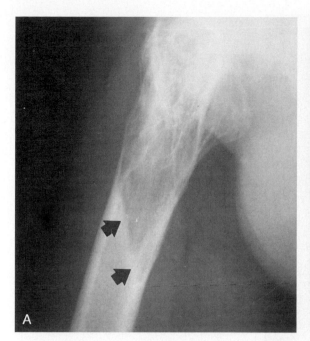 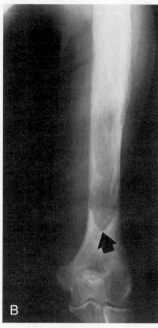

Fig. 4-19 Two examples of the blade of grass. **A,** Frog lateral view of the right proximal femur shows the mixed lytic and sclerotic phase in the proximal aspect of pagetic bone and the lytic phase in the distal portion of pagetic bone. This indicates that the advancing front of Paget's disease is in the distal aspect of Pagetic bone. The sharp, bladelike appearance of the margin between pagetic and normal bone (*arrows*) is shown, a feature that would be highly uncharacteristic for neoplasm. **B,** AP view of humerus shows a flame-shaped distal margin of Paget's disease with abrupt transition to normal bone (*arrow*). Note the mixed phase of Paget's disease in the more proximal humerus, where bone expansion, cortical bone thickening, and trabecular bone thickening is shown. At the flame-shaped margin, the appearance of Paget's disease is purely lytic.

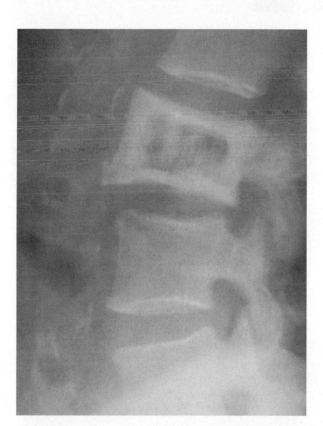

Fig. 4-20 AP view of lumbar spine shows picture frame appearance of L3 vertebral body. Note the increased density of the vertebral body, with greater density at the margins, trabecular bone thickening, and overall bone expansion. (Reprinted with permission from the ACR learning file.)

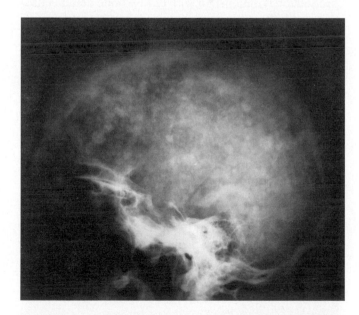

Fig. 4-21 Lateral radiograph of the skull shows a cotton-wool appearance due to the mixed lytic and sclerotic phase of Paget's disease.

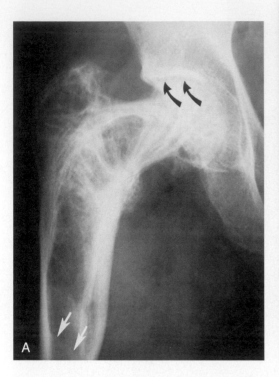

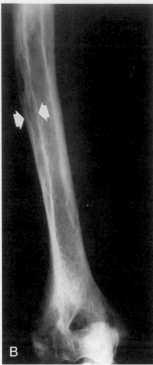

Fig. 4-22 The essential features of Paget's disease are bone expansion, cortical bone thickening and trabecular bone thickening. **A,** AP radiograph of the right hip shows bone expansion, cortical bone thickening, and trabecular bone thickening. Note also the abrupt transition to normal bone (*straight arrows*). In addition, there is moderate osteoarthritis of the hip (*curved arrows*), a common complication of Paget's disease adjacent to a joint. **B,** AP radiograph of humerus shows bone expansion, cortical bone thickening (*arrows*), and trabecular bone thickening.

Scurvy, a disease caused by low dietary intake of vitamin C is rarely encountered today. Vitamin C is required for collagen formation and therefore is needed for bone matrix, cartilage, tendon, and ligament synthesis. Without the vitamin, production of collagen and thus bone production is diminished with diffuse bone demineralization, and there is increased tendency toward insufficiency fracture. In children, bleeding risk can result in extensive pronounced subperiosteal hemorrhage and subsequent ossification. Other signs found in the immature skeleton are named and include Wimburger's sign, which is a sclerotic epiphyseal rim related to disorganized bone production at the epiphyseal center of ossification, Frankel's line, which is a dense metaphyseal line of similar pathophysiology, and Pelkin's fracture, which is a metaphyseal corner fracture.

Hypothryoidism manifests with mild osteoporosis, soft tissue edema and myopathy. The juvenile form manifests with severe delay in skeletal maturity, in which skeletal age lags markedly behind clinical age (Fig. 4-29A). Severely delayed dental development is also seen. Other characteristic findings in juvenile hypothyroidism include Wormian bones, a bullet-shaped vertebra at the thoracolumbar junction (Fig. 4-29B), and epiphyseal fragmentation which, in the proximal femur, can mimic Legg-Calve-Perthes disease.

Hypoparathyroidism is associated with end organ incapacity of the parathyroid glands to produce sufficient hormone for calcium homeostasis. This occurs most com-

---

Key Concepts	**Pseudo- and Pseudopseudo-Hypoparathyroidism**

- Share clinical features with hypoparathyroidism
- Added clinical features: short stature, obesity, brachydactyly, and small osteochondromas

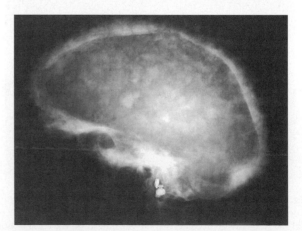

Fig. 4-23 Typical lateral radiograph of the skull in Paget's disease, showing basilar invagination, thickening of the skull, "cotton wool" sites of sclerosis, and the hearing aid for the patient's deafness due to otosclerosis.

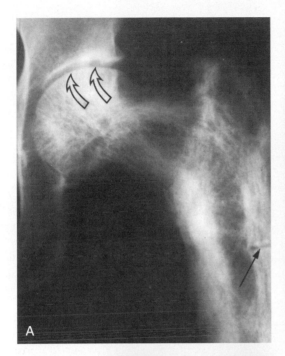

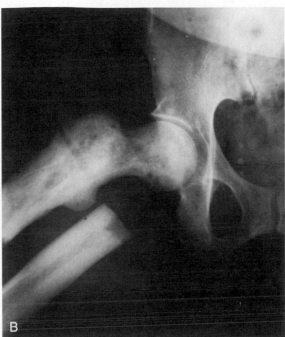

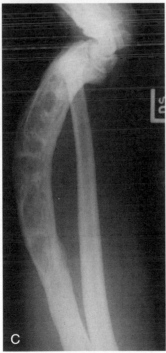

Fig 4-24 Complications of Paget's disease. **A,** AP radiograph of the left hip shows typical features of Paget's disease with bone expansion, cortical bone thickening, and trabecular bone thickening. Note the incomplete insufficiency fracture (*straight arrow*) at the extreme lateral margin of the radiograph in the subtrochanteric femur, mild varus deformity and moderate osteoarthritis of the hip (*curved arrows*). **B,** Frog lateral radiograph of the right hip shows insufficiency fracture of subtrochanteric femur and features of Paget's disease at and proximal to fracture site. **C,** Lateral radiograph of the left forearm shows substantial bone expansion in radius associated with cortical and trabecular bone thickening associated with angular deformity of radius due to multiple healed insufficiency fractures.

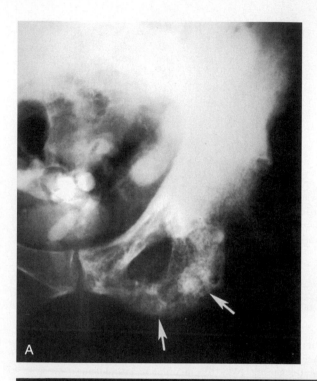

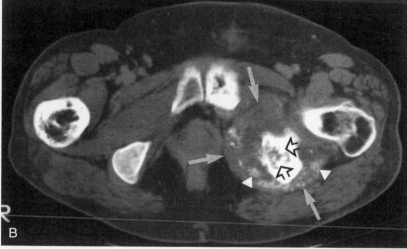

Fig. 4-25   Paget sarcoma. **A,** AP radiograph of left pelvis shows bone expansion, cortical bone thickening, and trabecular bone thickening in pubic bone diagnostic for Paget's disease. In the ischium, however, there is ill-defined mixed lysis and sclerosis (*arrows*) suspect for sarcomatous transformation. **B,** Axial CT image shows Pagetic left ischium with cortical bone thickening and slight bone expansion. However, the ischium is surrounded by a large soft tissue mass (*closed arrows*) with associated fluffy matrix calcifications (*arrowheads*). Similar calcifications are shown centrally in the ischium (*open arrows*). The diagnosis at surgery was osteosarcoma with background of Paget's disease.

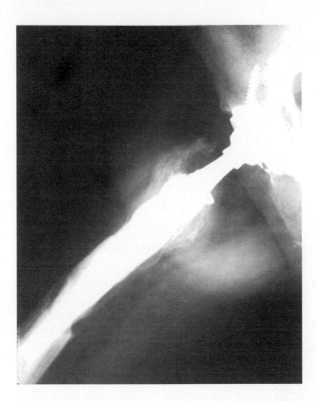

Fig. 4-26   Frog lateral radiograph of right proximal femur in patient with Paget's disease obtained 1 month after total hip replacement. In the interval, there has been rapid osteolysis of the Pagetic bone due to non-weightbearing in the perioperative period.

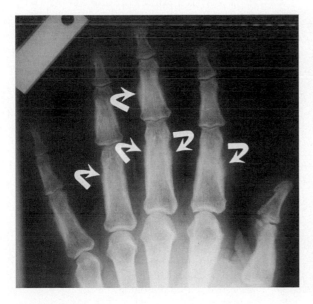

Fig. 4-27   PA radiograph of hand of woman with thyroid acropachy shows exhuberant fluffy periosteal new bone formation (*arrows*) in the proximal and middle phalanges and generalized swelling of the fingers.

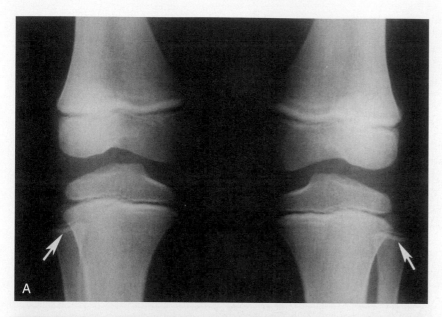

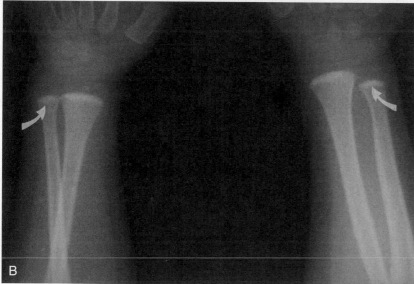

Fig. 4-28 Two patients with lead poisoning. **A,** AP radiograph of knees shows multiple dense metaphyseal bands bilaterally in the femur, tibia, and fibula (*arrows*). The presence of the increased density in the fibular metaphyses is highly suggestive of lead poisoning. Note mild metaphyseal undertubulation. **B,** AP radiograph of wrists shows dense metaphyseal bands in distal radius and ulna (*arrows*) bilaterally. The presence of the increased density in the distal ulnar metaphyses is highly suggestive of lead poisoning.

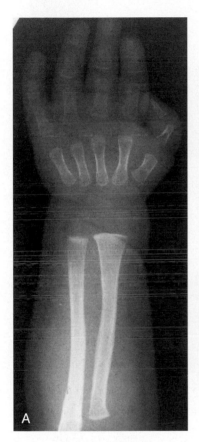

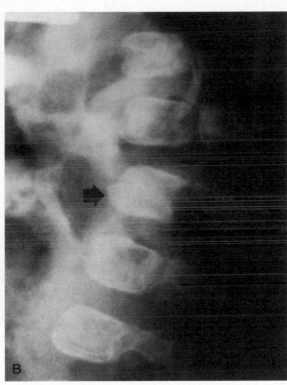

Fig. 4-29 Eleven-month-old girl with congenital hypothyroidism. **A,** PA radiograph of hand and forearm shows severe delay in skeletal maturity. Bone age is estimated as newborn. **B,** Lateral radiograph of thoracolumbar junction shows bullet-shaped vertebra (*arrow*).

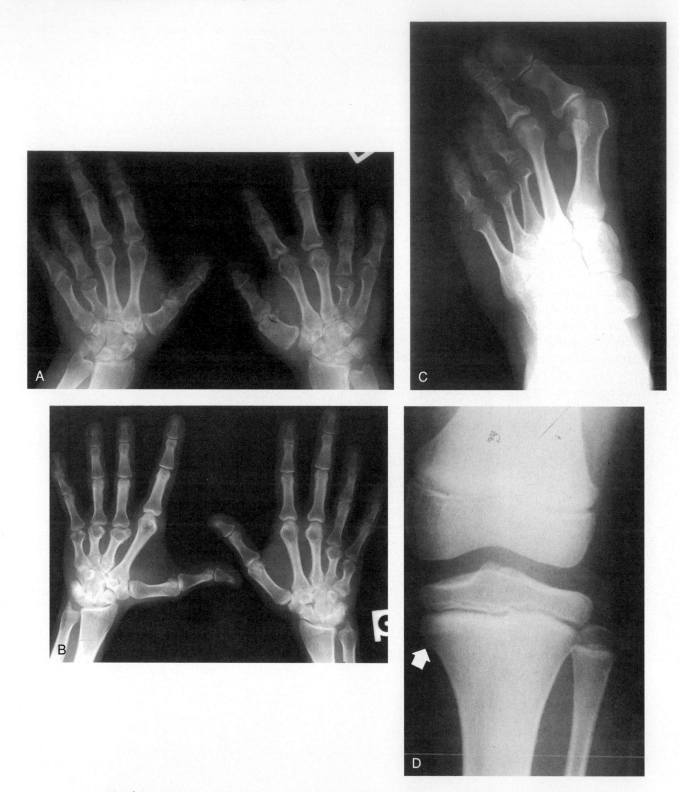

Fig. 4-30   Characteristic features of pseudohypoparathyroidism. **A,** PA radiograph of hands shows characteristic shortening and mild widening of multiple small tubular bones, particularly the first and fourth metacarpals in this patient. **B,** PA radiograph of hands in another patient shows pronounced shortening of the right third through fifth and the left fourth and fifth metacarpal bones. **C,** Frontal radiograph of foot shows third through fifth metatarsal shortening. **D,** AP radiograph of knee shows tiny osteochondroma (*arrow*) arising at right angle from medial aspect of proximal tibial metaphysis.

monly after parathyroid gland resection for hyperparathyroidism and results in hypocalcemia and hyperphosphatemia. Clinical manifestations predominate with irritability, seizures, and tetany. Radiographically, metastatic deposition of calcium phosphate salts can occur, often in subcutaneous locations or the basal ganglia of the brain, and osteosclerosis can be localized or generalized. Rarely osteoporosis is seen. *Pseudohypoparathyroidism* has similar clinical manifestations but represents target cell resistance to parathyroid hormone in which the patients are clinically hypocalcemic but serum levels of parathyroid hormone are high. These patients have a characteristic body type in that they are short and obese, with short metacarpals and metatarsals, especially in the first, fourth, and fifth (Fig. 4-30). Short stature and short metacarpals are due to accelerated, early growth plate closure. Thick calvaria and intracranial and soft tissue calcifications can be seen. Also seen are unusual small osteochondromas, projecting at right angles to the shafts of the bones (Fig. 4-30D). Radiographic features are otherwise similar to hypoparathyroidism. *Pseudopseudohypoparathyroidism* is clinically and radiologically the same as pseudohypoparathyroidism but serum hormone

levels of parathyroid hormone are normal and calcium levels are normal.

SUGGESTED READINGS

Holick MF, Krane SM, Potts JT: Calcium, phosphorus, and bone metabolism: calcium regulating hormones, In Fauci AS, Braunwald E, Isselbacher KJ, et al. *Harrison's principles of internal medicine,* ed. 14, New York, 1998, McGraw-Hill.

Knockel JP: Disorders of phosphorus metabolism, In Fauci AS, Braunwald E, Isselbacher KJ, et al. *Harrison's principles of internal medicine,* ed. 14, New York, 1998, McGraw-Hill.

Krane SM, Holick MF: Metabolic bone disease, In Fauci AS, Braunwald E, Isselbacher KJ, et al. *Harrison's principles of internal medicine,* ed. 14, New York, 1998, McGraw-Hill.

Lenchik L, Sartoris DJ: Current concepts in osteoporosis. *AJR* 1997;168:905–911.

Potts JT: Diseases of the parathyroid gland and other hyper- and hypocalcemic disorders, In Fauci AS, Braunwald E, Isselbacher KJ, et al. *Harrison's principles of internal medicine,* ed. 14, New York, 1998, McGraw-Hill.

Resnick D: Thyroid disorders. In Resnick D. *Diagnosis of bone and joint disorders,* ed. 3, W.B. Saunders Company, 1995.

Resnick D, Niwayama G: Paget's disease. In Resnick D. *Diagnosis of bone and joint disorders,* ed. 3, W.B. Saunders Company, 1995.

CHAPTER 5

Congenital and Developmental Skeletal Conditions

DAVID A. MAY, M.D.

INTRODUCTION

Development of the skeleton begins during the first trimester of gestation with aggregation of mesenchymal cells that subsequently become the bones and joints. A variety of disease processes and conditions may alter bone formation and growth and result in bone or joint deformity. This chapter begins with a review of normal skeletal growth and development, followed by a discussion of several of the more common, distinctive, or otherwise important congenital and developmental musculoskeletal abnormalities. A complete review of this topic is beyond the scope of this book. When more information is needed, excellent sources include Taybi and Lachman's *Radiology of Syndromes, Metabolic Disorders, and Skeletal Dysplasias,* and the major Pediatric Radiology textbooks. Resnick's *Radiology of Bone and Joint Disorders* provides an encyclopedic discussion of many congenital and developmental conditions reviewed in this chapter. Keats' *An Atlas of Normal Roentgen Variants that May Simulate Disease,* and Keats and Smith's *An Atlas of Normal Developmental Roentgen Anatomy* review many developmental variants, some seen only transiently during development, that may simulate pathologic conditions.

NORMAL SKELETAL GROWTH AND DEVELOPMENT

The bones are formed by two processes, both of which involve replacement of connective tissues by bone. The calvaria of the skull, the mandible, most of the facial bones, and the central portion of the clavicles are formed by direct transformation of primitive mesenchyme into bone by a process termed *intramembranous ossification.* The remainder of the skeleton, including the skull base, the spine, the pelvis, and the extremities are preceded by a continuously growing cartilage model that is continuously replaced by bone in a process termed *enchondral ossification.* The bone formed by either process is woven (immature) bone. The immature bone is

Key Concepts	Normal Skeletal Growth and Development

- Bone formation is formed by intramembranous ossification (direct conversion from mesenchyme to bone in most of the skull and facial bones and mandible, central portion of clavicle) or by enchondral ossification (conversion of a cartilage model into bone in skull base, spine, pelvis, extremities).
- The physis is responsible for longitudinal growth of long bones by enchondral ossification. Physeal injury can cause focal growth arrest and deformity.
- Tubulation is the process of remodeling the shaft of a long bone into normal configuration. Overtubulation occurs when the cylindrical portion of shaft is too long, with a short and narrowed metaphysis. (Causes include: absent weight bearing, neuromuscular conditions). Undertubulation occurs when the cylindrical portion of shaft is too short, with a wide and long metaphysis (Example: osteopetrosis)

subsequently extensively remodeled in a coordinated process of bone resorption by osteoclasts and bone formation by osteoblasts into the mature adult skeleton, which is composed of lamellar bone. After skeletal maturity is reached, further bone resorption and formation occur in response to mechanical stresses, hormonal regulation related to calcium homeostasis, or alterations in thyroid or sex hormones.

Longitudinal growth of long bones occurs by enchondral ossification at the *physis* (growth plate, epiphyseal growth plate; Fig. 5-1). The physis may be thought of as a rolling assembly line that pushes the epiphysis away from the metaphysis and diaphysis as it manufactures new bone. The process of new bone formation is initiated by chondrocytes located along the epiphyseal margin of the physis ("resting zone") that proliferate and produce a cartilage template that becomes calcified, and subsequently invaded by osteocytes, finally to be ossified at the metaphyseal side of the physis. The new bone deposited along the metaphyseal side of the physis is immature and undergoes extensive remodeling to become mature trabecular bone. New cartilage is produced along the epiphyseal side of the physis at the same rate that it is converted to bone along the metaphyseal side. This equilibrium results in uniform width of the healthy physis throughout growth. Note that only the uncalcified portion of the cartilage is radiolucent. This is often thought of as representing the entire physis on radiographs, although the metaphyseal margin of the physis is calcified.

Direct trauma to the physis can result in osseous healing across the physis or injury to the chondrocytes that are needed to produce the cartilage model. Either complication can cause growth arrest or growth deformity (see Fig. 3-22). Intact metaphyseal blood vessels adjacent to the physis are essential to convert the cartilage model into bone. Loss of integrity of these vessels by trauma, infection, or other insults can result in widening of the physis because the newly produced cartilage cannot be transformed into bone. Growth disturbance and deformity may result.

The rate at which a long bone is lengthened depends on circulating hormones, notably growth hormone, and poorly understood local factors that maintain proportional skeletal growth. The fastest longitudinal growth in the appendicular skeleton occurs at the distal femoral physis, where new bone is formed at up to 1 to 1.5 cm per year. As skeletal maturity is reached around puberty, the chondrocytes in the resting zone of the physis stop dividing. As a result, no new cartilage is formed and longitudinal growth ceases. The remaining cartilage is converted to bone as the physis closes. A dense transverse line on radiographs, sometimes termed a physeal scar, marks the final position of the physis. The timing of physeal closure varies at different sites. The medial clavicle physes are among the last to close, typically in the third decade, years after adult stature has been achieved.

Stress lines, also termed *growth recovery lines,* or *Park or Harris lines* are thin sclerotic lines within the metaphysis that are parallel to the physis (Fig. 5-2). They are associated with periods of childhood stress such as illness or trauma. The lines appear to be formed during the recovery phase after such episodes. Stress lines often persist into adulthood, but are eventually removed by routine bone remodeling. Stress lines are narrow and sharply defined, and do not abut the physis. In contrast, broader, less well-defined sclerotic transverse metaphyseal bands that abut the physis can be seen as a normal finding when found only in weightbearing bones, or as an abnormal finding when found in all bones as a consequence of heavy-metal poisoning (Fig. 5-3). Lucent metaphyseal bands can occur in rickets, leukemia, and metastatic neuroblastoma.

Long bones also undergo lateral growth and remodeling that is due primarily to periosteal new bone formation and remodeling of the metaphysis into an approximately tubular shape. This process, termed tubulation, is mediated by coordinated function of osteoclasts and osteoblasts. Disorders of tubulation may result in a wide metaphysis (undertubulation, *"Erlenmeyer flask deformity,"* Fig. 5-4 and Table 5-1), or a narrow, tubular metaphysis (*overtubulation,* Fig. 5-5 and Table 5-2). For example, the diminished osteoclastic activity associated with osteopetrosis and marrow packing in storage diseases result in undertubulation. Overtubulation is seen most commonly in neuromuscular syndromes with absent or diminished weight bearing such as cerebral palsy.

The process of skeletal maturation tends to follow an orderly progression, even when accelerated or delayed

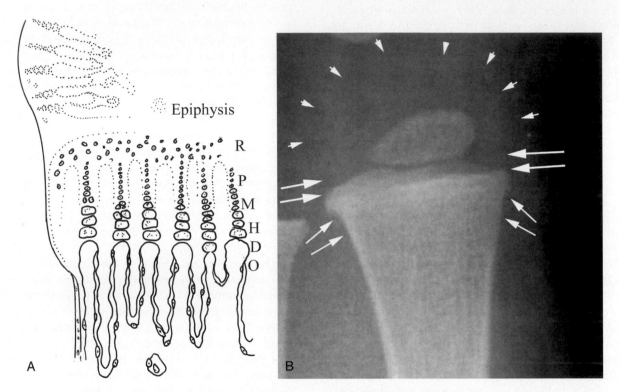

Fig. 5-1   The physis. **A,** Diagram shows the histologic organization of the physis. The *resting zone (R)* adjacent to the epiphysis contains small clusters of cartilage cells. The *proliferation zone (P)* contains dividing and enlarging cartilage cells organized into longitudinal columns. Cell division ceases in the *maturation zone (M)*, but the cartilage cells continue to enlarge. The cells greatly enlarge in the *hypertrophic zone (H)* and the surrounding cartilage becomes calcified (termed *provisional calcification* because it is not yet bone). The cartilage cells degenerate and die in the *cartilage degeneration zone (D)* and are replaced by osteoblasts. In the *osteogenic zone (O)*, the osteoblasts begin the process of conversion of the calcified cartilage into bone. This zone marks the transition from the physis to the metaphysis. **B,** Radiograph of a child's distal radius shows the corresponding radiographic anatomy. The large arrows mark the physis. The convex contour of the metaphysis (*small long arrows*) is the result of bone remodeling by osteoclasts and osteoblasts. If osteoclast activity is diminished, then this concave contour is not produced (*undertubulation,* see text and Fig. 5-4). The small, short arrows mark the true margins of the epiphysis, which is composed mostly of cartilage in this young child.

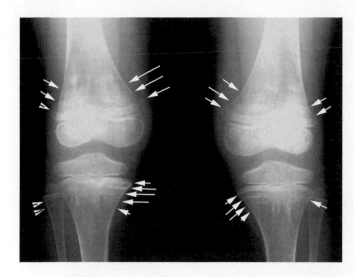

Fig. 5-2 Growth recovery lines (*Parke Lines, Harris Lines*). Note the bilaterally symmetric, thin, sharp lines parallel to the physes of both femurs, tibias and fibulas (*arrows*). The growth recovery lines are more widely spaced in the femurs than in the tibias because the femurs grow more rapidly.

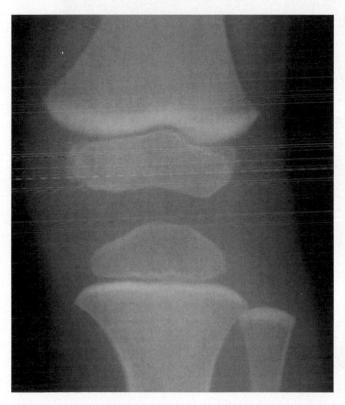

Fig. 5-3 Dense metaphyseal bands. Note the broad, fuzzy sclerotic bands adjacent to each physis. Dense metaphyseal bands can be seen as a physiologic finding when confined to load bearing bones, a finding most often seen between the ages of 2 and 6 years. However, the important clue in this case is the presence of fibular involvement. The fibula is not a load bearing bone, so heavy metal intoxication is more likely. The findings in this case were due to lead poisoning.

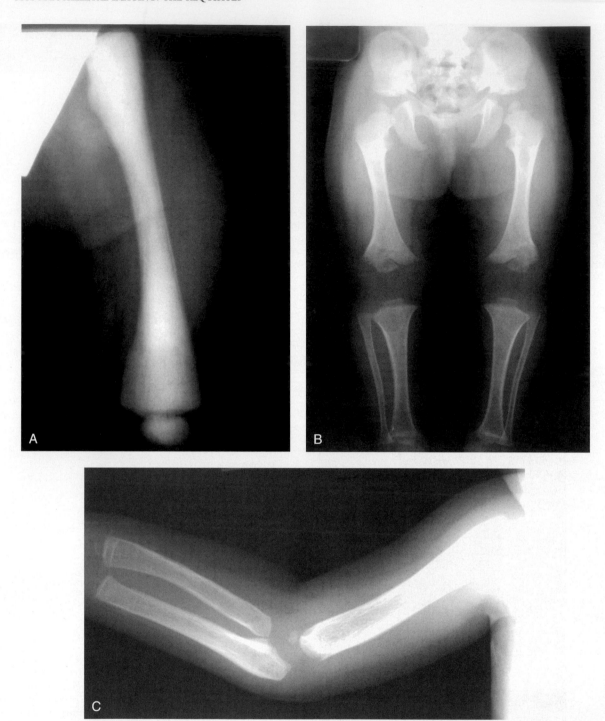

Fig. 5-4   Undertubulation. **A,** Osteopetrosis. Failure of osteoclast function results in wide metaphyses. **B,** Achondroplasia. Note the short, squat bones with wide metaphyses. **C,** Hurler's syndrome (mucopolysaccharidosis 1H). The marrow is packed with abnormal metabolites, causing expansion of the diaphyses and metaphyses. (B, Courtesy of Stephanie Spottswood, M.D., Medical College of Virginia, Richmond, VA.)

Table 5-1   Common causes of undertubulation
BONES OF NORMAL LENGTH Rickets Osteopetrosis Fibrous dysplasia Multiple osteochondromas **SHORT, OFTEN SQUAT BONES** Dwarfs (numerous types, achondroplasia most common) Storage diseases Multiple osteochondromas

Table 5-2   Common causes of overtubulation (long, thin bones)
Neuromuscular conditions (e.g., cerebral palsy, myelomenigocele) Osteogenesis imperfecta Juvenile rheumatoid arthritis Marfan syndrome Homocystinuria Arthrogryposis

by endocrine conditions, nutritional deficiencies, or other disease states. *Gruelich and Pyle's atlas* has been widely adopted as the standard reference for determining the skeletal age of children over one year of age. The

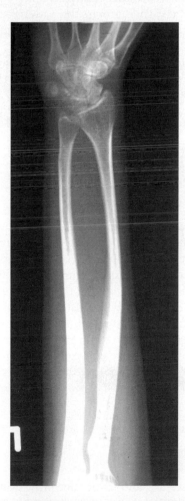

Fig. 5-5   Overtubulation. Note the short transition from epiphysis to diaphysis in the forearm of this child with osteogenesis imperfecta. Also note the long, narrow diaphyses. This overall appearance is often described as "gracile bones," and is most commonly seen in neuromuscular conditions with chronic absence of weight bearing such as cerebral palsy.

standard images of the maturing left hand used in this atlas were derived from a longitudinal study of healthy children of northern European decent living in the Cleveland area during the 1930s. This may not represent an optimal data set, but current appreciation of the potential harm of ionizing radiation makes it unlikely that a similar study will ever be performed in other racial or ethnic groups. When using Gruelich and Pyle's atlas, it is important to focus on the thumb and the distal phalanges of the other fingers in order to achieve the best estimate of skeletal age.

In infants and very young children up to about one year of age, the *method of Sontag, Snell, and Anderson* is a useful technique for determining skeletal age (Table 5-3). This method is based on tabulation of the number of secondary growth centers (epiphyses and apophyses) that have started to ossify and thus are visible on AP radiographs of one upper and one lower extremity. The appeal of this method is that it relies on a yes-or-no determination of the presence of visible ossification in each secondary growth center.

Table 5-3   Skeletal age in infants: the method of Sontag, Snell, and Anderson

Mean total number of centers on the left side of body ossified at given age levels*

AGE (MO)	Boys		Girls	
	MEAN NO.	SD	MEAN NO.	SD
1	4.11	1.41	4.58	1.76
3	6.63	1.86	7.78	2.16
6	9.61	1.95	11.44	2.53
9	11.88	2.66	15.36	4.92
12	13.96	3.96	22.40	6.93
18	19.27	6.61	34.10	8.44
24	29.21	8.10	43.44	6.65

* SD=Standard deviation.
Technique: Anteroposterior radiographs are taken of the left upper and lower extremities. The number of visible secondary growth centers is counted.
From: Sontag LW, Snell D, Anderson M. Rate of appearance of ossification centers from birth to the age of five years. *Am J Dis Child* 58:949-956, 1939, and Keats TE, Smith TH. *An Atlas of Normal Developmental Roentgen Anatomy.* 2nd ed. Chicago: Year Book Medical Publishers

The *Risser technique* is used to estimate skeletal maturity of the spine in adolescents with scoliosis. It is based on the radiographic appearance of the iliac crest apophyses (Fig. 5-6). This is wonderfully convenient, because the iliac crests are easily included on frontal spinal radiographs. The iliac crest apophyses ossify in an orderly sequence from lateral to medial that begins roughly 4 years before spinal growth is complete. Soon after becoming completely ossified, the apophyses fuse with the iliac crests. This fusion is synchronous with completion of spinal growth.

The appearance of the bone marrow on MR images also undergoes predictable changes during growth and development that reflect shifting distribution of hematopoietic elements. Hematopoietic marrow may be present in all portions of the marrow in neonates. MR images display hematopoietic marrow as intermediate signal intensity on T1-weighted images and intermediate to slightly high signal intensity on T2-weighted images with or without fat suppression. By age 6 months, the marrow of the epiphyses and apophyses normally completely and permanently converts to fatty marrow. Fatty marrow has high signal intensity on T1-weighted images and intermediate signal intensity on T2-weighted images. Anything other than fat signal intensity in the epiphyses and apophyses after age 6 months should be considered abnormal, with the exception for the medial humeral head, where hematopoietic marrow may be normally seen well into middle age. Conditions that may cause abnormal signal

Table 5-4   Abnormal epiphyseal marrow signal
Hematopoietic marrow
chronic anemia
marrow reconversion after chemotherapy
Neoplasm
Child: chondroblastoma, eosinophilic granuloma
Infection
Marrow packing with abnormal metabolites (e.g., Gaucher's disease)
Trauma (fracture, hemorrhage, edema)
Osteoarthritis (subchondral cyst, sclerosis, metaplasia)
Osteonecrosis
Bone island (low signal intensity on all sequences)
Orthopedic hardware

intensity in the secondary growth centers are listed in Table 5-4. As the child grows, the pattern of hematopoietic marrow distribution shifts towards the axial skeleton and the metaphyses (Fig. 5-7). Hematopoietic marrow is often seen in routine extremity MR images in adults, especially in menstruating women and cigarette smokers. Hematopoietic marrow may have a "wispy," ill-defined configuration, or may be occasionally rounded and well circumscribed, simulating a metastasis.

SPINE DISORDERS

Scoliosis

The normal infant spine is straight. The adult pattern of cervical lordosis, thoracic kyphosis, and lumbar lordosis develops after infancy. *Scoliosis* is lateral curvature of the spine in the coronal plane. Rotatory deformity (vertebral rotation along the long axis of the spine) and abnormal kyphosis or lordosis may coexist. Abnormal spinal alignment can cause cosmetic deformities, and severe scoliosis may decrease the size of the thorax with consequent restriction of pulmonary and cardiac function. Management decisions are complex, but generally depend on the cause of the scoliosis (the single most important

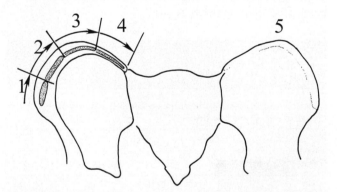

Fig. 5-6   Risser classification for estimation of spinal maturity. This system is based on the ossification of the iliac crest apophysis. Stage 0: no ossification of the iliac crest apophysis. Stage 1: ossification of the lateral one-fourth of the iliac crest apophysis. Stage 2: ossification of the lateral one-half of the iliac crest apophysis. Stage 3: ossification of the lateral three-fourths of the iliac crest apophysis. Stage 4: ossification of the entire iliac crest apophysis, without fusion to the iliac crest. Stage 5: fusion of the iliac crest apophysis (coincides with completion of spinal growth). (From: Scoles PV, Salvagno R, Villalba K, Riew D. Relationship of iliac crest maturation to skeletal and chronologic age, *J Pedatr Orthop* 8:639, 1988, and Ozonoff MB *Pediatric orthopaedic radiology,* ed 2, Philadelphia: WB Saunders, 1992.)

Key Concepts   Scoliosis
• Most cases are idiopathic, but must evaluate for other potential causes: vertebral body anomalies, neurofibromatosis, tumor, leg length discrepancy, and neuromuscular condition.
• Scoliosis in neurofibromatosis may progress rapidly and become unstable.

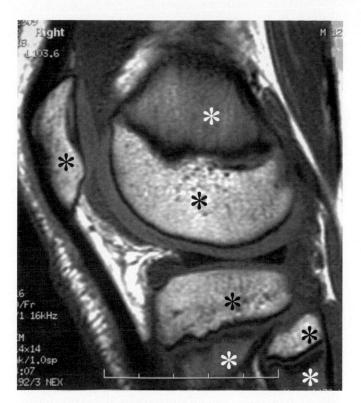

Fig. 5-7   Normal hematopoietic marrow distribution in an older child. Sagittal T1-weighted MR image of the lateral aspect of the knee in a 12-year-old boy shows uniform high signal intensity of fatty marrow in the epiphyses and the patella (*black asterisks*), and uniform intermediate signal intensity of hematopoietic marrow in the metaphyses (*white asterisks*). This amount of hematopoietic marrow would be unusual in an adult male, suggesting the presence of chronic anemia or a marrow infiltrating process such as leukemia.

issue), the degree of abnormal curvature, the child's age and how much further spinal growth may be expected, and whether the curvature is increasing over time. Radiographic assessment has an important role in each of these issues.

Causes of scoliosis are numerous (Tables 5-5, 5-6). Although idiopathic scoliosis is by far the most common

Table 5-5   Causes of scoliosis
Idiopathic (85%)
Leg length discrepancy
Congenital
Neuromuscular
Neurofibromatosis
Connective tissue disorders
Trauma
Tumors
Radiation therapy

Table 5-6   Clues that a scoliosis may not be idiopathic
Present at birth
Deformities of vertebral bodies
Multiple limb deformities (arthrogryposis, chromosomal abnormalities)
Convex left thoracic curve (associated with syringomyelia and spinal cord tumors)
Long, C-shaped curve (neuromuscular conditions)
Focal, sharp curve (trauma; focal bony bar; neurofibromatosis, often with kyphosis and vertebral body dysplasia)
History of radiation therapy
Pelvic tilt (leg length discrepancy)
Painful (osteoid osteoma or other tumor; fracture; infection)

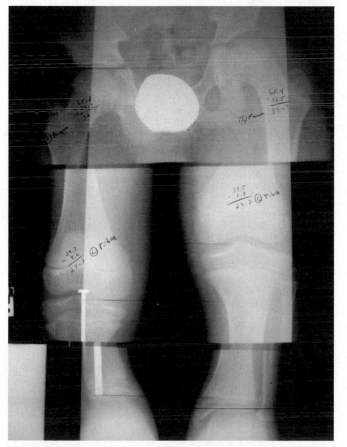

Fig. 5-8   Leg length discrepancy. Scanogram in a child with neurofibromatosis shows a short right tibia that causes a marked pelvic tilt, and also caused scoliosis (not shown). The annotations on the film were made by the orthopedic surgeon. The right tibia was short owing to a chronic pseudarthrosis that required resection of the pseudarthroses and pin fixation. The ends of the pin are visible in the right tibia, but the pseudarthrosis is not shown.

form of scoliosis (85%), it is a diagnosis of exclusion and therefore is discussed last.

Leg length discrepancy, that is unequal leg length, is considered to be significant if greater than 1 to 2 cm. A leg length discrepancy may be suggested by pelvic tilt on a standing radiograph. Unilateral leg shortening may be caused by trauma, especially if the physis was injured, or congenital conditions. Examples are slipped capital femoral epiphysis and infantile coxa vara. Conversely, unilateral leg lengthening may cause a leg length discrepancy. Any condition that causes hyperemia near a physis has the potential to accelerate growth at that physis.

Examples are inflammatory arthritis, high-flow vascular malformation, and fracture. Hemihypertrophy also may cause a leg length discrepancy. Radiographic assessment of leg length can be accomplished with "sliding table" radiographs (Fig. 5-8) or with a frontal CT scanogram. CT has the advantage of using less ionizing radiation. Regardless of the technique, radiographic assessment of leg length should be accomplished with gonadal shielding. The landmarks used for determination of the length of the femurs and tibia are the tops of the femoral heads, distal medial femoral condyles, and the tibial plafond. Orthopedic intervention for leg length discrepancy

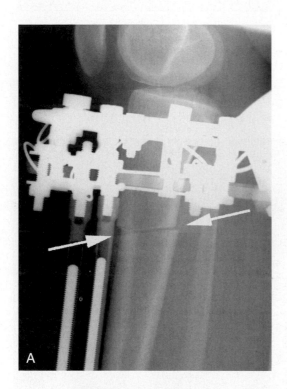

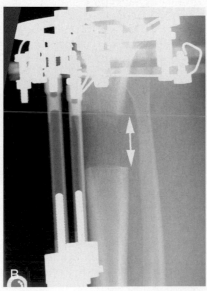

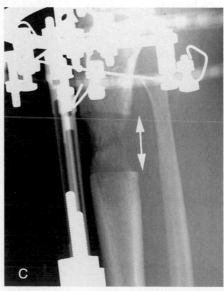

Fig. 5-9 Surgical leg lengthening. **A,** Initial study shows a proximal tibial osteotomy (*arrows*). The periosteum was not completely divided. Note the external hardware (only partially shown) that is designed to allow the fragments to be distracted each day by a small amount—usually 1 mm or less because this is the maximal rate of growth of the nerves that are also being elongated. **B, C,** Follow-up views 4 months (**B**) and 7 months (**C**) later show new bone formed by the perisosteum that will eventually thicken and remodel into normal cortex. Arrows mark the amount of bone lengthening. (Courtesy of Tim Sanders, M.D., San Antonio, TX.)

can be accomplished by unilateral lengthening of the short leg (Fig. 5-9) or shortening of the longer leg by *epiphysodesis* (fusion of the physis to prevent further growth, Fig. 5-10).

Congenital scoliosis is due to abnormalities of the formation or segmentation of the vertebral bodies during the first trimester of gestation. Each vertebra (segment) is normally formed from 3 ossification centers: one for the vertebral body and one for each side of the posterior elements. One of these ossification centers may fail to form or may aberrantly fuse to a center from an adjacent segment. The resulting deformities include misshapen vertebrae such as hemivertebrae, or a bone or fibrous bar that tethers part of one vertebral body to another (Fig. 5-11). The presence of vertebral body anomalies in a neonate warrants a careful search for associated abnormalities in the VACTERL spectrum (Vertebral, Anorectal, Cardiac, TracheoEsophageal fistula, Renal, and Limb anomalies, Fig. 5-11B) and spinal cord anomalies such as tethered cord or diastematomyelia. Spine MRI evaluation should be considered. Treatment of congenital scoliosis is frequently surgical, in order to provide stabilization and to prevent further deformity due to asymmetric growth.

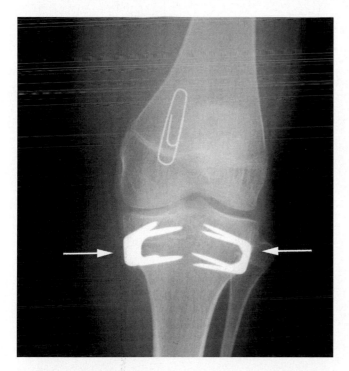

Fig. 5-10 Leg shortening by epiphyseodesis. The proximal tibial physis was fused (epiphyseodesis) by fixation with staples (*arrows*) over one year previously to allow the shorter contralateral leg (not shown) to catch up. (The paper clip is an artifact.) Note that the distal femoral physis is closing, indicating the completion of growth of both legs. Limb shortening can also be accomplished by resection of a segment of a long bone with plate fixation.

A variety of *neuromuscular conditions* cause paraspinal muscle imbalance due to spasticity or flaccidity with resulting scoliosis. Neuromuscular scoliosis tends to be long and C-shaped without compensatory curves above or below (Fig. 5-12). Cerebral palsy, muscular dystrophy, paralysis and arthrogryposis are frequent causes of neuromuscular scoliosis. Dysplasia or dislocation of one or both hips is a frequently seen association.

Scoliosis associated with *neurofibromatosis* (Fig. 5-13) deserves special mention because of its potential for devastating rapid progression to severe angulation and subluxation that can lead to paralysis. These curves frequently include a kyphotic component and are most frequently seen in the mid-thoracic spine. Clues to the diagnosis include associated findings of dural ectasia (posterior vertebral body scalloping, enlarged neural foramina) and rib abnormalities (twisted, narrow "ribbon ribs"). The musculoskeletal manifestations of neurofibromatosis are further discussed later in this chapter.

Connective tissue disorders such as Marfan syndrome and Ehlers-Danlos Syndrome frequently cause scoliosis. These conditions are further discussed later in this chapter in the section on connective tissue disorders.

Spine trauma may result in scoliosis. Instrumentation may be required to maintain stability.

Painful scoliosis should prompt a search for an underlying tumor of the spine or spinal cord, stress fracture, or infection. Although a variety of tumors of the vertebrae or spinal canal may cause scoliosis, *osteoid osteoma* is the most common. Vertebral osteoid osteoma usually occurs in the posterior elements. The scoliosis is concave towards the side of the nidus due to ipsilateral muscle spasm. Associated sclerosis may be detected on radiographs or CT. A radionuclide bone scan will reveal intense tracer uptake around the tumor. CT is the preferred technique for characterization and precise localization of the nidus before resection.

Radiation therapy has the potential to arrest the growth of any portion of the spine included in the radiation field. If only one side of the vertebral column is included in a radiation field in a child, the non-irradiated side will continue to grow, and vertebral body deformity with scoliosis convex away from the radiated side will develop. Associated findings may include hypoplastic ribs on the concave (radiated) side of the curve and a previous history of a childhood Wilms tumor or other neoplasm. Postradiation scoliosis is fortunately becoming rare, as careful attention to radiation ports and effective alternative treatments for childhood tumors have become more common.

Idiopathic scoliosis is by far the most common form of scoliosis, but, as mentioned earlier, is a diagnosis of exclusion. This is a fairly common condition, as it has been estimated that nearly 5% of the population has a curve of 10° or greater. Fortunately, the large majority

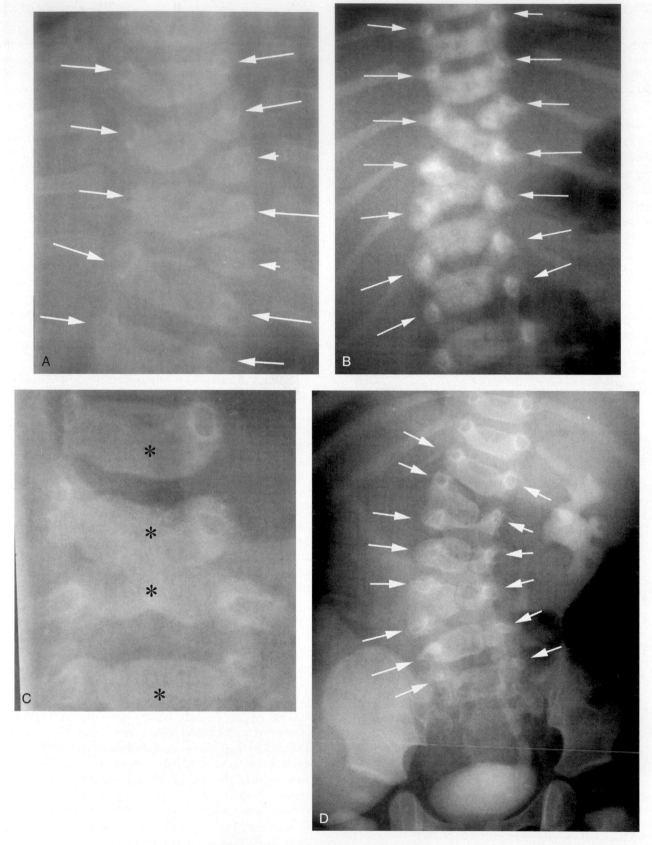

Fig. 5-11   For legend see opposite page

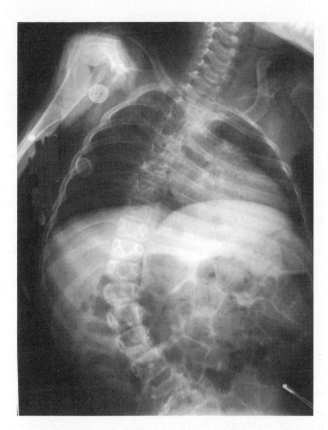

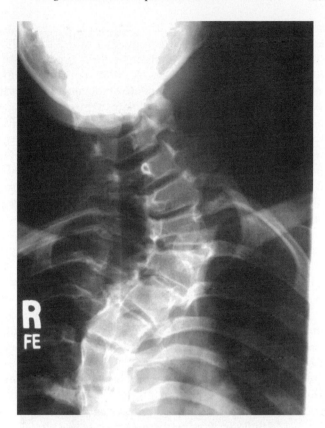

Fig. 5-12   Long C-shaped scoliosis due to a neuromuscular condition. (Courtesy of L. Das Narla, M.D., Richmond, VA.)

Fig. 5-13   Scoliosis in neurofibromatosis.

of these curves are less than 20°. Idiopathic scoliosis is more common in girls (7 : 1), and also tends to be more severe in girls. The cause is unknown, although a genetic component has been noted in many cases and muscular imbalance is thought to play a role.

The spinal curvature is usually composed of a primary ("major") curve that may be thoracic, thoracolumbar, or lumbar. Secondary compensatory ("minor") curves are seen above and below the primary curve. A double major "S"-shaped thoracolumbar curve is seen in many cases (Fig. 5-14). Long cassette radiographs are a cornerstone of diagnosis and surveillance. Scoliotic curves are mea-

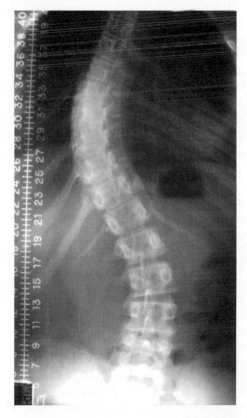

Fig. 5-11   Vertebral segmentation anomalies. **A,** Hemivertebrae. The pedicles are marked with arrows. Note the hemivertebrae (*short arrows*) with associated scoliosis. **B,** Segmentation anomalies with fusion abnormalities, hemivertebrae, and scoliosis. The pedicles are marked with arrows. **C,** Failure of segmentation. The vertebral bodies are marked with asterisks. Note the fusion of the two bodies at the center of the image. **D,** Failure of formation and the VACTERL association. The pedicles are marked with arrows. Note the greater number of pedicles on the right than the left, with associated scoliosis. The intravenous urogram shows unilateral right renal agenesis. (Courtesy of Stephanie Spottswood, M.D., Richmond, VA.)

Fig. 5-14   Idiopathic scoliosis with a double major curve.

sured by the Cobb method. The scoliosis is divided into individual components that are convex towards the right (dextroscoliosis, or simply "right scoliosis") or convex towards the left (levoscoliosis, or "left scoliosis"). The angle formed by the upper endplate of the most cephalad vertebral body and the lower endplate of the most caudad body of the curve is measured for each component. If the endplates are not well seen, then the pedicles are used. The vertebral body or disk space at the apex (midpoint of the angular deformity) of the curve is also noted. It is important to document whether a radiograph was obtained while the child was wearing a body brace, especially when comparing with previous radiographs, because the brace will tend to reduce the scoliotic curvature. Frontal radiographs, obtained with left and right lateral bending, demonstrate how much of a curve is fixed ("structural") from how much is flexible ("functional") and hence correctable by surgery (Fig. 5-15).

The initial radiograph may be obtained anteroposterior (AP) to allow for better assessment for underlying vertebral anomalies or tumors. (The vertebral bodies are closer to the film cassette on an AP radiograph and thus are more sharply rendered.) Follow-up radiographs should be obtained posteroanterior (PA), because the breast and thyroid radiation dose is dramatically reduced by this technique. Routine breast and gonadal shielding should also be used. By optimizing these techniques, radiation dose to the breast and thyroid may be reduced over 50-fold when compared to conventional AP radiographs. This is an important consideration because many children will require dozens of radiographs during the course of their treatment.

Management options in idiopathic scoliosis include observation, bracing, and surgical instrumentation and fusion. Important management decisions require knowledge of the skeletal maturity of the spine and specifically the anticipated completion of spinal growth. Because the ring apophyses of the spine (Fig. 5-16) do not contribute significantly to vertebral growth, their fusion is not a reliable indicator of completion of growth of the spine. Thus, the Risser method described earlier in this chapter is a preferred method for the determination of spinal maturity in adolescents (Fig. 5-6). Many surgeons will also use bone age determination by Gruelich and Pyle's technique. Less severe curvature tends not to progress after skeletal maturity is attained, and thus is often managed successfully with observation or bracing. A brace is used for a scoliosis of about 25° or greater, or in a younger child with less severe curvature that is rapidly progressing. The goal of bracing is to halt progression of the scoliosis until spinal maturity is reached. Severe curves of greater than 50° generally require surgery to prevent respiratory and other complications. It is often preferred to delay surgery until after spinal growth is complete, but very severe or rapidly progressing curves

that are not responding adequately to bracing may require earlier surgical intervention.

There are several surgical options, each designed to improve alignment and prevent further growth. The popular techniques combine fixation hardware with fusion of either the posterior elements (posterior fusion) or across the disc spaces (anterior fusion). The importance of the bony fusion must be emphasized, because the hardware eventually may fail if spinal fusion is unsuccessful.

The basic hardware elements used in posterior fusion are rods or plates, hooks, and wires. The famous, early application of orthopedic fixation in management of scoliosis was the Harrington rod (Fig. 5-17). In this technique, a single straight spinal rod was placed along the concave side of the curve. The rod was fixed to the spine by two hooks: one under the inferior margin of the vertebral lamina at the upper end of the curve, and one over the superior margin of the vertebral lamina at the lower end of the curve. The hooks were distracted (spread apart) resulting in straightening of the curve, and fixed to the Harrington spinal rod. This system is simple, but it is limited by the amount of force that can be safely applied to just two laminae. In addition, the early Harrington rods were vulnerable to rod fracture owing to their distinctive shape. Current applications of the distracting rod technique tend to employ smooth or threaded distracting rods that are less vulnerable to rod failure. Some techniques employ custom fitted spinal rods, often in pairs, that are fixed to the posterior elements at multiple points. Spinal rods may be fixed to multiple laminae by wires (Luque, Fig. 5-18) or hooks (Cotrel-Dubousset, Fig. 5-15, and Texas Scottish Rite), or they may be fixed to the spinous processes by wires (Drummond-Wisconsin). These techniques distribute forces more widely than can be achieved with a single distracting rod, thereby allowing better correction of the curve, better fixation, and reduced risk of laminar fracture. The basic hardware elements used in anterior spinal fusion are vertebral body screws and a cable or rod linkage. The screws are placed transversely in the vertebral bodies, with portions projecting laterally along the convex side of the scoliotic curve. The screws are linked

Fig. 5-15 Idiopathic scoliosis: the surgeon's perspective. Orthopedic surgeons prefer to view spine radiographs the same way they examine the spine—from the back. Thus, they will view and mark the radiographs with the patient's right to the right. **A,** Standing view in an adolescent girl shows a convex right curve from T5 to L1 that measures 25°. The child was treated with a brace. **B,** Standing PA view obtained three years later shows that the curve has progressed despite the bracing and now measures almost 50°. **C, D,** Right (**C**) and left (**D**) bending views reveal that the primary curve is partially but not completely correctable.

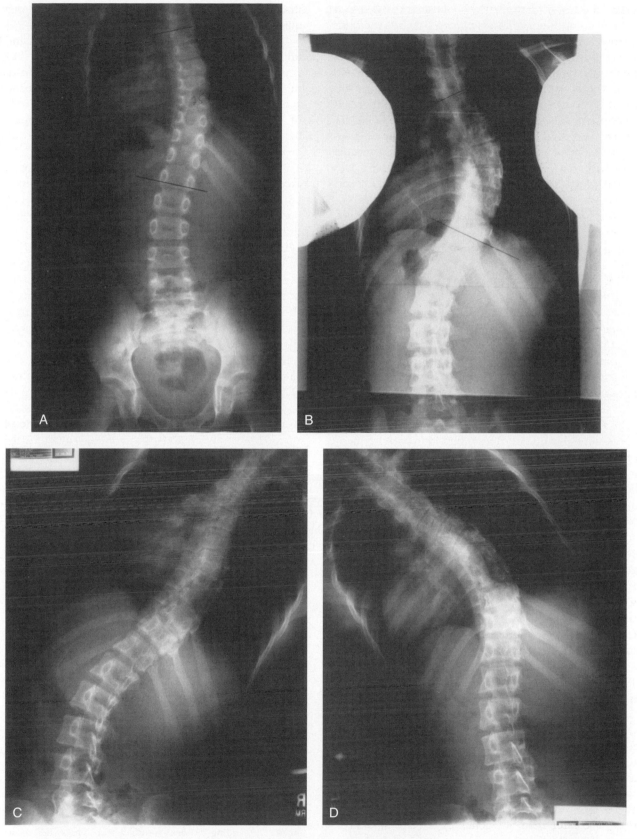

Fig. 5-15   For legend see opposite page

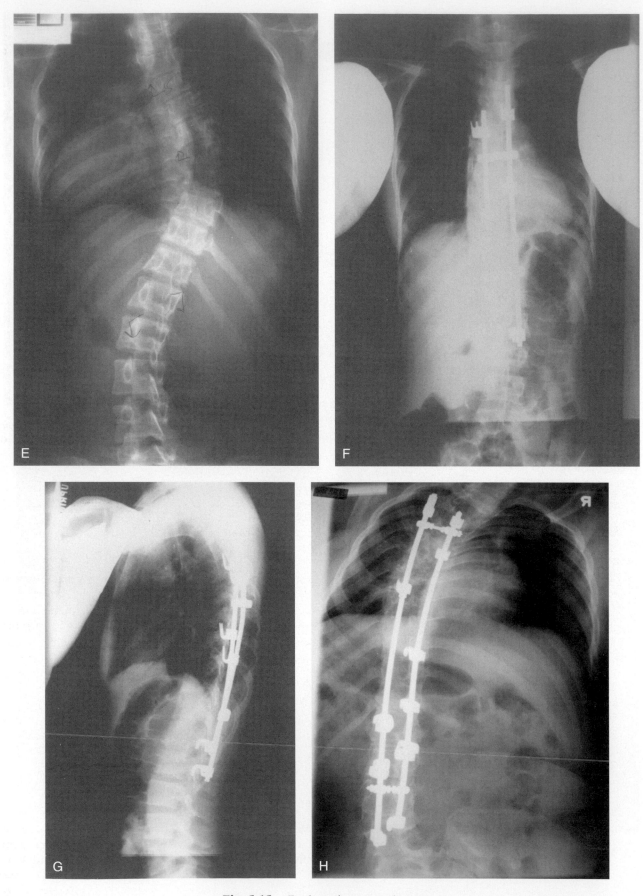

Fig. 5-15   For legend see opposite page

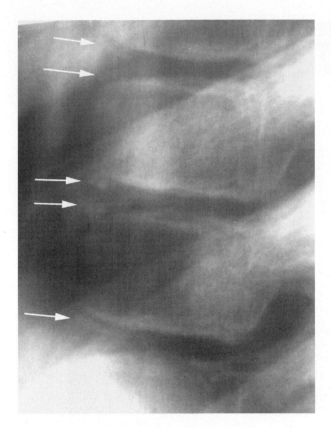

Fig. 5-16   Spinal ring apophyses (*arrows*).

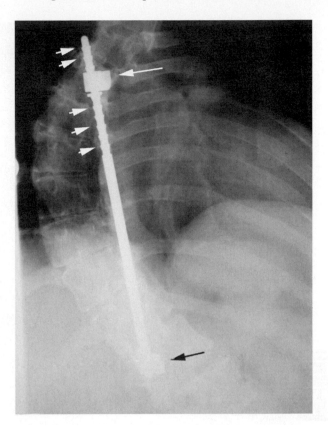

Fig. 5-17   Harrington rod. Note the laminar hooks (*long arrows*) and the distinctive serrated contour of the superior portion of the rod (*short arrows*).

together by a rod (Zielke) or a cable (Dwyer). These systems are employed most often when treating neuromuscular or congenital scoliosis.

Each system has advantages and disadvantages, and the surgeon's preference often determines which system is used. Because surgical hardware and technique are constantly evolving, the reader is cautioned not to be dogmatic in naming the hardware system seen when interpreting radiographs. In particular, not all rods are Harrington rods! In fact, most are not. It is preferable to use generic terms such as "spinal rod" unless the radiologist is certain of the system that has been implanted.

Fig. 5-15, cont'd   **E,** Preoperative standing radiograph shows the surgeon's planned placement of laminar hooks (*arrows drawn on the radiograph*) as part of spinal fixation. **F, G,** Postoperative AP (**F**) and lateral (**G**) views show Cotrel-Dubousset hardware with significant improvement in the scoliosis. Note that the primary curve was not corrected beyond the alignment revealed in the preoperative bending views (**C**). This is because further straightening of the spine would injure the paraspinal supporting soft tissues. **H,** Cotrel-Dubousset instrumentation in a different patient better demonstrates the appearance of this hardware.

Juvenile Kyphosis and Scheuerman's Disease

Juvenile kyphosis is greater than 40° of kyphotic curvature from T3 to T12. Juvenile kyphosis may be caused by any of the many causes of scoliosis (Table 5-5), or may be idiopathic. Idiopathic forms include postural kyphosis, in which case there are no associated abnormalities, and *Scheuerman's disease* (Fig. 5-19). In the latter condition, thoracic vertebral body wedging, disc space narrowing, and frequently pain and multiple Schmorl's nodes (focal areas of endplate collapse due to herniation of the nucleus pulposis or fibrous or cartilagenous metaplasia) are present. Some authorities consider Scheuerman's disease to be a type of osteochondritis (see "Osteochondroses" in Chapter 2).

Spondylolysis

Spondylolysis is interruption of the pars interarticularis of the posterior elements (Fig. 5-20). Although the rare cervical spondylolysis likely is congenital, it is generally thought that the more common lumbar spondylolysis is acquired during childhood as a form of stress fracture. These fractures occur more frequently in children who

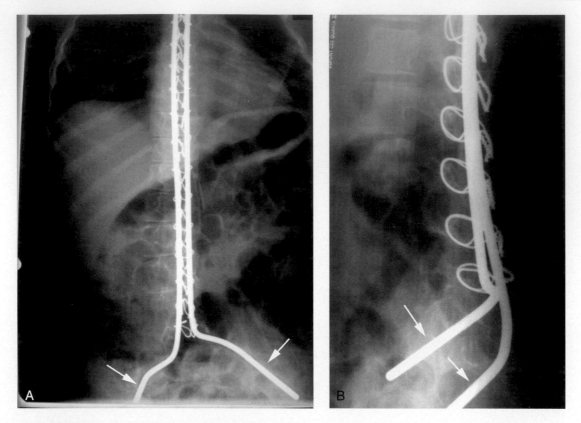

Fig. 5-18   Luque fixation. **A,** AP. **B,** lateral. The spinal rods are fixed to the laminae at multiple levels by wires. Note the extension of the spinal rods into the iliac bones (*arrows*), termed the "Galveston technique."

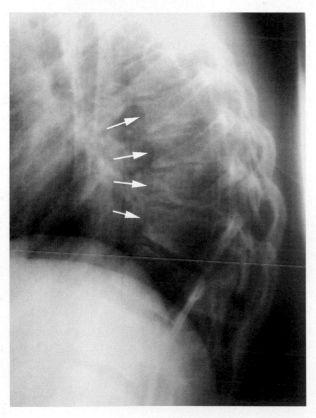

Fig. 5-19   Scheuerman's disease. This teenage boy had painful, clinically evident kyphosis. Note the wedging of several adjacent mid thoracic vertebral bodies (*arrows*) with irregular vertebral body endplates.

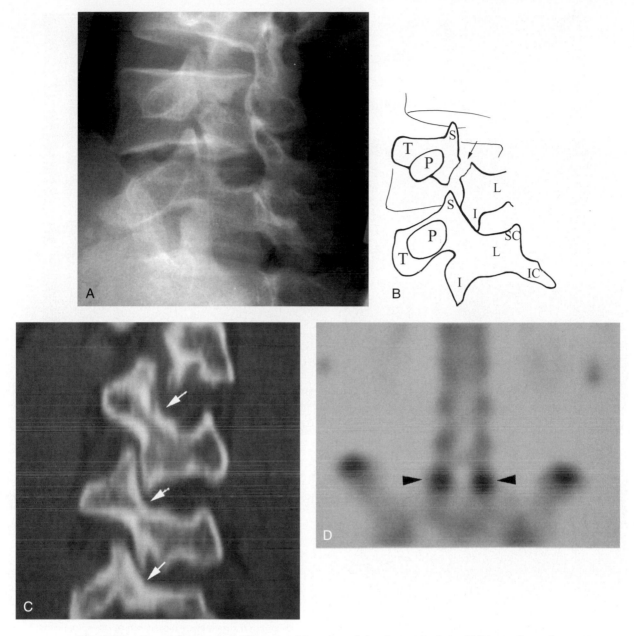

Fig. 5-20   Spondylolysis. **A, B,** Normal and interrupted pars interarticularis. Oblique radiograph (**A**) and corresponding line drawing (**B**) show an intact pars interarticularis at L5 and a pars defect with a collar around the "Scottie dog's" neck at L4 (*arrow* in B). P = pedicle (the Scottie dog's eye), T = transverse process (nose), S = superior articulating facet (ear), I = inferior articulating facet (front leg), L = lamina (body), IC = contralateral inferior articulating facet (rear leg), SC = contralateral superior articulating facet (tail). **C,** Oblique sagittal CT reconstruction in a normal patient. Note the intact pars interarticularis (*arrows*). **D,** Radionuclide bone scan of bilateral L5 pars defects. Coronal SPECT image through the posterior elements shows increased tracer bilaterally at L5 (*arrowheads*). CT (not shown) was needed to confirm bilateral defects, as a unilateral defect with adaptive hypertrophy on the contralateral side could have similar bone scan findings.

Continued

participate in activities with extreme lumbar spine extension such as gymnastics. There also appears to be a genetic predisposition in some cases. L5 is the most commonly affected level. Bilateral spondylolysis may result in *spondylolisthesis* (anterior displacement of the affected

vertebral body relative to the body below) that is graded by the degree of displacement. Grade 1 spondylolisthesis is anterior displacement of the superior vertebral body by up to 25% of the anteroposterior dimension of the endplate. Grade 2 spondylolisthesis is displacement of

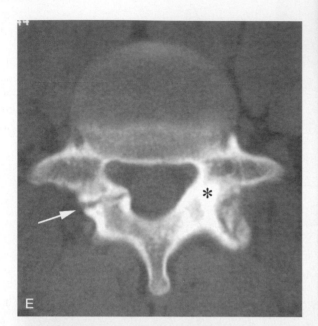

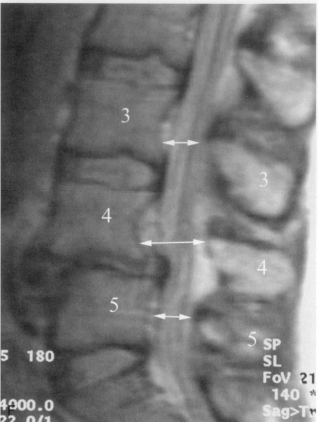

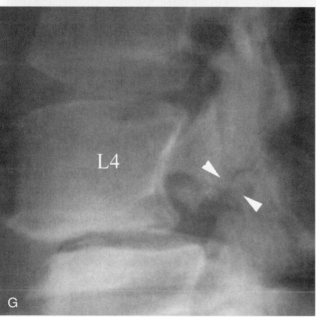

Fig. 5-20, cont'd **E,** CT of unilateral spondylolysis. Axial CT image. Note the spondylolysis on the right (*arrow*). Also note the sclerosis of the contralateral pars interarticularis (*astrick*). This nonspecific finding may reflect left-sided adaptive changes caused increased stress due to the right sided pars defect, or an impending left pars stress fracture. **F, G,** Bilateral L4 spondylolysis with grade 1 spondylolisthesis at L4–5. The sagittal proton density weighted MR image (**F**) shows the spondylolisthesis, but, as is often the case, the pars defects could not be seen on the MR images. Because the most common cause of mild spondylolisthesis is disc degeneration, which is present in this case, it would be easy to overlook the pars defects. However, note the greater anteroposterior dimension of the spinal canal at L4 compared with the levels above and below (*arrows;* the numbers mark the vertebral bodies anteriorly and the corresponding spinous processes posteriorly). This focal widening is an important clue to the correct diagnosis of spondylolysis with spondylolisthesis. The lateral radiograph (*G*) clearly reveals the pars defects (*arrowheads*). Bilateral pars defects are often easy to see on a lateral view. (C and E, Courtesy of Fred Laine, M.D., Richmond, VA.)

25% to 50%. Grade 3 is displacement by 50% to 75%, and grade 4, 75%–100%. Spondylolithesis tends not to progress after about age 20, but may become painful after that age. Spinal fusion is sometimes required.

Spondylolysis may be detected with oblique radiographs, where the defect is seen as a break in the neck of the famous "scottie dog" (Fig. 5-20). Bilateral spondy-

lolysis often may be appreciated on a coned lateral radiograph. CT is the optimal method to detect and characterize these lesions (Fig. 5-20E). Radionuclide bone scanning may reveal increased tracer uptake at the affected side in a subacute or healing defect, at the contralateral side due to increased mechanical stress or an additional impending spondylolysis, or bilaterally. SPECT imaging helps to localize the tracer uptake to the posterior elements. These lesions may be difficult to detect on routine MRI scans unless spondylolisthesis is present.

Transitional Segmentation and Klippel-Fiel

A spectrum of spinal abnormalities may result from abnormal formation and segmentation of the vertebral bodies, as noted earlier in the discussion of congenital scoliosis. Two common variations of congenital spinal segmentation anomalies that merit further discussion are transitional segmentation of the lumbosacral spine and the Klippel-Feil syndrome.

Transitional segmentation refers to congenital variation from the standard arrangement of 7 cervical, 12 thoracic, and 5 lumbar vertebrae and 5 sacral segments. Transitional segmentation occurs most frequently in the lumbosacral spine. A wide variety of variations may be seen. A common form of transitional segmentation is a transitional lumbosacral segment, with morphologic features intermediate between a lumbar vertebra and a sacral segment (Fig. 5-21). Assigning a numeric level to each vertebra (L1, L2, etc.) can be somewhat arbitrary. Consistency is essential when correlating different studies, in order to to direct spine surgery to the intended level. Guidelines to assist in assigning numbers to lumbar vertebra are based on findings in "normal" spines: a chest radiograph usually shows 12 rib pairs but may show 11 or 13 rib pairs; a line connecting the top of the iliac crests usually passes through L4–5; the widest transverse processes usually occur at L3, and, on MR images, the left renal vein is usually located anterior to L1–2.

Klippel-Feil refers to a syndrome of failure of cervical segmentation at multiple levels, with a short neck with low hairline (Fig. 5-22). Cervical motion is limited owing to the paucity of normally formed disks and facet joints. Associated findings may include renal, spinal cord, and inner, middle and outer ear abnormalities. The term Klippel-Fiel is also often used less restrictively to describe any congenital fusion anomaly encountered in the cervical spine (Fig. 5-23). Such abnormalities most frequently are isolated to a single disk level and are asymptomatic. The congenitally fused segments tend to be short in the anteroposterior dimension.

Approximately one-third of patients with Klippel-Feil syndrome have *Sprengel deformity* (Fig. 5-24). Sprengel deformity is tethering of the scapula to the cervical spine by a fibrous band or an anomalous bone (*omovertebral bone*) that results in a high position of the scapula and reduced shoulder mobility.

Caudal Regression Syndrome

The *caudal regression syndrome* is a spectrum of caudal axial skeletal and associated neurologic and soft tissue defects caused by an insult to the caudal mesoderm and ectoderm early in the first trimester. A wide spectrum of spinal defects may result, ranging from subtle partial sacral agenesis to complete absence of the sacrum, lumbar spine, and caudal thoracic spine (Fig. 5-25). Other axial skeletal findings may include spina bifida, spinal stenosis, an angular, wedge shaped conus medullaris, and presacral (anterior) meningocele. Clinical findings also are highly varied, ranging from mild leg weakness to bowel and bladder control difficulties to anorectal atresia, renal aplasia, and pulmonary hypoplasia. Sagittal MR images reveal a characteristic angular contour of the malformed conus medullaris (Fig. 5-25B). The caudal regression syndrome is much more frequent in children of diabetic mothers, but most cases are sporadic. The association between the caudal regression syndrome and congenital fusion of the lower extremities (*sirenomelia,* Fig. 5-26) is controversial. They likely are unrelated conditions. Sirenomelia is associated with severe oligohydramnios. This condition is named after the mythical creatures called Sirens or Mermaids who, with their sweet songs, lured sailors to their deaths on rocky reefs and coastlines.

HIP DISORDERS

Developmental Dysplasia of the Hip (DDH)

Developmental dysplasia of the hip (DDH), congenital hip dislocation (CHD), and congenital dislocation of the hip (CDH) are terms that are often used interchangeably, although each term reflects different nuances of what may be thought of as a diverse group of abnormalities of the newborn and infant hip. These conditions have

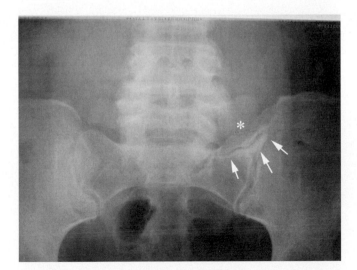

Fig. 5-21 Transitional lumbosacral segmentation. AP view of the lower lumbar spine shows wide transverse process of the lowest lumbar segment (*asterisk*), with a false joint formation with the sacrum. Note the sclerosis along this joint (*arrows*).

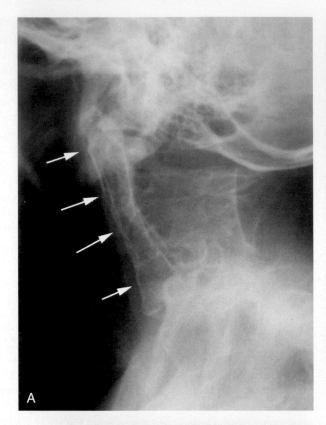

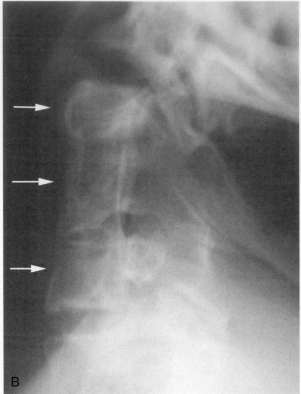

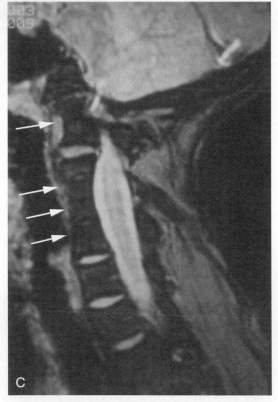

Fig. 5-22   Klippel-Feil. **A,** Lateral cervical spine radiograph shows absent segmentation of several cervical segments (*arrows*). **B, C,** Different patient with similar findings (*arrows*) on a lateral radiograph (*B*) and a sagittal T2-weighted MR image (*C*) (*arrows*).

Key Concepts	Developmental Dysplasia of the Hip

- Deformity and subluxation of the hip, usually developmental rather than congenital. Generally completely curable if diagnosed and treated early.
- Delayed diagnosis leads to loss of mobility, pain, and early osteoarthritis.
- Radiographs are of limited utility in neonates.
- Ultrasound is highly sensitive, but usually is best performed after age 4–6 weeks due to false positives in neonates.

in common hip dysplasia or dislocation at birth, or more frequently *the potential to develop dysplasia and possibly dislocation later in infancy and childhood.* True congenital hip dislocation is relatively infrequent. It may occur in association with severe congenital defects such as Chiari II malformation or arthrogryposis, in which case it is termed *teratogenic* or *pathologic dislocation.* Pathologic dislocations are usually readily detected at birth by physical examination and confirmed with radiographs. Congenital hip dislocation may also occur as an isolated abnormality in otherwise normal neonates due to severe hip laxity. The hip dislocation in such neonates may be intermittent, and easy to reduce and redislocate. An experienced clinician usually reliably detects this con-

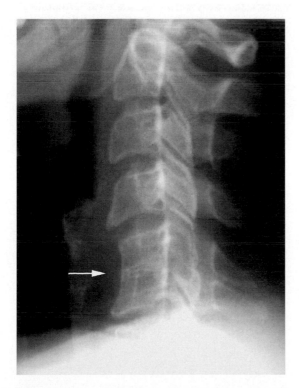

Fig. 5-23 Absent segmentation at C5–6 (*arrow*). Note the narrow anteroposterior dimension of the fused vertebral bodies, which distinguishes this finding from a mature surgical fusion.

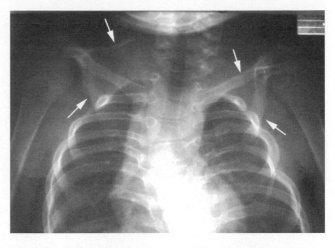

Fig. 5-24 Sprengel deformity. Compare the position of the scapulae (*arrows*), with the right higher than the left. Also note the upper thoracic spinal segmentation anomalies with associated scoliosis.

dition, but radiographs are occasionally of some use, for example, in excluding an underlying teratogenic condition. The most insidious and most frequent form of neonatal hip dysplasia is merely mild hip laxity and/or a shallow acetabulum at birth. This seemingly innocuous situation has the potential to progress over a period of months and years to significant hip dysplasia, hip dislocation, and early osteoarthritis. Because the initial abnormalities are so minimal, they may not be detected by physical examination or by radiographs. The term *developmental dysplasia of the hip* (DDH) is generally preferred to describe this progressive condition, as it emphasizes that dislocation was not present a birth.

DDH is a frequent condition (1:1000), and is bilateral in one third of cases. Several risk factors have been identified (Table 5-7). These include female gender (6:1, due to increased sensitivity to maternal hormones that relax ligaments), intrauterine positioning such as breech presentation that tends to lever the femoral head out of the acetabulum, and genetic and cultural factors. The left hip is more frequently affected, because the fetal spine is usually to the maternal left in a fetus in vertex presentation. This places the fetal left knee against the unyielding maternal spine, which tends to displace the left knee anteriorly relative to the mother and medially relative to the fetus and lever the femoral head out of the acetabulum. The practice in some cultures of papoosing infants with the hips adducted and extended increases the risk of DDH. (In contrast, the popular backpack-style child carriers promote healthy hip development because they hold the hips in flexion and abduction.)

The ligamentous laxity that initiates DDH results in abnormal femoral head mobility. The acetabulum adapts to the abnormal femoral head mobility by becoming wider and shallower ("acetabular dysplasia") as it at-

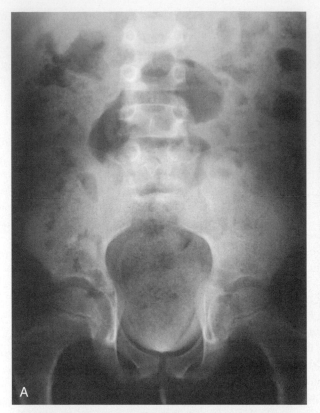

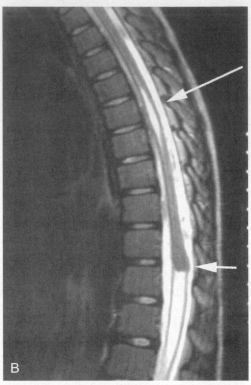

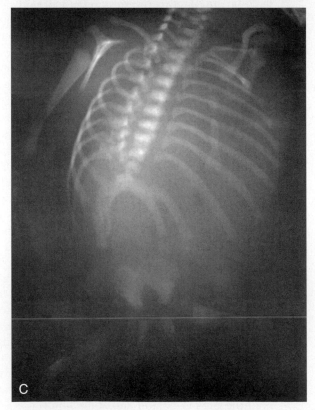

Fig. 5-25 Sacral Agenesis (caudal regression syndrome). **A,** This radiograph was obtained after an intravenous urogram (note the contrast in the bladder). Note the absence of the mid and lower sacrum. **B,** Sagittal T2-weighted MR image shows the characteristic angular contour of the conus medullaris (*short arrow*). Also note the syrinx (*long arrow*), a finding that can occur in association with caudal regression. **C,** Severe case. Note the complete absence of the lumbar spine and sacrum.

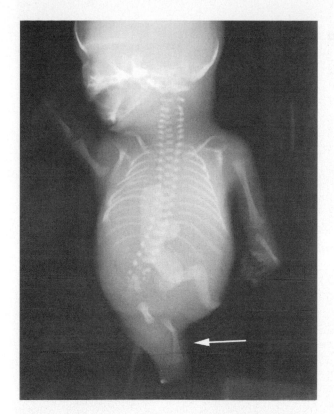

Fig. 5-26   Sirenomelia. Note the fused, dysplastic lower extremities (*arrow*).

tempts to accommodate the abnormal range of motion of the femoral head. A vicious cycle may ensue of worsening ligamentous laxity, femoral head subluxation, and acetabular dysplasia. Muscle pull and weight bearing tend to direct the femoral head out of the acetabulum in a superior and lateral direction. In advanced cases, the femoral head dislocates completely and flattens along its superomedial margin as it abuts the lateral aspect of the ilium.

A variety of soft tissue changes may occur in chronic hip subluxation that can impede or completely block hip reduction (Fig. 5-27). Fibrofatty tissue, termed *pulvinar,* can fill the acetabulum. The acetabular labrum may flip inferiorly against the medial margin of the subluxed femoral head, termed an *inverted limbus.* A tight psoas tendon may stretch across the hip joint medial to the laterally displaced femoral head, resulting in an hourglass configuration of the joint capsule. The adductor muscles also are shortened by the superior migration of the femoral head. The ligamentum teres, which extends from the femoral head to the center of the acetabulum, becomes elongated and redundant.

Superior femoral head migration is eventually halted by tightening of the surrounding connective tissues, which helps to alleviate the hip instability but with loss of hip joint mobility. A broad shallow depression can develop in the lateral ilium adjacent to the dislocated femoral head, termed a *pseudoacetabulum,* as the body attempts to adapt to the abnormal position of the femoral head and form a stable hip joint (Fig. 5-28). Pain and early osteoarthritis are late complications, even in com-

Table 5-7   Risk factors for developmental dysplasia of the hip (DDH)

MECHANICAL (IN UTERO "PACKAGING PROBLEMS")

Breech
Oligohydramnios
First born ("unstretched" uterus)
Large birth weight

GENETICS

Females
Family history
Native Americans (may be entirely cultural)
Caucasian

CULTURAL: PAPOOSING, SWADDLING

Native Americans
Lapps

MUSCULOSKELETAL ASSOCIATIONS

Contralateral DDH
Torticollis
Scoliosis
Ehlers-Danlos (generalized joint laxity)
Neuromuscular imbalance (e.g., cerebral palsy)

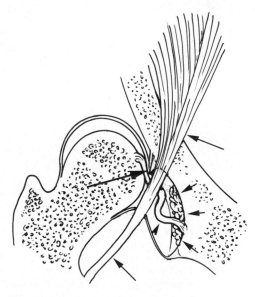

Fig. 5-27   Chronic hip subluxation: associated soft tissue changes. Pulvinar (*short arrows*). Elongated ligamentum teres (*arrowhead*). Labrum flipped medially ("inverted limbus," *large long arrow*). Tight psoas tendon stretched across the anterior joint capsule (*small long arrows*).

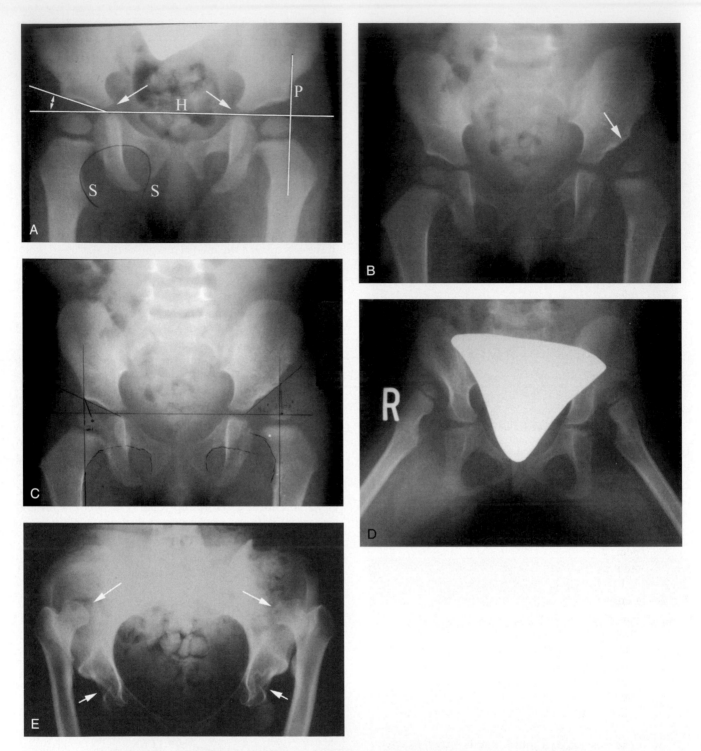

Fig. 5-28 Radiography of DDH. **A,** Normal hips. H = Hilgenreinner's line, P = Perkin's line, S = Shenton's arc (arc drawn in black). Arrows mark the triradiate cartilages. Double arrow marks the acetabular angle (acetabular index). Note that the femoral heads are symmetric in size and are nearly completely covered by the acetabular roofs. The acetabular angle is less than 30°. **B,** Left DDH. Note the shallow acetabular roof, early pseudoacetabulum (*arrow*), superolateral subluxation of the left femoral head, and small size of the left femoral epiphysis compared with the normal right side. **C,** Same radiograph as B, after review by an orthopedic surgeon. The lines listed in **A** have been marked on the film, as well as the center-edge angle. The normal right acetabular angle is 24°. The dysplastic left hip acetabular angle is 42°. The right center-edge angle is 21° (normal), and the left is −3°. Also note the discontinuity of Shenton's arc on the left. **D,** Bilateral hip dislocations in a child with cerebral palsy. **E,** Untreated DDH: late sequellae. 35-year-old woman with bilateral, severe, untreated DDH. Note the superior bilateral femoral head dislocations (*long arrows*). Also note the dysplastic acetabula (*short arrows*). This patient was able to ambulate, but was developing progressive hip pain that required bilateral hip arthroplasties.

paratively mild cases. Hip replacement surgery may be required as early as the fourth decade.

Imaging of DDH   Radiographs and ultrasound are the cornerstones of imaging of DDH. Ultrasound is ideally suited to assessment of the neonatal hip because it provides excellent visualization of the cartilaginous femoral head without exposure to ionizing radiation, and it allows for dynamic assessment of hip joint stability. Radiographs are of limited value in the newborn period because the capital femoral epiphyses are not ossified at birth. In infants older than about 3 months of age, the capital femoral epiphyses begin to ossify and both techniques are useful. After about 6 months of age, shadowing from the increasing ossification of the capital femoral epiphyses obscures the acetabulum and limits the role of ultrasound to selected cases. Arthrography, CT, and MRI can be highly useful in specific situations that are discussed below.

Radiography   Radiographic evaluation of DDH requires a well-positioned anteroposterior radiograph (Fig. 5-28). The symphysis pubis and coccyx should be superimposed or very nearly superimposed on a properly positioned AP radiograph (assuming that neither is deformed). A series of lines and curves are drawn on the radiograph as part of the assessment of DDH. *Hilgenreiner's line* (think "H for horizontal," also called the Y-Y line) is drawn horizontally through the center or top of the bilateral radiolucent triradiate cartilages. The triradiate cartilage marks the center of the acetabulum. It is formed by cartilage of the three bones that comprise the pelvis, hence its name. *Perkins' line* is drawn perpendicular to Hilgenreiner's line (think "P for perpendicular") through the superolateral corner of the acetabular roof. The ossified portion of the capital femoral epiphysis should be entirely or nearly entirely medial to this line. Compare each side. A difference in acetabular coverage of the ossified portion of the femoral heads by as little as 2–3 mm is considered by some authors to be significant. Lateral femoral head subluxation may also be quantified by measuring the *center-edge angle* that is formed by Perkins' line and a line drawn through anterior inferior iliac spine and the center of the capital femoral epiphysis. A normal center edge-angle is about 20° in infancy and 26°–30° in adolescence. A fourth line is drawn between the triradiate cartilage and the anterior inferior iliac spine of each hip. The angle formed by this line and Hilgenreiner's line is the *acetabular angle* or *acetabular index*. A *useful rule of thumb is that the acetabular angle should be 30° or less.* The reader should note that 30° is a useful oversimplification. In fact, the acetabular angle normally decreases with increasing age, and, on average, is about 2° greater in normal girls than boys. Also note that a nearly horizontal acetabular roof is abnormal. A nearly horizontal acetabular roof is seen in several syndromes and skeletal dysplasias, and is further discussed later in

this chapter. *Shenton's arc* is drawn along the medial and superior obturator foramen and medial-proximal femur. This arc is interrupted or elongated if the femoral head is subluxed. Finally, some hips with DDH have a smaller ossified capital femoral epiphysis on the affected side. This is a nonspecific finding, as some asymmetry may be normal.

Limitations of radiography in DDH include limited assessment of the hips of neonates because the capital femoral epiphyses are not ossified at birth, potential for incorrect acetabular angle measurements if the radiograph is improperly positioned, static rather than dynamic imaging, and the use of ionizing radiation.

Ultrasound   The initial application of ultrasound to infants with DDH emphasized static coronal imaging, simulating an anteroposterior radiograph. An elaborate system of measurements and categories was developed, termed the Graf system in honor of the Austrian orthopedic surgeon Reinhard Graf, M.D., who developed this approach. The subsequent application of real time sonography by the American radiologist H. Theodore Harcke, M.D., and others pioneered the dynamic assessment of hip stability. Posteriorly oriented stress, similar to the Barlow maneuver used in screening newborns for hip dislocation, can detect hip laxity in infants with a subluxable or a dislocatable hip that might be normally located on static images. Current practice of hip ultrasound incorporates features of both approaches (Figs. 5-29 and 5-30), although some institutions prefer to emphasize the detailed morphologic assessment of the Graf system, while others emphasize the dynamic assessment of hip stability. An overview of a popular hybrid approach is described in Appendix 2.

Regardless of the radiologist's preferred technique, complete sonographic assessment of the infant hip always includes documentation of the position of the femoral head relative to the acetabulum, the contour of the acetabular roof, hip stability, and the alpha angle. The osseous portion of the acetabular roof should cover at least half of the cartilaginous femoral head. The contour of the osseous acetabular roof should be straight or gently concave, matching the contour of the cartilaginous femoral head. The cortex of the roof of the acetabulum and the lateral ilium should meet at a sharp angle that is not rounded. The angle formed by the acetabular roof and the lateral ilium is the *alpha angle* (Fig. 5-29D). *A normal alpha angle is 60 degrees or greater,* although lower values as low as 55° may be accepted in newborns if no other findings to suggest DDH are present. The *beta angle,* a component of the Graf system, is the angle formed by the osseous acetabular roof and the inferior surface of the labrum (Fig. 5-29D). A normal beta angle is roughly ≤55°. If the femoral head is subluxed laterally, the beta angle will be greater than 55°. The beta angle

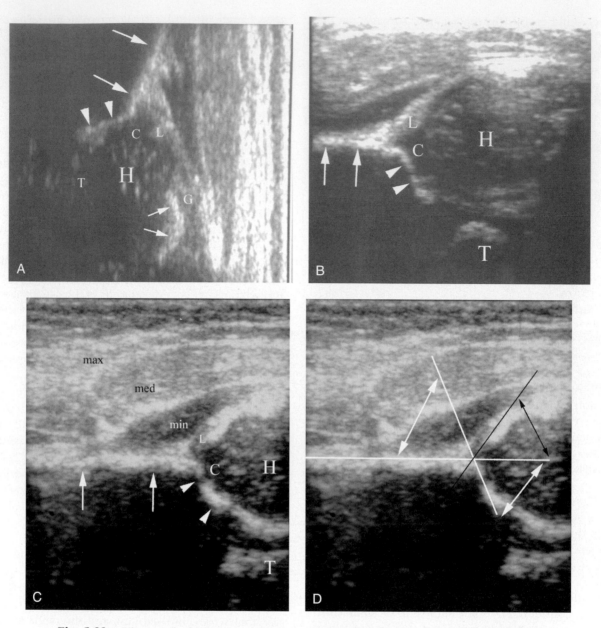

Fig. 5-29   Ultrasound of DDH: Coronal images. **A,** Coronal image of the left hip oriented to simulate an AP radiograph. The lateral margin of the ilium (*large arrows*) is seen as an echogenic line with posterior acoustic shadowing. Note the osseous roof of the acetabulum (*arrowheads*), the unossified (cartilaginous) portion of the acetabular roof (*C*), and adjacent hyperechoic labrum (L), and the cartilaginous femoral head (*H*). The hypoechoic triradiate cartilage (*T*) is located at the center of the acetabulum. This image was obtained with the hip extended; note the lateral margin of the ossified portion of the proximal femur (*small arrows*) and a portion of the cartilaginous greater tuberosity (*G*). **B, C,** Normal standard coronal image (two different infants). Superior is to the viewer's left and lateral is towards the transducer. The transducer has been positioned to display the lateral margin of the ilium as a straight line parallel to the transducer (*long arrows*), with the center of the cartilagenous femoral head (*H*) and the triradiate cartilage (*T*) toward the right side of the image. Note that the osseous portion of the acetabular roof (*arrowheads*), which is straight in **B** and slightly concave in **C**, covers at least 50% of the femoral head (just barely in **A**). Note the hypoechoic cartilaginous acetabular roof (*C*) and the echogenic laburm and capsule (*L*). Also note the overlying muscle layers, labeled in **C**: gluteus maximus (max), gluteus medius (med), and gluteus minimus (min). **D,** Alpha and beta angles. Same image as **C.** The alpha angle is formed by the osseous acetabular roof and the lateral ilium (*white lines and arrows*). The beta angle is formed by the lateral ilium and the inferior surface of the labrum (*black line, black arrows*). The beta angle is not widely used.

Continued

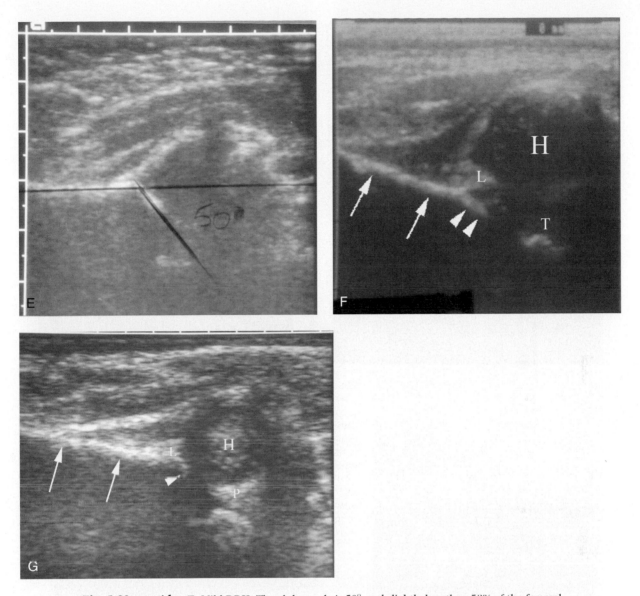

Fig. 5-29, cont'd   E, Mild DDH. The alpha angle is 50°, and slightly less than 50% of the femoral head is covered by the acetabulum. **F, G,** Severe DDH (different infants). In both cases, the humeral head (*H*) is subluxed superiorly and laterally (i.e., towards the transducer). Note the very shallow angle formed by the ilium (*arrows*) and the steep osseous acetabular roof (*arrowheads*). **F,** demonstrates an inverted limbus (*L*): the echogenic capsule and labrum are interposed between the femoral head and the acetabulum (*T,* triradiate cartilage). **G,** demonstrates pulvinar (*P*) as echogenic tissue filling the acetabulum medial to the femoral head (*H*).

is not routinely measured unless the complete Graf system is used.

Limitations of ultrasound include operator dependence, limited visualization of the acetabulum in older infants due to shadowing from the ossifying capital femoral epiphysis, and potential for false positive examinations in the immediate neonatal period. The latter is due to transient, physiologic hip ligamentous laxity in neonates caused by residual maternal hormonal effects. False positive neonatal scans can result in unnecessary follow-up examinations and over treatment. Therefore, it is generally recommended that the first ultrasound examination be delayed until the child is 4 to 6 weeks old in order to avoid such false positive examinations. However, if clinical findings are suggestive of a dislocated or unstable hip, then earlier ultrasound may be appropriate.

Other modalities: Arthrography, MRI and CT Arthrography and MRI allow visualization of the

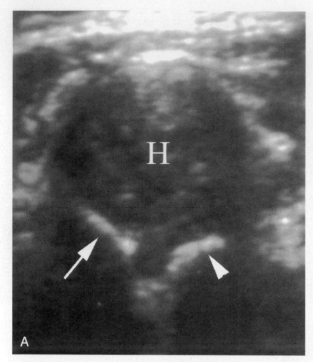

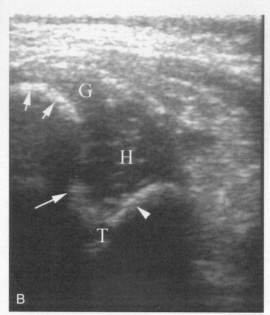

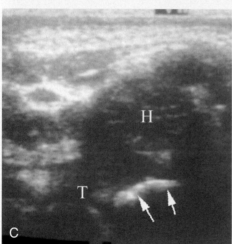

Fig. 5-30 Ultrasound of DDH: Axial images. **A, B,** Normal axial image (two different infants). The transducer is positioned to display the center of the femoral head (*H*) centered over the triradiate cartilage (*T*), between the pubis anteriorly (*arrow*) and the ischium posteriorly (*arrowhead*). **B,** was obtained approximately parallel to the flexed femur; note the cartilaginous apophysis of the greater tuberosity (*G*) and the ossified portion of the proximal femur (*short arrows*). **C,** Severe DDH, oblique axial image. The transducer was angled to include the triradiate cartilage (*T*) at the center of the acetabulum, and the subluxed femoral head (*H*). The femoral head is subluxed superiorly, laterally, and posteriorly over the ilium (*arrows*).

femoral head, acetabular cartilage, and potential soft tissue impediments to reduction such as pulvinar, inverted limbus, tight psoas tendon, and redundant ligamentum teres. Arthrography is usually performed by an orthopedic surgeon at the time of reduction of a chronically subluxed or dislocated hip (Fig. 5-31). CT is often used to determine whether reduction with casting has successfully aligned the femoral head and acetabulum (Fig. 5-32). Low dose technique should be used in this setting by obtaining only 4 or 5 slices with a low mA technique (30 mAs). Ultrasound and MRI may also be used to document hip joint alignment in this setting (Fig. 5-32C). In addition, gadolinium enhanced MRI and possibly ultrasound may also allow

assessment of the integrity of the femoral head blood supply after closed reduction. This is not a trivial matter, as AVN of the femoral head is an infrequent but potentially catastrophic complication of hip reduction with casting. Early identification of femoral head ischemia allows this complication to be avoided. Finally, CT with 3-dimensional reconstruction can be used to assist the orthopedic surgeon in assessing the shape of a dysplastic acetabulum before surgical modification of the acetabulum (acetabuloplasty, see discussion below).

Management of DDH Management of DDH depends on the age of the patient and the severity of the dysplasia. Very mild dysplasia may resolve spontaneously. A harness

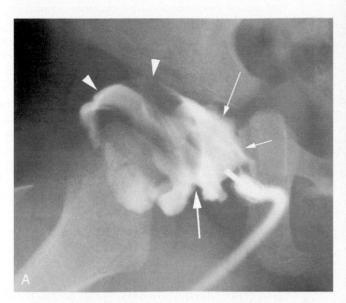

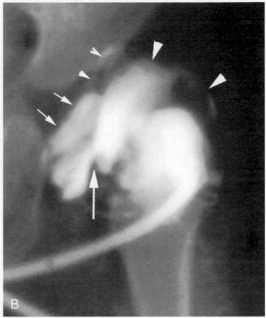

Fig. 5-31 DDH: arthrography. Compare to Figure 5-27. **A, B,** Both studies show the radiolucent cartilaginous femoral head (*arrowheads*), filling defect from pulvinar (*small arrows*) and hourglass shape of the capsule (*large arrow*). **B,** also shows an inverted limbus (*small arrowheads*).

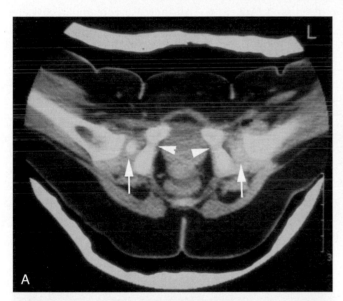

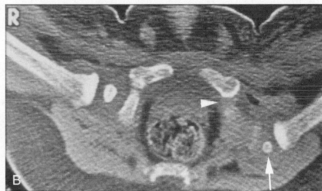

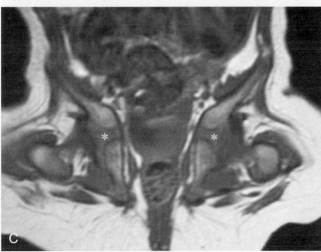

Fig. 5-32 DDH: imaging after reduction and casting. **A,** Good reduction of left DDH. Axial CT through the hip joints shows both femoral heads (*arrows*) to be adjacent to the triradiate cartilages (*arrowheads*). The left capital femoral epiphysis ossification center is smaller than the normal right side, a frequent finding in DDH. **B,** Poor reduction of left DDH. The left femoral head (*arrow*) is subluxed posteriorly relative to the triradiate cartilage (*arrowhead*). The right hip is normal. **C,** Poor reduction of bilateral DDH. Coronal T1-weighted MR image through the triradiate cartilages (*asterisks*) should also show both femoral heads, but neither is seen. Axial images (not shown) revealed both femoral heads to be posteriorly dislocated.

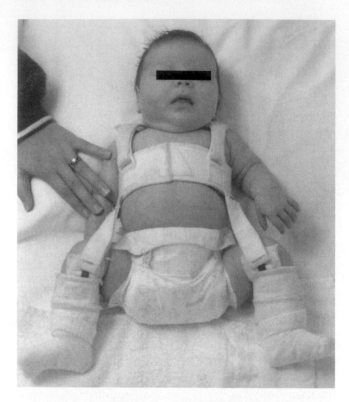

Fig. 5-33   Pavlik harness.

that holds the hips in flexion, mild abduction, and mild external rotation may be used (Pavlik Harness, Fig. 5-33). This position keeps the femoral head within the center of the acetabulum, allowing healthy acetabular growth. The infants and their parents tolerate this treatment well, and follow-up ultrasound scans can be obtained with the harness in place. After a few months, the acetabulum will deepen and the hip joint capsule will tighten (Fig. 5-34). No further intervention will be needed.

Advanced dysplasia in older children requires aggressive therapy, and a completely normal outcome is often impossible. The main goal of the orthopedic surgeon is to return the femoral head to the center of the acetabulum and keep it there with a brace, cast, or surgical modification of the femoral neck and/or acetabulum. Closed reduction may be combined with casting or skeletal traction. Soft-tissue impediments to closed reduction may require correction, including releasing tight adductor or psoas tendons. *Varus osteotomy* of the proximal femur, that is, an osteotomy of the proximal shaft that produces varus alignment of the femoral neck, tends to enhance hip reduction and stability. Excessive femoral anteversion is a frequent complication of advanced DDH. Anteversion is defined and discussed further in the section on torsion at the end of this chapter. A "derotation osteotomy," also performed through the proximal femoral shaft, corrects excessive femoral anteversion and results in better containment of the femoral head within the acetabulum. These procedures are frequently combined (*varus derotation osteotomy,* VDRO; Fig. 5-35). A variety of surgical modifications of the acetabulum have been developed (Fig. 5-36). All increase acetabular coverage of the femoral head and are used variably, depending on the patient age, morphology of the acetabulum, and preference of the surgeon.

Proximal Focal Femoral Deficiency

Proximal focal femoral deficiency (PFFD) refers to a spectrum of congenital hypoplasia or aplasia (deficiency) of the proximal femur (Fig. 5-37). PFFD may be bilateral. Curiously, the abnormalities in PFFD tend to be centered roughly at the intertrochanteric femur. Mild cases have only hypoplasia of a short segment of intertrochanteric

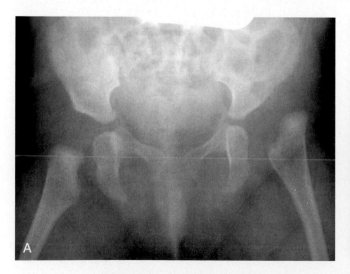
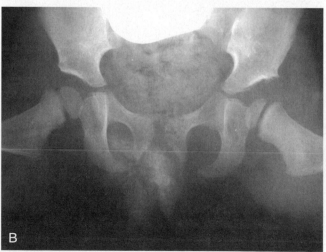

Fig. 5-34   Successful treatment with a Pavlik harness. **A,** Radiograph during the first week of life shows a left hip dislocation and shallow left acetabulum. The right is normal. **B,** Radiograph at approximately age 8 months shows near-normal left hip.

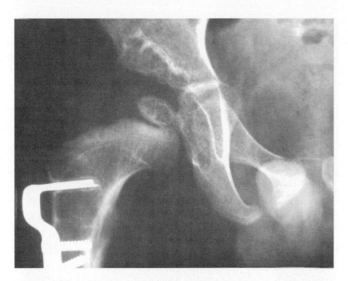

Fig. 5-35 Varus derotation osteotomy (VDRO). A blade plate and screws (not completely shown) were used to fix the varus producing osteotomy.

femur, with a normal femoral head and hip joint. The hypoplastic segment may be composed of uncalcified cartilage or bone. More severe cases have hypoplasia of the femoral head with resulting acetabular dysplasia, or absence of the proximal femoral shaft, resulting in a gap (deficiency) in the femur between the head and shaft with overall femoral shortening. The most severe cases of PFFD involve absence of nearly the entire femur (Fig. 5-37C). Sonography and MRI can assist in characterizing the femoral deficiency and the status of the hip joint. Associated abnormalities include congenital absence of

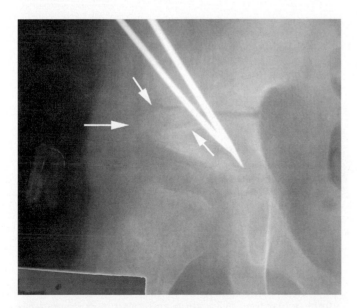

Fig. 5-36 Salter osteotomy for DDH. An osteotomy has been performed through the innominate bone and a wedge opened and fixed with a bone plug (*arrows*), resulting in a more horizontal alignment of the acetabular roof.

the ipsilateral fibula and foot deformities. Most cases are evident at birth because the affected leg is short. The goal of treatment is to maximize function of the affected limb. Mild cases do not benefit from surgery.

Coxa Vara and Coxa Valga

The angle formed by the femoral neck and shaft is normally 150° at birth. This angle decreases throughout development to reach an average angle of about 125° in normal adults. Increase in this angle is coxa valga, and decrease is coxa vara.

Coxa vara in children may be divided into congenital, infantile, and acquired forms. *Congenital coxa vara* likely results from a limb bud insult in the first trimester of gestation. In this manner it is similar to proximal focal femoral deficiency and both may occur in the same patient. Congenital coxa vara tends to worsen little, if at all, after birth (Fig. 5-38). In contrast, *infantile coxa vara* (also termed developmental coxa vara) progresses as the child grows, with resulting limb length discrepancy. Infantile coxa vara is often bilateral (up to 50%), but otherwise usually occurs as an isolated abnormality. Surgery is often required to manage this progressive condition. *Acquired coxa vara* may be caused by trauma to the proximal femoral physis, notably slipped capital femoral epiphysis, metabolic conditions that cause bone softening, notably rickets and osteomalacia, and tumors, skeletal dysplasias, and fibrous dysplasia and Paget's disease in adults.

Coxa valga in children usually reflects decreased tone of the muscles that cross the hip and decreased ambulation. Neuromuscular conditions such as cerebral palsy are the most frequent cause of coxa valga (Fig. 5-39).

Primary Protrusio of the Acetabulum (Otto Pelvis)

Protrusio acetabuli is abnormal medial position of the femoral head compared to the pelvis. Protrusio acetabuli is present if the medial margin of the femoral head touches or crosses a line connecting the lateral margins of the pelvic inlet and the obturator foramen on an AP radiograph of the pelvis (Fig. 5-40). Unilateral or bilateral protrusio acetabuli can occur *secondary to* RA and rheumatoid variants, OA, Turner's syndrome, pelvic fracture, and "bone softening" conditions such as Paget's disease, fibrous dysplasia, osteomalacia, and renal osteodystrophy.

In contrast, *primary protrusio of the acetabulum* (Otto pelvis) refers to severe bilateral protrusio acetabuli that appears to occur as a developmental malformation (Fig. 5-41). The cause is unknown, but abnormal acetabular remodeling appears to contribute. Otto pelvis is more frequent in women and is often familial. It may not be discovered until adulthood. Complications include pain,

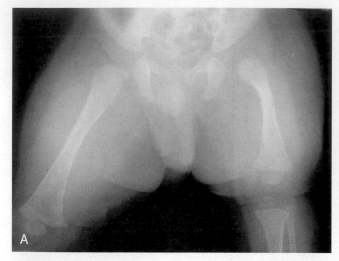

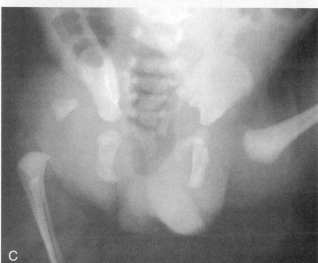

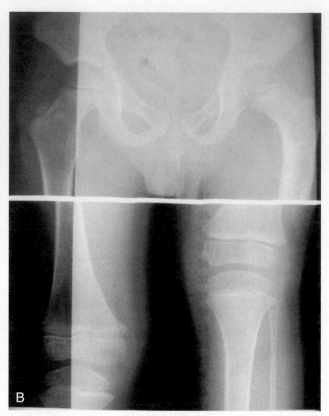

Fig. 5-37   Proximal focal femoral deficiency: spectrum of abnormalities. **A,** Mild case in a 2-month-old. Note the normal left acetabulum, which indicates that the femoral head is present. **B,** Same patient at age 4 years. The proximal femur has ossified but is short and dysplastic. **C,** Severe case with presence only of the most distal right femur. Note the shallow acetabulum, which indicates that there is no right femoral head.

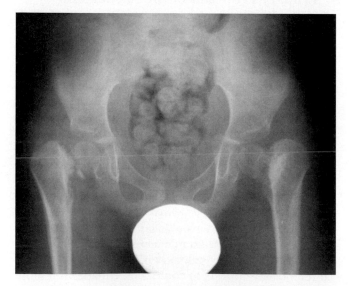

Fig. 5-38   Congential coxa vara. The findings in this 4-year-old were unchanged from birth.

decreased range of motion, secondary OA, and, when severe, interference with childbirth.

CONNECTIVE TISSUE DISORDERS

Marfan syndrome is a connective tissue defect of unknown cause, possibly due to abnormal cross-linking of collagen fibers. Patients with Marfan syndrome are tall and have disproportionate lengthening of the distal aspects of the extremities (arachnodactyly; Fig. 5-42). Skeletal manifestations include kyphoscoliosis, joint hypermobility, early OA, protrusio acetabuli, spondylolysis of L5, posterior scalloping of the vertebral bodies due to dural ectasia, and pectus excavatum. Bone mineral density is normal. Important extraosseous complications include ocular lens dislocation and cystic medial necrosis of the proximal ascending aorta and pulmonary artery. The cardiovascular lesions may lead to aortic dissection or rupture, or to aortic or pulmonic valve insufficiency.

| Key Concepts | Connective Tissue Disorders |

- Marfan syndrome: unknown defect, autosomal dominant with variable expression that causes abnormal collagen. Findings include arachnodactyly, scoliosis, posterior vertebral body scalloping, lens dislocations, ascending aorta dissection, aortic and pulmonic valve insufficiency.
- Homocystinuria: an autosomal recessive inborn error of metabolism that causes abnormal collagen. Findings are similar to Marfan syndrome, but also with osteoporosis and fractures.
- Ehlers-Danlos syndrome: family of clinically similar, mostly autosomal dominant conditions with marked skin and joint laxity, and easy bleeding. Ehlers-Danlos syndrome shares many features in common with Marfan syndrome and homocystinuria, but also with phlebolith-like subcutaneous calcifications, especially in the shins and forearms, due to subcutaneous hemorrhages.

Marfan syndrome is an autosomal dominant disorder with high penetrance but variable expression. Spontaneous mutations account for a minority of cases.

Homocystinuria is an autosomal recessive condition caused by an inborn error in metabolism (cystathionine synthetase deficiency) that leads to accumulation of homocystine in the serum and urine and causes defective collagen synthesis. Many of the morphologic and radiographic features of homocystinuria resemble those seen in Marfan syndrome. Both conditions are associated with scoliosis, posterior vertebral body scalloping, pectus ex-

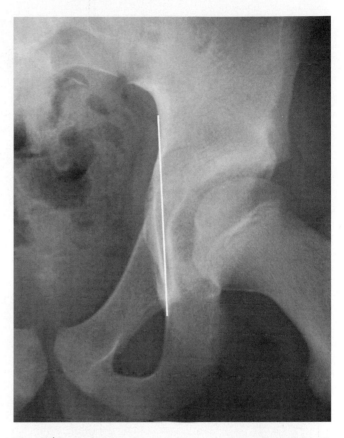

Fig. 5-40 Reference line for diagnosis of protrusio acetabuli. The femoral head should not touch or cross the line drawn between the lateral margins of the pelvic inlet and the obturator foramen. This example is normal.

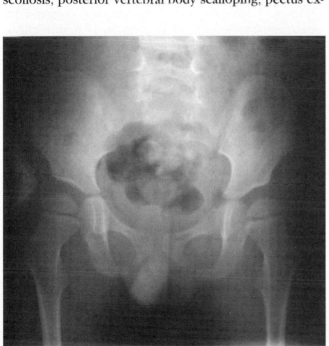

Fig. 5-39 Bilateral coxa valga.

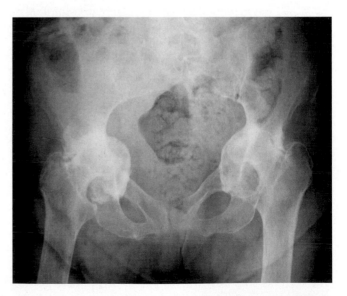

Fig. 5-41 Primary protrusio of the acetabulum (Otto Pelvis) in an adult with bilateral secondary osteoarthritis.

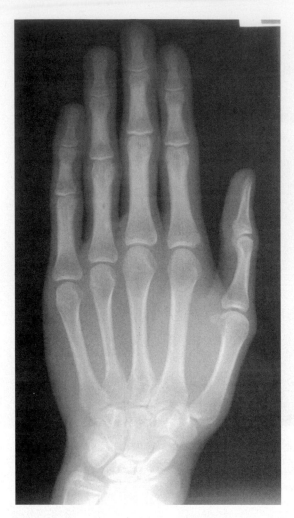

Fig. 5-42   Marfan syndrome. Note the long, slender fingers (arachnodactyly).

cavatum, and arachnodactyly (uniformly present in Marfan syndrome, variably present in homocystinuria). However, patients with homocystinuria have osteopenia with associated vertebral compression fractures, which are not typical features of Marfan syndrome. In addition, patients with homocystinuria also suffer from mental retardation, seizures, and joint contractures, which are not usual clinical features of Marfan syndrome.

Ehlers-Danlos Syndrome is a spectrum of mostly autosomal dominant familial conditions each caused by a defect in collagen synthesis, that have in common exceptionally lax skin that is easily injured and heals poorly, hypermobile joints that are prone to contractures in old age, and easy bleeding due to fragile blood vessels. Musculoskeletal features overlap with those seen in Marfan syndrome and homocystinuria. Kyphoscoliosis, posterior vertebral scalloping, arachnodactyly, and spondylolysis are seen, as well as marked joint hypermobility leading to dislocations, flat feet, and early OA. Hemarthroses may occur after minimal trauma. The great vessels are prone

to aneurysm, dissection, and tortuosity. Angiography is dangerous owing to the fragility of the vessels. Patients with Ehlers-Danlos syndrome are vulnerable to subcutaneous bleeding and fat necrosis from minimal trauma, resulting in phlebolith-like subcutaneous calcifications, especially in the forearms and shins. The presence of such calcifications combined with a history of skin hyperelasticity help to make the diagnosis of Ehlers-Danlos syndrome.

NEUROFIBROMATOSIS

The large majority of patients with *neurofibromatosis type 1* (NF1, von Recklinhausen disease) have skeletal involvement (Fig. 5-43) in addition to the characteristic central and peripheral neurologic findings. The skeletal findings are largely due to a diffuse mesodermal dysplasia, although extrinsic compression by a neurofibroma may also cause bone deformity. Perhaps the most important skeletal manifestation of NF1 is scoliosis (Fig. 5-13). Scoliosis in NF1 may resemble idiopathic scoliosis, but may also present as a short segment, sharply angulated thoracic kyphoscoliosis most frequently centered at T3 to T7. These focal thoracic curves are prone to rapid progression and instability that can result in paralysis. Thus, scoliosis in a patient with neurofibromatosis should be closely monitored. Other spinal abnormalities seen in neurofibromatosis include enlarged neural foramina and posterior vertebral body scalloping due to dural ectasia (Fig. 5-43C). Cranial abnormalities include hypoplastic or absent cranial bones (sphenoid wing, posterosuperior orbital wall, mastoid), macrocranium, and enlarged cranial neural foramina due to neurofibromas. Anterior distal tibial bowing, often with pseudarthrosis that may develop characteristic tapered margins may be seen at birth or develop during childhood (Fig. 5-43, Tables 5-8 and 5-9). These pseudarthroses are frequently resistant to healing despite orthopedic fixation, and a short leg can result (Fig. 5-8). Multiple nonossifying fibromas may be present. In fact, a finding of multiple nonossifying fibromas in any patient should suggest the diagnosis of neurofibromatosis. Twisted, narrow, irregular "ribbon ribs" reflect the mesodermal dysplasia more frequently than extrinsic compression from adjacent neurofibromas. The plexiform neurofibromas found in NF 1 often reveal a "target sign" appearance on T2-weighted MRI, with low signal intensity centrally and high signal intensity peripherally (Fig. 1-71).

Skeletal manifestations are prominent in phakomatoses other than NF. The findings of Klippel-Trenaunay-Weber syndrome are discussed below with focal gigantism. Tuberous sclerosis causes patchy bone sclerosis and cystlike changes in the bones of the hands and feet. Gorlin syndrome (basal cell nevus syndrome) of basal

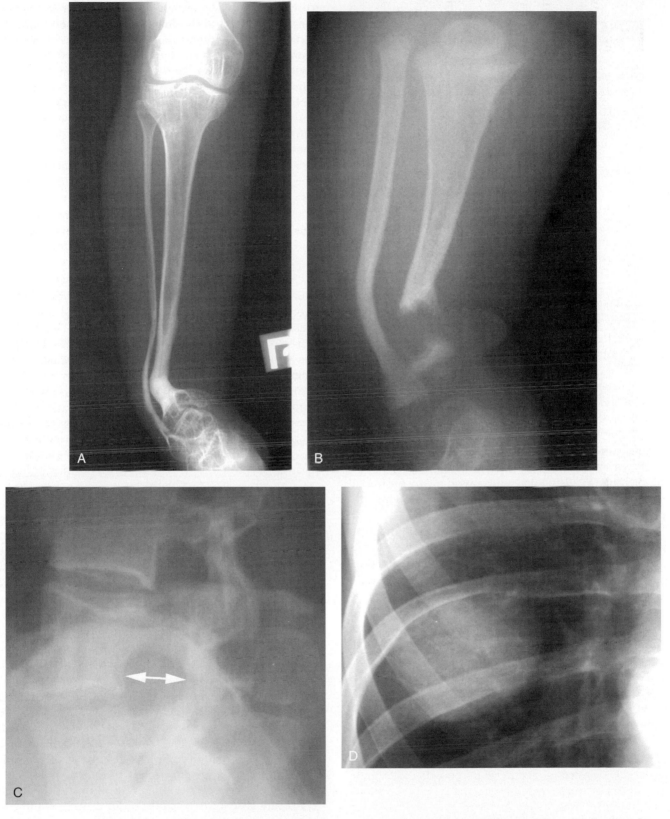

Fig. 5-43   Neurofibromatosis type 1. **A,** Tibial bowing. Note the characteristic anterolateral curve of the distal tibia and fibula. **B,** Distal tibial pseudarthrosis. **C,** Dural ectasia with posterior vertebral body scalloping and wide neural foramina (*arrow*). **D,** Pressure erosion of a rib due to a neurofibroma.

Table 5-8 Bowed long bones in children: common causes

MULTIPLE BONES

Rickets
Osteogenesis imperfecta

LOCALIZED

Trauma (plastic bowing type fracture)
Posttraumatic
Madclung's deformity (radius)
Neurofibromatosis

cell carcinomas and palmar skin pits also causes mandible cysts, patchy and bone-island-like bone sclerosis, and scoliosis.

CHROMOSOMAL ABNORMALITIES

Skeletal manifestations of *trisomy 21* (Down Syndrome, Fig. 5-44) include numerous cervical spine anomalies, most importantly atlantoaxial subluxation in 10%–20%. The posterior arch of C1 is often hypoplastic. Other skeletal abnormalities may include 11 rib pairs, two manubrial ossification centers rather than the normal single ossification center, short tubular bones of the hands and fingers with *clinodactyly* (abnormal angulation of a finger in the coronal plane) due to a short and broad fifth finger middle phalanx, flared iliac wings with nearly horizontal acetabular roofs, hip dysplasia, patellar dislocations, and a variety of foot anomalies.

Trisomy 18 results in abnormalities of multiple organ systems, notably severe congenital heart disease. Characteristic skeletal manifestations that may be detected on prenatal US include rocker bottom feet and a clenched hand with an adducted thumb and a short first metacarpal. Postnatal radiographic findings also include hypoplasia of the mandible and maxilla, and 11 rib pairs with thin, hypoplastic ribs. The fingers are in ulnar deviation. Stippled epiphyses may be seen. Survival beyond one year is unusual.

Turner Syndrome (45X0, deletion of one X chromosome) is associated with short stature, webbed neck, and abnormalities of many organ systems including congeni-

Table 5-9 Pseudoarthrosis

Fracture nonunion
Fibrous dysplasia
Neurofibromatosis (especially tibia)
Osteogenesis imperfecta
Congenital (clavicle, tibia)

tal heart disease, horseshoe kidney, and streak ovaries. The most characteristic skeletal findings are short fourth metacarpals (a finding that is also seen in pseudohypoparathyroidism and pseudopseudohypoparathyroidism), depression of the medial tibial plateau, tarsal coalitions, diffuse osteopenia, and Madelung deformity.

Madelung deformity (Fig. 5-45) is caused by distal radius bowing that displaces the distal radius in a volar and ulnar direction. The radial curvature effectively shortens the radius when compared to the ulna, and the articular surface of the radius is oriented abnormally medially. The ulna is often dorsally dislocated. Madelung deformity also can be seen as a consequence of previous trauma or growth disturbance caused by multiple osteochondromas or enchondromas, as part of the rare skeletal dysplasia dyschondrosteosis (discussed below), and as a sporadic finding.

SKELETAL DYSPLASIAS

Dozens of distinct skeletal dysplasias, or more precisely *osteochondrodysplasias*, have been identified. These are constitutional diseases of bones, caused by errors in bone formation and/or remodeling. This section emphasizes many of the more common or distinctive skeletal dysplasias, and includes a limited review of the more esoteric topics of dwarfism and the storage diseases.

Cleidocranial Dysplasia

Cleidocranial dysplasia (cleidocranial dysostosis, pelvicocleidocranial dysplasia) results from abnormal development of membranous bones. This condition is inherited in an autosomal dominant pattern, with about one-third of cases due to spontaneous mutations. Clinical and radiographic manifestations are often evident at birth. Clinical manifestations include a small face, wide head with hypertelorism, and generalized joint laxity. After the newborn period, dental dysplasia (too many or too few teeth, abnormal teeth), drooping shoulders, and an abnormal gait may become evident. Radiographic findings reflect the abnormal development of membranous bone (Fig. 5-46). These may include delayed closure of the cranial sutures and fontenelles including a persistent metopic suture, wormian bones (sutural ossicles, Fig. 5-46D), and partial or complete absence of the clavicle with occasional apparent pseudarthroses due to discontinuous ossification. The middle third of the clavicle is classically absent, as that portion of clavicle is thought to be formed by intramembranous ossification (Fig. 5-46A). However, it is the lateral third of the clavicle that is often absent, a finding that may simulate other causes of an absent distal clavicle (Table 5-10). Coxa vara due

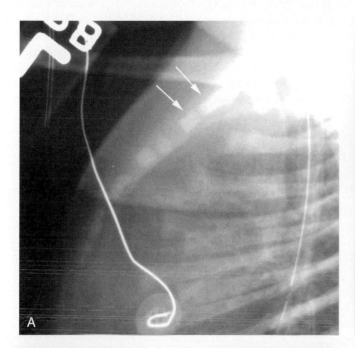

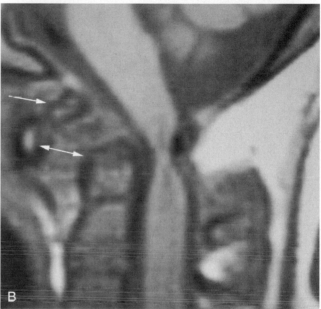

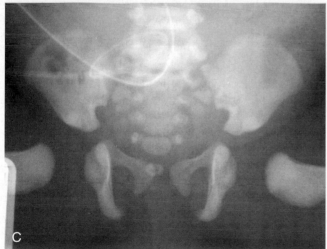

Fig. 5-44   Trisomy 21. **A,** Lateral sternum shows multiple ossification centers, including two manubrial ossification centers (*arrows*). **B,** Atlantoaxial subluxation. Sagittal T1-weighted MR image obtained with voluntary neck flexion shows severe cord compression. Note the ununited ossiculum terminale (*arrow*) and the wide interval between the anterior arch of C1 and C2 (*double arrow*). Atlantoaxial instability is present in 10%–20% of children with Trisomy 21. **C,** Pelvis in an infant shows low acetabular angles, rounded iliac wings, and inferior tapering of the ischia.

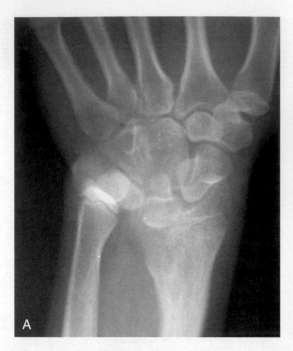
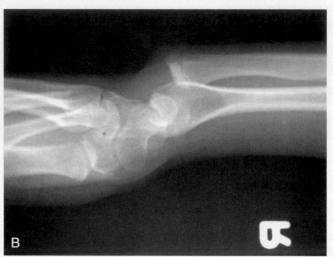

Fig. 5-45 Madelung deformity. (**A**) Note the short radius and (**B**) wide distal radioulnar joint.

to dysplasia of the femoral neck also may occur (Fig. 5-46C), perhaps reflecting the fact that portions of the long bones are partially formed by intramembranous ossification. Cleidocranial dysplasia is also in the differential diagnoses of a wide symphysis pubis (Fig. 5-46B and C, Table 5-11), and Wormian bones (Table 5-12).

Osteogenesis Imperfecta

Osteogenesis imperfecta refers to a group of disorders of collagen synthesis that result in abnormal bone formation with radiolucent bones that are easily fractured (Figs. 5-5 and 5-47, Table 5-13). The severity of skeletal manifestations is varied. Severe forms result in multiple fractures *in utero* and are incompatible with life. Mild forms have only relatively mild bone fragility that may not be diagnosed until adulthood. Intermediate forms result in multiple fractures that can cause deformity manifesting as short-limbed dwarfism. Healing fractures often exhibit exuberant callus formation (Table 5-14). Hearing loss due to otic bone fractures, gray teeth (dentinogenesis imperfecta), and blue sclerae are seen in 90% of cases. Basilar invagination with brainstem compression may occur.

Key Concepts	**Osteogenesis Imperfecta**

- A group of heritable, debilitating conditions characterized by weak bones with frequent fractures that often result in severe deformity.
- Blue sclerae, osteoporosis, and Wormian bones are frequently present.

A large number of genetic defects have been identified that cause abnormal collagen synthesis leading to osteogenesis imperfecta. Most forms are heritable in an autosomal dominant pattern, but autosomal recessive patterns are seen. Spontaneous mutations account for many cases. Sillence and colleagues have developed a widely accepted classification system that organizes osteogenesis imperfecta into four major groups based on clinical and genetic features (Table 5-13). Type I is the most frequent form of osteogenesis imperfecta (1 : 30,000). Types I and IV may be subtyped by the absence (subtype A) or presence (subtype B) of dentinogenesis imperfecta. Type II, the most severe form, is lethal in the neonatal period owing to extensive rib fractures and associated pulmonary hypoplasia and pulmonary infections. Type II may be divided into three subtypes, A–C, based on specific features of the osseous abnormalities. The distinction is important for genetic counseling of the parents. Type A has broad, crumpled long bones likened to an accordion, as well as rib fractures so numerous that the ribs have a beaded appearance. Type B has similar appearance of the long bones, but with less severe rib involvement. Type C has thin long bones and ribs, with multiple fractures.

The main differential diagnosis in an infant or child with multiple fractures is child abuse or osteogenesis imperfecta. (Several very rare conditions such as Caffey disease and Menke syndrome also may resemble child abuse.) Note that child abuse is much more frequent than all forms of osteogenesis imperfecta combined. Osteogenesis imperfecta can usually be diagnosed or ex-

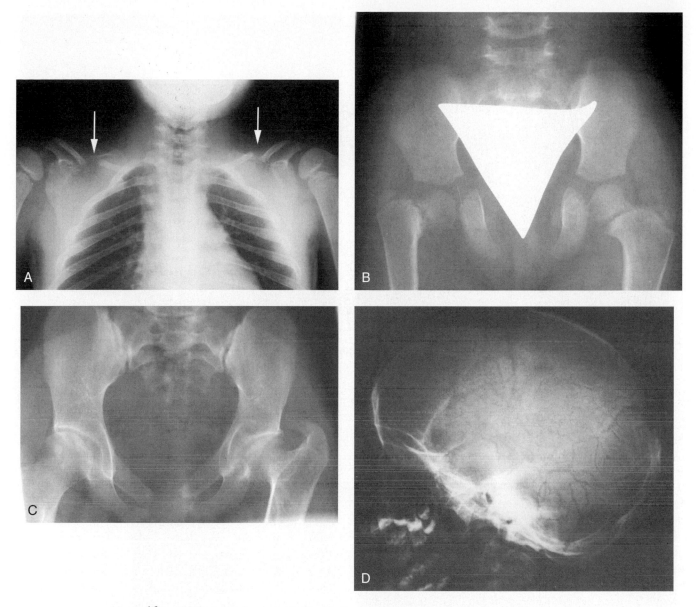

Fig. 5-46   Cleidocranial dysplasia. **A,** Dysplastic clavicles with absent middle segments (*arrows*). **B,** Pelvis in a child shows no pubis ossification, and unusually shaped capital femoral epiphyses. **C,** Pelvis in an adult shows absence of ossification around the symphysis pubis and bilateral hip dysplasia with early secondary osteoarthritis. **D,** Wormian bones (sutural ossicles).

Table 5-10   Absent distal clavicle
Trauma: posttraumatic osteolysis (weightlifters)
Mets/myeloma
Infection
Surgery
Rheumatoid arthritis
Hyperparathyroidism
Cleidocranial dysplasia

Table 5-11   Wide symphysis pubis
Trauma
Mets/myeloma
Infection
Surgery
Hyperparathyroidism
Cleidocranial dysplasia
Epispadius/bladder extrophy/prune belly syndrome spectrum

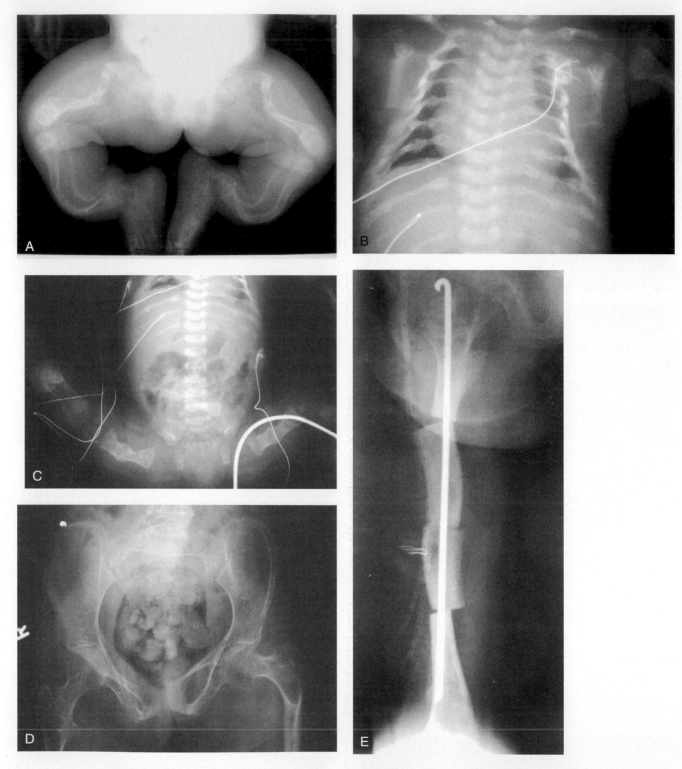

Fig. 5-47   Osteogenesis imperfecta. **A,** Osteogenesis imperfecta, type 3, with severe bowing. **B,** Osteogenesis imperfecta, type 2, in a newborn, with multiple rib fractures. **C,** Lower body in same patient as B. There are numerous fractures but the bones are not bowed. **D,** Pelvis in an older child shows osteopenia, deformity due to prior fractures, and gracile and deformed proximal femurs. **E,** Surgical intervention for a bowed femur. Multiple osteotomies were performed with intramedullary pin fixation. (E, Courtesy of Stephanie Spottswood, M.D., Richmond, VA.)

Table 5-12   Wormian bones (sutural bones)*
Hypothyroidism
Hypophosphatasia
Cleidocranial dysplasia
Pycnodysostosis
Osteogenesis imperfecta
Zellweger syndrome (autosomal recessive, seizures, mental retardation, microcystic renal disease, death in infancy)
Menke's syndrome (males. Fragile bones, abnormal copper metabolism)

*This is a partial listing. See Taybi H, Lachman RS. *Radiology of syndromes, metabolic disorders, and skeletal dysplasias,* ed 4. St. Louis: Mosby, 1996 for more complete differential diagnosis.

cluded by a combination of clinical and radiographic findings. Note that a very small subset of children with osteogenesis imperfecta has neither blue sclerae, abnormal dentition, nor juvenile hearing loss. The correct diagnosis of osteogenesis imperfecta can occasionally be difficult to establish in this very rare situation. The pattern and extensiveness of fractures in osteogenesis imperfecta tends to differ from child abuse. Certain fracture patterns are highly specific for child abuse, including posterior rib fractures and metaphyseal corner fractures. Fractures in osteogenesis imperfecta more typically involve the shafts of long bones and result in deformity. Biochemical assessment for osteogenesis imperfecta also can assist in establishing this diagnosis in unusual cases.

Sclerosing Bone Dysplasias

A large and heterogeneous group of conditions have radiographically dense bones as a cardinal feature. Several dozen are listed in Taybi and Lachman's textbook. Many of these conditions result from a failure of osteoclasts to resorb bone during remodeling. Several of the most common or distinctive sclerosing bone dysplasias are discussed in this section. Other potential causes of diffusely increased bone density that are not reviewed in this section include renal osteodystrophy, and less commonly myelofibrosis, hypothyroidism, chronic infections (including intrauterine infections, notably rubella and syphilis), and heavy metal poisoning (Fig. 5-3). *Caffey disease* (infantile cortical hyperostosis) is an unusual condition that causes exuberant periosteal new bone in infants, especially around the mandible (Fig. 5-48). Both sporadic

Key Concepts   Sclerosing Bone Dysplasias
• A varied group of conditions that have in common various patterns of increased bone density. Some are incidental and asymptomatic, while others have fragile bones that are easily fractured.

(possibly infectious) and familial forms have been described.

Osteopetrosis   *Osteopetrosis* is a group of conditions characterized by diffusely very dense but brittle bones, caused by diminished osteoclast function. The osteoclast dysfunction is theorized to be variable over time, with periods of more normal function alternating with periods of diminished function. This pattern results in broad, dense metaphyseal bands or a bone-with-a-bone appearance on radiographs (Figs. 5-4A and 5-49). The metaphyses are wide owing to failure of remodeling by the impaired osteoclasts (undertubulation). Vertebral bodies tend to have dense endplates with prominent posterior vascular notches, resulting in a "sandwich" appearance on radiographs. Failure to remodel around cranial foramina during growth causes stenosis with blindness and hearing loss in the more severe forms. Dental dysplasia and infections are frequent. Long bone fractures in osteopetrosis tend to be transverse, as do many pathologic fractures.

Four clinically and radiographically distinct subtypes of osteopetrosis are recognized (Table 5-15). Radiographs of the *precocious* or *infantile form* of osteopetrosis reveal absent corticomedullary differentiation, that is the cortical thickening is so severe that there is virtually no medullary space. This has profound consequences, as normal marrow components are displaced and diminished. The resulting pancytopenia is often lethal in infancy or early childhood. Hepatosplenomegaly is usually present. The *delayed* or *adult type* (*Albers-Schönberg disease*) is clinically much less severe, and may not be discovered until later in life owing to a fracture or mild anemia, or as an incidental finding on a chest radiograph. Radiographs of this form reveal dense bones with markedly thickened cortices. Corticomedullary differentiation is preserved, in contrast with the precocious form. A rare *intermediate autosomal recessive type* with clinical and radiographic features intermediate between the precocious and adult types is recognized. Finally, *osteopetrosis associated with renal tubular acidosis* is a fourth distinct subtype. These patients develop cerebral calcifications and are often mentally retarded. The skeletal abnormalities tend to improve during the patient's life, in contrast with the other forms of osteopetrosis.

The radiographic finding of "bone within a bone" is not specific to osteopetrosis, and may be seen as a transient normal finding during periods of rapid growth, especially in very young children (Fig. 5-50).

Pycnodysostosis   *Pycnodysostosis* (pyknodysostosis, Toulouse-Lautrec syndrome, Fig. 5-51) is a rare autosomal recessive short-limbed dwarfism with diffuse osteosclerosis, frequent transverse fractures, wormian bones (sutural ossicles, Table 5-12), and progressive resorption and occasionally fragmentation of the distal phalanges. The distal clavicles also may be resorbed (Table 5-10). The

Table 5-13   Osteogenesis imperfecta

Type	Relative bone fragility	Bone deformity	Stature	Blue sclerae	Dentinogenesis imperfecta	Hearing loss	Inheritance
I	+	+ −> ++	Normal or short	+	IA:−	+	AD
					IB:+	+	
II	++++ (crumbled)	++++ (accordion)	No long-term survival	+	−	−	AD (new mutation) AR (rare)
III	+++	+++ −>++++ (bowing)	Very short	birth: + adolescence: −	−	−	AD (new mutation) AR (rare)
IV	+ −> +++	+ > ++	Short	birth: ± adolescence: −	IV A: − IV B: +	− −	AD

From Sillence DO, Senn A, Danks DM: Genetic heterogeneity in osteogenesis imperfecta. *J Med Genetics* 16:101–116;1979; Laor T, Jarmillo D, Oestereich AE: Musculoskeletal system. In Kirks DR, Griscom NT, eds. *Practical pediatric imaging* ed 3. Philadelphia: Lippincott-Raven, 1998; Goldman AB. Heritable diseases of connective tissue, epiphyseal dysplasias, and related conditions. In Resnick D, *Bone and Joint Disorders* 3rd ed. Philadelphia: Saunders, 1995.

long bone findings can resemble the adult form of os-teopetrosis. The French painter Toulouse-Lautrec is be-lieved to have had pycnodysostosis.

Progressive Diaphyseal Dysplasia   *Progressive dia-physeal dysplasia* (diaphyseal dysplasia Englemann type, Camurati-Englemann disease) is an autosomal dominant condition that results in symmetric thickening of the diaphyseal cortices of long bones, especially in the legs (Fig. 5-52). The cortical thickening is both periosteal and endosteal, and the bones are remarkably expanded. The epiphyses are spared. The ribs and pelvis may rarely be involved. Clinical features appear during childhood and include an abnormal gait, muscle weakness, and leg pain. Clinical and radiographic penetrance is highly variable.

Ribbing Disease   *Ribbing disease* (hereditary multi-ple diaphyseal sclerosis) is most likely a variant form of progressive diaphyseal dysplasia. This condition is named in honor of the person who first described it; it has nothing specifically to do with the ribs. The radiographic findings are similar to progressive diaphyseal dysplasia except that the abnormalities are asymmetric and are less widely distributed, and clinical manifestations do not appear until the third or fourth decade. The tibia is the most frequently involved bone. This condition is painful and familial.

Table 5-14   Excessive callus formation

Corticosteroids (exogenous, Cushing's)
Neuropathic joint
Congenital insensitivity to pain
Paralysis
Osteogenesis imperfecta
Renal osteodystrophy
Burn patients
Subperiosteal bleed in scurvy

Osteopoikilosis   *Osteopoikilosis* is a generally be-nign familial condition consisting of multiple bone islands clustered around joints (Fig. 5-53). A minority of patients also has small subcutaneous fibrous nodules. Osteopoi-

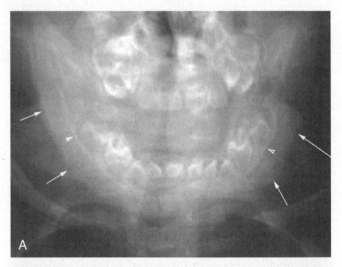

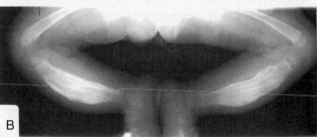

Fig. 5-48   Caffey disease (infantile cortical hyperostosis). **A,** Man-dible shows prominent expansion of the mandible due periosteal new bone formation (*arrows*). Note the underlying mandible cor-tex (*arrowheads*). **B,** Legs show bilateral prominent periosteal new bone formation in the tibias. (B, Courtesy of L. Das Narla, M.D., Richmond, VA.)

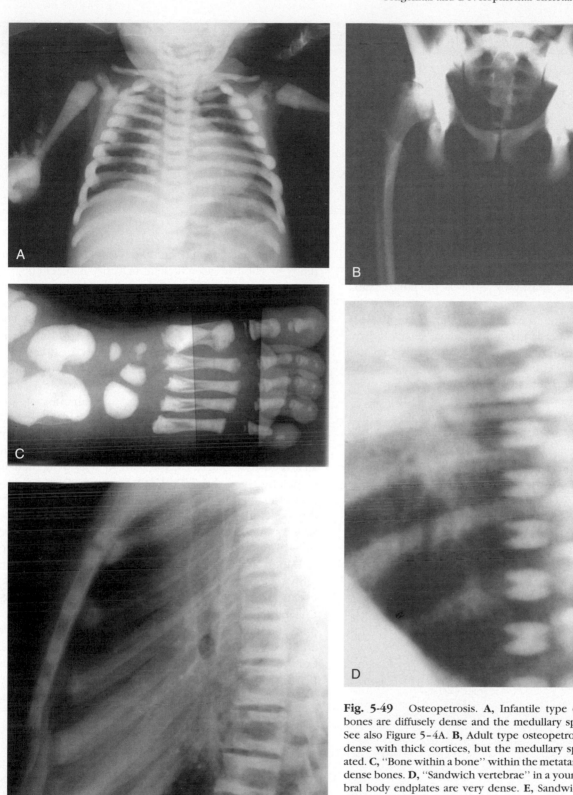

Fig. 5-49   Osteopetrosis. **A,** Infantile type osteopetrosis. The bones are diffusely dense and the medullary space is obliterated. See also Figure 5-4A. **B,** Adult type osteopetrosis. The bones are dense with thick cortices, but the medullary space is not obliterated. **C,** "Bone within a bone" within the metatarsals, with diffusely dense bones. **D,** "Sandwich vertebrae" in a young child. The vertebral body endplates are very dense. **E,** Sandwich vertebrae in an adult.

Table 5-15　Osteopetrosis

Type	Clinical severity	Inheritance	Comments
Precocious (infantile)	++++	AR (Rarely AD)	Often lethal early in life due to infections and anemia
Delayed (adult, Albers-Schonberg disease)	+	AD	Mild anemia Cranial nerve palsies
Intermediate	++ −> +++	AR	Short stature Hip AVN
OP with renal tubular acidosis	++ −> +++	AR	Cerebral calcification, mental retardation, hypotonia, long survival

kilosis in adults is easily distinguished from multiple blastic metastases by the distribution of the lesions: metastases tend to spare the epiphyses, whereas the bone islands of osteopoikilosis are most densely concentrated in the epiphyses. In addition, the individual "lesions" of osteopoikilosis are bone islands, which have characteristic findings of uniform density, continuity with the surrounding bony trabeculae, and orientation parallel to the alignment of the surrounding bony trabeculae. The number of bone islands may increase during childhood, but tends to stabilize after skeletal maturity is reached.

Osteopatha Striata *Osteopatha Striata* (Voorhoeve's disease) refers to a finding of uniform, dense linear striations in the metaphyses of the long bones. The striations are oriented parallel to the long axis of the long bones (Fig. 5-54). If the striations occur in the ilium, they radiate from the acetabulum in a "sunburst" pattern. This condition is benign.

Melorrheostosis *Melorrheostosis* is an unusual, sporadic condition with highly distinctive radiographic findings. Dense bone is deposited along the cortex of otherwise normal bones, usually along a single extremity, in an irregular, elongate, wavy pattern that is likened to dripping candle wax (Fig. 5-55). The pattern of distribution tends to follow a sclerotome, that is, a portion of the skeleton innervated by a single spinal nerve. The added bone is usually periosteal but may be endosteal. It is histologically similar to cortical (compact) bone. Although life expectancy is not shortened in patients with melorrheostosis, significant morbidity can occur, especially when the condition presents in childhood. Clinical features include pain, contractures, and limited joint mobility. Premature physeal closure can occur in an affected limb, resulting in growth disturbance and limb length discrepancy. Orthopedic intervention may be required to manage these complications.

Mixed Sclerosing Bone Dysplasia Melorrheostosis, osteopatha striata, and osteopoikilosis have been observed to occur simultaneously in some patients. This observation probably provides a clue to the etiology of these curious conditions, although each remains incompletely understood. The term "mixed sclerosing bone dysplasia" refers specifically to the simultaneous occurrence of these three conditions, acknowledging the possible association between them.

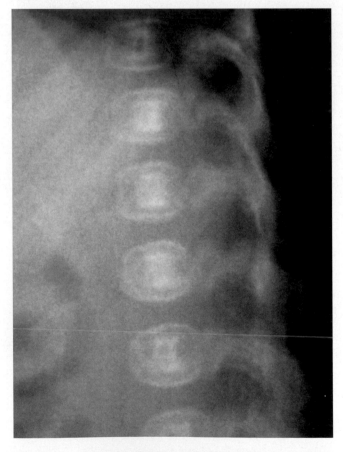

Fig. 5-50 "Bone within a bone" of thoracic and lumbar vertebral bodies as a normal finding in a former premature infant. Nutritional and metabolic factors associated with prematurity often lead to this appearance, which will eventually remodel to a normal appearance.

Dwarfism

Dwarfisms are skeletal dysplasias with disproportionate limb or spine shortening that results in short stature.

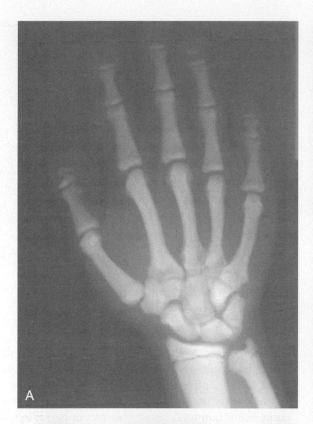

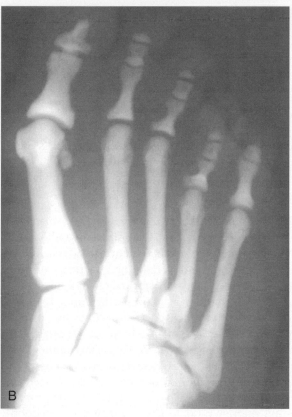

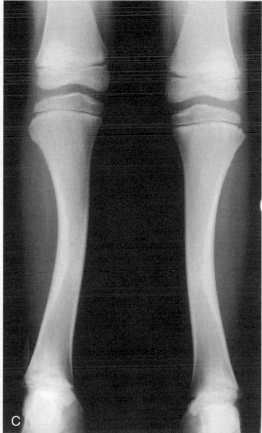

Fig. 5-51   Pycnodysostosis. **A,** Hand. **B,** Foot. **C,** Legs. Note the diffuse osteosclerosis, short, tapered distal phalanges with acroosteolysis, and mild bowing deformity of the tibias due to prior insufficiency fractures.

Key Concepts | Dwarfism

- Dwarfisms are a large and very heterogeneous group of skeletal dysplasias with short stature and disproportionate limb and/or spine shortening.
- Classification is based on clinical, genetic, laboratory and radiologic features.
- Achondroplasia is the most common dwarfism.
- Radiologic features of achondroplasia include a large cranium, short, squat long bones, spinal stenosis, and horizontal acetabular roofs.

Several types of dwarfism have been identified, many of which are extraordinarily rare. The role of the radiologist has diminished with the advancement of understanding of the genetic and pathophysiologic features of the dwarfisms. However, all dwarfisms have radiologic manifestations, and the radiologist may be called upon to assist in the diagnosis of these cases. Establishing the correct diagnosis is important for management of the child and genetic counseling of the parents. This is an intimidating prospect for most radiologists, as dwarfisms are complex to describe and are seen infrequently outside of specialized centers. But don't despair. An organized approach and a good reference book are invaluable. This section will provide a brief overview of the terminology used to describe dwarfisms, and review a few of the more common forms. Taybi and Lachman's *Radiology of Syndromes, Metabolic Disorders, and Skeletal Dysplasias,* and Spranger, Langer, and Wiedemann's *Bone Dysplasias* are excellent sources when more information is needed. Shultz's algorithmic approach in Manaster's *Handbook of Skeletal Radiology* provides a useful practical approach to diagnosing dwarfisms.

A dwarfism may affect all or only parts of the skeleton. Try to identify which of the following categories of bones are abnormal: skull, spine, thorax, pelvis, and the limbs. (If the spine is abnormal, the syndrome's name may con-

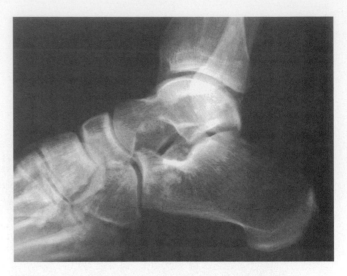

Fig. 5-53 Osteopoikilosis. Multiple bone islands are centered around the joints.

tain the prefix "spondylo," Table 5-16.) If the limbs are abnormal, try to localize the findings to the epiphyses, metaphyses, and/or the diaphyses. If the limbs are short, identify whether the shortening is most severe in the humeri and femurs (rhizomelic shortening; *rhizo,* root), forearms and legs (mesomelic shortening), or hands and feet (acromelic shortening) (Table 5-17). Are the abnormal bones narrow or wide? Are the epiphyses fragmented into small "punctate" or irregular ossicles? Are the ribs

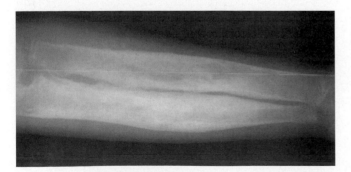

Fig. 5-52 Progressive diaphyseal dysplasia. Forearm shows expansion and cortical thickening of the diaphyses of both bones. The opposite forearm and lower extremities had an identical appearance (not shown).

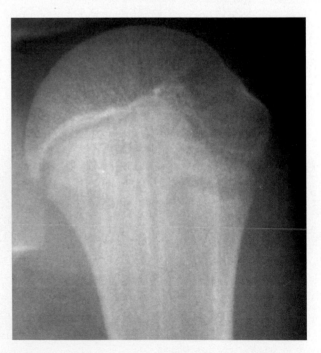

Fig. 5-54 Osteopatha striata. Note the longitudinally oriented dense striations in the metaphysis of the proximal humerus.

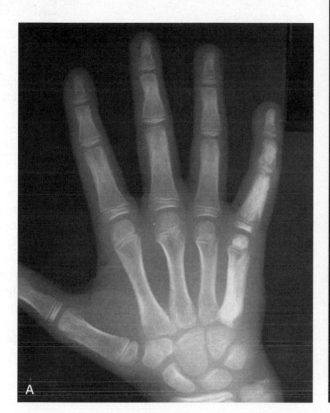

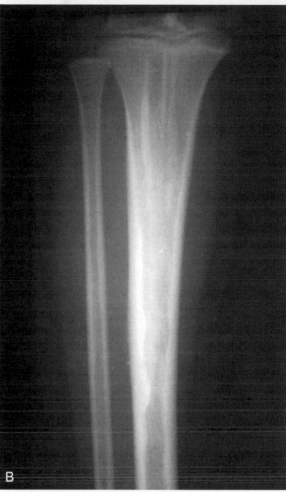

Fig. 5-55 Melorrheostosis. **A,** Hand. **B,** Tibia (different patient). Note the new bone formation in a pattern similar to "candle wax dripping" of the fifth ray of the hand and the tibia.

Table 5-16 Dwarfism with major spine involvement (partial listing)

NORMAL SPINE LENGTH

Chondrodysplasia punctata

SHORT SPINE

Achondroplasia
Campomelic dysplasia
Diastrophic dysplasia
Metatrophic dysplasia
Spondyloepiphyseal dysplasia
Spondylometaphyseal dysplasia
Thanatophoric dysplasia

Table 5-17 Dwarfism with short extremities (partial listing)

RHIZOMELIC SHORTENING

Achondroplasia
Pseudachondroplasia
Achondrogenesis
Thanatophoric dwarfism
Chondrodysplasia punctata
Diastrophic dwarfism

MESOMELIC SHORTENING

Dyschondrosteosis
Mesomelic dysplasia (numerous subtypes)

ACROMELIC SHORTENING

Chondroectodermal dysplasia (Ellis-van Creveld syndrome)
Asphyxiating thoracic dysplasia (Jeune syndrome)

Table 5-18   Dwarfism with short ribs (partial listing)
Achondroplasia
Achondrogenesis
Asphyxiating thoracic dysplasia (Jeune syndrome)
Chondroectodermal dysplasia (Ellis-van Creveld syndrome)
Campomelic dysplasia
Metatrophic dysplasia
Spondyloepiphyseal dysplasia congenita

short (Table 5-18)? Are the acetabular roofs horizontal or nearly horizontally oriented (Table 5-19)?

Screening radiographs in a child with a dwarfism should include a lateral skull, AP and lateral thoracolumbar spine, frontal chest (including the shoulders), AP pelvis and hips, AP view of a single upper extremity, AP view of a single lower extremity, and a PA hand detail view. The radiographic findings can be correlated with a series of gamuts listed in Tables 5-16 to 5-19. The following paragraphs provide a brief review of the major clinical and radiographic findings in the dwarfisms listed in the gamuts. Neither the conditions covered nor the descriptions are exhaustive (although you may find this topic to be *exhausting*!), but the information provided extends well beyond material routinely covered in the board exams.

Achondroplasia and clinical mimickers *Achondroplasia* is an autosomal dominant, rhizomelic short-limbed dwarfism (Fig. 5-56). Most cases are due to spontaneous mutations. Intelligence and life span are normal. Achondroplasia is one of the most common dwarfisms (1 : 26,000 live births). Clinical features include a protuberant forehead, normal intelligence, lumbar kyphosis in infancy that progresses to exaggerated lordosis in adulthood, and limited elbow extension. The skull is enlarged with narrowing of the foramen magnum and the jugular foramina. The vertebral bodies are bullet shaped in infancy, and become mildly flattened in adulthood. The interpediculate distance narrows in the lumber spine, and the pedicles are short. The ribs are shortened. The pelvis has squared iliac wings, horizontal acetabular

Table 5-19   Dwarfism with horizontal acetabular roofs*
Achondroplasia
Metatrophic dysplasia
Thanatophoric dysplasia
Spondyloepiphyseal dysplasia
Chondorectodermal dysplasia
Asphyxiating thoracic dysplasia

* Horizontal acetabular roofs also seen in Down syndrome and Cleidocranial dysplasia.

roofs, and a narrow pelvic inlet that has been likened to a champagne glass (Fig. 5-56D). The long bones are short and wide, with flared metaphyses (see Fig. 5-4B). The hands have a "trident" configuration due to equal length of the second, third and fourth fingers. The major cause of morbidity is neurologic impingement caused by the spinal and cranial stenosis.

Hypochondroplasia is nearly identical to achondroplasia in clinical and radiographic features, except that the skull is relatively spared in hypochondroplasia.

Pseudoachondroplasia is an autosomal dominant dwarfism that shares a few clinical features with achondroplasia, but is a distinct condition. It is usually not detected until the second to fourth years of life. Clinical features include short limbs *and* a short trunk, short hands and feet, and a normal facial appearance. The skull is normal. The spine is variably affected. The vertebral bodies may be flattened and irregular with anterior beaking, or may be normal. The ribs are broad and flat, and may be likened to a spatula. The acetabular roofs are irregular and horizontal. The epiphyses are markedly abnormal, with fragmentation and deformity. The metaphyses are widened. The proximal ends of the metacarpal bones are rounded. The carpal and tarsal bones are hypoplastic. Life expectancy in pseudoachondroplasia is normal, but early osteoarthritis can be disabling.

Dwarfisms that are uniformly lethal at birth *Achondrogenesis Types I and II* are lethal autosomal recessive dwarfisms with extremely short limbs and a large head (Fig. 5-57). The vertebral bodies are unossified or only minimally ossified. The ribs are short and may be fractured. The pelvis is poorly ossified. Type II achondrogenesis has similar but less severe radiographic findings, but also is lethal.

Thanataphoric dwarfism is a lethal rhizomelic short-limbed dwarfism that may be diagnosed by prenatal ultrasound. The heritance pattern is uncertain. The skull has a cloverleaf deformity due to global synostosis. The ribs are severely shortened and the chest is small. The spine has platyspondyly (flat verteral bodies) with U shaped vertebral bodies, and narrow interpediculate distance (Fig. 5-58). Overall spine length is normal because the disc spaces are wide. The iliac wings are squared and the acetabular roofs are horizontal. The limbs are severely shortened and the femurs are characteristically curved ("telephone-receiver femurs").

Dwarfisms with short ribs as a main finding *Asphyxiating thoracic dysplasia* (Jeune syndrome) is an autosomal recessive dwarfism with a small thorax and short ribs with bulbous ends (Fig. 5-59A,B). This leads to pulmonary hypoplasia and poor ventilation that is most prominent during the first year of life. The clavicles project far above the ribs on an AP chest radiograph. The pelvis has inferiorly oriented spurlike excrescences at the triradiate cartilage ("trident pelvis," Fig. 5-59C) and

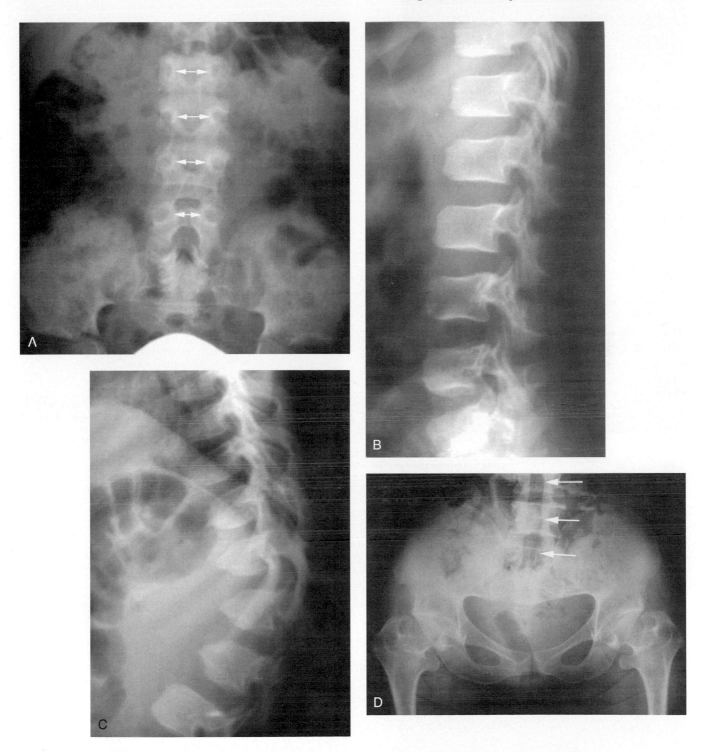

Fig. 5-56   Achondroplasia. **A,** AP spine shows narrow interpediculate distance in the lower lumbar spine (*arrows*). **B,** Lateral lumbar spine. Note the posterior vertebral body scalloping, mild anterior beaking, and the short pedicles. **C,** Lateral spine, more severe dysplasia. Note the thoracolumbar kyphosis with prominent anterior beaking. **D,** Pelvis in an adult. Note the prior lumbar laminectomy (*arrows*) performed to relieve spinal stenosis. See also Figure 5-4B. (B, Courtesy of Stephanie Spottswood, M.D., Richmond, VA.)

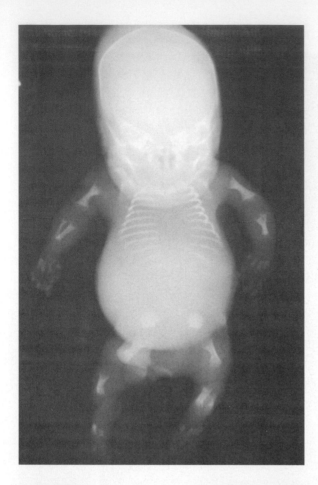

Fig. 5-57 Achondrogenesis. The spine is not mineralized. Also note the shortened limbs and ribs, and the large head. (Courtesy of Stephanie Spottswood, M.D., Richmond, VA.)

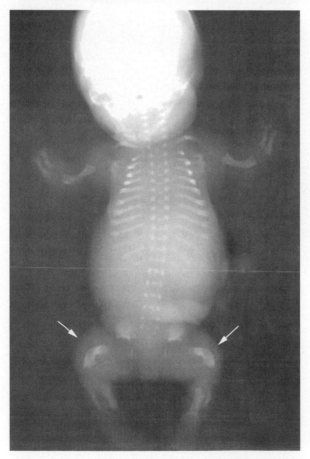

Fig. 5-58 Thanatophoric dwarfism. Note the short, bowed femurs (*arrows*) and the flat, U-shaped vertebral bodies with wide disc spaces.

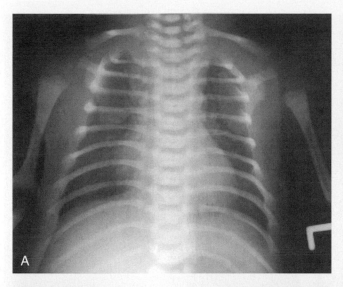

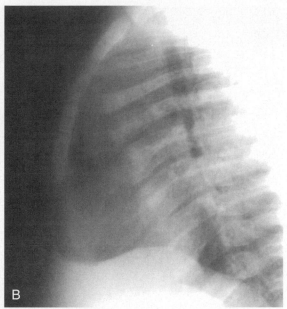

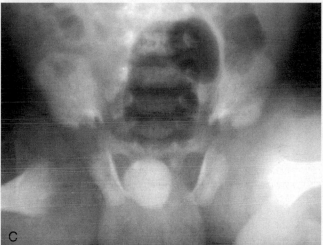

Fig. 5-59   Asphyxiating thoracic dysplasia (Jeune syndrome) in a newborn. **A, B,** Chest. Note the short ribs and small thorax with high position of the clavicles. **C,** Pelvis. The ilia are small and there are downward projecting spurs at the triradiate cartilage. The acetabular roofs are horizontal. This case does not have the classic finding of premature ossification of the capital femoral epiphyses.

often at the lateral margins of the acetabular roof as well. Ossification of the capital femoral epiphyses may be seen at birth. These centers do not normally begin to ossify until about age 3 months. The limbs are shortened, usually in an acromelic pattern, with irregular metaphyses. The hands have short middle and distal phalanges. If the child survives the pulmonary complications of the first year, many of the clinical and osseous abnormalities improve with age. However, progressive renal disease develops during childhood and consequently the lifespan is shortened.

Chondroectodermal dysplasia (Ellis-van Creveld syndrome) is an autosomal recessive dwarfism that occurs most frequently in the Amish (Fig. 5-60). Clinical features include sparse hair, polydactyly with an ulnar sided supernumerary finger, abnormal teeth and hypoplastic nails, and frequent congenital heart disease (usually atrial septal defect or common atrium). The skull and spine are generally spared. The ribs usually are short and the thorax

long and narrow in infancy. These abnormalities resolve during growth. The pelvis has flat acetabular roofs with medial spurlike projections ("trident pelvis") and hypoplastic iliac wings. The capital femoral epiphyses are ossified at birth. The limbs are shortened, especially distally, and the metaphyses are wide and irregular. The distal ulna and the proximal radius are especially widened. The hamate and capitate may be fused. The proximal tibial epiphyses are hypoplastic, resulting in genu valgum. Prognosis depends on the presence and severity of congenital heart disease, and complications of the small thorax. Overall mortality during infancy is 50%. Chondroectodermal dysplasia shares many features with asphyxiating thoracic dystrophy in the newborn period, but asphyxiating thoracic dystrophy does not have nail hypoplasia.

Campomelic (*camptomelic*) *dysplasia* (*campomelic,* "bent limb") is a dwarfism with uncertain genetics. Cleft palate is frequently present. The cervical spine

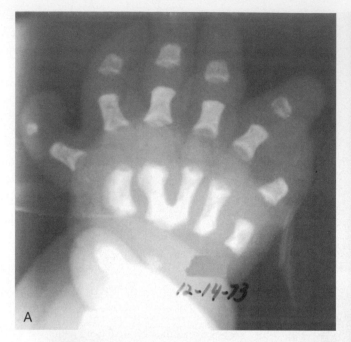

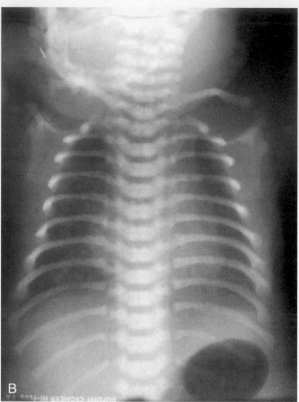

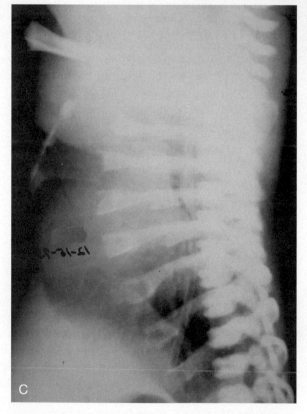

Fig. 5-60   Chondroectodermal dysplasia (Ellis-van Creveld syndrome). **A,** Hand. Note the polydactyly (extra digit in the hand) and the fused metacarpals. **B, C,** Chest. The findings are essentially identical to asphyxiating thoracic dysplasia (Fig. 5-59) with short ribs, small thorax, and high clavicles. The hand findings and other clinical features of these syndromes allow them to be differentiated. (Courtesy of Stephanie Spottswood, M.D., Richmond, VA.)

and the posterior elements of the thoracic spine are poorly mineralized. The thoracic cage is small and has 11 rib pairs, and the scapulae are hypoplastic. The pelvis is dysplastic and poorly mineralized. The long bones of the lower extremity have characteristic anterior and lateral bowing. Skin dimples are present over the shins. Neonatal death due to pulmonary insufficiency and infection is common.

Metatrophic dysplasia is a rare dwarfism with *a distinctive taillike appendage* or cutaneous fold over the sacrococcygeal region. Inheritance is heterogeneous, with lethal and nonlethal types. The skull is spared. The spine is relatively normal in length at birth, but platyspon-dyly and development of kyphoscoliosis lead to spine shortening as the child grows. C1–C2 instability due to dens hypoplasia may occur. The ribs are short. The pelvis has horizontal, irregular acetabular roofs. The long bones are disproportionately short at birth, but with subsequent growth the limbs attain a more normal length whereas the spine becomes markedly shortened. (The term *"met-atrophic"* means *changing*.) The long bones have wide, club-shaped metaphyses.

Dwarfism with stippled epiphyses as a main find-ing *Chondrodysplasia punctata* is a short-limbed dwarfism, usually rhizomelic, with stippled epiphyses (Fig. 5-61). Several subtypes are recognized, but the two main subtypes are an autosomal dominant form also known as *Conradi disease,* and a rhizomelic recessive form. Clinical features include cataracts, joint con-tractures, and ichthyosiform (fishscale-like) skin rash. The long bone epiphyses and the spine ossify in a punctate pattern during childhood. The epiphyses in adults are no longer stippled, but they are not normally shaped. The long bones are shortened, usually unilaterally in the domi-nant form, and symmetrically and severely in the reces-sive form. The ribs and pelvis are spared. The dominant

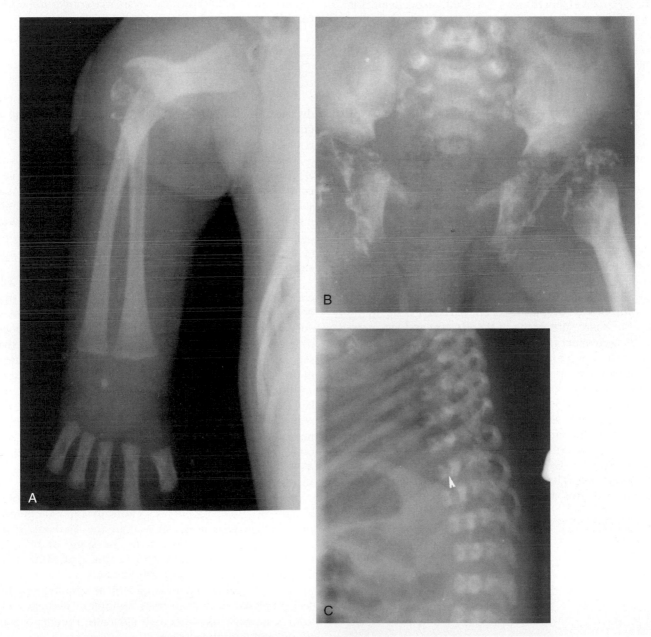

Fig. 5-61   Chondrodysplasia punctata. **A,** Upper extremity. Note the short humerus (rhizomelic dwarf) and stippled epiphyses. **B,** Pelvis. **C,** Lateral spine shows coronal vertebral body clefts (*ar-rowhead*).

form also may have coronal vertebral body clefts. Severe cases of the dominant type are fatal in the first week of life, but milder cases may survive for years. The recessive type is fatal in infancy.

In addition to chondrodysplasia punctata, stippled epiphyses also occur in spondyloepiphyseal dysplasia and diastrophic dysplasia (both described in the following section), and in children of mothers who used coumadin or excessive alcohol during pregnancy.

Miscellaneous other dwarfisms *Pycnodysostosis* (Fig. 5-51) was discussed earlier with the sclerosing bone dysplasias. *Diastrophic dysplasia (diastrophic, "twisted")* is an autosomal recessive dwarfism that may resemble arthrogryposis in severe cases. The skull and pelvis are normal. The spine has narrowing of the lumbar interpediculate distance (potentially simulating achondroplasia), and may also have scoliosis, cervical kyphosis, and/or vertebral body posterior scalloping. The long bones of the extremities are short and club-shaped, and the epiphyses may be stippled. The hand has a distinctive "hitchhiker's thumb" deformity with a short first metacarpal. Clubfeet are a typical feature. The earlobes are swollen.

Mesomelic dysplasias are a group of dwarfisms characterized by mesomelic limb shortening. Over 20 types are recognized. *Dyschondrosteosis* (Leri-Weill disease) presents in late childhood with Madelung deformity (Fig. 5-62) as the primary finding. The Madelung deformity results in diminished forearm mobility and may be painful. The tibias and fibulas may be mildly shortened. Dyschondrosteosis is inherited in an autosomal dominant pattern. Distinction from Turner syndrome, which also may have Madelung deformity, is easily made by the other clinical findings in Turner syndrome. The numerous other mesomelic dysplasias do not have Madelung deformity, but share shortening of the forearm and leg bones as a distinguishing feature. The mesomelic dysplasias are otherwise a heterogeneous group of conditions, with varying severity of skeletal dysplasia and abnormalities of other organ systems. Enumeration of these conditions is beyond the scope of this discussion.

Spondyloepiphyseal dysplasia congenita (SEDC) is an autosomal dominant dwarfism with marked abnormalities of the spine and epiphyses. Clinical features include a short spine, C1–C2 instability, muscular hypotonia, and a waddling gait. The face is flat and cleft palate may be present. The ribs are normal in length, but the chest is barrel shaped with pectus carinatum ("bird chest," protruding sternum). Spinal manifestations at birth include ovoid or pear shaped vertebral bodies and dens hypoplasia (Fig. 5-63). In childhood and later life, the vertebral bodies become flattened (platyspondyly) and irregular. Scoliosis is frequent. The long bones are mildly shortened. Ossification of the pelvis and the epiphyses of the long bones are delayed, and the epiphyses often are irregular and fragmented. These abnormalities consistently lead to early osteoarthritis, especially of the hips. Note that the term *spondyloepiphyseal dysplasia* is also applied to a number of other, less frequent skeletal dysplasias that have different clinical and radiologic manifestations. Spondyloepiphyseal dysplasia *congenita* refers to the specific condition described here.

Other Skeletal Dysplasias with Short Stature

The following conditions are distinguished from the dwarfisms because they do not become clinically apparent until late childhood or adolescence, and loss of stature is milder than in the dwarfisms.

Spondyloepiphyseal dysplasia tarda (SED-tarda) is an X-linked recessive form of SED that presents in adolescence with back and hip pain, limited joint motion, and short stature due to a short spine. The radiographic findings include platyspondyly with anterior disc space widening but central and posterior disc space narrowing (Fig. 5-64). The epiphyses are small and irregular, and early OA is a typical feature.

Multiple epiphyseal dysplasia (MED, *Fairbank disease*) is an autosomal dominant skeletal dysplasia that does not manifest clinically until late childhood or adolescence with joint pain and limp, and a mildly short limbed dysplasia (Fig. 5-65). The primary abnormality is defective secondary growth centers. The abnormalities are greatest in the secondary ossification centers of the tubular bones and the bones of the wrists and ankles, which have delayed ossification and are small and fragmented. The endplates of the spine may also be affected, with Schmorl's nodes and mild vertebral body flattening. Osteoarthritis before the fourth decade is characteristic. Clinically silent AVN occurs frequently in MED, but does not appear to accelerate the secondary degenerative changes.

Ribbing type MED (not to be confused with Ribbing disease, discussed earlier) is a clinically and radiographically milder variant of MED than the Fairbank type. Involvement may be limited to the spine or hips, or may be more diffuse. As with Fairbank type MED, early osteoarthritis is the main complication.

The differential diagnosis of MED is spondyloepiphyseal dysplasia, early dysostosis multiplex (discussed below), extensive osteonecrosis, juvenile rheumatoid arthritis, and hypothyroidism.

Metaphyseal chondrodysplasia (MChD) is a collection of dysplasias with metaphyseal deformity as a primary ab-

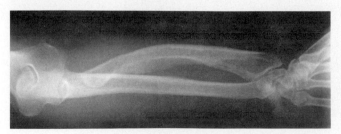

Fig. 5-62 Dyschondrosteosis: Madelung deformity. Note the bowed radius and associated wrist deformity.

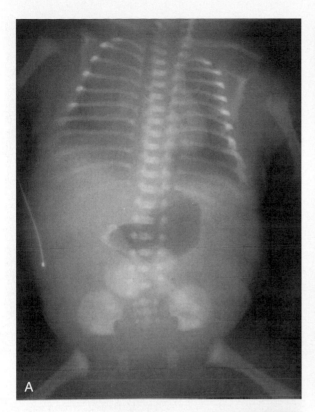

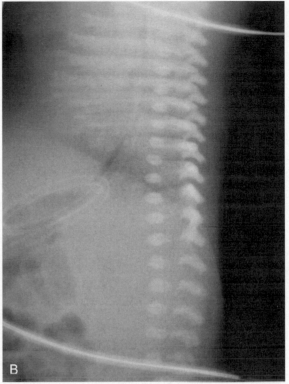

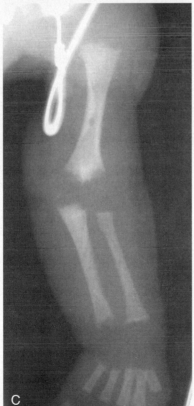

Fig. 5-63   Spondyloepiphyseal dysplasia congenita. **A, B,** Spine shows platyspondyly (flat vertebral bodies) with many oval vertebral bodies. There is no pubis ossification. **C,** Note normally shaped but short bones of the upper extremity. Note the absence of ossification centers. Delayed appearance of ossification centers is a typical feature of spondyloepiphyseal dysplasia congenita. (Courtesy of L. Das Narla, M.D., Richmond, VA.)

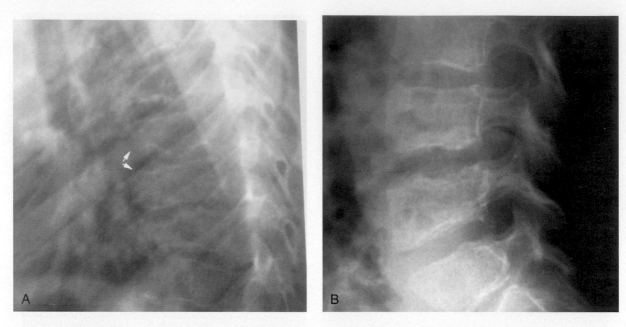

Fig. 5-64   Spondyloepiphyseal dysplasia tarda. **A, B,** Lateral thoracic and lumbar spine. Note the irregular endplates with widened disc spaces anteriorly (*arrows in A*). (Courtesy of Stephanie Spottswood, M.D., Richmond, VA.)

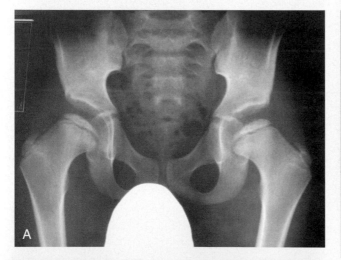

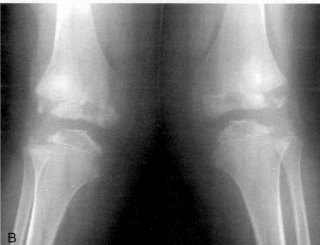

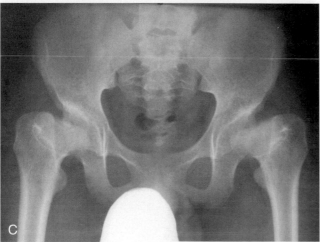

Fig. 5-65   Multiple epiphyseal dysplasia, Fairbank type. **A, B,** Pelvis and knees in a child show flattening and irregularity of the epiphyses. **C,** Pelvis in a young adult shows bilateral coxa vara, a frequent consequence of Fairbank disease.

normality. All are characterized by short stature. The most common type is the autosomal dominant *Schmid type,* which presents during the second year with short stature, bowed legs, and a waddling gait. Radiographs reveal findings suggestive of rickets, with metaphyseal flaring, physeal widening, and irregularity and wide, cupped anterior rib ends (Fig. 5-66). However, the zone of provisional calcification has normal density, in contrast with rickets in which this region is radiolucent. The autosomal recessive *McKusick type* MChD has more pronounced metaphyseal abnormalities, resulting in cone-shaped epiphyses, especially in the hands. Children with McKusick type MChD have sparse hair, and this condition is also known as cartilage hair syndrome. Like chondroectodermal dysplasia, this condition is more common in the Amish. The autosomal recessive *Shwachman type* MChD (Shwachman-Diamond syndrome) combines metaphyseal dysplasia with exocrine pancreatic insufficiency and neutrophil dysfunction. The rare autosomal dominant *Jansen type* MChD causes severe short stature.

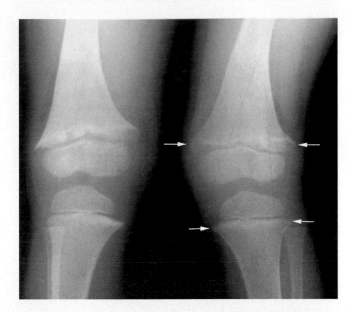

Fig. 5-66   Schmid type Metaphyseal chondrodysplasia. Physeal widening and metaphyseal fraying suggest rickets, but the density of the zone of provisional calcification (*arrows*) is not diminished.

Mucopolysaccharidoses and Other Storage Diseases

The mucopolysaccharidoses are a group of conditions caused by inborn errors of mucopolysaccharide metabolism that result in accumulation of mucopolysaccharides in the bone marrow, brain, liver, and other organs. The MPS are distinguished by differences in clinical manifestations, biochemistry, and inheritance, outlined in Table 5-20. (*Do not* memorize this table. Your friends will worry about you.)

The mucopolysaccharidoses have in common a group of skeletal manifestations that are collectively termed *dysostosis multiplex* (Fig. 5-67). Short stature is universal, and the long bones are shortened with wide metaphyses and diaphyses. The bridge of the nose is flattened. There is focal kyphosis at the thoracolumbar junction, with an L1 or adjacent vertebral body that is small, retrolisthesed, and oval in shape with a central anterior beak. Several vertebral bodies may have this finding. The hands have short wide metacarpals, with narrowed proximal ends resulting in a fanlike configuration of the hands. The pelvis has constricted (narrow) inferior iliac bones with flared iliac wings, and femoral heads are dysplastic. Additional features of dysostosis multiplex include osteopenia

with coarse trabeculae, macrocranium with a J shaped sella tursica, and "oar shaped" ribs with focal constriction at the costovertebral junction (Fig. 5-67C).

The mucopolysaccharidoses are unusual conditions. Hurler syndrome (MPS IH) and Morquio syndrome are the most common mucopolysaccharidoses (both 1 : 100,000 at birth). Hurler syndrome deserves special mention as it causes early and severe appearance of dysostosis multiplex beginning by about one year of age. Morquio syndrome (MPS IV) deserves special mention because it is the only (relatively) common MPS that does not cause mental retardation. Radiographic findings of Morquio syndrome include those of dysostosis multiplex, as well as several important or distinctive additional findings. Dens hypoplasia with atlantoaxial instability, expansion of C2, and displacement of the posterior arch of C1 into the foramen magnum can cause spinal cord compression. Surgical stabilization may be required. The vertebral bodies have mid-anterior beaking. The vertebral bodies can flatten ("platyspondyly"), especially in the lumbar spine, in contrast to Hurler syndrome in which this finding is not present. Delayed appearance of the epiphyses, with fragmented epiphyses may be seen.

Dysostosis multiplex is also caused by other storage diseases such as the mucolipidoses and Gaucher disease. As with the mucopolysaccharidoses, the clinical and radiographic changes caused by these conditions are not present at birth, but rather take years to develop as the abnormal metabolites accumulate. Also similar to the mucopolysaccharidoses, diagnosis of these conditions is based primarily on clinical and laboratory findings.

Key Concepts	**Mucopolysaccharidoses**

- A group of conditions caused by inborn errors of mucopolysaccharide metabolism that result in accumulation of mucopolysaccharides in the bone marrow, brain, liver, and other organs, resulting in dwarfism and a distinctive set of skeletal abnormalities (dysostosis multiplex).

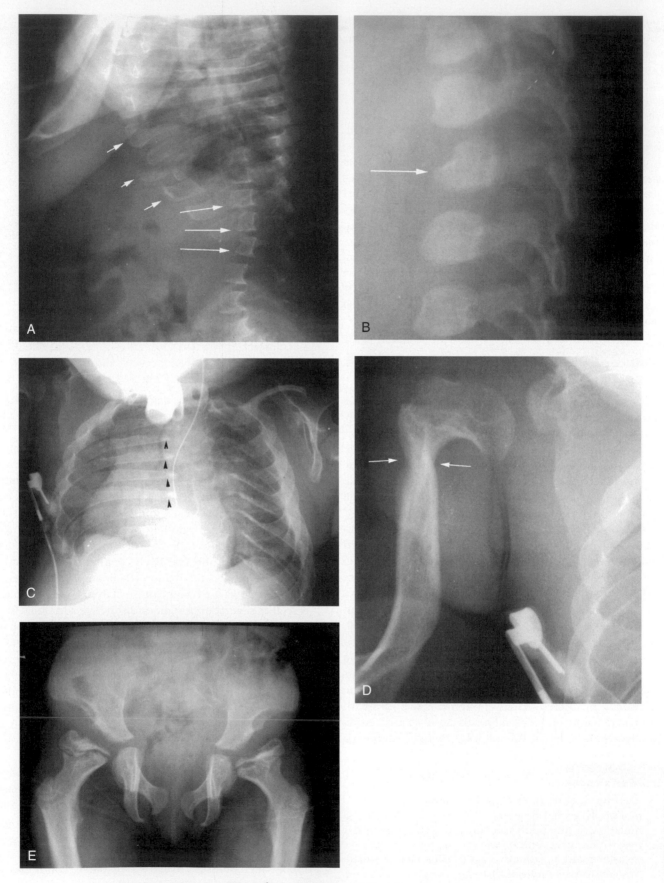

Fig. 5-67   For legend see opposite page

Table 5-20   Classification of the mucopolysaccharidoses

Type	Eponym	Heritance	MPS stored and excreted	Features
1H	Hurler	AR	DS, HS	DO (severe), C1-C2 subluxation, MR, HSM, corneal clouding
1S	Scheie	AR	DS, HS	DO, stiff joints, cardiac disease, corneal clouding
II	Hunter	XR	DS, HS	DO, often MR, HSM
III	San Filipo	AR	HS	DO, neurologic impairment
IV	Morquio	AR	KS	DO, C1-C2 subluxation, organomegaly, corneal clouding, no MR
V	none (formerly Scheie)			
VI	Maroteaux-Lamy	AR	DS	Very rare. Variable expression. DO, C1-C2 subluxation, organomegaly, corneal clouding, no MR
VII	Sly	AR	CS,DS,HS	Very rare. Variable expression. DO, MR, corneal clouding

AR = autosomal recessive; XR = X-linked recessive
DS = dermatan sulfate; KS = keratan sulfate; HS = heparan sulfate; CS = chondroitin sulfate
DO = dysostosis multiplex; MR = mental retardation; HSM = hepatosplenomegaly
From: Taybi H, Lachman RS. *Radiology of Syndromes, Metabolic Disorders, and Skeletal Dysplasias.* 1996 4th ed. Mosby St. Louis

MISCELLANEOUS CONDITIONS

Amniotic Band Syndrome

Amniotic band syndrome (Fig. 5-68) refers to congenital amputations and soft tissue defects caused by entanglement of the fetus by aberrant bands of amniotic membrane that traverse the gestational sac. Abnormalities range from minimal amputations or focal syndactyly to major cranial or body wall defects. Focal soft-tissue constrictions may occur that may result in chronic lymphedema. Surgery is often required to minimize loss of function and to improve appearance.

Arthrogryposis Multiplex Congenita

Arthrogryposis multiplex congenita (Fig. 5-69) is a rare, sporadic condition characterized by severe joint abnormalities that include fixed flexion deformities, dislocations, radiographically dense joint capsules, long scoliosis (neuromuscular pattern), muscle and soft tissue atro-

Fig. 5-67 Dysostosis multiplex. **A,** Lateral thoracic and lumbar spine and ribs (MPS VI). Note the broad "oar-like" ribs (*short arrows*) and the thoracolumbar kyphosis with small inferior beaks (*long arrows*). **B,** Lateral thoracolumbar spine (MPS 1H). The vertebral bodies are shaped differently than MPS VI in **A,** but also have a short anteroposterior size and an inferior beak in a thoracolumbar junction vertebral body (*arrow*). **C,** Chest (MPS VI). Note the wide ribs, with focal constrictions at the costovertebral junctions (*arrowheads*). **D,** Humerus (MPS VI). The long bones are generally expanded and may be bowed. Note the characteristic focal constriction in the proximal diaphyses (*arrows*). **E,** Pelvis (MPS 1H). The iliac wings are narrowed inferiorly. The femoral heads are flat and the hips are dysplastic.

phy, and osteoporotic bones (from disuse) that are prone to insufficiency fracture. Clubfeet and hands may be present. Soft-tissue webs may be seen across joints fixed in flexion. The lower extremities are almost always involved, particularly the distal limbs, but the distribution is variable. The upper extremities may be involved. Intelligence is normal. The cause is unknown, but severely restricted fetal motion as can result from chronic oligohydramnios is suspected.

Gigantism and Hypoplasia

Abnormalities of size and shape may affect only a small portion of the body (focal gigantism), an entire extremity (macromelia), or even half of the body. Only one or two organ systems may be affected, for example, the lymphatics or the blood vessels, or every tissue may be involved. *Hemihypertrophy* is overgrowth of half (or nearly half) of the body. A variety of syndromes and malignancies are associated with hemihypertrophy, most notably the Beckwith-Wiedemann syndrome and Wilms tumor. *Hemiatrophy* is usually an acquired condition caused by asymmetric neurologic and neuromuscular conditions that cause severe unilateral muscle atrophy. *Hemihypotrophy* may be thought of as congenital hemiatrophy. Hemihypotrophy is rare. It is associated with intrauterine growth retardation and chromosomal abnormalities. A leg length discrepancy resulting from any of these conditions may require orthopedic intervention.

Macrodystrophia lipomatosa is a distinctive form of localized gigantism of unknown etiology characterized histologically by overgrowth of adipose and periosteal osteoblasts (see Fig. 1-66). Fingers and toes are most frequently involved with this condition.

Klippel-Trenaunay-Weber syndrome is macromelia associated with a cutaneous capillary hemangioma (port-

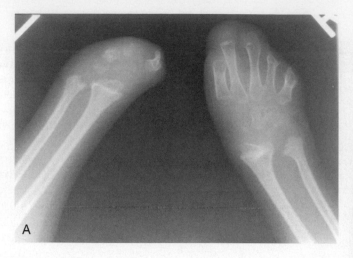

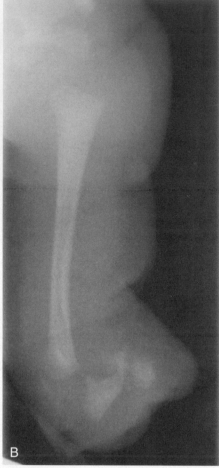

Fig. 5-68   A, B, Amniotic band syndrome. Note the amputations of the extremities.

wine nevus) and dilated and tortuous superficial veins. A lower extremity is the usual site of involvement (Fig. 5-70). Occasionally, hemangiomas also occur in the liver, spleen, bowel, and bladder wall. The limb overgrowth becomes most apparent during the growth spurt at puberty. It is speculated that the vascular abnormalities are

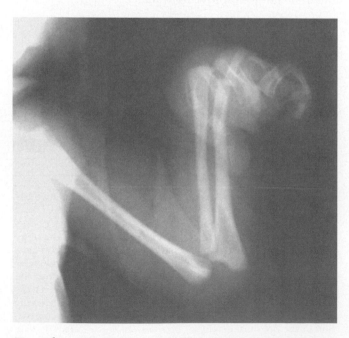

Fig. 5-69   Arthrogryposis multiplex congenita. The upper extremity was fixed in this position.

Key Concepts   Focal Gigantism

- Chronically increased blood flow, regardless of the cause, causes accelerated growth in adjacent physes.
- Potential causes include vascular malformation, chronic inflammation as in juvenile rheumatoid arthritis, and chronic low-grade infection.
- Macrodystrophia lipomatosa is idiopathic overgrowth of fingers or toes with fibrofatty proliferation.
- Klippel-Trenaunay-Weber syndrome is overgrowth of a limb, usually a lower extremity, related to congenital absence of a normal deep venous system and increased flow through an abnormal subcutaneous venous system.

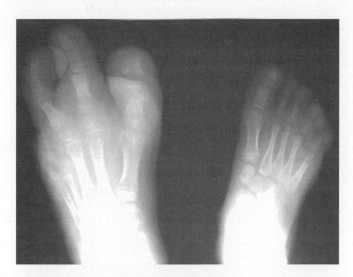

Fig. 5-70   Klippel-Trenaunay-Weber syndrome. In addition to the foot overgrowth evident on this image, most of the right lower extremity was overgrown (not shown).

due to failure of primitive superficial vascular channels to regress during gestation, resulting in or from failure of development of a normal deep venous system of the affected extremity. The resulting vascular abnormalities cause chronically increased blood flow that is the cause of the limb overgrowth. (Remember that chronically increased blood flow causes accelerated growth in adjacent physes, regardless of the cause. Examples include vascular malformation, chronic inflammation as in juvenile RA, and chronic low-grade infection.)

Fibromatosis Coli

Fibromatosis coli (Fig. 5-71) refers to a nonneoplastic masslike focal or diffuse enlargement of a sternocleido-

mastoid muscle in an infant. This condition probably results from birth injury to the sternocleidomastoid muscle, and not surprisingly, is associated with forceps delivery. The affected sternocleidomastoid muscle often shortens, which may result in torticollis. Imaging studies reveal nonspecific enlargement of the affected muscle, but are especially useful in excluding another cause of a neck mass such as adenopathy, neoplasm, branchial cleft cyst, or cystic hygroma. Fibromatosis coli typically presents at about two weeks of age and may enlarge before spontaneously resolving over a period of months. Most cases require no specific treatment, but passive stretching of the shortened sternocleidomastoid muscle is often helpful in relieving torticollis. Surgery is occasionally required for refractory torticollis.

Radial Dysplasias

Congenital absence, partial aplasia, or hypoplasia of the radius occurs in association with numerous syndromes and as part of the VACTERL spectrum.

Holt-Oram syndrome is an association of congenital heart disease (classically atrial septal defect) and thumb or radius abnormalities. The classic osseous finding is triphalangeal thumbs (Fig. 5-72A), but a spectrum of thumb abnormalities can occur, ranging from absence to hypoplasia to bifid. The radius may be absent, hypoplastic, or normal. Inheritance is autosomal dominant.

TAR syndrome (thrombocytopenia-absent radius) is an association of congenital radial anomalies and severe thrombocytopenia. The classic skeletal findings are absence of the radius and shortening of the ulna when the hand is held at a 90° angle to the forearm (Fig. 5-72B). The radii are often absent bilaterally, but the thumbs are typically present. There is evidence for autosomal recessive inheritance.

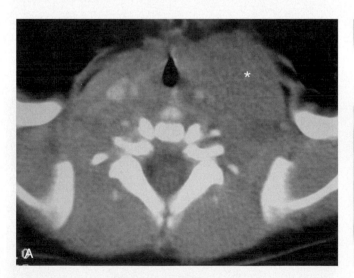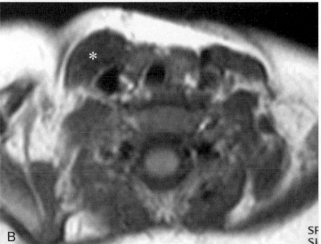

Fig. 5-71   Fibromatosis coli. CT image (**A**) and axial T1-weighted MR image in a different patient (**B**) show unilateral enlargement of a sternocleidomastoid muscle (*asterisks*). No CT attenuation or MR signal intensity alterations are present. (Courtesy of Fred Lainc, M.D., Richmond, VA.)

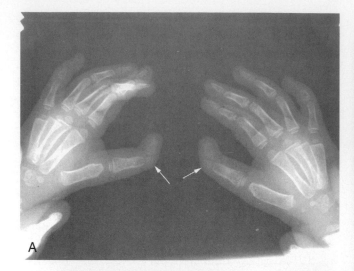

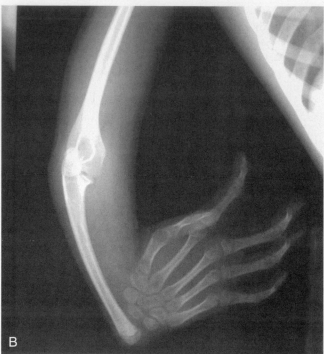

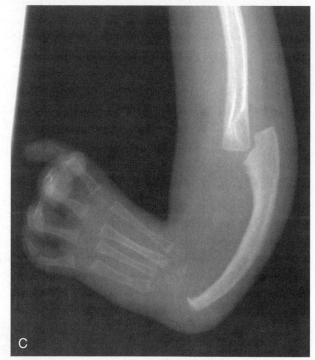

Fig. 5-72   Radial ray dysplasias. **A,** Holt-Oram syndrome. Note the triphalangeal thumbs (*arrows*). **B,** TAR syndrome (thrombocytopenia absent radius). The radius is absent, but the thumb and scaphoid are present. **C,** Radial club hand. In contrast with **B,** the thumb is absent.

Radial club hand is similar to the deformity just described in the TAR syndrome, but the term usually also implies that the thumb and scaphoid are also absent (Fig. 5-72C).

Fanconi anemia is an association of brown pigmentation of the skin and late childhood pancytopenia. Congenital radial ray and thumb anomalies are present in about half of cases, classically a hypoplastic thumb. A variety of congenital renal anomalies may occur as well.

Congenital radioulnar synostosis is caused by failure of segmentation of the proximal radius and ulna (Fig. 5-73). The proximal radius is often posteriorly displaced, and the radius is often bowed laterally. Radioulnar synostosis can occur as an isolated abnormality, as a familial condition, or in association with a variety of rare syn-

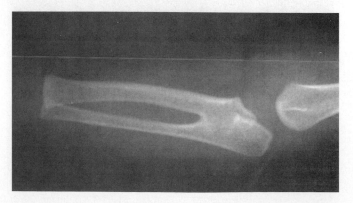

Fig. 5-73   Congenital radioulnar synostosis. The proximal fusion is typical.

dromes such as abnormal karyotypes (XXXY, XXYY). Acquired radioulnar synostosis can occur after infection or Caffey disease (infantile cortical hyperostosis).

Madelung deformity was described earlier in the discussions of Turner syndrome and the skeletal dysplasia dyschondrosteosis (Figs. 5-45 and 5-62).

Congenital radial head dislocation (see Fig. 3-93) is discussed in the upper extremity trauma chapter.

Symphalangism *Symphalangism* is congential coalition of metacarpals and phalanges (Fig. 5-74). The condition is variable and frequently is familial.

Torsion of the Femur and Tibia

Torsion is rotation measured around the long axis of a bone. The term torsion is most frequently applied to describe abnormal twisting along the long axis of the femur or tibia. Imagine that you are looking down the long axis of a lower extremity. Femoral alignment is determined by comparing the angle formed by the femoral neck and the condyles. If the femoral head projects anterior to the plane containing the femoral condyles, then antetorsion is present. The synonymous term *anteversion* is more frequently used. If the femoral head projects posterior to this plane, then retrotorsion, or retroversion is present. The terminology used to characterize tibial torsion is slightly different, but less confusing. *Medial* or *internal tibial torsion* results in internal rotation-like twisting of the distal tibia (pigeon-toed). *Lateral* or *external tibial torsion* is the opposite (penguin-footed). Femoral anteversion is best assessed by limited CT scan. A few slices are obtained through the femoral neck and the femoral condyles, and their relative angle

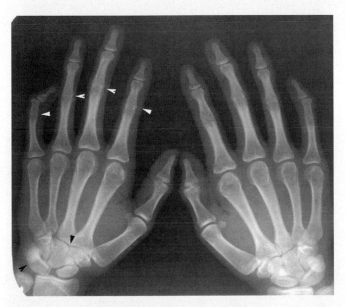

Fig. 5-74   Symphalangism. This mild case involves only the PIP joints (*white arrowheads*). Also note the lunotriquetral and trapezoid-capitate carpal coalitions (*black arrowheads*).

is determined (Fig. 5-75). Radiographs can easily estimate tibial torsion, but CT is occasionally used when a high degree of precision is needed.

Normal femoral torsion is 30° anteversion at birth, decreasing to 10° by adulthood. Excessive femoral anteversion causes gait and hindfoot abnormalities and contributes to hip dysplasia. Excessive anteversion occurs in DDH, Legg-Perthes, and neurologic and neuromuscular conditions. Excessive anteversion frequently resolves spontaneously during growth, but surgery may be needed. Surgical treatment is accomplished by femoral osteotomy: The femur is divided into two pieces, alignment is improved, and the fragments are fixed with orthopedic hardware and allowed to heal with casting. A proximal osteotomy is preferred when excessive valgus and/or hip instability and dysplasia are present to correct both problems (varus derotation osteotomy, VDRO, see Fig. 5-35). A distal femoral osteotomy is preferred when genu valgum or varus is also present to simultaneously correct the abnormal knee alignment (Fig. 5-76).

Abnormal tibial torsion usually resolves during growth. Excessive internal torsion frequently occurs in association with congenital foot deformities or genu varum. Toddlers will have bowlegs and a pigeon-toed gait. Excessive lateral torsion causes a penguin-footed gait.

Osteo-onychodysostosis

Osteo-onychodysostosis (nail-patella syndrome, Fong syndrome) is a rare autosomal dominant condition with multiple skeletal abnormalities. The most distinctive feature is posterior iliac horns, a pathognomonic finding that is present in most cases (Fig. 5-77A). The knees are dysplastic with absent or hypoplastic patellae (Fig. 5-77B), hypoplastic lateral femoral condyles and associated valgus alignment (genu valgum). The elbows also are dysplastic with a hypoplastic capitellum and associated radial head dislocation. The fifth metacarpals may be short. Clinical features include dysplastic fingernails, especially of the thumb and index fingers, clinodactyly, and renal disease.

Common Congenital Foot Deformities and Tarsal Coalitions

B. J. MANASTER, M.D., Ph.D.

Foot deformities seem to confound radiologists. They seem to be described in multiple different ways and to require too many measurements of angles. However, the common foot deformities can be described in a straightforward manner, using descriptors and occasional measurement of only three parameters. This section will first

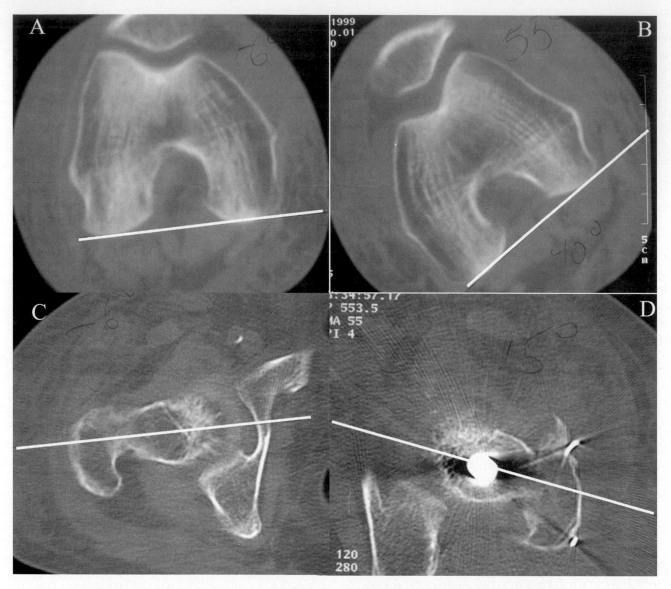

Fig. 5-75   Femoral anteversion. Adult patient who had a left femur fracture fixed with an intramedullary rod. Limited CT slices were obtained through the knees, then the couch was moved *without moving the patient* and limited slices were obtained through the proximal femurs. Representative images are shown. **A** = right knee, **B** = left knee, **C** = right femoral neck, **D** = left femoral neck. The uninjured right side has 0° of anteversion. On the left, the fragments had twisted around the rod, resulting in 55° of femoral anteversion. Corrective surgery was required.

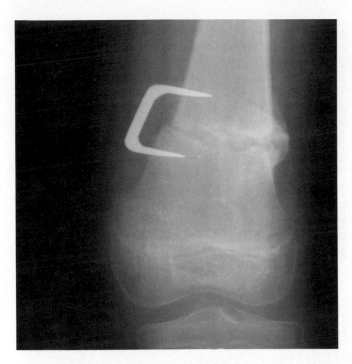

Fig. 5-76   Distal femoral osteotomy performed to correct excessive anteversion in a child.

describe these parameters, and then relate these to the common foot deformities.

First, it is most important to note that evaluation of foot deformities should only be made on weight bearing films. AP and lateral weight bearing films are used to

evaluate hindfoot equinus, hindfoot varus or valgus, and forefoot varus or valgus.

Hindfoot equinus is the easiest concept of the three. It is evaluated only on a lateral weight-bearing film. Normally, the calcaneus is dorsiflexed. This is simple enough to evaluate without measurement. However, if measurement is desired, the angle between the longitudinal axis of the tibia and the calcaneus (measured along its base) ranges between 60° and 90° (Fig. 5-78). Another way of measuring the dorsi or plantarflexion of the calcaneus is "calcaneal pitch" where on a lateral view a line drawn along the base of the calcaneus should slant upward from the horizontal surface by 20°–30°. The relationship of the calcaneus is abnormal either if it is plantarflexed or if it is excessively dorsiflexed. Plantarflexion of the calcaneus such that the calcaneal-tibial angle is greater than 90° represents hindfoot equinus (Fig. 5-78B). Hindfoot equinus is seen in clubfoot and congenital vertical talus. The opposite occurs with hindfoot calcaneus, where the calcaneus is excessively dorsiflexed such that the calcaneal-tibial angle is less than 60° (Fig. 5-78C). Hindfoot calcaneus is seen in cavus and spastic deformities.

The second parameter in evaluating a foot deformity is the presence of hindfoot varus or valgus. Both the AP and lateral weight-bearing radiographs are used for this evaluation. Conceptually, the talus may be considered the point of reference as it may be assumed to be fixed relative to the lower leg. Although this is not exactly correct, for the purpose of this discussion, let us assume

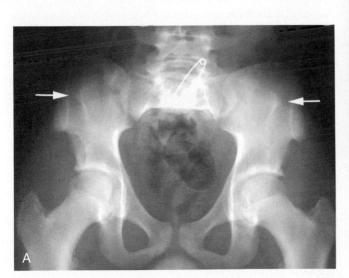

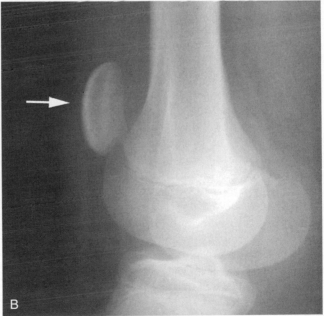

Fig. 5-77   Osteo-onychodysostosis (Fong syndrome). **A,** Pelvis shows characteristic laterally oriented posterior iliac horns (*arrows*). **B,** Lateral knee shows hypoplastic patella (*arrow*).

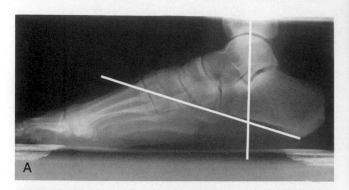

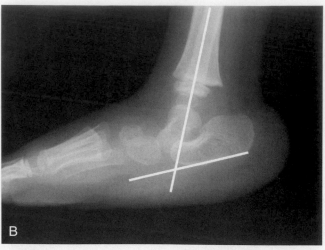

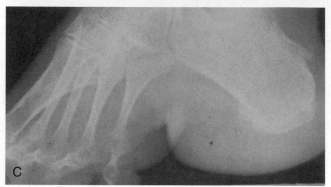

Fig. 5-78   Evaluation of equinus. **A,** Normal tibiocalcaneal angle, with normal dorsiflexion of the calcaneous. **B,** Equinus with calcanotibial angle greater than 90° and plantar flexion of the calcaneus. **C,** Hind foot calcaneus, with abnormal dorsiflexion of the calcaneus (in this case due to a bound foot in a Chinese woman).

that the calcaneus rotates medially or laterally with respect to a fixed talus. On an AP view, the talocalcaneal angle is described by lines drawn through the longitudinal axis of the talus and calcaneus. The AP talocalcaneal angle normally measures 15°–40° (30°–50° in newborns). You might note also that in the normal foot the mid-talar line passes through or slightly medial to the base of the first metatarsal. The mid-calcaneal line passes through the base of the fourth metatarsal (Fig. 5-79). If you presume then that the talus is fixed and the calcaneus adducts, the talocalcaneal angle decreases to less than 15°, to the point that in some cases the talocalcaneal angle may approach 0° or parallelism of those bones. A decreased talocalcaneal angle describes a hindfoot varus deformity (Fig. 5-79B). You might note that in a hindfoot varus deformity the talus ends up pointing lateral to the first metatarsal because the entire foot is swung medially. The opposite occurs when the calcaneus abducts relative to the talus. With calcaneal abduction, the talocalcaneal angle is increased greater than 40°. Note also that with this increased talocalcaneal angle, the talus points medial to the first metatarsal because the calcaneus and the entire foot swings laterally. This is hindfoot valgus (Fig. 5-79C).

As noted above, hindfoot varus or valgus is also evaluated on the lateral view. Normally, the lateral talocalcaneal (also termed Kite's) angle is measured by a line bisecting

the talus and a line along the base of the calcaneus, measuring 25° to 45° (50° in newborns). The calcaneus is dorsiflexed, as already discussed, and the talus is mildly plantarflexed to produce this angle (Fig. 5-80). Consider now the case when the calcaneus adducts (hindfoot varus). With the anterior portion of the calcaneus moving into a position beneath the head of the talus, the talus can no longer be as plantarflexed. This results in a decrease in the talocalcaneal angle on the lateral view, with the two bones approaching parallelism (Fig. 5-80B). This is the appearance on the lateral view of a hindfoot varus. Thus, on both the AP and lateral views, with a hindfoot varus deformity the talocalcaneal angles decrease and the bones approach parallelism. Consider now the situation where the calcaneus abducts, hindfoot valgus as seen on the AP view in Fig. 5-79C. With abduction of the calcaneus, the anterior calcaneus no longer supports the head of the talus at all and the talus is allowed to further plantar flex. On the lateral view then, we see increased plantarflexion of the talus, which results in an increased talocalcaneal angle (Fig. 5-80C). This is the appearance of hindfoot valgus on the lateral view. Thus, with hindfoot valgus there is an increased talocalcaneal angle on both the AP and lateral films.

Radiologists seem to have a difficult time remembering whether the talocalcaneal angle is increased or decreased in varus or valgus. It is worth remembering that in most

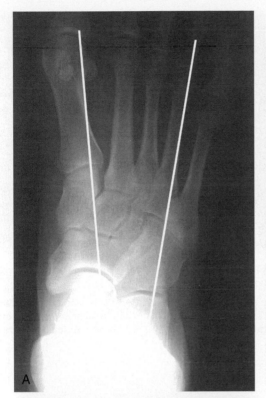

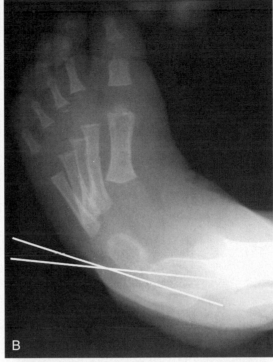

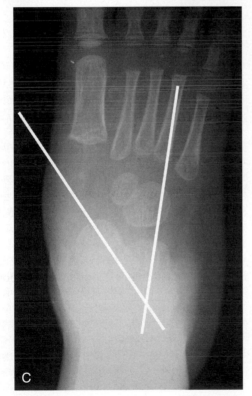

Fig. 5-79   AP hind foot evaluation. **A,** The normal AP talocalcaneal angle, with the mid talar line passing through the base of the first metatarsal and the mid-calcaneal line passing through the base of the fourth metatarsal. **B,** The AP evaluation of hindfoot varus, with a decreased talocalcaneal angle and the talus pointing lateral to the first metatarsal base. **C,** AP evaluation of hindfoot valgus, with an increased talocalcaneal angle and the talus pointing medially to the first metatarsal base.

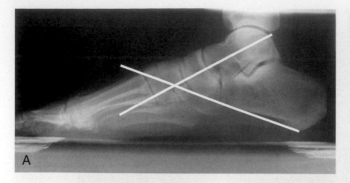

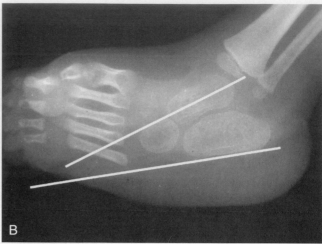

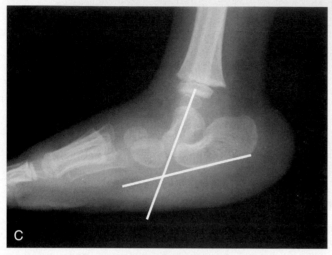

Fig. 5-80 Evaluation of the hindfoot on the lateral film. **A,** A normal hindfoot, with a normal lateral talocalcaneal angle. **B,** A varus hindfoot, with a decreased talocalcaneal angle. **C,** A valgus hindfoot, with an increased talocalcaneal angle.

congenital abnormalities, the talocalcaneal angle is increased on both AP and lateral films or decreased on both AP and lateral films. One additional hint is given by one radiologist educator who suggests that hindfoot valgus can be remembered because it has an increased angle as well as an increased number of letters relative to hindfoot varus.[1]

Having described hindfoot equinus and hindfoot varus or valgus, that leaves forefoot varus or valgus to be understood. This is a much more qualitative and subjective evaluation. On the AP radiograph, the metatarsals normally converge proximally with slight overlap at the bases (Fig. 5-81A). With forefoot varus, the forefoot is inverted and often slightly supinated. On the AP film then, the forefoot would appear narrowed, with an increased convergence at the bases of the metatarsals (Fig. 5-81B). With forefoot valgus, the forefoot is everted and often pronated. With this change in position, on the AP film the forefoot is seen to be broadened with a decrease of overlap at the bases (Fig. 5-81C). Consider now the appearance of the forefoot on the lateral view. Normally, the metatarsals are partially superimposed, with the fifth metatarsal in the most plantar position (Fig. 5-82A). With forefoot varus (inversion, often with supination), the metatarsals on the lateral view have a more ladderlike arrangement, with the first metatarsal in the most dorsal position and the fifth metatarsal in the most plantar position (Fig. 5-82B). On the other hand, with fore-

foot valgus (eversion and pronation), the metatarsals are usually more superimposed on one another on the lateral film, and the first metatarsal is in the most plantar position (Fig. 5-82C).

We are now in a position to discuss the common foot deformities. The one which is most commonly filmed is clubfoot (talipes equinovarus; *talipes,* any deformity of the foot involving the talus). Clubfoot is seen in 1 in 1000 births, more frequently in males than females (2–3:1 ratio). The etiology of the clubfoot deformity is unclear, but possible contributing factors include ligamentous laxity, muscle imbalance, intrauterine position deformity, and persistence of an early normal fetal relationship. The radiographic findings of a clubfoot deformity are hindfoot equinus, hindfoot varus, and forefoot varus (Fig. 5-83).

Congenital vertical talus (rocker bottom foot) is a deformity in which the talus is in extreme plantarflexion with dorsal dislocation of the navicular, locking the talus into plantarflexion. Radiographically, one sees an equinus deformity, valgus hindfoot, dorsiflexed and valgus forefoot, and an abnormal talus with dislocated navicular (Fig. 5-84). Congenital vertical talus clinically presents as a rigid flat foot and may occur in either isolation or part of a variety of syndromes, and frequently is associated with myelomeningocele.

Flexible flatfoot deformity (pes planovalgus) is relatively common, affecting 4% of the population. An impor-

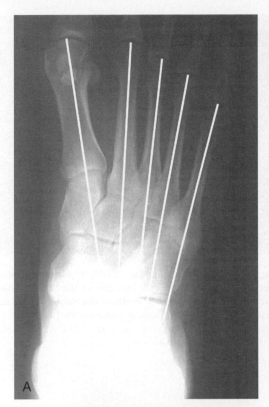

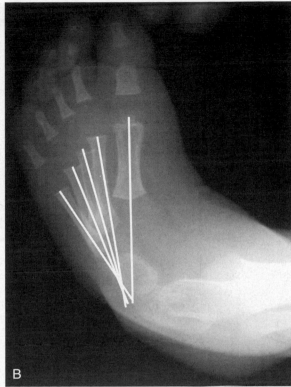

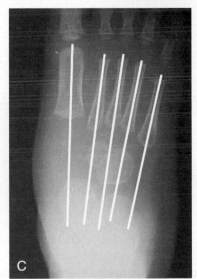

Fig. 5-81   AP evaluation of the forefoot. **A,** The normal appearance of convergence with slight overlap at the bases of the metatarsals. **B,** Forefoot varus, with abnormally increased convergence at the bases of the metatarsals. **C,** Forefoot valgus, with divergence or at least a decrease in the overlap at the bases of the metatarsals.

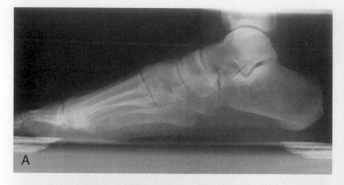

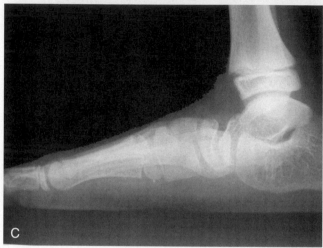

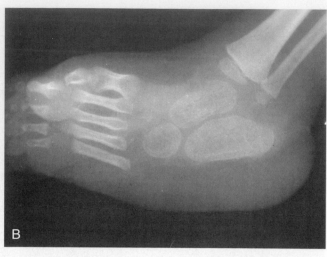

Fig. 5-82   Lateral evaluation of the forefoot. **A,** Normal, with partial superimposition of the metatarsals and the fifth in the plantar position. **B,** Varus forefoot, with a ladderlike configuration of the metatarsals, fifth in the plantar position. **C,** Forefoot valgus, with superimposition of the metatarsals on the lateral view and the first in the most plantar position.

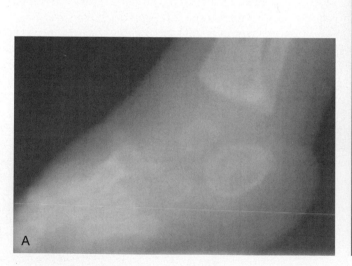

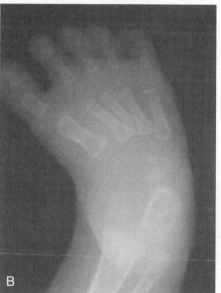

Fig. 5-83   Clubfoot. The lateral view (**A**) demonstrates equinus of the hindfoot. Both the AP (**B**) and lateral views show a varus hindfoot (decreased talocalcaneal angle, with the bones approaching parallelism). AP and lateral views show a varus forefoot.

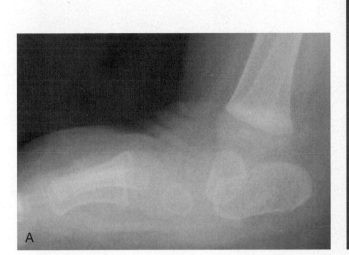

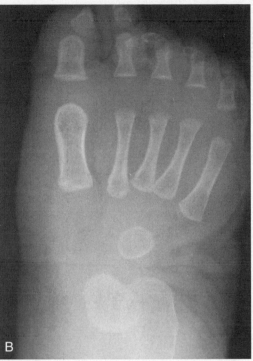

Fig. 5-84 Congenital vertical talus (rocker bottom foot). The lateral view (**A**) shows equinus of the hindfoot. The AP (**B**) and lateral views show a valgus hindfoot (increased talocalcaneal angle), with the talus being nearly vertical on the lateral view. The AP and lateral show a valgus forefoot.

tant part of the diagnosis is that it is indeed flexible; the abnormality is seen only on weight-bearing radiographs and the deformity is reduced with nonweight-bearing radiographs. The flexible flatfoot deformity has a hindfoot valgus and forefoot valgus, but no equinus (Fig. 5-85). The valgus deformities are usually subtler than those of a congenital vertical talus.

Pes cavus is a high arched foot (hindfoot calcaneus) with compensatory plantarflexion of the forefoot. It is seen in patients with upper motor neuron lesions (Friedreich's ataxia), lower motor neuron lesions (polio), vascular ischemia as in Volkmann's contracture, and muscular dystrophy of the peroneal type (Charcot-Marie-Tooth disease).

Metatarsus adductus is the most common structural abnormality of the foot, seen in infancy (10 times as frequently as clubfoot). Radiologists do not see it as frequently, as it usually is not imaged. Metatarsus adductus is usually bilateral and more common in females than males. The radiographic findings are of forefoot adductus, with a normal hindfoot.

Foot deformities that combine varus and valgus hindfoot and forefoot deformities are usually spastic in nature, such as might be seen in polio or cerebral palsy.

Tarsal coalition (peroneal spastic flatfoot) is a painful flatfoot deformity that occurs in 1% of the population. The vast majority are congenital, due to a failure of seg-

mentation of the bones of the foot in utero. More rarely, tarsal coalitions may be seen as a part of various syndromes, including hereditary symphalangism, Apert's acrocephalosyndactyly, and hand-foot-uterus syndrome. Males are more commonly affected, and tarsal coalitions are found to be bilateral in 25% of cases.

Symptoms of a tarsal coalition are generally first noted in the second or third decade. A teenager or young adult who presents with limited subtalar motion, pes planus, and shortening or persistent or intermittent spasm of the peroneal muscles should be imaged for tarsal coalition. The coalition may be fibrous, cartilaginous, or osseous. Therefore, one may not demonstrate bony bridging in all cases. However, in the absence of bony bridging, abnormally close approximation of the bones with cortical irregularity, broadening, or sclerosis suggests fibrous or cartilaginous bridging.

Any or all of the hindfoot and hindfoot/midfoot joints may be fused. When there is a substantial coalition, with multiple fusions, the patient may develop a ball and socket ankle as seen on the AP radiograph (Fig. 5-86). Converting the tibiotalar joint from a hinge joint to a ball and socket joint provides an inversion-eversion function that is restricted at the coalesced talocalcaneal joint.

Calcaneonavicular and talocalcaneal coalitions are the two most common varieties. They may both show a secondary sign of talar "beaking," a reactive process to ex-

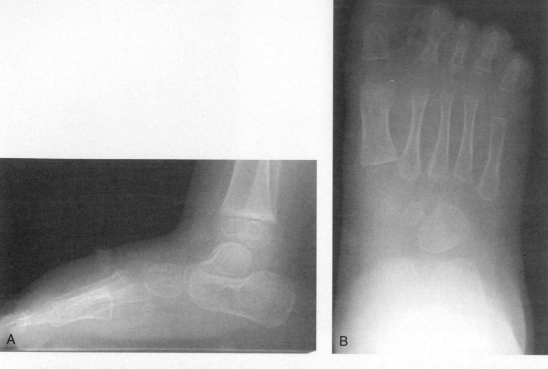

Fig. 5-85 Flexible flat foot deformity. The lateral and AP weight-bearing views (**A** and **B**, respectively) demonstrate no hindfoot equinus but hindfoot and forefoot valgus. Nonweight-bearing films (not shown) would show a normal alignment of both the hindfoot and forefoot. (Reprinted with permission from the ACR learning file.)

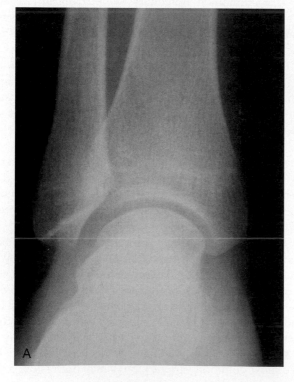

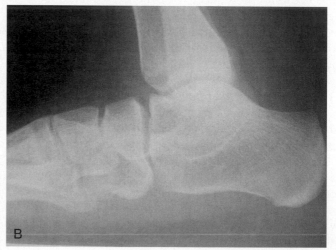

Fig. 5-86 Tarsal coalition: ball and socket joint. The AP radiograph, **A**, shows that the ankle has assumed a more rounded appearance at the tibiotalar joint, allowing a ball and socket type of motion. This indicates lack of motion in the other joints of the hindfoot, confirmed on the lateral view, which shows complete fusion of all the facets of the talocalcaneal joint (**B**).

cess motion at the talonavicular joint resulting from restricted in the other hindfoot/midfoot joints. Talar beaking is more frequently seen with talocalcaneal coalitions than calcaneonavicular coalitions, due to the greater mechanical restriction in the former type.

A calcaneonavicular coalition is not seen reliably on an AP radiograph, and is seen only indirectly on a lateral film with an "anteater" sign of a bony extension arising from the anterior calcaneus toward the navicular (Fig. 5-87). A calcaneonavicular coalition is seen directly and much more reliably on an oblique film, where either the solid osseous coalition or the fragmented sclerotic abnormal joint is noted. CT is generally not required to prove a calcaneonavicular coalition, but if it is employed, must be positioned such that the cuts project perpendicu-

larly to the calcanconavicular joint. On CT, the broadening of the articulation is noted on a coalition (Fig. 5-88).

Talocalcaneal (subtalar) coalition may be more complex than calcaneonavicular coalition. It is not seen on an AP radiograph and is seen only indirectly as an increase in sclerosis in the subtalar region on a lateral view. CT or MRI directly demonstrate the three facets of the talocalcaneal joint: the posterior (lateral facet), the middle (medial facet) formed with the sustentaculum tali inferiorly, and the anterior facet (Fig. 5-89). A talocalcaneal coalition usually occurs at the middle facet between the talus and the sustentaculum tali (Fig. 5-89). Ankylosis of the posterior or anterior facets is far less common, but may occur and is best diagnosed by CT or MRI (Fig. 5-90). We routinely image both feet, because tarsal coalitions of any

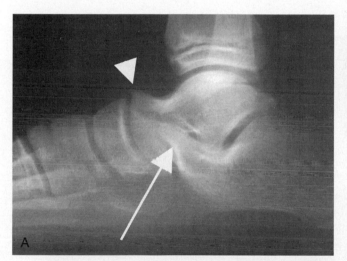

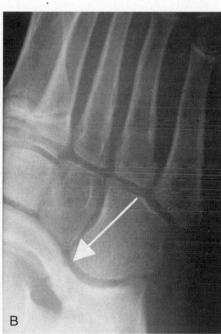

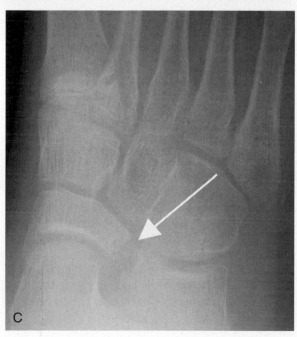

Fig. 5-87   Tarsal coalition: calcaneonavicular. **A,** A lateral view of the foot in a 14-year-old male, demonstrating a small talar beak (*arrowhead*) and an elongated anterior extension of the calcaneus (*arrow,* "anteater" sign). The oblique view (**B**), shows the calcaneonavicular coalition to be osseus (*arrow*). **C,** An oblique of a different patient, showing irregularity and fragmentation at the calcaneonavicular joint (*arrow*). This is a fibrous coalition.

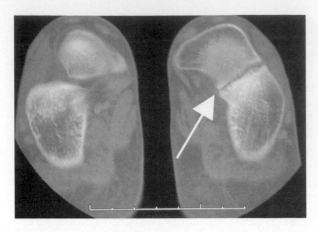

Fig. 5-88   Tarsal coalition: calcaneonavicular. CT demonstrates a normal calcaneonavicular joint on the right and broad and irregular calcaneonavicular joint on the left (*arrow*). This represents a fibrous or cartilaginous coalition.

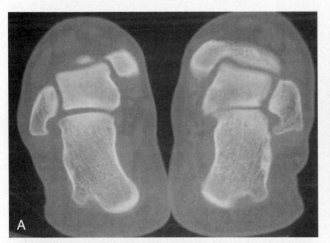

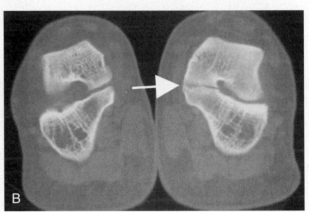

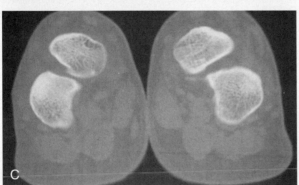

Fig. 5-89   Tarsal coalition: talocalcaneal. **A,** The normal posterior facets. **B,** The normal middle or medial facet on the right foot, but a broadened irregular coalition of the medial facet on the left (*arrow*). **C,** The normal bilateral anterior facets. The middle facet is the most frequently involved facet in a talocalcaneal coalition.

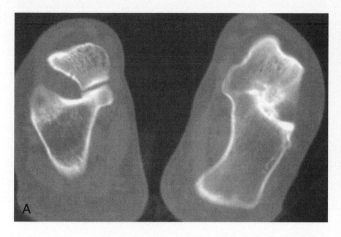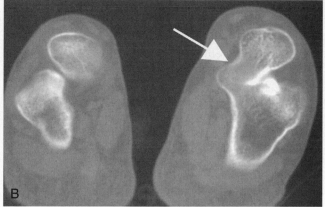

Fig. 5-90   Tarsal coalition: talocalcaneal. This is an example of an unusually extensive talocalcaneal coalition. The posterior facets (not shown) are normal bilaterally. The middle facet shows an osseus fusion on the left and is normal on the right (**A**). This is the expected site of coalition. However, we also see coalition of the anterior facet on the left (**B**, *arrow*).

type can be bilateral. All three facets of the talocalcaneal joint are seen with adequate positioning for CT. Optimum positioning is obtained with the feet flat on the table, knees flexed, and gantry tilted slightly away from the knees. This results in cuts perpendicular to the talocalcaneal joint. If a spiral or multidetector CT scanner is available, then 1 mm or 0.5 mm cuts can be obtained, with the feet taped together to minimize motion, in any position that the patient finds comfortable. The thin slices allow for satisfactory reformats in any desired plane.

REFERENCE

1. Kilcoyne R, Rych S, Gloch H: Radiological measurement of congenital and acquired foot deformities. *Applied Radiology* 1993;(December):35-41.

SOURCES AND SUGGESTED READINGS

Gerscovich EO: Practical approach to ultrasound of the hip in developmental dysplasia. *Radiologist* 1998;5:23-33.

Graf R: *Guide to sonography of the infant hip* New York: Thieme, 1987.

Greenspan A: Sclerosing bone dysplasias: a target sign approach. *Skeletal Radiology* 1991;20:561.

Greulich WW, Pyle SI: *Radiographic atlas of skeletal development of the hand and wrist.* 2nd ed. Stanford: Stanford University Press, 1959.

Harcke HT: Screening newborns for developmental dysplasia of the hip: the role of sonography. *AJR* 1994;162:395-397.

Harcke HT, Grisson LE: Performing dynamic sonography of the infant hip. *AJR* 1990;155:834-844.

Keats TE: *An atlas of roentgen variants that may simulate disease.* 5th ed. St. Louis. Mosby, 1992.

Keats TE, Smith TH: *An atlas of normal developmental roentgen anatomy.* 2nd ed. Chicago: Year Book Medical Publishers, 1988.

Kleinman P: *Diagnostic imaging of child abuse.* St. Louis: Mosby, 1998.

Laor T, Jarmillo D, and Oestereich AE: Musculoskeletal system. In Kirks DR, Griscom NT, eds. *Practical pediatric imaging* 3rd ed. Philadelphia: Lippincott-Raven, 1998.

McAlister WH, Heman TE: Osteochondrodysplasias, dysostoses, chromosonal abberations, mucopolysaccharidoses, and mucolipidoses. In Resnick D, ed. *Diagnosis of bone and joint disorders.* 3rd ed. Philadelphia: WB Saunders 1995 4163-4244.

Ozonoff MB: *Pediatric orthopaedic radiology* 2nd ed. Philadelphia: WB Saunders 1992.

Sontag LW, Snell, D, Anderson M: Rate of appearance of ossification centers from birth to the age of five years. *Am J Dis Child* 1939;58:949-956.

Spranger J: International classification of osteochondrodysplasias. The International Working Group on Constitutional Diseases of Bone. *Eur J Pediatrics* 1992;151:407-415.

Spranger JW, Langer LO, Wiedemann HR: *Bone dysplasias.* Philadelphia: WB Saunders, 1974.

Swischuck LE, John SD: *Differential diagnosis in pediatric radiology* 2nd ed. Baltimore: Williams and Wilkins, 1995.

Taybi H, Lachman RS: *Radiology of syndromes, metabolic disorders, and skeletal dysplasias.* 4th ed. St. Louis: Mosby, 1996.

Teele RL, Share JC: *Ultrasonography of infants and children.* Philadelphia: WB Saunders, 1991.

CHAPTER 6

Miscellaneous, Including Hematogenous Disorders and Infection

B.J. MANASTER, M.D., Ph.D.

HEMATOGENOUS DISORDERS

Hemophilia

Hemophilia is a bleeding disorder resulting from a clotting factor deficiency. From a musculoskeletal standpoint, it results in hemarthroses, deformity, and arthropa-

Key Concepts	Hemophilia

- Gender specific for males
- Joints:
    Effusions may appear dense.
    Erosive disease may be severe.
    Overgrowth due to hyperemia results in "ballooning" of the joints
    Early osseous fusion due to hyperemia.
    Knees, elbows, ankles most common locations.
- Pseudotumor:
    Shows extrinsic scalloping.
    Occurs most frequently in the femur, pelvis, and calcaneus.
    Bizarre masses arising in bone or soft tissue with evidence of products of hemorrhage.

thy. The two most common varieties of hemophilia, hemophilia A (factor VIII deficiency) and hemophilia B (factor IX deficiency, Christmas disease) are inherited through an X-linked recessive pattern and therefore are only found in males.

Hemarthroses may occur in several joints, but are often asymmetric and are related to trivial trauma. The most commonly involved joints are the knee, elbow, and ankle, followed by less frequent occurrences in the hip and shoulder. Chronic, recurrent hemarthroses often result in flexion contractures and arthropathy. The arthropathy occurs only after multiple episodes of hemarthrosis. The hemarthrosis results in hypertrophied synovium, which often contains hemosiderin deposits. The hemosiderin deposits may be seen on radiographs as an unusually dense effusion (Fig. 6-1), and is seen on MR as having a low signal intensity on T1 and intermediate to low signal intensity on T2 imaging, often with a "blooming" effect on gradient echo imaging (Fig. 6-2). The synovial inflammation in turn causes hyperemia. With hyperemia, the adjacent bones become osteoporotic. Because hemarthroses usually occur in skeletally immature patients, the hyperemia also results in epiphyseal overgrowth, which is seen radiographically as flared, enlarged epiphyses, with comparatively gracile diaphyses (Fig. 6-1). The hyperemia can also result in early epiphyseal fusion and resultant skeletal shortening. With the synovitis, cartilage destruction ensues, along with erosions and subarticular cysts. Eventually, secondary degenerative joint disease develops. Thus, the joints appear quite distinctive, with the metaphases and epiphyses themselves being enlarged, notches being enlarged (such as the intercondylar notch in the knee and trochlear notch in the elbow) and variable articular destruction. The elbow and knee both show these features well, but the elbow often seems to have a distinctively enlarged radial head (Fig. 6-3). Although these features seem quite distinctive, it should be remembered that patients with juvenile rheumatoid arthritis (JRA) have a similar pattern of overgrowth and

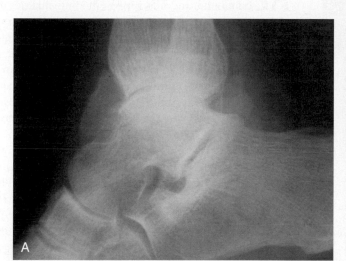

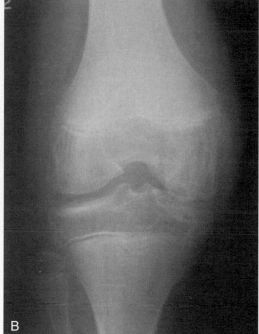

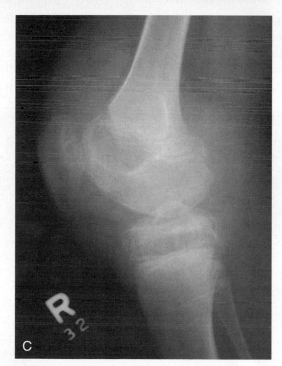

Fig. 6-1   Hemophilia. **A,** A lateral radiograph showing the dense effusions that can occur in hemophilia owing to repeated episodes of hemarthrosis and hemosiderin deposition. **B,** and **C** AP and lateral radiographs, respectively, of a knee in a 13-year-old hemophilic patient. They demonstrate the large dense effusions, overgrown epiphyses and metaphyses, widened intercondylar notch, and erosive change seen typically in these patients.

destructive change as the pathology relates to inflammatory change in a growing skeleton. The two processes may not be distinguishable radiographically.

Pseudotumor of hemophilia is a nonneoplastic mass lesion that occurs with an intraosseous, subperiosteal, or soft-tissue bleed. With repeated bleeding in the same area, extrinsic and/or intrinsic scalloping and pressure erosion occurs at the cortical margin of bone. The area of destruction may be extremely large, but the margins

are generally sharply circumscribed and sclerotic. Periosteal reaction may be extensive. There may be a large soft tissue mass. The appearance may be quite bizarre (Fig. 6-4). MRI of the mass may show a hypointense rim due to the hematoma's fibrous capsule and to hemosiderin deposits, whereas the central signal will vary according to the age of the hematoma and the presence of clot contained therein. Usually, many different combinations of signal intensities are seen, reflecting the process of

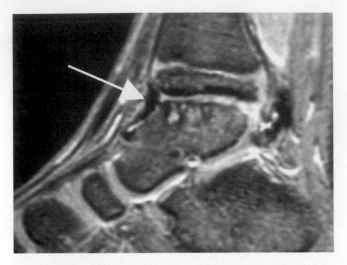

Fig. 6-2 MRI hemophilia. The sagittal gradient echo images of the ankle in a 7-year-old male with hemophilia demonstrates erosive change, as well as the ankle effusion (*arrows*). Note that the ankle effusion is low signal intensity, and shows the "blooming" effect on gradient echo imaging due to the hemosiderin deposits. (Courtesy of Ray Kilcoyne, M.D.)

remote and recurrent bleeding as well as clot organiza tion. The size and extent of the pseudotumor may simulate neoplasm, but the sclerotic margins with scalloping may suggest the correct diagnosis. Similarly, location may suggest the correct diagnosis, as pseudotumor of hemo-

philia is found most frequently in the femur, pelvis, tibia, and calcaneus.

Sickle Cell Anemia and Thallasemia

The congenital anemias represent abnormalities in one of the chains comprising hemoglobin, with the abnormality affecting the shape and/or function of hemoglobin. Nonmusculoskeletal radiographic findings include renal papillary necrosis, cholelithiasis, splenic autoinfarction, cardiomegaly, and pulmonary infarction. Three major osseous radiographic abnormalities can occur in each of the anemias. However, each of the anemias seems to have unique features. The three radiographic abnormalities are marrow hyperplasia, infarction, and osteomyelitis. Marrow hyperplasia occurs because of long-term anemia. Radiographically, it is manifest as osteopenia with coarsened trabeculae, which may give an overall appearance of sclerosis of the tubular bones. In addition, the tubular bones may be widened from marrow expansion, as may be the mandible and diploic spaces of the skull (Fig. 6-5).

Patients with congenital anemias have a predilection for osteomyelitis, which radiographically may be indistinguishable from osseous infarction. Specialized radionuclide scanning, MR imaging, and sometimes biopsy are necessary to distinguish between the two diagnoses. Although salmonella osteomyelitis is seen more frequently

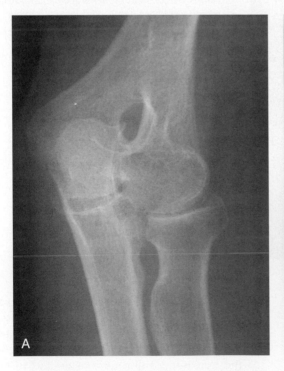

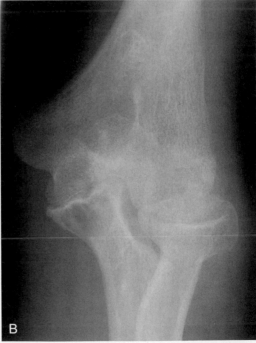

Fig. 6-3 Hemophilia: elbow. **A,** An oblique radiograph of the elbow in an 18-year-old male. It demonstrates modest changes of hemophilia, with a wide trochlear notch and mild cartilage narrowing as well as relatively overgrown radial head. A more severe case is seen in **B.** This is a different patient, a 34-year-old male, who shows an even more exaggerated size of the radial head and much more advanced erosive change.

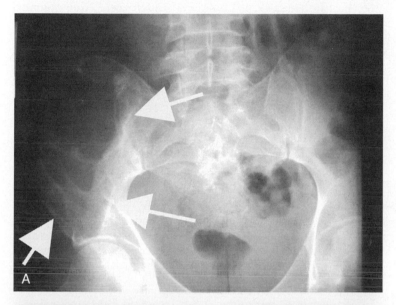

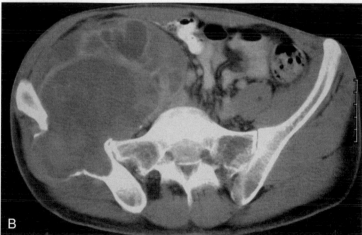

Fig. 6-4 Pseudotumor of hemophilia. **A,** An AP radiograph of the pelvis in a 35-year-old male. It demonstrates a well-defined lesion in the right iliac wing (*arrows*). There is pseudo-trabeculation of the lesion and no other characterizing feature. **B,** CT demonstrates the lesion to be large, to have broken through the cortex, but to have smoothly scalloped the bone. There are different densities within the lesion, and the rim enhances.

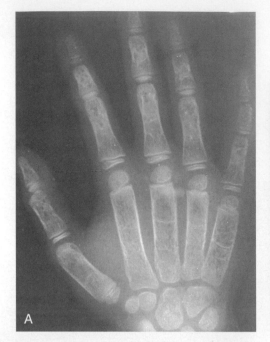

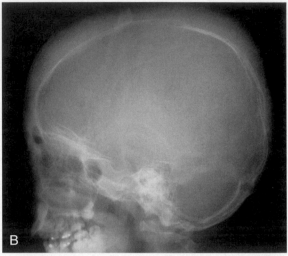

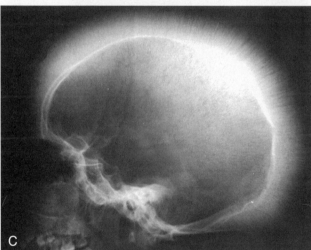

Fig. 6-5 Marrow hyperplasia: thalassemia. **A,** A PA radiograph of a hand demonstrating diffuse osteopenia and both widening and squaring of the metacarpals and phalanges. These features are seen in diseases where there is severe marrow hyperplasia. Thalassemia is the most pronounced of these disease processes. The skull can also accommodate marrow hyperplasia. **B,** shows widened diploic space in the calvarium and replacement of air in the maxillary sinuses by marrow. These findings are exaggerated in the lateral skull film of another patient, (**C**). (C, reprinted with permission of the ACR learning file.)

in these patients than in the normal population, staphylococcus is still the most common causative organism for osteomyelitis in patients with congenital anemia.

Osseous infarction is due to vascular occlusion. It is seen in the very young as "dactylitis." This is also called hand-foot syndrome, where ambient cold temperatures result in vasoconstriction in the persistent hematopoietic marrow of the digits. Radiographically, dactylitis is seen as periosteal reaction and soft tissue swelling (Fig. 6-6). In the adult patient, infarcts occur in the diaphyses and metaphyses of long bones, seen radiographically as patchy sclerosis or serpiginous calcified densities (Fig. 6-7). There may rarely be associated periosteal reaction. Infarcts can also occur in the vertebral body endplate. This may result in sclerosis and endplate depression, sometimes resulting in a more specific appearance termed "H-shaped vertebrae." This distinct appearance

of the endplate occurs because of the distribution of small vessel arcades at the endplates in which the sickled cells sludge, resulting in necrosis at this specific site (Fig. 6-8). Infarction also occurs in the femoral and humeral heads, manifest as the typical appearance of avascular necrosis (Fig. 6-9).

Sickle cell anemia (Hb SS) is found in 1% of the black population in North America. Dactylitis is a common feature, occurring in 10%–20% of children with sickle cell disease. Avascular necrosis of the femoral and humeral heads is extremely common. H-shaped vertebrae due to avascular necrosis of the vertebral body endplates is seen as well.

Sickle cell trait (Hb AS) causes very few musculoskeletal findings. Bone infarcts are occasionally seen. Sickle cell hemoglobin C (Hb SC) predominately shows marrow hyperplasia of the skull and subchondral avascular necro-

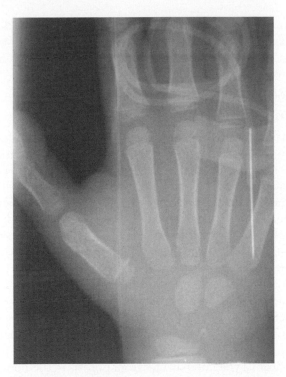

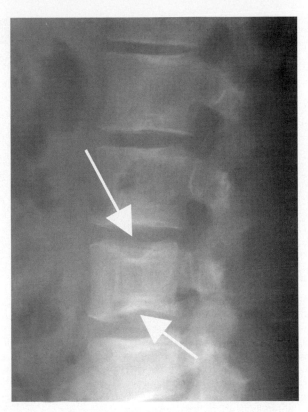

Fig. 6-6   Sickle cell dactylitis. The radiograph of the thumb in this 3-year-old female with sickle cell disease demonstrates abnormal density and periosteal reaction in the first metacarpal. The changes are subtle, and could represent other disease processes, such as infection, but in this case represent the early changes of the bone infarct in this youngster with the clinical findings of hand/foot syndrome. (Reprinted with permission from the ACR learning file.)

Fig. 6-8   Sickle cell: spine. The patchy increased density in all the vertebral bodies is typical of sickle cell disease. Additionally, the sickled cells may sludge in the looping arcades at the end plates of the vertebral bodies, causing them to collapse in their central portion. This is seen on this radiograph (*arrows*), where L4 is approaching what has been termed an "H shaped" vertebra.

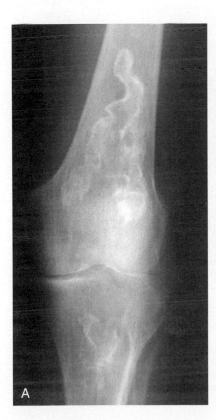

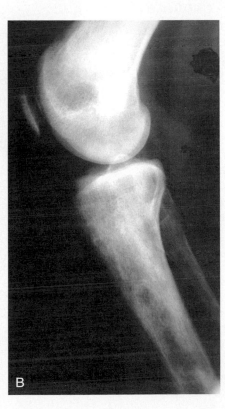

Fig. 6-7   Bone infarct. **A,** Bone infarct can be seen either as a serpiginous calcification, or (**B**) as a generalized but patchy increase in bone density. The latter is the more common appearance of bone infarct in sickle cell patients.

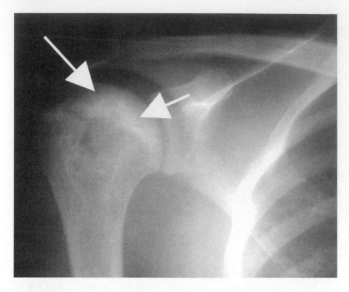

Fig. 6-9 Sickle cell: avascular necrosis. Avascular necrosis, particularly of the humeral head and femoral head, are typical findings of sickle cell disease. In this case, the patchy sclerosis of the bone, suggesting multiple infarcts, is seen. Superimposed on this is a more concentrated sclerosis of the humeral head (*arrows*) in its superior weight-bearing portion. This is the typical location for avascular necrosis of the humeral head. There is no collapse at this time in this patient. Please refer to Fig. 2-90 to see avascular necrosis in the hip in a patient with sickle cell.

sis, without featuring other metadiaphyseal bone infarcts. Splenomegaly rather than splenic infarction is also a feature of this disease.

Thalassemia major (Cooley's anemia) has features that are distinct from those of sickle cell anemia. Thalassemia major is clinically manifested early in life, and death often occurs by young adulthood. Marrow hyperplasia is the major radiographic feature, and may be spectacular. The skull may show dense striations within a very widened diploic space, to the point that they have been described as having a hair-on-end appearance (Fig. 6-5). In addition, the paranasal sinuses are obliterated. To accommodate marrow hyperplasia, the tubular bones are often squared and the distal femera may show an Erlenmeyer flask deformity. Avascular necrosis is much less common in thalassemia than in sickle cell disease. Finally, sickle cell-thalassemia has a radiographic appearance that ranges from normal to typical sickle cell, with infarcts overshadowing hyperplastic marrow changes.

Mastocytosis

Mastocytosis is a proliferative disorder of mast cells, which results in the clinical symptoms of flushing, nausea, vomiting, and skin lesions resembling urticaria pigmentosa. The radiographic abnormalities are not distinct, as bones may show either osteoporosis or sclerosis. It seems that histamine release from mast cells can result

in osteoporosis which is usually generalized (Fig. 6-10) although occasionally may be focal. On the other hand, host reaction to marrow infiltration by mast cells may result in bony sclerosis (Fig. 6-11).

Myelofibrosis

Myelofibrosis results in fibrosis in areas of the skeleton that are normally involved in hematopoiesis. Because of the resultant restriction in hematopoiesis in the usual locations (axial skeleton and proximal femoral and humeral diaphyses), patients develop compensatory hematopoiesis in the fatty marrow of large tubular bones and extramedullary hematopoiesis. These latter osseous sites, in turn, may become fibrotic. The patients who develop extramedullary hematopoiesis show hepatosplenomegaly and paraspinous masses. Radiographic findings include sclerotic bone marrow (either diffusely or as a patchy increased density with cortical thickening) in the hematopoietic bones (vertebrae, pelvis, ribs, and the long tubular bones) (Fig. 6-12). MR shows low signal on both T1- and T2-weighted images from fibrosis in the hematopoietic bones, with reconversion of fatty marrow to red marrow in the shafts and more distal portions of the large tubular bones. The appearance varies based on the severity and stage of the disease.

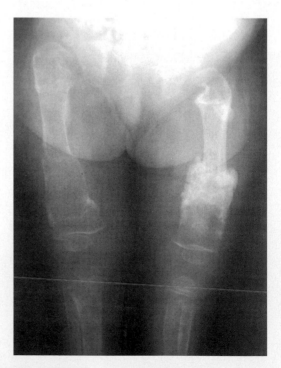

Fig. 6-10 Mastocytosis. Radiographic manifestations of mastocytosis include diffuse osteopenia, as seen in this 4-month-old child who has already sustained multiple fractures. (Reprinted with permission from the ACR learning file.)

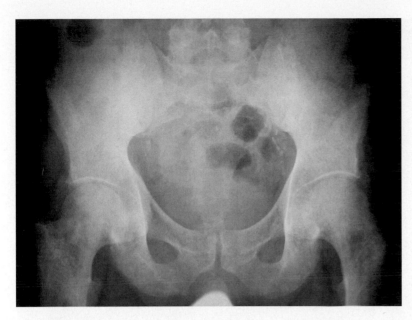

Fig. 6-11   Mastocytosis. Mastocytosis can present with mixed osteopenia and sclerosis as in this 50-year-old male. The sclerosis can be either diffuse as in this patient or focal.

Gaucher's Disease

Gaucher's disease is a familial sphingolipid storage disorder, with accumulation of lipid laden macrophages called Gaucher cells in the reticuloendothelial system including the marrow. There are infantile and juvenile forms that involve the central nervous system and produce mental retardation and early death. The more common form shows an onset in later childhood or young adulthood and normal life span. The most frequently noted radiographic osseous abnormality is expansion of the distal femur, termed the Erlenmeyer flask deformity (Fig. 6-13). This expansion is due to marrow infiltration, and is present in 40%–50% of patients. The same percentage of patients develop avascular necrosis (Figs. 2-91 and 6-13), especially of the femoral head. Because of the marrow replacement, the patients may show generalized osteoporosis and be susceptible both to fracture and osteomyelitis. The vertebral endplates may fracture in an H-shaped pattern, as is seen in sickle cell disease. Less frequent radiographic findings of Gaucher's disease include bone infarction with focal sclerosis and occasional bone-within-bone appearance, or focal "cystic" lesions.

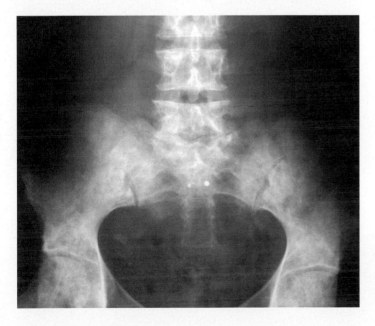

Fig. 6-12   Myelofibrosis. Myelofibrosis presents in the skeleton with fibrosis in the regions normally involved in hemopoiesis (axial skeleton), with subsequent compensatory hematopoiesis in the fatty marrow of the large tubular bones. The latter sites may in turn become fibrotic. The involved bones show mixed sclerosis and lucency, as do all the bones on this AP radiograph.

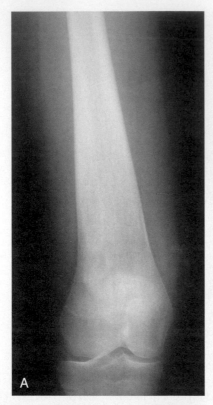

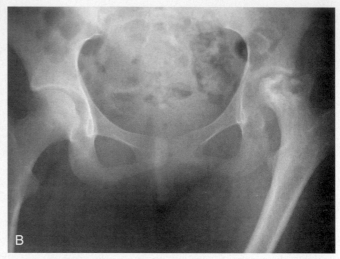

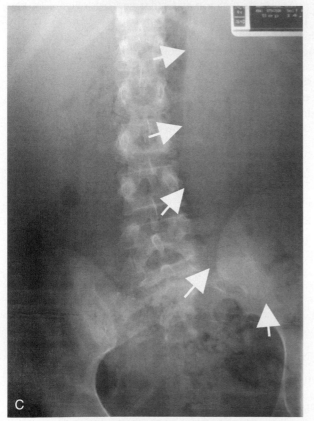

Fig. 6-13   Gaucher's disease. **A,** An AP radiograph of the femur in an 18-year-old female with Gaucher's disease. Note the minimal abnormality in density, as well as the slight widening of the distal metadiaphysis of the femur. This change in morphology to accommodate deposition within the marrow has been termed an Erlenmeyer flask deformity. **B,** The same patient had severe avascular necrosis of the left hip, a common problem in Gaucher's disease. **C,** An AP view of the lumbar spine in this patient. The spine itself is normal, but the film demonstrates a tremendous hepatosplenomegaly seen in Gaucher's disease, with the bowel gas concentrated in the center of the abdomen and the spleen outlined (*arrowheads*).

Any of the above abnormalities, seen in conjunction with hepatosplenomegaly, should suggest the diagnosis of Gaucher's disease.

There is a differential diagnosis for the Erlenmeyer flask deformity of the distal femurs. Many of the anemias may repopulate marrow with expansion like this. In Niemann-Pick disease, sphingomyelin may accumulate with similar infiltrative bony findings, as well as hepatosplenomegaly. Finally, Pyle's disease is a metaphyseal dysplasia that results in expanded metaphyses of the tubular bones, especially about the knee, with normal diaphyses. Pyle's disease, however, does not show a true marrow infiltration.

BONE MARROW

The marrow is a highly dynamic part of the musculoskeletal system that can be very difficult to understand. There is normally a predictable pattern of conversion from red (hematopoietic) marrow to fatty marrow. The earliest conversion to fatty marrow occurs in the epiphyses and apophyses. After that, there is progressive conversion to fatty marrow, which begins in the peripheral appendicular skeleton, and extends toward the central axial skeleton. The terminal phalanges convert first. In the long bones, conversion begins in the diaphysis and progresses toward the metaphyses. Conversion of marrow in the flat bones lags behind that of the long bones. Marrow in the spine is typically the last to convert from hematopoietic to fatty elements. Conversion to fatty marrow is mostly complete by age 25, when red marrow remains only in the axial skeleton and proximal humeral and femoral metaphyses. However, women often retain residual spotty red marrow in the femurs and the pelvis, likely related to the demands of menstruation. With further aging beyond 25 years, there is a slower continuation of the fatty conversion process. By the eighth decade, even the pedicles and posterior elements of the vertebrae contain fatty marrow.

Fatty marrow is quite labile and reconverts to hematopoietic marrow with any stress. Like the initial conversion, re-conversion to hematopoietic marrow follows an orderly pattern, beginning in the spine and flat bones and extending towards the appendicular skeleton. Reconversion may be spotty or complete, especially in the femora and humeri. Reconversion is often seen incidentally on MR examinations. Conditions in which one sees marrow reconversion include anemias (Fig. 6-14) (whether hemolytic, related to chronic disease, or chronic blood loss), obesity, smoking, hypoventilation hypoxia, poorly compensated heart disease, AIDS, and "sports anemia," most frequently seen in endurance athletes such as marathon runners. Pathologic processes can mimic marrow reconversion. These include polycythe-

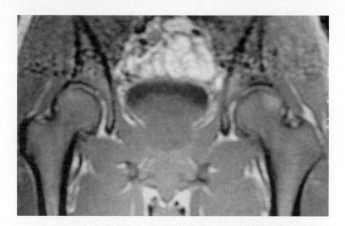

Fig. 6-14   Marrow reconversion. This coronal T1-weighted MRI (600/16) in a 23-year-old male with sickle cell disease demonstrates lower than normal signal abnormality in the femoral heads, necks, and greater trochanters. By this age, there should be fatty marrow (high signal) in the femoral heads and greater trochanters, with a patchier pattern in the femoral necks. This marrow abnormality represents marrow reconversion in this patient with abnormal red blood cell production.

mia vera, hemochromatosis, amyloidosis, Gaucher's disease, lymphoma, myelofibrosis, myeloma, and metastases. One valuable hint that can be used to differentiate an infiltrative marrow pathology from hematopoietic marrow in the spine on MRI examination is as follows: With T1-weighted SE imaging, marrow signal alteration that is lower than skeletal muscle or normal disk should not be attributed to hematopoietic marrow alone (Fig. 6-15). An infiltrative process should be assumed. Exceptions to this include TR weighting that is greater than 700 ms (not a true T1), the spine in infants, and patients with profound anemia such as sickle cell, bone marrow transplant, and transfused AIDS patients.

Myeloid depletion occurs when the marrow space is devoid of hematopoietic elements. The marrow signal is that of fat on all sequences. Myeloid depletion is seen in patients with aplastic anemia, radiation therapy, and with some chemotherapy regimens.

Marrow edema is seen in a variety of clinical settings including trauma, infection, transient osteoporosis, and at the periphery of tumors. Edematous marrow shows low signal intensity on T1 and high signal intensity on T2-weighted MR imaging.

Osteonecrosis tends to occur more frequently in fatty marrow rather than hematopoietic marrow. (For a more in depth discussion of osteonecrosis, please see the section on avascular necrosis in the arthritis chapter.) Osteonecrosis has many different etiologies, but the pattern of injury and osseous response is predictable. Following ischemic insult, myeloid cell death occurs within the first 12 hours. The bone responds with increased blood flow and inflammation. Granulation tissue forms and fibrosis develops in the area of injury. Bone resorption follows,

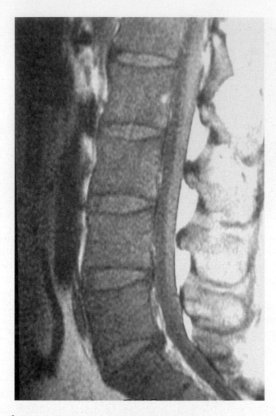

Fig. 6-15   Marrow replacement, AML. This is a sagittal T1-weighted MRI (600/16) in a 30-year-old male who had severe low back pain but normal plain films. No focal lesion is seen. However, there is diffuse low signal abnormality in the vertebral bodies. The rule of thumb is that on a T1 image the vertebral body should have higher signal than the disk that has been violated. Blood smear showed early acute myelogenous leukemia.

itself followed by osteoblastic reinforcement. At a stage where an interface is formed between areas of osseous resorption and healing, the MR "double-line" sign may be seen. This consists of a high signal intensity line of hyperemic tissue immediately adjacent to a low signal intensity line of sclerotic bone as seen on T2-weighted MR imaging.

Marrow infiltration occurs with neoplastic processes, infection, or marrow packing disorders. With the marrow packing disorders there may be a significant amount of fibrous content and signal intensity may be intermediate on T1- and T2-weighted images. With infection or neoplastic infiltration, T1-weighted images are low signal and T2 weighted images usually have high signal.

Evaluation of marrow after treatment for tumor can be complex. Some chemotherapeutic agents are given to promote hematopoiesis to prevent or ameliorate anemia. Distinguishing recurrent metastatic disease from reconversion (rebound) hematopoietic marrow may be difficult, because both tend to have intermediate signal intensity on T1-weighted images and high signal intensity on T2-weighted images. Opposed-phase gradient echo im-

aging has been described as being useful in the evaluation of treated marrow.[1]

After radiation of an osseous tumor, the marrow may retain abnormal signal of the tumor for an undetermined amount of time. To compound the difficulty of evaluation, normal hematopoietic marrow (spine and pelvis in adults) that is irradiated shows cell death and partial conversion to fatty marrow as early as 8 days posttreatment, and complete fatty replacement by 8 weeks.[2]

Finally, the bone marrow signal can be difficult to evaluate following bone marrow transplant. In the vertebral body, marrow regeneration appears to have a T1-weighted MRI pattern which shows a peripheral zone of intermediate signal intensity and central zone of bright signal intensity, with the peripheral zone relating to regenerating hematopoietic cells.[3]

INFECTION

Infections, whether they involve the soft tissues, osseous structures, or joints, can be both highly aggressive and extremely subtle to diagnose clinically and radiologically.

Soft-Tissue Infections

Radiographic signs of soft tissue infections are generally nonspecific, showing only a mass, often with blurring or obliteration of the soft-tissue fat planes. CT can be more specific in appearance if used in conjunction with contrast administration. An enhancing rim surrounding a water density mass may be diagnostic. However, it should be noted that in parts of the extremities where the muscles are tightly packed, without loose fascial planes surrounding them (particularly the forearm and leg), soft-tissue infections can be difficult to diagnose with CT, even with contrast administration. MRI of an infection in the soft tissues may be nonspecific with T1- and T2-weighted imaging, but if an abscess is present, post contrast T1-weighted MRI imaging demonstrates an enhancing rim around a lesion which is of lower signal intensity than muscle. Sinus tracts, the presence of multiple abscesses, and extensive inflammatory change may contribute greater specificity in diagnosing soft-tissue infection. There may be associated reactive change seen in adjacent osseous structures (Fig. 6-16). Occasionally, necrotic tumors may have a similar appearance. However, cases of tumor with necrosis usually show some mural nodularity to differentiate them from abscess.

Osteomyelitis

The radiographic appearance of osteomyelitis varies, depending on the clinical timing and the time of imaging

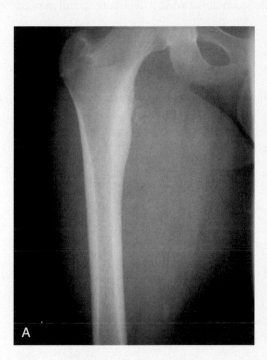
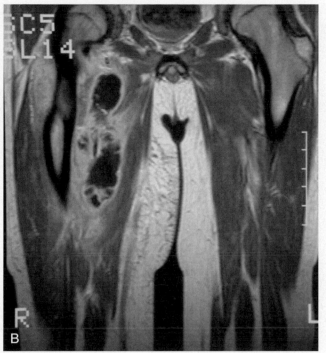

Fig. 6-16   Soft tissue infection. **A,** An AP radiograph of the thigh in a 16-year-old patient who had complained of pain for 6 months. The film demonstrates diffuse soft tissue swelling and thick bone reaction in the medial subtrochanteric region. T1-weighted MRI (500/15) following IV gadolinium demonstrates a multiloculated abscess with thick enhancing rim and nearby edema (**B**). The underlying bone was normal with the exception of thick cortical reaction as seen on the radiograph. This is the usual appearance of a soft tissue abscess, but the bone reaction is more exaggerated than we usually see because the condition was ignored for so lengthy a time.

during the course of the infection. Acute osteomyelitis is first demonstrated radiographically by blurring or obliteration of soft-tissue fat planes. Even this radiographic change lags behind the clinical onset of infection by 1 to 2 weeks. Soft-tissue changes are followed by signs of intramedullary destruction. This can be seen as an extremely subtle permeative pattern within the bone or even a mere indistinctness of the cortex (Fig. 6-17). If the permeative pattern is serpiginous, it assures the diagnosis of osteomyelitis (Fig. 6-18). These early changes are then followed by cortical destruction, endosteal scalloping, and periosteal as well as occasional endosteal reaction. These osseous changes may appear highly aggressive in the acute phase of osteomyelitis and may be difficult to differentiate from tumor (Fig. 6-19). Knowing the time course of the disease may be helpful, as an acute osteomyelitis will cause osseous destruction much more rapidly than does tumor. Eventually, if the infection is not treated, a sequestrum and involucrum may develop. A sequestrum is necrotic bone isolated from living bone by granulation tissue. It appears relatively dense because it has no blood supply, whereas the surrounding bone is hyperemic and loses its mineralization (Fig. 6-20). A sequestrum may harbor bacteria, leading to chronic osteomyelitis.

Subacute or chronic osteomyelitis may be seen as a Brodie's abscess. This type of infection is usually found in the metaphysis of a child. It is seen as a lucent focus of osteomyelitis, sharply delineated by a sclerotic margin (Fig. 6-21). It is usually oval, with the long axis oriented to the length of the bone and borders the growth plate. Thus, a Brodie's abscess appears much less aggressive than does acute osteomyelitis. Clinically, patients with Brodie's abcess may not have associated fever or elevated sedimentation rate. One might consider esinophilic granuloma and other benign metaphyseal lesions in the differential diagnosis. Brodie's abcess may be located in the epiphysis in a young child. Occasionally, a Brodie's abcess is cortically based, and elicits significant sclerosis and periosteal reaction. These cortically based infections with significant reactive bone formation can have a similar appearance to a cortically based osteoid osteoma or reactive bone formation around a subacute stress fracture (see Fig. 1-10).

Chronic osteomyelitis may demonstrate a prominent host reaction, including thickened cortices and variable mixtures of lucency and density. Sequestra may or may not be apparent. The radiographic appearance may remain stable over a period of several years, yet chronic osteomyelitis may reactivate. Chronic osteomyelitis is

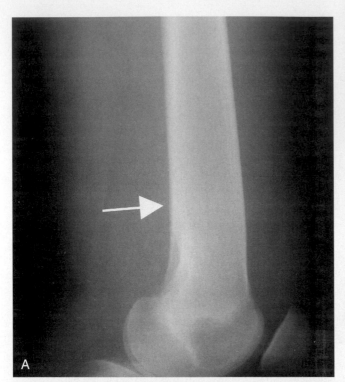

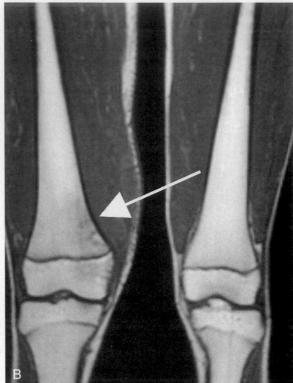

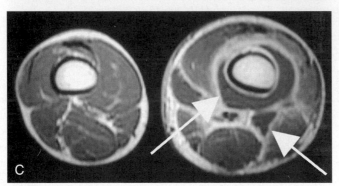

Fig. 6-17   Osteomyelitis. **A,** A lateral radiograph of the thigh in a 16-year-old male which has the subtle abnormalities of diffuse soft tissue swelling, obliteration of fat planes, and periosteal reaction at the posterior cortex (*arrows*). There is no convincing permeative change in the bone at this time. **B,** T1-weighted MR, however, shows a subtle marrow abnormality involving predominantly the metaphysis of the left thigh (*arrow*). **C,** The post gadolinium T1-weighted axial MR (566/10) shows a thick enhancing rim surrounding the cortex of the bone, as well as a multiloculated abscess with thick enhancing rim surrounding each site (*arrows*). This was a staphylococcus osteomyelitis.

evaluated by serial radiographs, searching for change in bone density or development of periosteal reaction. If serial films are not helpful, a four-phase bone scan or white blood cell scan may improve specificity.

Cross sectional modalities are useful in the diagnosis of osteomyelitis. CT imaging usually mirrors the appearance of the plain film, but destructive osseous changes with serpigenous tracking may be more apparent. As with radiographs, the soft-tissue fat planes are obliterated on CT and the soft-tissue abnormality may involve several muscle groups and be less discrete than many soft-tissue tumor masses. Contrast enhancement may be nonuniform, but a thin enhancing rim helps make the diagnosis of abscess. MR is even more sensitive than CT in diagnosing osteomyelitis. STIR and T1 imaging are highly sensi-

tive in diagnosing the presence and extent of osteomyelitis, whereas T1 with contrast administration can demonstrate the presence of abscess. Specificity however is limited in the absence of abscess or sinus tract formation.

The location of osteomyelitis relates to the route of involvement. A direct penetrating wound can result in osteomyelitis at any site. On the other hand, osteomyelitis resulting from hemotogenous spread is more site specific and strongly influenced by vascular anatomy. Thus, in infants (up to 12 months of age), some of the metaphyseal vessels penetrate the epiphyseal plate to anastamose with epiphyseal vessels. Therefore, metaphyseal infections in infants not uncommonly involve the epiphysis and joint, and may result in slipped epiphyses and growth defor-

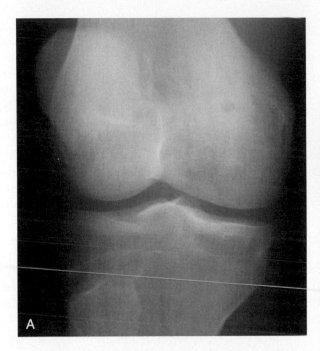

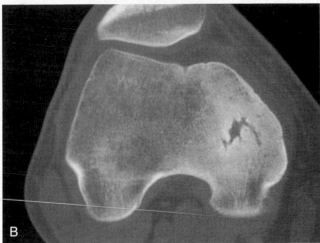

Fig. 6-18   Serpiginous tracking of osteomyelitis. **A,** An oblique radiograph demonstrating a lytic, ill-defined lesion with surrounding sclerosis in the medial femoral condyle. **B,** The CT demonstrates the serpiginous branching pattern of the lytic area, again surrounded by reactive bone. This pattern is typical for osteomyelitis.

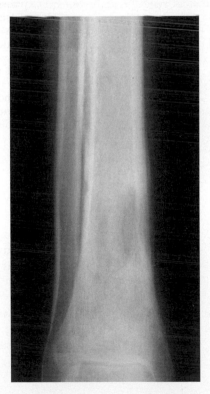

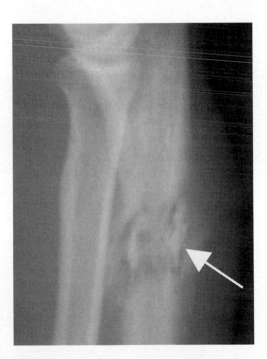

Fig. 6-19   Osteomyelitis. The osseus destruction is highly aggressive in appearance in this case, with a permeative pattern involving both the marrow and cortex, and periosteal reaction. Remember that osteomyelitis can have a radiographic appearance that is highly aggressive, and not always differentiable from tumor.

Fig. 6-20   Sequestrum in osteomyelitis. The lateral radiograph of a proximal ulna demonstrates osteomyelitis that has developed following a night-stick fracture. There is bone destruction in a permeative pattern, as well as the presence of a dense piece of necrotic bone (*arrow*), termed a sequestrum. (Reprinted with permission from the ACR learning file.)

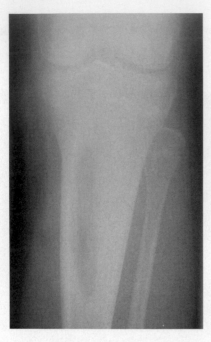

Fig. 6-21   Brodie's abscess. This well-defined, oval, metaphyseal lytic lesion with a sclerotic margin and thick periosteal reaction represents a chronic osteomyelitis, sometimes also termed Brodie's abscess.

mity (Fig. 6-22). In older children, terminal vessels occur as loops with sluggish blood flow in the metaphases and do not cross into the epiphyses. This vascular anatomy, combined with the relative lack of phagocytes in the metaphyseal region, results in the metaphases being the most common site of infection in the child (Fig. 6-23). Epiphyseal and joint involvement are much less common in children than in infants, but MR imaging may demonstrate extension of infection from the metaphysis to the epiphysis which may not be suspected on radiograpic evaluation alone. The most common site of osteomyelitis in the child is the tubular bones of the lower extremities. Finally, in the adult, one has closure of the epiphyseal plate and the terminal metaphyseal vessels anastamose with epiphyseal vessels. Thus, joint involvement secondary to osteomyelitis is more common in the adult than in the child. In addition, adults tend to have osteomyelitis involving the spine and small bones more frequently than the large tubular bones.

There are some specific types of osteomyelitis, which deserve separate mention. Tuberculosis and fungal infections tend to have a slower course and less host reaction than does pyogenic osteomyelitis. In the child, tuberculosis may be demonstrated first as dactylitis, termed spina ventosa, where the tubular bones of the hands and feet show periosteal reaction followed by expansion of the

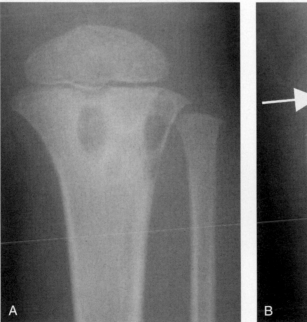

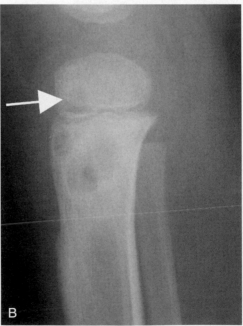

Fig. 6-22   Osteomyelitis in a toddler. **A,** AP and **(B)** lateral radiographs demonstrate multiple rather well defined lytic lesions predominantly in the metaphysis, but also involving the epiphysis (*arrow*) in this toddler. Epiphyseal involvement with osteomyelitis can be seen, particularly in infants and toddlers.

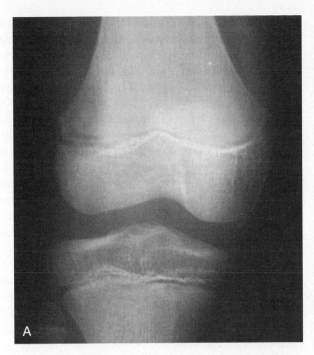
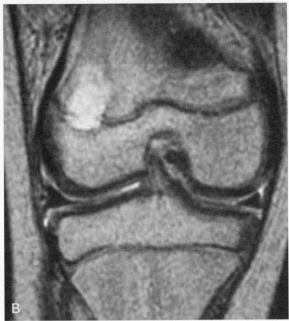

Fig. 6-23   Osteomyelitis in an adolescent. **A,** The AP radiograph and (**B**) T2-weighted MR (*B*, 2500/80), demonstrate a typically located focus of osteomyelitis in the metaphysis of the lateral femoral condyle, not crossing into the epiphysis, in this 8-year-old child.

bone. The differential diagnosis for this appearance includes juvenile rheumatoid arthritis, sickle cell dactylitis, and other infections.

Syphilis osteomyelitis, in its congenital form, initially demonstrates metaphyseal irregularity and a widened zone of provisional calcification, occasionally resulting in slipped epiphyses. It may progress to invade the diaphysis and elicit periosteal reaction. Congenital syphilis is in the extensive differential for infants with periosteal reaction (Fig. 6-24), with the differential diagnosis including nonaccidental trauma, tumor, other infections, and metabolic diseases. Acquired syphilis presents as a chronic osteomyelitis, with periostitis and endosteal reaction resulting in an enlarged bowed bone with mixed lytic and sclerotic areas. The flat bones and cranium may be involved with syphilis osteomyelitis. When the tibia is involved, it tends to develop an anterior bowing deformity that has been termed the "saber shin" deformity. Another manifestation of syphilis is neuropathic arthropathy, especially involving the knees.

Diagnosing osteomyelitis in the diabetic foot can be fraught with difficulty. Ulcerations and underlying osteopenia are routinely present even in the absence of osteomyelitis. Therefore, there is heavy reliance on soft-tissue ulceration, tracking of air, periosteal reaction, cortical destruction, and progression on serial films to diagnose osteomyelitis. MRI with IV contrast can be very useful and improve specificity. However, diabetic patients also may have neuropathic joints in the foot. Neuro-

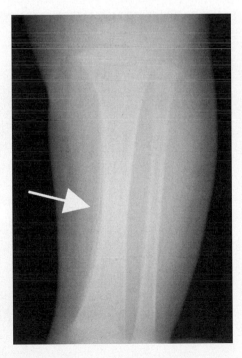

Fig. 6-24   Congenital syphilis. This AP radiograph shows one of the manifestations of congenital syphilis, periosteal reaction (*arrow*). The child's other long bones showed a similar periosteal reaction. Other radiographic manifestations of congenital syphilis, not shown here, include metaphyseal defects. This child's periosteal reaction is not a specific indicator of congenital infection, but could also represent multiple other abnormalities, including child abuse and physiologic bone formation.

pathic joints result in cortical destruction, fragmentation, loss of cartilage, and effusion, which may not be differentiable from infection. The presence of osseous or soft tissue abscesses, ulcers extending to the bone, and sinus tracts extending between bone and ulcers or abscesses helps to differentiate osteomyelitis from neuropathic changes (Fig. 6-25).

In the hand, metacarpals and phalanges are at risk for infection from a human bite, usually acquired by punching an adversary in the mouth. A finger or toe may develop a felon or infection in the terminal pulp which may progress to osteomyelitis of the tuft. Furthermore, a stubbed toe with a nail-bed injury may result in osteomyelitis of the distal phalanx as the periosteum is immediately adjacent to the nail bed (Fig. 6-26). Soft tissue infection may spread along tendon sheaths and fascial planes of the hand or foot, so that the site of bone involvement may actually be distant from the initial site of injury. The presence of foreign bodies in the hand or foot may not be known to the patient and may of course lead to infection (Fig. 6-27).

It is important to be familiar with the radiographic appearance of infection of the spine. Genitourinary infections can be a frequent source of spine infection as there is communication between the pelvic and thorocolumbar venous systems via the epidural venous plexus of Batson. In the spine, the infection starts in the subendplate region of the vertebral body and subsequently extends to the adjacent vertebral endplate and disk. The pathognomonic appearance of a disk space infection is irregularity and loss of cortex in two adjacent endplates, with decrease in the height of the corresponding disk (Fig. 6-28). A paravertebral mass or displaced psoas shadow in the lumbar region may be seen. Later, a sclerotic host reaction may evolve. A less significant and often self-limited disk space infection may be seen in skeletally immature patients and is termed discitis. This condition usually represents a hematogenous infection of the disk and is seen in patients who present with back pain, low-grade fever, elevated sedimentation rate, and preexisting minor infections such as upper respiratory infection. The radiographic changes are delayed but include a decrease in disk height, mild endplate irregularities, and eburnation of the endplates. Paravertebral soft-tissue mass is minimal and organisms are often not cultured, either from blood or biopsy of the disk.

Tuberculosis of the spine (Pott's disease) can be specific in appearance. It tends to involve the thorocolumbar region. Tuberculosis shows a slow progression of the disease process, with relative preservation of the disk

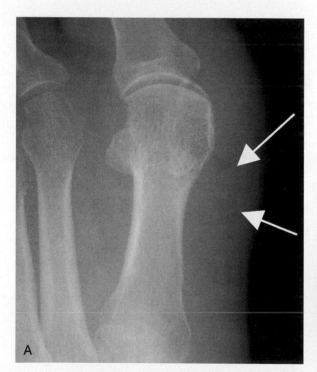
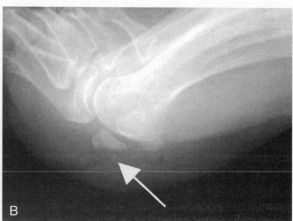

Fig. 6-25 Osteomyelitis in the diabetic foot. **A,** Soft tissue swelling about the first MTP, with air in the soft tissues that seems to approach the osseus structures and joint (*arrows*). **B,** The lateral view shows that the air arises from a plantar ulcer, and extends to the sesamoid, which is partially destroyed (*arrow*). This patient had osteomyelitis of the sesamoid, and the sinus tract extending to the bone helps to substantiate that diagnosis. Not shown on this film are the calcifications in the small arteries of the foot and fractures in the metatarsals of the other foot, not noticed by this patient with diabetes and associated decrease in proprioception.

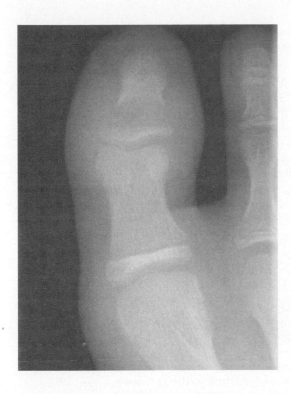

Fig. 6-26   Osteomyelitis in the stubbed toe. This AP radiograph demonstrates soft-tissue swelling about the great toe, and destructive change in the distal phalanx. This 13-year-old had a history of stubbed toe and nail bed injury, which resulted in osteomyelitis due to the attachment of the nail bed to the periosteum at the level of the proximal aspect of the distal phalanx. (Reprinted with permission from the ACR learning file.)

height and lack of sclerotic response. Late in the disease process, the patient may develop an acute angular kyphosis, termed a gibbus deformity. In addition, a calcified psoas abcess may develop (Fig. 6-29). The infection may spread under the anterior longitudinal ligament to involve several disk levels.

Septic Arthritis

Joint effusion is the first radiographic sign of septic arthritis. With time, hyperemia may lead to osteoporosis, and cartilage destruction is seen as a decreasing joint space width. Bone erosion and destruction may follow rapidly (Fig. 6-30) and osteomyelitis may develop by means of contiguous spread. The patient may show sclerotic host reaction if the septic arthritis is bacterial in

origin. Eventually, ankylosis may occur. In the child, the hip is a common site of septic arthritis as the hematogenous focus of osseous infection in the metaphysis is within the hip joint capsule. Soft tissue signs of effusion in the hip, seen as an increased distance between the teardrop and the femoral metaphysis or as bulging fat planes may be helpful in a perfectly aligned AP radiograph (Fig. 6-31). Producing a vacuum phenomenon in the joint with traction on the hip rules out an effusion and septic hip but is less sensitive than ultrasound. However, if there is any real clinical suspicion of septic hip, it should be regarded as an emergency and hip aspiration should be performed.

Tuberculosis and fungal septic arthritides are more chronic processes than bacterial arthritis. They therefore may elicit little or no host bone reaction. Cartilage de-

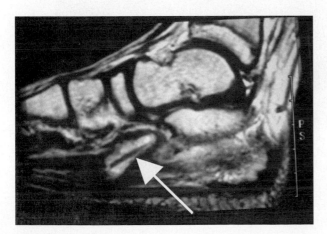

Fig. 6-27   Foreign body with infection. T2-weighted sagittal MR of the foot in this child demonstrates a long and thin foreign body surrounded by high signal (*arrow*). This proved to be a toothpick that this child was unaware he had stepped on. STIR imaging (not shown) demonstrated osteomyelitis in the navicular and cuneiform. (Case courtesy of Carol Andrews, M.D.)

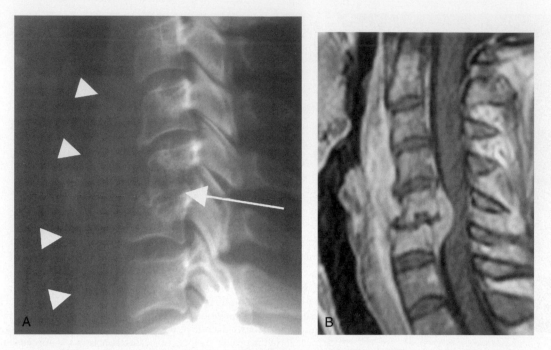

Fig. 6-28   Disk space infection. **A,** Lateral radiograph demonstrates prevertebral soft tissue swelling (*arrowheads*) and destruction of the disk space and end plates at C5-6 (*arrow*). This is a classic radiographic appearance of a disk space infection. **B,** Post-gadolinium T1-weighted MR (500/11) shows enhancement of C5 and C6, as well as the epidural mass and prevertebral abscess. There is cord compression.

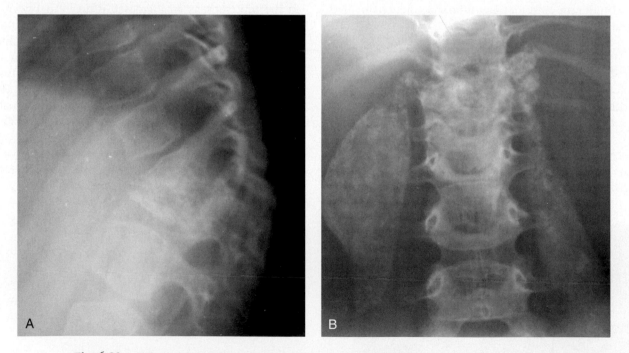

Fig. 6-29   Tuberculosis of the spine. **A,** Lateral and (**B**) AP radiographs demonstrate destruction of much of the vertebral bodies and disk spaces of T11, T12, and L1. There is a gibbous deformity, as well as densely calcified abscesses in the psoas muscles bilaterally as seen on the AP view. (Reprinted with permission from the ACR learning file.)

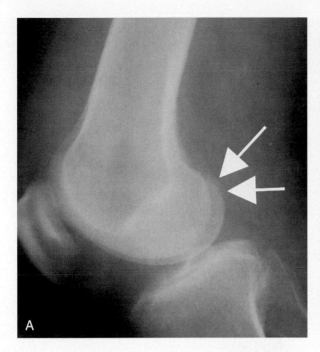 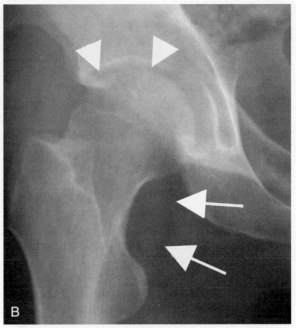

Fig. 6-30   Septic joint. **A,** A lateral radiograph of the knee, which demonstrates very early findings of septic arthritis. There is a knee effusion. There is also an extremely subtle disruption of the posterior cortex of the femoral condyle (*arrow*). **B,** In a different case of septic arthritis, this is an AP radiograph of the hip which shows not only distention of the hip joint with bulging gluteal and psoas fat pads (*arrow*), but also loss of cortical distinctness of the femoral head (*arrowheads*).

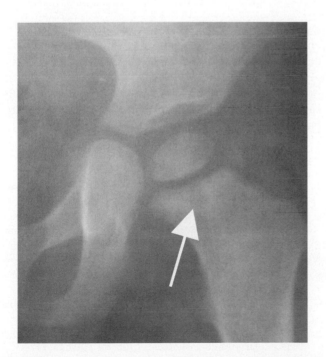

Fig. 6-31   Septic hip in a child. The AP radiograph demonstrates bulging fat pads, indicating an effusion of the hip. In addition, there is a faint lucency seen in the metaphysis (*arrow*). This indicates that the septic hip has already progressed to osteomyelitis. (Reprinted with permission from the ACR learning file.)

struction is often much slower and joint space width remains normal. The joint may demonstrate osteoporosis with minimal cartilage destruction. Erosions are slow to progress and may appear particularly well-delineated (Fig. 6-32). The hip and knee are the most common sites of TB and fungal septic arthritis, followed by the wrist and elbow.

MISCELLANEOUS

Sarcoidosis

Sarcoidosis is a systemic granulomatous disorder that shows osseous involvement in 1%–15% of cases.[4] If bone lesions are present, skin lesions usually are present as well (in up to 90% of cases). Lung abnormalities, including hilar adenopathy, pulmonary infiltrates, fibrosis, and apical bullous disease, are also usually present (80%–90%). Nodular liver disease with hepatosplenomegaly may be present as well, as may ocular abnormalities such as uvitis and iritis.

Sarcoidosis is seen in young adults without gender predominance. Black patients are affected more frequently than either Caucasians or Asians. The most frequently noted osseous abnormality is a lytic lesion or lesions with lacey trabeculae, usually found in the middle or distal phalanges, due to granulamatous infiltration (Fig.

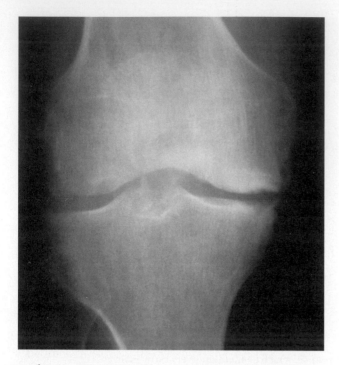

Fig. 6-32   TB arthritis. This AP radiograph demonstrates osteopenia and small cortical erosions but nearly normal cartilage width. This combination is typical of TB or fungal arthritis.

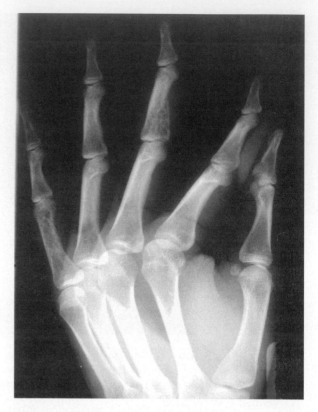

Fig. 6-33   Sarcoid. The lacy appearing lytic lesions seen here in the proximal phalanx of the fifth digit and the middle phalanx of the third give the typical radiographic appearance of osseus sarcoid. (Reprinted with permission from the ACR learning file.)

6-33). Other, less frequent, osseous manifestations include generalized osteopenia, sclerosis of phalangeal tufts, and focal or generalized sclerosis. The patients experience polyarticular arthralgias, but usually show no radiographic joint abnormality.

Muscular sarcoidosis is common but rarely symptomatic.[5] The early myositic type is controlled by steroids and shows no abnormality on MR imaging. The chronic myopathic type is seen as a nonspecific atrophy on MR imaging. The nodular type presents as a palpable mass but is least common. On MR images one sees a mass with central low signal on T1 as well as T2-weighted images due to granulomatous material, surrounded by nonspecific low signal on T1 and high signal intensity on T2 imaging.

AIDS

Patients with AIDS may demonstrate a variety of musculoskeletal abnormalities.[6] These include development of lymphoma or Kaposi sarcoma, either in bone or soft tissue. Infection can be common and opportunistic. In addition, bacillary angiomatosis may be seen. This is usually a multi-focal bacterial infection that may produce osteolytic lesions with periosteal reaction as well as markedly increased T2 signal intensity when muscle is involved. Patients with AIDS also may demonstrate a low

signal intensity in the marrow related to anemia of chronic disease as well as chronic transfusions. MRI may demonstrate and differentiate between septic or aseptic myositis. Finally, arthritic-like changes may be seen in patients with AIDS, resembling psoriatic and Reiter's disease, as well as secondary hypertrophic osteoarthropathy.

REFERENCES

1. Andrews C: Evaluation of the marrow space in the adult hip. *Radiographics* 2000;20:s27-s42.
2. Blomlie V, Rofstad E, Skjonsberg A, Tvera K, Lien H: Female pelvic bone marrow: Serial MR imaging before, during, and after radiation therapy. *Radiology* 1995;194:537-543.
3. Stevens S, Moore S, Amylon M: Repopulation of marrow after transplantation: MR imaging with pathologic correlation. *Radiology* 1990;175:213-218.
4. Sartoris D, Resnick D, Resnik C, et al: Musculoskeletal manifestations of sarcoidosis. Sem Roentgen 1985;20:376-386.
5. Matsuo M, Ehara S, Tomakawa Y, Chida E, Nischida J, Sugai T: Muscular sarcoidosis. *Skeletal Radiol* 1995;24:535-537.
6. Steinbach L, Tehrawzadeh J, Fleckenstein J, Vanarthos W, Pais M: Human immunodeficiency virus infection: musculoskeletal manifestations. *Radiology* 1993;186:833-838.

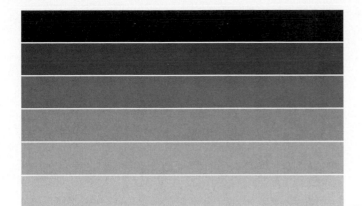

Appendices

DAVID A. MAY, M.D. and B.J. MANASTER, M.D., Ph.D.

APPENDIX 1: ARTHROGRAPHY TECHNIQUE

Generalizations

Contrast

1. For conventional or CT arthrography, iodinated contrast (Omnipaque 300, Hypaque 60, or equivalent) is injected. For larger joints, a specified amount of undiluted ("full strength") contrast is followed by enough room air to distend the joint capsule. For smaller joints, no air is used, but the contrast is diluted with saline, lidocaine, or both.

2. MR arthrography can be performed after intraarticular injection of saline, with emphasis on T2-weighted images, or with intraarticular gadolinium, with emphasis on T1-weighted images. With either contrast agent, the goal is to distend the joint capsule. We prefer gadolinium because T1-weighted MR images have slightly better spatial resolution. Also, we prefer fat suppressed images in at least some planes. Remember that any MR imaging study of a joint, with or without arthrography, benefits from at least one fat suppressed T2-weighted or inversion recovery sequence to enhance detection of edema, and at least one non-fat suppressed T1-weighted sequence to assess fat signal.

An intraarticular gadolinium concentration of 1–2 mmol/l maximizes signal intensity on T1-weighted images. This concentration is achieved by dilution of the gadolinium contrast agent by a factor of 1 : 125 to 1 : 250. The gadolinium is measured in a tuberculin syringe, then added to normal saline, iodinated contrast, or a combination to form the injected solution.

Two different strategies may be used during joint injection prior to MR arthrography. The specific volumes listed are appropriate for shoulder or hip arthrography.

Use the same proportions, but smaller amounts may be prepared for a small joint injection.

Strategy 1. Two syringes are prepared. Syringe #1 contains only full strength iodinated contrast. Syringe #2 contains gadolinium (0.1–0.2 ml), saline (10 ml), and iodinated contrast (4 ml). After the needle is placed, full strength contrast is injected from syringe #1 to confirm satisfactory intraarticular needle position, followed by the dilute gadolinium and contrast solution in syringe #2. This approach avoids extraarticular injection of gadolinium, which increases the likelihood that aesthetically pleasing T1-weighted MR images will be obtained.

Strategy 2. A single syringe is prepared that contains gadolinium (0.2 ml), normal saline (10 ml), and iodinated contrast (10 ml). This approach is simpler and is appropriate if you are confident in your ability to properly place the needle on the first try.

With either strategy, *do not inject air bubbles of any size,* as they may mimic an intraarticular body on MR images.

Analgesia *Skin:* 1%–2% lidocaine, buffered with sodium bicarbonate to enhance patient comfort (10 : 1 ratio of lidocaine to bicarbonate).

Intraarticular: This is controversial. Adding lidocaine to the injected contrast enhances patient comfort, and can be useful as a diagnostic test to confirm that the source of the patient's pain is from the joint. However, intraarticular lidocaine can rapidly enter the bloodstream, with potential for seizure or arrhythmia in some patients if a large amount is injected. Thus, some caution is appropriate. We routinely add lidocaine to the injected contrast when performing arthrography in small joints such as the wrist, because this procedure is fairly painful and the amount of injected lidocaine is small.

Epinephrine Adding about 0.1–0.3 ml of 1 : 1000 epinephrine per 5–10 ml of total injected solution causes synovial vasoconstriction, which results in longer retention of contrast within the joint. This can be helpful if a

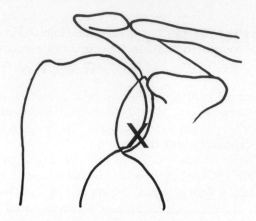

Fig. A1-1   Shoulder. "X" marks the injection site.

CT or MR to follow the injection might be delayed. It can be argued that the use of epinephrine is otherwise a matter of personal preference.

Shoulder

Patient position: supine with palm up at patient's side, sandbag on hand.

Approach: straight down to inferomedial humeral head at or 2 mm lateral to junction of middle and inferior thirds of the glenohumeral joint using a 22 g spinal needle ("X" in Fig. A1-1).

1. For conventional arthrography or CT arthrography, inject approximately 5 cc of full strength contrast, followed by enough room air to distend the joint capsule. Total injection volume usually is from 10 to 15 cc. Overdistension causes shoulder "achiness," "heaviness," or frank pain, and may result in unaesthetic (but harmless) contrast extravasation, typically along the anterior cortex of the scapula. Gently exercise the shoulder before imaging.

2. MR arthrography: same total volume as conventional, but with dilute gadolinium solution and no air. Gently exercise the shoulder before imaging.

Elbow

Patient position: prone with arm above head and elbow flexed 90°.

Approach: Straight down (lateral approach) to radiocapitellar joint with a 25g 1½-inch needle (center of the "O" in Fig. A1-2). This needle can be used for analgesia as well.

If the patient cannot tolerate the prone position, an alternative approach is easily performed with the patient supine, with his hand on his abdomen and elbow flexed, at his side. Palpate the lateral epicondyle, olecranon process, and radial head. These landmarks form a triangle on the posterolateral region of the elbow. Place the needle in the center of the triangle and advance towards the joint.

1. For conventional arthrography or CT arthrography, inject approx 2–3 cc of 60% strength contrast (e.g., Hypaque 60 or Omnipaque 300), followed by enough room air to distend the joint capsule (total injection volume usually is about 10–12 cc).

2. For MR arthrography, inject about 6–8 cc of the dilute gadolinium solution. Gently exercise the elbow before imaging.

Wrist

Begin with fluoroscopy. Observe the wrist during ulnar and radial deviation in PA and lateral projections, and any maneuver that might elicit a click or reproduce the patient's symptoms. Videotaping for later review can be helpful.

Specific provocative maneuvers can be used to reveal instability patterns that may not be evident on standard radiographs:

Scapholunate dissociation: widening of scapholunate interval with a clenched fist or ulnar deviation. Widening greater than 2 mm is more likely to be significant. In the lateral projection, the scaphoid and lunate bones should move in unison during wrist flexion and extension and radial and ulnar deviation.

Capitolunate instability ("CLIP maneuver"): in the lateral projection, stabilize the patient's forearm with his wrist in slight ulnar deviation. With your other hand, grasp the patient's hand at the metacarpals and apply alternating dorsal and volar oriented force while observing for subluxation at the capitolunate articulation. An alternative technique, also in the lateral projection, is to apply volar and dorsal pressure to the distal lateral scaphoid at the scaphoid tuberosity rather than to the metacarpals.

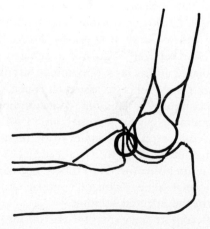

Fig. A1-2   Elbow. Inject at the center of the "O" if using a lateral approach.

Triquetrum-hamate instability: during radial to ulnar deviation, the proximal carpal row abruptly shifts from palmar flexion to dosiflexion just before extreme ulnar flexion is achieved. The hamate may be seen to slide against the triquetrum. Watch for this in both the frontal and lateral projections.

Wrist arthrography is more complex than at other joints because the wrist has three major synovial compartments (distal radioulnar joint, radiocarpal joint, and midcarpal joint). Arthrography can be tailored to the region of concern, or all three compartments may be routinely injected. We generally prefer the former approach, as it is simpler and easier for the patient. For example, if the clinical concern is limited to the triangular fibrocartilage complex, there is no need to inject the midcarpal joint. Injection of the radiocarpal joint theoretically should diagnose all communicating tears, but "one-way" tears can *occasionally* be present that could escape detection with injection of only one compartment.

During contrast injection, observe for passage of contrast from one compartment to another ("communicating defect"). The site of the defect has important surgical implications. Videotaping, serial spot filming, or digital subtraction arthrography can be helpful in documenting the location of a communicating defect.

Patient position: supine with arm at side, palm down. A rolled washcloth is placed under the wrist to allow mild flexion. Adjust the position of the wrist as needed to profile the injection site (i.e., no overlap of the bones).

Approach (all are dorsal approach, needle straight down, injection sites marked with "X" in Fig. A1-3), using a 25g 1-inch or 1½-inch needle (this needle can also be used for analgesia):

Distal radioulnar joint (DRUJ): distal lateral ulnar metaphysis. Capacity is 1 cc.

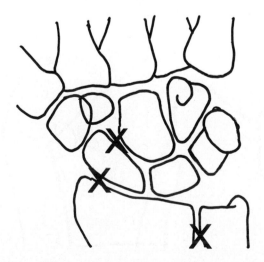

Fig. A1-3 Wrist. Each "X" marks injection sites for the three synovial compartments of the wrist.

Radiocarpal joint: lateral aspect of radioscaphoid joint. Capacity is 4 cc. Full volume should be injected in order to force contrast through small perforations. May communicate with the triquetrum-pisiform joint as a normal variant.

Midcarpal joint: space formed by the capitate, scaphoid and trapezoid. Capacity is 6 cc. Alternatively, an easy injection site is the "four corners," the junction of the lunate-capitate-hamate-triquetrum.

1. For conventional arthrography: If only a single compartment is to be injected, use full strength contrast mixed with an equal amount of 1 or 2% lidocaine.

   Often, two adjacent compartments need to be injected. For example, if a triangular fibrocartilage complex tear is suspected, both the radiocarpal joint and the DRUJ may need to be injected, as some communicating tears are "one-way" tears, that is, they may not allow the passage of contrast in both directions between the radiocarpal and DRUJ compartments. Also, an incomplete triangular fibrocartilage tear may extend only to one compartment.

   When injecting two adjacent compartments, one of three approaches may be used:

   A. Use iodinated contrast of different densities for each compartment. Specifically, the first compartment is injected with dilute iodinated contrast (one part contrast mixed with one part saline and one part lidocaine). If this injection is normal, but a one-way communicating defect must be excluded, then the adjacent compartment can be injected with near-full strength contrast (containing a small amount of lidocaine). If a one-way communicating defect is present, the dense contrast can be seen flowing into the dilute contrast. If all three compartments are to be injected, start with dilute contrast in either the radiocarpal joint or both the DRUJ and the midcarpal joint.

   B. Alternatively, the first injection is made with near full-strength contrast (diluted with lidocaine). The second injection is delayed by approximately 2 hours to allow resorption of most of the injected contrast.

   C. Digital subtraction arthrography.

2. For MR arthrography, one may inject gadolinium into only one compartment, usually the radiocarpal joint or into all three compartments simultaneously.

Hip

Patient position: supine with hip extended.

Approach: Palpate the femoral artery (to avoid it). Advance a 22 g spinal needle straight down to the junc-

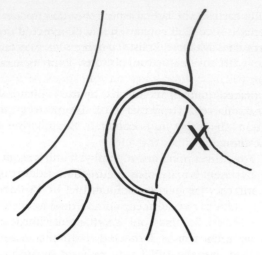

Fig. A1-4 Hip. "X" marks the injection site.

tion of lateral femoral head and neck ("X" in Fig. A1-4). Note: if aspirating for suspected infection, use an 18g or larger needle, because a thick exudate may not flow through a smaller needle.

Alternative approach: Anterolateral, with anterior fluoroscopy, aiming for the femoral neck.

1. Conventional arthrography: 60% strength contrast (e.g., Hypaque 60 or Omnipaque 300), to distend the joint capsule. Total injection volume usually is about 6-10 ml.
2. For MR arthrography: Inject 6-10 ml of gadolinium solution.
   Gently exercise the hip before imaging.
3. Arthrographic assessment for possible infection or loosening of a hip arthroplasty needs special mention. Careful attention to sterile technique is required. Because iodinated contrast is bacteriostatic, contrast is not injected until after fluid is aspirated from the joint. (Current research, not yet published, suggests that low strength nonionic contrast such as Omnipaque 180 may be injected to confirm intraarticular needle position before aspiration without decreasing the sensitivity for detection of joint infection.) A large bore (18 gauge) needle is used. An anterior or a lateral approach may be used. If using an anterior approach, advance straight down to the prosthetic head-neck junction ("X" in Fig. A1-5). A lateral approach begins with lateral palpation to identify the greater trochanter. The needle is advanced towards the prosthetic head from a lateral approach above the greater trochanter with frontal fluoroscopy. With either approach, the "metal-on-metal" sensation of touching the prosthesis with the needle is unmistakable. After placing the needle, attempt to aspirate fluid. If no fluid is returned, lavage the joint with 10 ml of nonbacteriostatic normal saline, then attempt to withdraw fluid. Internally rotating the hip may en-

hance return of fluid. Repeat if necessary, until fluid is returned. Contrast may now be injected. Pre- and post-injection images are compared. Flow of contrast around the intraosseous portions of the acetabular or femoral components indicates component loosening. This finding can be extremely subtle. Subtraction techniques such as digital subtraction can be useful. Exercising the patient also can be helpful.

Knee

Patient position: supine or seated with the knee extended.

Approach: Medial anterior, between the patella and medial femoral condyle, with a 22 gauge needle. Fluoroscopy is not needed for MR arthrography.

1. For conventional arthrography or if CT to follow, inject approximately 5-10 ml of full strength contrast followed by enough room air to distend the joint capsule. Total injection volume usually is about 20-40+ ml.
2. For MR arthrography: inject about 25 ml of dilute gadolinium solution. Gently exercise the knee before imaging.

Ankle (tibiotalar joint)

Ankle position: lateral position.

Approach: After palpating the dorsalis pedis artery and the anterior tendons (to avoid them), use an anterior

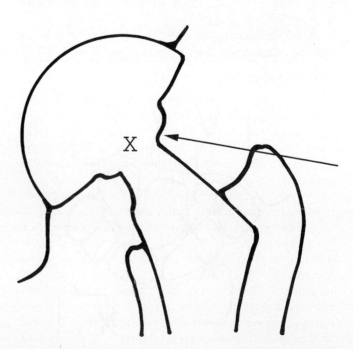

Fig. A1-5 Hip arthroplasty. "X" marks the injection site if an anterior approach is used. Arrow marks the needle tract using an anterolateral approach, aiming for the prosthetic femoral head.

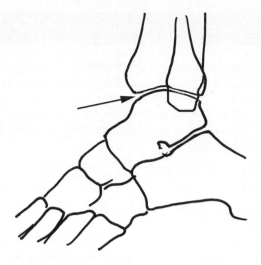

Fig. A1-6 Ankle. Arrow marks the needle tract using an anterior approach with lateral fluoroscopy.

approach with lateral fluoroscopy (arrow in Fig. A1-6). Use a 25g 1-inch or 1½-inch needle. This needle can also be used for analgesia.

1. Conventional arthrography or CT arthrography: approximately 2 cc of full strength contrast, followed by enough room air to distend the joint capsule (total injection volume usually is about 8 cc). The tibiotalar joint may communicate with the posterior subtalar joint as a normal variant.
2. MR arthrography: same volume as conventional. Gently exercise before imaging.

APPENDIX 2: SONOGRAPHY OF THE INFANT HIP: TECHNIQUE

Generalizations

This appendix briefly reviews how to obtain sonographic images of the infant hip. The pathophysiology and interpretation of sonographic findings of hip dysplasia are reviewed in Chapter 5. Review of that section is suggested prior to reading this appendix. The sonographic technique emphasized here is based on a popular and widely accepted approach to infant hip sonography. It must be emphasized that this is not the only way to reliably detect and follow DDH. Many experienced sonographers have developed slightly or even widely different approaches that have stood the test of time. For example, the Graf system (Table A2-1) of careful measurements of static coronal images is popular in many centers, at least as part of a hybrid approach. If your institution does it differently, this description is not intended as a criticism of your technique.

Scans are easiest to perform when the child is relaxed and quiet. The temperature and lighting should be comfortable for an infant, and the gel should be warmed.

Feeding the child before or during the examination helps the child to relax. Glucose water will suffice if no milk or formula is available. Enlist the parent's help in feeding, calming and positioning the baby. Beware of male infants, as they will invariably urinate on your shoes. An appropriately placed towel or washcloth can avoid this problem. Stress maneuvers are best left until the end of the examination, as the infant may become irritated by this forceful handling.

A high frequency linear array transducer, at least 5 MHz, is used. Occasionally, a curved transducer is used to obtain the "big picture" of a dislocated hip, and can better show the relationship of the dislocated femoral head and acetabulum. If the child is in a cast placed to maintain reduction of a previously dislocated hip, the available window may be too small for anything other than a small footprint sector array transducer. Be creative.

If the child is in a Pavlik harness, do not remove it. The harness will not impede the examination. Do not perform stress maneuvers on an infant in a harness, unless specifically requested to do so by the referring orthopedic surgeon. Stress maneuvers may redislocate a hip that was difficult for the surgeon to reduce.

A routine examination includes both hips. The examination is often easiest to perform from a lateral approach with the child in a decubitus or oblique decubitus position, scanning the upside hip. The hips may be flexed or extended, but infants usually prefer keeping their hips flexed.

Major landmarks of hip sonography include the femoral head, triradiate cartilage, lateral ilium, and the acetabular roof (see Figs. 5-29B,C, and 5-30A,B).

The *cartilaginous femoral head* is round, hypoechoic, and contains speckled internal echoes. Ossification of the femoral head begins as early as the third month as a central small, round hyperechoic focus with posterior acoustic shadowing (Figs. A2-1, A2-2). Such ossification provides a convenient landmark for localizing the center of the femoral head. In younger infants, adjust the transducer position to maximize the diameter of the femoral head on each image. This technique guarantees that the center of the femoral head is in the image.

The hypoechoic *triradiate cartilage* is located at the center of the acetabulum. A few echoes will project medial to the triradiate cartilage, assisting in locating this landmark (Fig. A2-1). On axial images, the triradiate cartilage is located between the pubic bone anteriorly and the slightly longer ischium posteriorly.

The *lateral cortex of the ilium,* like the other ossified bones, is seen as a well-defined hyperechoic line with dense posterior acoustic shadowing. The lateral ilium is continuous with the osseous *acetabular roof.* The angle formed by the lateral ilium and the acetabular roof is the *alpha angle* (Fig. 5-29D).

The *acetabular labrum* forms an echogenic triangle lateral to the acetabular roof (Fig. 5-29C).

Table A2-1 The Graf classification of infant hip dysplasia

Hip Type	Bony Roof*	Angle†	Alpha angle (degrees)	Beta angle (degrees)
Ia: mature hip	Good	Sharp	≥60	>55
Ib: transitional form	Good	Blunt	≤60	>55
IIa: physiologically immature (<3 mo of age)	Sufficient	Round	50–59	>55
IIb: delayed ossification (>3 mo of age)	Deficient	Round	50–59	>55
IIc: critical range (any age, normal labrum)	Deficient	Round or flat	43-49	70–77
IId: subluxed hip	Severely def.	Round or flat	43-49	>77
IIIa: dislocated hip (no structural alteration)	Poor	Flat	<43	>77
IIIb: dislocated hip (with structural alteration)	Poor	Flat	<43	>77
IV: severely dislocated hip	Poor	Flat	<43	>77

* Bony roof, coverage of femoral head. Good is ≥ 50%.
† Angle, junction of osseous ilium and osseous acetabular roof.
(Modified from Graf R, Wilson B. *Sonography of the infant hip and its therapeutic implications.* London: Chapman and Hall, 1995, and Laor T, Jarmillo D, and Oestereich AE. Musculoskeletal system. In Kirks DR, Griscom NT, eds. *Practical Pediatric Imaging* ed 3, Philadelphia, Lippincott-Raven, 1998.)

Scans are obtained in the coronal and transverse planes. The hips may be flexed or extended.

Optimal coronal images have the following features (Figs. 5-29B,C, A2-2A):

1. The lateral cortex of the ilium is displayed as a straight line parallel to the transducer.
2. The acetabular roof is clearly displayed. The alpha angle is formed by the lateral ilium and the acetabular roof (Fig. 5-29D)

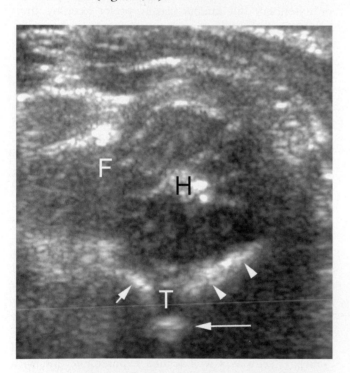

Fig. A2-1 Transverse image, with anterior to the viewer's left, in a 10 week old girl. Note the triradiate cartilage (T) with echoes medial to the cartilage (*long arrow*). Also note the early ossification at the center of the femoral head (H), ischium (*arrowheads*), and pubis (*short arrow*). The pubis is partially shadowed by the femoral shaft anteriorly (F).

3. The femoral head is on the right side of the image (inferiorly). The center of the femoral head is in the image.
4. The triadiate cartilage is in the image. In a normally aligned hip, the femoral head is centered over the triradiate cartilage. (The triradiate cartilage is so-named because it is at the center of the acetabulum, and includes portions of all three pelvic bones—the ilium, ischium, and pubis.)
5. The labrum is seen as an echogenic triangle lateral to the acetabular roof.

An image with these qualities is termed "the standard plane" in the Graf system, and is the only image that this system requires.

Displaying the lateral ilium as a straight line parallel to the transducer is usually straightforward. If the lateral ilium has a concave contour, then the transducer is too far posterior (Fig. A2-2B). If the lateral ilium flares laterally towards the transducer, then the transducer is too far anterior (Fig. A2-2C). Angling the transducer slightly is often needed to fine-tune the image.

Including both the center of the femoral head and the center of the triradiate cartilage in the image requires some dexterity. One approach is to first find the lateral ilium, then, while keeping the ilium in proper alignment, find the center of the femoral head. Next is the hard part: while keeping the ilium *and* femoral head in proper alignment, find the hypoechoic triradiate cartilage to complete the image. These maneuvers require sliding the transducer over the hip while constantly adjusting the angle. Slight rotation off of true coronal is often helpful.

Obtain the coronal image at least twice to document that the alpha angle is reproducible.

Transverse scans are obtained with and without posterior subluxing stress. The acetabulum is demarcated by the echogenic pubic bone anteriorly, the slightly longer, echogenic ischium posteriorly and the hypoechoic trira-

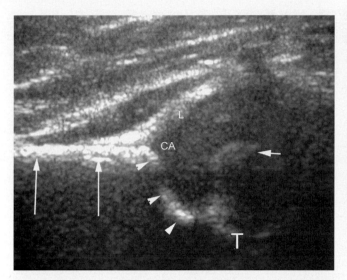

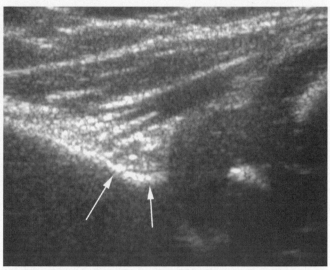

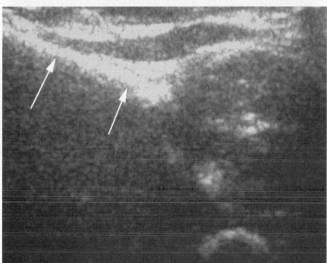

Fig. A2-2   Optimizing transducer position in the coronal plane. **A,** Standard coronal image displays the center of the femoral head (note short arrow on ossification at the center), triradiate cartilage (T), and lateral ilium (*long arrows*) as a straight line. Note the normal concave contour of the osseous acetabular roof. Also note the hypoechoic cartiagenous acetabulum (CA) and hyperechoic labrum (L). **B,** Transducer too far posterior. The lateral ilium has a concave contour (*arrows*). **C,** Transducer too far anterior. The lateral ilium flares towards the transducer (*arrows*).

diate cartilage between them. An optimal axial image in a normal hip will extend through both the center of the femoral head and the center of the triradiate cartilage. If the hip is flexed and the scan is obtained parallel to the femur, the ossified femoral shaft will obscure some of the pubis (Figs. 5-30B, A2-1). The greater trochanter and sometimes the femoral shaft will be included on routine transverse views with the hip in flexion. Obtaining axial scans with the hip flexed and extended also can be performed. A modified Barlow maneuver is performed with the hip flexed and adducted. Posterior force is applied to the femur and the relationship of the femoral head and acetabulum is observed. A subluxable hip is displaced posteriorly and laterally by this maneuver. When performing this stress maneuver, you may find it helpful to hold the transducer between your thumb and index and middle fingers while placing your remaining fingers against the infant's sacrum. This allows force to be directed to the hip joint, rather than simply displacing the entire infant posteriorly. Start gently and observe closely. If no subluxation is evident during application of light force, push a little more firmly. A mm or two of subluxation with firm pressure is normal in neonates. (How much force is enough? The amount of force to apply is somewhat subjective, and experience is helpful. Several experienced sonographers have demonstrated to me the amount of pressure they apply. I have attempted to reproduce this force on a scale. Most apply a force in the range of 2 to 5 kg, but sometimes more. Practice on your bathroom scale.)

A minimum set of images obtained in a routine screening examination will include at least two coronal images that document reproducible measurement of the alpha angle (and the beta angle if you use the Graf system), and axial images with and without stress. Remember to scan both hips. Compare the hips to each other, and with any prior studies. A complete examination will document the size and symmetry of the cartilaginous femoral heads and the ossific femoral nuclei (if present), the shape of the acetabular roof (concave is normal, straight is gray zone between normal and abnormal, wavy is abnormal), femoral head coverage by the osseous acetabular roof (should be at least 50% covered), the position of the femoral head (should be centered over the triradiate cartilage), the position of the labrum (should not be flipped medially), and hip stability if stress views were obtained.

Scans of a dislocated hip are different. If the femoral head is subluxed or frankly dislocated, it is important to document whether alignment was improved by altering the position of the femur. This can be assessed by moving the femur through a range of motion under direct sonographic observation. Note what you see, as this information will assist the orthopedic surgeon. Chronically subluxed or dislocated hips may demonstrate an inverted limbus, i.e., medial displacement of the hyperechoic superior labrum between the laterally and superiorly displaced femoral head and the acetabulum (Fig. 5-29F).

Interpretation of properly obtained images is relatively straightforward, except in the most dysplastic hips. In contrast, performing the study has a slow learning curve. There is no substitute for experience. Advice to residents: take advantage of any opportunity offered to perform the scan yourself, particularly under the direction of an experienced sonographer who can assist and guide you towards obtaining reproducible and accurate images.

APPENDIX 3: FRACTURES WITH EPONYMS

Bankart	glenoid anteroinferior rim chip from anterior humeral head dislocation
Barton's	unstable, intra-articular dorsal lip radius with dorsal subluxation of fragment and carpus
Baseball finger	avulsion dorsal base of finger distal phananx (same as mallet finger)
Bennett	intra-articular fracture base of thumb metacarpal
Boutonnière	flexion of finger PIP and extension of DIP
Boxer's	4th or 5th metacarpal shaft or neck
Chauffeur	radial styloid (same as Hutchinson)
Chopart	hindfoot-midfoot fracture-dislocation
Clay Shoveler's	avulsion of C7 or T1 spinous process
Colles	distal radius, apex volar angulation
Duputren	distal fibular
Duverney	iliac wing
Essex-Lopresti	proximal radial fracture with interosseous membrane tear and distal radioulnar dislocation
Galeazi	distal radial shaft fracture with distal ulnar dislocation
Gamekeeper's thumb	thumb MCP ulnar collateral ligament avulsion (same as skier's thumb)
Hill Sachs	impaction posterior humeral head from anterior shoulder dislocation
Hutchinson	radial styloid (same as Chauffeur)
Jefferson	C1 ring
Jones	proximal diaphysis 5th metatarsal
LisFranc	midfoot-forefoot fracture dislocation with LisFranc ligament tear
Little leaguer's elbow	acute or chronic elbow medial epicondyle avulsion
Maissoneuve	medial malleolus, proximal fibula and interosseous membrane tear
Malgaigne	vertical shear pelvic fracture through sacral ala and pubic bones
Mallet finger	avulsion dorsal base of finger distal phananx (same as baseball finger)
March	metatarsal stress fracture
Monteggia	proximal ulnar shaft fracture with radial head dislocation
Pouteau's	same as Colles
Rolando	comminuted Bennett
Segond	small avulsion lateral tibial plateau (high association with ACL tear)
Skier's thumb	thumb MCP ulnar collateral ligament avulsion (same as gamekeeper's thumb)
Smith	distal radius, apex dorsal angulation (reverse Colles)
Tilleaux	Salter Harris 3 distal lateral tibia

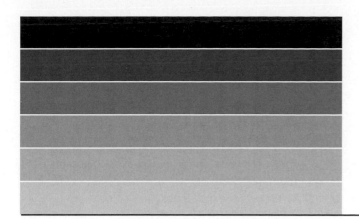

Index

Note: Page numbers followed by f refer to figures; page numbers followed by t refer to tables.